DOCTORS UNDER HITLER

DOCTORS UNDER HITLER

Michael H. Kater

The University of North Carolina Press

Chapel Hill and London

Manufactured in the United States of America

The paper in this book meets the guidelines for
permanence and durability of the Committee
on Production Guidelines for Book Longevity
of the Council on Library Resources.

04 03 02 01 00 6 5 4 3 2

Library of Congress Cataloging-in-Publication Data

Kater, Michael H., 1937–
Doctors under Hitler / by Michael H. Kater.
p. cm.
Bibliography: p.
Includes index.
ISBN 0-8078-1842-9 (alk. paper)
ISBN 0-8078-4851-1 (pbk.: alk. paper)
1. Medicine—Germany—History—20th century.
2. Physicians—Germany. 3. World War,
1939–1945—Atrocities. 4. World War,
1939–1945—Medical care. I. Title.
R510.K37 1989
610'.943—dc19
89-5466
CIP

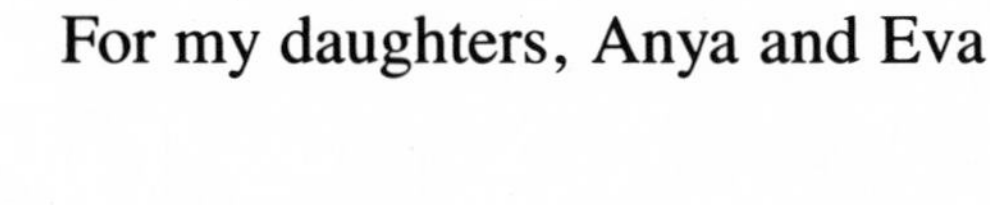

For my daughters, Anya and Eva

Contents

Acknowledgments

In researching and writing this book, I was generously assisted by many friends and colleagues. Foremost, I thank the staff of the Social Sciences and Humanities Research Council of Canada in Ottawa, who consistently helped me with financial grants and allotted me a leave fellowship in 1982–83. The council also enabled me to travel to meetings of the International Society for the History of Medicine to present papers on Nazi medicine: at Düsseldorf in 1986 and at Bologna in 1988. The Office of Research Administration and Atkinson College of York University granted me research fellowships to free me from teaching and administrative duties in 1984–85 and 1987–88 and made available additional funds for travel and research. In 1985–86 the Hannah Institute for the History of Medicine in Toronto, under its Executive Secretary Dr. G. R. Paterson, invited me to serve as Hannah Visiting Professor of the History of Medicine at McMaster University in Hamilton. This proved to be a rewarding experience especially because there I met two knowledgeable experts in the field of medicine and its history, Charles G. Roland, the resident Hannah Professor, and William E. Seidelman. Both not only initiated me to the rudiments of medicine and helped with bibliographical problems but also became close personal friends. I owe a special debt to Konrad H. Jarausch for having made rare documents available to me and offering sage advice along the way, and to Daniel P. Simon, the director of the Berlin Document Center, whose willingness to provide me with documentary records time and again defies any attempt at description.

Several other individuals assisted me in various ways. They include William Sheridan Allen, Wolfgang Benz, Gert Brieger, Henry Friedlander, Hans Halter, Hartmut Hanauske-Abel, H.-G. Herrlitz, Georg G. Iggers, Frederick H. Kasten, Eric D. Kohler, Fridolf Kudlien, Robert Jay Lifton, Gunter Mann, Howard Margolian, Sybil Milton, George L. Mosse, Benno Müller-Hill, Christian Pross, Mark Richardson, Ronald Schmalz, Rolf and Helga Steffensmeier, Lawrence D. Stokes, Achim Thom, and Hermann Weisert.

I am grateful to the University of North Carolina Press, in particular its executive editor, Lewis Bateman, for agreeing to publish the manuscript and carefully preparing it for print.

Last but not least I once again thank the expert staff at York University's interlibrary loan service, Mary Hudecki, Gary MacDonald, and John Carter, who procured books and articles for me from as far away as the shores of California and the German Democratic Republic.

Any mistakes the reader may encounter are of course entirely my own.

Abbreviations

The following abbreviations are used in the text. For abbreviations used in the appendix and notes, see page 263.

Adgo	Allgemeine deutsche Gebührenordnung
ANSt	Arbeitsgemeinschaft Nationalsozialistischer Studentinnen; Working Community of Nazi Women Students
BDÄ	Bund Deutscher Ärztinnen; League of German Woman Doctors
BDM	Bund Deutscher Mädel; League of German Girls (=female Hitler Youth)
CDU	Christlich-Demokratische Union; Christian Democratic Union
CIA	Central Intelligence Agency
DAF	Deutsche Arbeitsfront; German Labor Front
DDR	Deutsche Demokratische Republik; German Democratic Republic
DFW	Deutsches Frauenwerk; German Women's Front
Dr. med.	doctor of medicine (=M.D.)
Dr. phil.	doctor of philosophy (=Ph.D.)
HJ	Hitlerjugend; Hitler Youth
IPPNW	International Physicians for the Prevention of Nuclear War
KPD	Kommunistische Partei Deutschlands; Communist Party of Germany
KVD	Kassenärztliche Vereinigung Deutschlands; Association of German Health-Insurance Physicians
Napola	Nationalpolitische Erziehungsanstalten; (SS elite schools)
NDH	Neue Deutsche Heilkunde
NS	Nationalsozialistisch; National Socialist
NSÄB (or) NS-Ärztebund	Nationalsozialistischer Deutscher Ärztebund; Nazi Physicians' League
NSDAP	Nationalsozialistische Deutsche Arbeiterpartei; National Socialist German Workers' Party

NSD-Dozentenbund	Nationalsozialistischer Deutscher Dozentenbund; Nazi Lecturers' League
NSDStB	Nationalsozialistischer Deutscher Studentenbund; Nazi Student League
NSF	NS-Frauenschaft; Nazi Women's Organization
NSFK	Nationalsozialistisches Fliegerkorps; Nazi Aviation Corps
NSKK	Nationalsozialistisches Kraftfahrkorps; Nazi Motor Corps
NS-Kulturgemeinde	Nazi Cultural Community
NSV	Nationalsozialistische Volkswohlfahrt; Nazi People's Welfare
OKH	Oberkommando des Heeres; Army High Command
POW	Prisoner of War
Preugo	Preussische Gebührenordnung
RÄK	Reichsärztekammer; Reich Physicians' Chamber
REM	Reichserziehungsministerium; Reich Education Ministry
RM	Reichsmark
RSHA	Reichssicherheitshauptamt; SS Security Main Office
RSW	Reichsstudentenwerk; Reich Student Services
SA	Sturmabteilungen; Storm Troopers (Brown Shirts)
SD	(SS-) Sicherheitsdienst; SS Security Service
SPD	Sozialdemokratische Partei Deutschlands; Social Democratic Party of Germany
SS	Schutzstaffel; Black Shirts
tb	tuberculosis
TH	Technische Hochschule; technical university
uk-Stellung	unabkömmlich-Stellung; status of indispensability
VDI	Verein Deutscher Ingenieure; Association of German Engineers

DOCTORS UNDER HITLER

Introduction

Before us are the individual case histories of seven German men and women, all of them physicians. The gynecologist Professor Carl Clauberg, responsible for cruel experiments on concentration camp inmates during the Nazi era, was captured by the Russians in June 1945. Sentenced to twenty-five years in a penitentiary in the Soviet Union, he was repatriated to West Germany in 1955. Clauberg immediately looked for a new secretary to reestablish a medical office. The West German Federal Physicians' Chamber (Bundesärztekammer) did nothing to stop him; it decertified him as a doctor only after the application of severe outside pressure. Clauberg died in prison in 1957 awaiting a new trial for his crimes.[1]

Rupprecht Bernbeck was a student of various academic disciplines in the Third Reich, a veritable Renaissance man. Before World War II was over, the young Nazi earned three doctorates. One was in philosophy; the dissertation was called "Race-Psychological Observations on the Sea and Seafaring with Especial Consideration of the German People." Another was in medicine; whenever Bernbeck was not traveling the oceans in one of Adolf Hitler's submarines he worked toward becoming a surgeon. After 1945, Bernbeck began an orthopedic career; he was appointed adjunct professor, first in Munich and then in Hamburg. In 1984 this chief surgeon, now sixty-seven, was being charged with malpractice by hundreds of patients; allegedly he had crippled young men and women for the sake of private experimentation. In many cases, Bernbeck had operated needlessly and with great gusto. He was known for his black humor. One patient, who was to have had his spine operated on, awoke from anesthetics with his leg in a cast. When asked why, Bernbeck answered: "So you won't run away from me!" By early 1988, Bernbeck was facing trial.[2]

Dr. Ilse Szagunn was a seasoned physician in 1941 when she took over the editorship of *Die Ärztin*, a magazine for female doctors controlled by the Nazi medical administration. She published and edited profusely in the National Socialist spirit.[3] In 1951, now sixty-four years old, Szagunn was allowed to print an article in a German professional journal in which she spoke about changes in the conception of illness in the past five decades. Not only did she fail to mention changes that might have occurred in 1933 and again in 1945, but Szagunn cited the name of Professor Werner Catel, a "euthanasia" killer of hundreds of children, who was himself in the process of adjusting to a "change" in political circumstances just as noiselessly as Szagunn had.[4]

Walter Kreienberg was born in 1911, the son of a general practitioner. After receiving a Gymnasium diploma in 1931, he commenced the study of medicine at the venerated universities of Würzburg, Hamburg, Düsseldorf, and Erlangen. In Erlangen, he graduated in medicine in 1937, publishing as his thesis ruminations on the new Nazi law regarding the hereditarily diseased. He endorsed the "race-hygienic" stipulations of the law, touting them as a "moral victory for Germany." He scoffed at its non-German critics, who wished only to use "every measure decreed by the new Germany in a political manner, to vent their fanatical hatred against the new regime leadership."[5] That same year Kreienberg became a Nazi party member; he already was a fellow of the National Socialist Motor Corps and the Nazi Physicians' League.[6] Politically unassailable, Kreienberg was a university lecturer in physiology by 1943, and one year later the credentials of that young scientist, who was now occupied with pressure-chamber (high-altitude) research in the air force, were reviewed before a reallocation of university chairs.[7] Although no academic appointment resulted while the war was on, Kreienberg was invested with a professorship in physiology at the newly founded University of Mainz in 1948. In 1971 he received his first West German national award (Bundesverdienstkreuz), in 1977 an upgraded one, and in 1984 the highest possible citation of that order.[8] Finally, in spring 1987 the physiologist was the recipient of the Paracelsus-Medaille, awarded to him, as it had been to Albert Schweitzer earlier, by the German medical establishment. Ironically, the very medical congress that honored him for his "exemplary attitude as a physician in the service of his patients" was also charged with deliberating a motion calling for the annulment of the sterilization law of 1933 that earned the laureate his doctorate.[9]

Ernst Rodenwaldt began his career as a physician as a twenty-five-year-old medical officer active in the imperial German army in 1903; between 1910 and 1913 he served in Togo, one of Germany's four African colonies. After several years in the Dutch East Indies in the 1920s and early 1930s, during which time he intermittently belonged to the Nazi party, Rodenwaldt returned to Germany in 1934 to assume the duties of a full professor of hygienics and bacteriology at Kiel; in 1935 he was in Heidelberg. Throughout World War II, he assisted the Nazis as head of a tropical-medical institute within the military medical academy.[10] Rodenwaldt was an enthusiastic convert to the specifically Nazi discipline of *Rassenkunde*, or race science. In Heidelberg, he lectured on people and race, and in his publications he condemned the "mixing of the races" in colonial territories because of its repercussions in the mother countries. He polemicized against the "liberalistic-Jewish, race-negating spirit of the system [Weimar republican] period" and, emphasizing the "racial contrast with Jewry," welcomed the Nuremberg race legislation of September 1935.[11] By 1944, now a physician-general, he prided himself on his research into racial hybrids and touted his expertise as an assessor in Nazi "hereditary biology" (*Erbbiologie*).[12] After 1945 the professor was denounced by his students for Nazi connections and consequently lost his chair. Nonetheless, the Western Allies in 1947 mandated him to author a comprehensive report about hygiene in the Third Reich—which lacked any references to race hygienics. Rodenwaldt also set to work on an epidemiological world atlas, commissioned by the Academy of Sciences. The Institute of War Medicine and Hygienics of the West German Bundeswehr in Koblenz was named after Rodenwaldt in 1967.[13]

Gerhard Jungmann was born in Elberfeld in 1910. He studied medicine at Munich, Bonn, and Kiel and received his doctorate in 1935. In May 1933, still a student, he joined the Nazi party; by 1936, he was in the brown-shirted SA and the Nazi Physicians' League. By June 1938, he had established himself as a general practitioner in Markoldendorf, in the Hanoverian countryside, but between 1939 and 1945 service in the Nazi air force claimed him.[14] After 1945, his halcyon days had arrived. In 1953, he was deputy president for Lower Saxony of the Hartmannbund, West Germany's professional physicians' association; after 1955, he acted as a medical functionary at the federal level for many years. Heavily committed to the aims of Konrad Adenauer's right-wing Christian Democratic Union (CDU), Jungmann first became a councilman in Markoldendorf and then entered the Bonn parliament in 1961. In 1968 this doctor, too, was awarded the democracy's Bundesverdienstkreuz.[15] But he well remembered the Nazi period and some of the medical dogma he learned as a student. In 1972 he published an article in the main professional journal, *Deutsches Ärzteblatt*, espousing the ideal of preventive rather than curative medicine (*Vorsorge* as opposed to *Fürsorge*). His arguments sounded suspiciously National Socialist, based as they were on the tenets of an old Nazi naturalist physician and professor, Karl Kötschau, to whom Jungmann had dedicated his paper and whom he highly lauded throughout.[16]

At the age of eighteen Hans Joachim Sewering was already a medical student when he entered the SS in November 1933. Nine months later he joined the Nazi Student League and the party. In 1941 he graduated as a physician from Munich University. After a few months in the army, from which he was released on medical grounds, he took up the post of a Munich municipal doctor at the tubercular clinic of Schönbrunn near Dachau, in summer 1942.[17] This clinic also sheltered handicapped patients, feeble-minded ones, and epileptics, many of them children. At least one such child, fourteen-year-old Babette Fröwis, on October 26, 1943, was pronounced by Dr. Sewering to be "no longer suitable for Schönbrunn; she will be sent to Eglfing-Haar, the healing institution responsible for her."[18] That "healing institution" was one of the Reich's notorious killing centers for Germans deemed not worthy of life, and there, on November 16, Babette died, probably after systematic overdoses of a painkiller.[19] The referring doctor, subsequently described by admiring colleagues as a "*homo politicus* of rare talent,"[20] embarked upon a grandiose career in postwar medical politics:

president of the Bavarian Physicians' Chamber (1955); vice-president of the Federal Physicians' Chamber (1959); board member of the World Medical Association (1966); adjunct professor for social medicine (1968).[21] Finally, in 1973, internist Sewering became president of the Federal Physicians' Chamber and hence top doctor in the country. He was forced to resign this post five years later, not for his Nazi past but because of questionable billing practices. Nevertheless, in 1988 he still headed the Bavarian regional organization.[22]

If the biographies of these seven individuals suggest the continuation beyond 1945 of an unwholesome trend in a medical culture that could have started, for some of them, even before Hitler's rise to power in January 1933, certain phenomena in West Germany's broader medical history reinforce that impression. It has been claimed that a restructuring of the German panel physicians' law (Kassenarztrecht) after 1945 was prevented by the corporation of doctors for ten years because they were afraid social reforms would result in economic disadvantages.[23] Sterilization of disabled persons, one of the medical abuses of the Nazi era, was reportedly practiced in West Berlin's university clinic in the early 1980s.[24] And in 1986, when the law courts were investigating these cases, victims of the original acts of sterilization had still not been recognized as sufferers from National Socialist oppression and had received no appropriate compensation.[25] Nor had such recognition been extended to the victims of medical experiments in concentration camps, such as Dr. Josef Mengele's in Auschwitz.[26]

Such glimpses of anomalies in the German health care system over the last few decades make one curious to learn more about the medical profession during the time of its greatest crisis—National Socialist rule—which both brought earlier negative developments to a head and created new ones. Indeed, the fate of doctors under Hitler is unique for a variety of reasons. One might assume the Führer himself had something to do with the problem, but closer examination shows that he did not. Notwithstanding his private relationship to a bevy of physicians to whom the dictator was beholden and who would find him increasingly hypochondriac as time wore on, Hitler had no special sympathy for the medical profession.[27] It does not necessarily follow that the converse was true. Actually, representative members of the German healing profession imputed to Hitler a value that accorded with their novel racial view of the medical cosmology. As Dr. Dietrich Amende, a well-established early National Socialist doctor, put it in 1937, not only was Adolf Hitler a natural genius to have written from scratch such an important book as *Mein Kampf*, but he was also "the great physician of his people."[28]

What exactly Amende meant will become clearer in the chapters that follow. His statement touches on a further compelling reason for studying doctors in the Third Reich: physicians became Nazified more thoroughly and much sooner than any other profession, and as Nazis they did more in the service of the nefarious regime than any of their extraprofessional peers. To confirm the former assertion, for the decennial of Hitler's rise to power in 1943 Dr. Leonardo Conti, then the highest medical administrator and an "Old Fighter" for the Hitler cause, stated that physicians in Germany had surpassed all other academic professions in the timing and the extensiveness of their commitment to the National Socialist movement.[29] To verify the latter notion, another inside witness may be quoted, Professor Hans Reiter, who was a leading public health expert. As early as September 1933 he forecast that National Socialist *Weltanschauung* would reshape the guidelines for medicine more than any other field.[30]

The extreme manifestation of this prophecy was to be attested to later by victims of Nazi terror, oppression, and liquidation, in "euthanasia" wards, concentration camps, and on the selection ramp of Auschwitz. In the early 1960s, Louis Falstein corroborated Reiter from hindsight when he wrote that in no other sector of professional life had the Nazi force of destruction "demonstrated greater power for evil than in the medical profession. The Nazis prostituted law, perverted education and corrupted civil service, but they made killers out of physicians."[31] Extracting the demonological quality that occluded so many interpretations of immediate post-1945 historiography, Robert Jay Lifton has more recently specified this argument from the sobering vantage point of the psychoanalyst by divining that "*as a profession* German physicians offered themselves to the regime. So also did most other professions; but with doctors, that gift included using their intellectual authority to justify and carry out medicalized killing," which meant "practicing therapy via mass murder."[32]

One may ask whether physicians in Germany had a choice in the matter of Nazification and collaboration with a treacherous regime. For a historian, this could perhaps be an unfair question. But postulating that medicine automatically predisposed a doctor to fascism is simplistic in light of the Dutch situation under German occupation. In Holland in the early 1940s the physicians resisted Nazi attempts to co-opt them for oppression, mutilation, and destruction. A hundred doctors were sent to concentration camps and many died, but the remaining colleagues' attitude did not change. The eminent medical scientist Leo Alexander concluded: "It is obvious that if the medical profession of a small nation under the conqueror's heel could resist so effectively, the German medical profession could likewise have resisted had they not taken the fatal first step."[33]

Alexander's judgment implies the need to scrutinize physicians in related fascist environments, including Italy's. Mária Kovács is conducting such work on fascist Hungary; little is known as yet about doctors under Mussolini.[34] Japanese historians have been discouraged by their government from telling the story of Unit 731, the germ-warfare experimental station in Manchuria that abused prisoners of war as human guinea pigs. The daily life of medical practitioners in Hirohito's empire would have to be analyzed in comparison to such transgressions.[35]

Physicians under Hitler cannot be viewed in total isolation from similar professional groups in the German dictatorship. Dentists, lawyers, and perhaps pharmacists could serve for facile comparisons and as members of control groups, inasmuch as information on those subgroups is available. This has posed a problem for my research because it has been known that dentists, pharmacists, and even lawyers did not excel in Hitler's killing machine; hence few pioneering studies have been done. And yet lawyers, for example, experienced processes in the development of their profession very similar to those of physicians, particularly "Aryanization," that is, ridding the peer group of its Jewish members.[36] Only lately has research on the lawyers under Hitler made strides, chiefly because of the pathbreaking work of Konrad Jarausch.[37]

All this is not to infer that *every* doctor in the Hitler era was perverted to the point of executing murder. Assuredly, the vast majority were not. Indeed, the vast majority carried on as they had before and would again. Those who changed and the forces behind those changes in the atmosphere of the post-1933 horror constitute the exceedingly difficult subject of this book. Certain pitfalls ought to but cannot always be avoided. For instance, one has to be cautious not to speak of "National Socialist medicine" when describing medicine under National Socialism.[38] The automatic equation of medicine with Nazism from 1933 to 1945 is too easy a formula and obviously will not do in ascertaining the degree to which ordinary medicine in Germany became acculturated to Nazi ideas and, reciprocally, in what strength political ideology and practice under the Nazis became "medicalized" even before 1933. To find answers to such questions is a long and tedious procedure. The historian has to deal with ideas from very different realms, with the gray zones resulting from the collusion of these ideas, carefully weighing the evidence to reach a balanced verdict. Not the least of the obstacles is inherent in the interdisciplinary approach necessitated by generic discrepancies potentially leading to cognitive confusion: the course of politics on one side and the development of medicine on the other, both tempered by notions of ethos or morality.

It is a legitimate question whether the fate of doctors and medicine under Hitler, the most twisted aspects of which were revealed at the so-called Doctors' Trial at Nuremberg, has had a salutary effect on the practice of medicine in our modern world. The not altogether heartening answer could partially be the result of the immutability of human nature, but also because a study dealing with the gradual decline of a culturally developed nation's medicine has never been presented before and certainly not for universal dissemination.

Because of what happened with the German medical profession, a "Nuremberg Code" was created and endorsed for international adoption in the late 1940s, condemning medical abuses in experimentation on humans. Its clauses were refined by the World Medical Association in 1954 and again by the association's Declaration of Helsinki in 1964.[39] Scientific torture, with the help of medical personnel, was not generally associated with Nazi doctors, but its kinship with medical experimentation was obvious. Torture was expressly censured in the United Nations Universal Declaration of Human Rights of 1948.[40] There were follow-up pronouncements in 1975 (Declaration of Tokyo) and 1982 (United Nations Principles of Medical Ethics); infractions today are closely watched by Amnesty International.[41] To this day, that organization's observations in regard to basic human rights have not been very encouraging, and it appears that few lessons have been learned from the Nazi medical past. The routine torture of political prisoners, notably in Latin American dictatorships such as Chile, Colombia, Brazil, and, until a few years ago, Argentina and Uruguay, was and is a daily occurrence. By personally monitoring such practices, physicians are again violating the Hippocratic Oath. They make sure the victims do not die so they will remain useful, and they advise in interrogation and in the kinds and degrees of torture to be employed. President Alfredo Stroessner of Paraguay, who was host to Mengele for many years, is said to have reserved an entire story in Asunción's police hospital for the medical revival of unconscious torture victims.[42] Only Uruguayan, Argentinean, and Chilean doctors, the latter still under dictator Augusto Pinochet's iron fist, have deplored their previous complicity in crime; in Chile the Council of Physicians (Colegio Medico) has done so at great risk to the safety of its members.[43] Unlawful acts on prisoners, aided by physicians, are still reported from Iraq, Lebanon, Turkey, Syria, South Africa (the Steve Biko case), such African countries as Uganda and Tanzania, and even Israel.[44] In the Soviet Union, the use of pharmachemicals in psychiatric mind manipulation has become notorious.[45]

Nor are the so-called civilized nations exempt from charges of medical inhumanity, even though abuses may take place there less systematically. Britain has been reprimanded by the Compton Committee for hooding militants of the Irish Republican Army and exposing them to "white noise."[46] In France in early 1988, "a comatose patient was made the object of an experiment to shed light on the trial of two doctors charged with killing another patient."[47] In Canada the specter of forcible sterilization loomed as late as 1986; coincidentally, a medical practitioner was found guilty by the Ontario College of Physicians and Surgeons "after he hired two men to beat someone up and oversaw the administration of certain drugs to the victim."[48] Both for Canada and the United States, whose Central Intelligence Agency (CIA) stood to benefit, unflattering reference could also be made to the ignominious "de-patterning" experiments by psychiatrist Dr. Ewen Cameron at Montreal's Allan Memorial Institute in the 1950s and 1960s, in which the confidence of trusting patients was betrayed in memory-loss experiments.[49]

There is, then, a need to show the dangerous straits a medical profession under totalitarianism and dictatorship may get itself into. To a certain extent, of course, this need has already been filled. Nearly a dozen substantial books have been published on various aspects of physicians and medicine in the Nazi Reich, one or two of which are truly outstanding. The first one to appear, in the late 1940s, was superb and today is regarded as a classic. It is the sagaciously annotated documentation of the Doctors' Trial at Nuremberg, at which twenty-three defendants were accused, twenty of them physicians, and it was written by the young lecturer in psychiatry Alexander Mitscherlich in collaboration with a medical student, Fred Mielke.[50] These two authors concentrated on illicit human experimentation. The next monograph to make an impact, by Alice Platen-Hallermund, dealt with the killing of the handicapped, which the Nazis mendaciously termed "euthanasia."[51]

In the first two decades after the war, only books (and some articles) on the perverted physicians of the Third Reich came forth because the connection between their activities and the "normalcy" of ordinary doctors had not yet been forged. Moreover, because historians generally were not interested in wider issues of social history, the regular medical profession under Hitler did not interest them. Hence the first book on the general health administration of the Third Reich, composed by Frenchmen Yves Ternon and Socrate Helman and published in the early 1970s, still lacked any social or psychological dimension, but at least it had moved away from the purely pathological. This volume, largely based on secondary works and Nazi journal literature, albeit—apart from a few Nuremberg Trial documents—not on archival sources, was revealing in its day but is of limited value at present.[52] Walter Wuttke-Groneberg, then of Tübingen, in 1980 published the first work showing the intersections between Nazi medical crimes and everyday medicine in the Third Reich. His book contained well-chosen primary documents, although they were not always satisfactorily analyzed because of the editor's strong Marxist bias.[53] Knowing of the potential complicity of "good" medical practitioners and medicine professors in crimes against humanity, Ernst Klee, a Frankfurt journalist and social worker, returned to the theme of "euthanasia" in the early 1980s. He produced a monograph to show that this perverted form of mercy killing occurred in the most ordinary medical venues and was perpetrated by many more people than the handful of doctors indicted after 1945 in West German courts.[54] Klee's book has now been superseded by the Bielefeld University dissertation of Hans-Walter Schmuhl, which not only details "euthanasia" but also probes its cultural and ideological depths in German race hygiene.[55] In 1985, finally, the first comprehensive volume treating regular and criminal physicians alike came out, edited by the Kiel historian of medicine Fridolf Kudlien. The anthology marked the entry of the West German university establishment into this thematic orbit, and for that reason alone it is significant. Its weakness, however, is its obsession with facts and its relative lack of overall analysis and coherence, for its chapters were composed not by Kudlien alone but also by colleagues of his, few of them genuine physicians.[56]

A spate of books appeared in 1985 and 1986. In 1985 the young American historian Geoffrey Cocks published his dissertation on Martin Göring's institute of psychotherapy. Though this volume affords insights into the workings of applied psychology in the Third Reich, it says little about the public or private health delivery system and not enough about classical psychiatry.[57] In East Germany, the Leipzig medical historian Achim Thom, assisted by his Berlin colleague Horst Spaar, edited a collection of essays, most of which are knowledgeable, particularly those by nondogmatic Marxists from countries other than the German Democratic Republic, but some too obviously follow the Communist party line.[58] In West Germany, the noted Cologne geneticist Benno Müller-Hill wrote a small but revealing volume on "deathly science," pointing to the intricate interrelations between medical research and medical crime. The undisputed highlight of this monograph is a demonstration of the working relationship between Josef Mengele and his teacher, Professor Otmar Freiherr von Verschuer, which may have lasted beyond the catastrophe of 1945.[59]

Probably the most important work since Mitscherlich's and Mielke's, and surely the most significant in recent times, is that by the American psychoanalyst Robert Jay Lifton, who has also written on the survivors of Hiroshima and brainwashing in Communist China. In *The Nazi Doctors* (1986), Lifton examines the role of physicians on the selection ramps of Auschwitz, their obsession with human experimentation, but also their ordinary roles in the nexus of their formal university education and as *patres familias*. One of the most valuable of Lifton's many findings for the present study is that physicians trained in the SS converted their healing into killing without changing the meaning of their original (medical) function. Lifton ties this insight to the demystification of SS physicians as exotic, morally depraved brutes, thus contributing to a further understanding of the banal, the "ordinary" quality of evil, which Hannah Arendt had already exposed so brilliantly. Lifton reduces the demonological side of all the German Mengeles, be their names Sigmund Rascher (Dachau) or Karl Gebhardt (Ravensbrück), making them look more like the average. In so doing, he moves all the other normal German physicians much closer to the standard that was Mengele's—perhaps a somewhat shocking consequence of "humanizing" the "Angel of Death," but a necessary one for comprehending what took place, and certainly one that is incorporated into this study.[60]

Lifton's antidemonological treatment is not likely to find much favor in the West German medical scene, for the official establishment, for apologetic reasons and, one presumes, professional self-preservation, prefers to cling to the notion that killer-physicians were an aberration, a deplorable accident of German history. Early on this view led to a closing of eyes and denial of what a few brave young scholars detected right after the German collapse in 1945: that Nazi medical crimes, as unique as they may have appeared, were repeatable, had become an integral part of German medical history, and—Mitscherlich and Mielke could but imply—that German physicians of the future would have a responsibility to own up to their past. That, however, was precisely what the German medical establishment was not prepared to do, and in punishment, Mitscherlich long was ostracized from the profession in the academic echelons.[61] With this distasteful Freudian analyst safely removed from any major university chair in the Federal Republic's higher education system, there was no need for the formally invested historians of medicine to rewrite the recent chronicle of their profession or even to write it at all.

To this day, this situation has barely changed. Wuttke-Groneberg, the Marxist, lost his position as a budding historian of medicine at the University of Tübingen after his critical stance had become known, even though personal problems and formal irregularities may have played a part in his failure.[62] Peer pressure today is as immense as ever. When Müller-Hill embarked on his revelationary study, he was reminded by a colleague to be thankful for the shelter of his tenured chair.[63]

The potential for professional self-damage for West German medical historians of conscience was once again painfully demonstrated when in August of 1986 Dr. Hartmut Hanauske-Abel, a young biogeneticist from Mainz, published an article in the prestigious British journal *Lancet*, in which he alluded to Nazi medical crimes as a moral responsibility for present-day West German doctors.[64] Only three weeks later, this gifted scientist, who already had an international research reputation and was affiliated with the Nobel Prize-winning IPPNW, was dismissed on a pretext from his post as emergency physician in Rhenish Hesse. Since then on the staff of Children's Hospital, Harvard Medical School in Boston, the thirty-six-year-old doctor sued the West German Panel Physicians' Association in Mainz, hoping to be reinstated. Although he won his case in May 1987, the association appealed, placing Hanauske-Abel in indefinite limbo.[65]

This is one side of the story. The other is of more direct concern. Not only did the establishment take formal steps to destroy Hanauske-Abel professionally, its arcane representatives used his case as an occasion to brand the truth-seeking physician as a man without honor, without a country, a man of total ignorance, thus to discredit his objective of enlightenment. In a construed interview published by the official organ of the Bundesärztekammer in Cologne, Dr. Karsten Vilmar, Sewering's successor as president, accused Hanauske-Abel of historiographic sloppiness while himself minimizing the significance of the corporate Nazi medical past for West German physicianship.[66] So far, the result has been a vigorous and well-informed rebuttal on the part of the Boston-based doctor and fresh legal action, with which he is fighting the obstructively reactionary Cologne mandarins, if at astronomical cost.[67] Yet also, clearly, one can discern a wave of sympathy for him within progressive German circles, especially younger doctors, as several letters to the editor attest.[68]

Thus Hanauske-Abel no longer stands alone in his altruistic quest, and this bodes well for the future. Yet there is room for a more comprehensive study to retrace the path of doctors in the Third Reich—the good ones, who ended up on the gallows, the bad ones, who went to work in Auschwitz, and the ordinary ones, who simply survived. My attempt to write this monograph fundamentally rests on my earlier studies analyzing the course of doctors and their profession from Wilhelm II to Hitler. The main data base for this book is the wealth of documents in the Federal Archive of Koblenz and in the Berlin Document Center. Much primary material was obtained from the student archive in Würzburg and several regional West German archives. Of great importance were papers of the former panel physicians' association (KVD), which were located in West Berlin, almost by accident, and are now said by the Cologne establishment to have been "destroyed."[69] A number of representative samples were drawn of medical students from mass data in the Koblenz holdings and of practicing physicians in the Berlin Center. Beyond that, the predominant professional journals and tabloids of the period were perused, such as *Deutsches Ärzteblatt*, *Ärztliche Mitteilungen*, and *Ziel und Weg*. Several representative medical journals were also screened, including *Münchener Medizinische Wochenschrift* and *Deutsche medizinische Wochenschrift*. Of the extant memoirs of physicians who lived beyond 1945, probably all were read, and most were found to be useful in some way. The same cannot be claimed for the secondary literature, which, despite the significant lacunae that I indicated, in its smaller and greater ramifications of the central topic today is huge. But keeping in mind that this book purports to be a sociohistorical study, if not a sociological one, the reader can be fairly assured that anything regarding the doctors as a social unit, in the context of the society they lived in, has been critically noted.

Chapter 1

Organizational and Socioeconomic Setting

1. Supply, Demand, and Deployment of Physicians

When the Third Reich was ushered in on January 30, 1933, it inherited a surplus of physicians from the republican era.[1] Even though published statistics on the number of medical doctors are inconsistent and spotty, it is now possible to reconstruct the picture. There were just over 48,000 independently practicing physicians in Germany by the end of 1931. This number had fallen to somewhat over 47,000 by 1934 but rose to more than 49,000 in 1937.[2] By a different count the number of physicians in Germany increased from somewhat over 52,000 in 1935 to above 55,000 in 1937, but the number of independently practicing ones declined from 38,000 to over 37,000, suggesting that more doctors were entering private employ and government services, as indeed they were.[3]

Yet another set of figures illustrates the transition in the supply of doctors from peacetime to wartime. The total number of German physicians jumped from over 59,000 just before World War II to nearly 76,000 in 1942, a gain of more than 25 percent, but the number of independently established practitioners rose only about 10 percent, from around 33,000 to just under 37,000.[4] By this time, the general shortage of physicians was a much discussed national issue, with critical repercussions for the civilian population. For the period after 1942, the figures are very sparse. By spring of 1944, 79,462 doctors were said to exist, including 32,000 at the fronts.[5]

For the entire period of the Third Reich, there can be no doubt that the ratio of medical doctors per capita decreased. One public health insurance panel doctor was practicing for 1,344 medically insured patients in 1935, but this ratio slipped to 1 for 1,370 in 1936. In 1939, there were 1,432 health-insured and other (privately paying) patients for every doctor, compared to 1,380 in 1938 and 1,351 at the start of the regime. By July 1943, 2,543 civilians were looked after by one medical practitioner, and that figure was on the upswing as the war drew to a close.[6]

In February 1933, most German physicians greeted the new regime with high hopes, expecting it to redress anomalies left over from the health administration of the Weimar Republic. Third Reich officials, however, enacted new policies gradually. At the end of the Weimar Republic, young doctors straight out of medical school found it almost impossible to establish independent practices honored by the panel insurance fund system, which allowed only one new doctor per six hundred patients. The medical graduate was compelled to spend three years as an assistant physician (*Assistenzarzt*) in a hospital.[7] These provisions were moderated slowly. The medical internship was shortened to one year (*Medizinalpraktikum*), but the doctor still had to spend two years as helper or deputy for an already established colleague. War veterans were given credit for a year's practice of the two years spent as helper. After June 1935, three months of this preparatory period had to be in a country doctor's office, in keeping with the regime's "blood and soil" ideology. In summer 1939, with war in the offing and a pronounced scarcity of doctors, this long period of training after final university examinations was reduced.[8]

Under demographic pressures, the distribution ratio per capita was also altered. The limit of six hundred insurance fund patients per doctor, originally set to guarantee minimum earnings to a practitioner, was a reality only in Berlin, which had more doctors than anywhere else, and possibly Munich. Vast stretches of countryside, such as in East Prussia or Thuringia, had been understaffed by physicians even since republican times. As younger doctors attempted to establish themselves, they were to find that Nazi health administrators discouraged them from settling in the cities, exhorting them instead to move to rural areas. It became a policy to make certification of fund insurance doctors (*Kassenzulassung*) contingent on the candidates' willingness to endure such regimentation.[9] As of March 1, 1937, Berlin and Munich were declared special-permit territories.[10] Eighteen months later the government promulgated an emergency decree allowing the regional health administrations to deploy physicians solely according to supply and demand. This measure was not implemented at the time, but it was premonitory of wartime practices and, to the wary, a signal of the imminent curtailment of the medical profession's traditional freedoms.[11]

Younger doctors, many of whom were at the compulsory three-year waiting stage, harbored special grievances as the Third Reich began. Economically, they were badly off, for either as municipal employees, in a polyclinic, for example, or as state servants, perhaps in a university teaching hospital, they never earned more than 250 marks per month, a share of which was automatically deducted for room and board. If they decided to forgo the latter, they received no remuneration. These conditions prevented most young doctors, who usually underwent their professional licensure (*Approbation*) around the age of twenty-seven, from getting married and founding families, and their contracts allowed for their dismissal from their positions if they married even against such financial odds. Very few of their superiors, commonly well-entrenched medicine professors, tolerated or protected them. Customarily, no provisions existed for married doctors to be housed and fed in hospitals. Furthermore, these junior physicians were not entitled to more than four weeks of vacation per year at the most, and they were forbidden to undertake extracurricular medical activities to increase their incomes.[12]

Spokesmen for this group began early in the Third Reich to clamor for a change in this demeaning situation, arguing, more or less sincerely, on the basis of racial politics, that a nation that cut off its life stream by hampering biologically sound progenitors was mortgaging its future.[13] Specifically, it was claimed that medical institutions should stop advertising junior positions for bachelors only, and it was emphasized that the physicians constituted, after public school teachers, high school teachers, and jurists, the fourth largest group of academically trained professionals of the younger generation, those born after December 31, 1900.[14]

Changes were slow in coming, however, because the interim periods young doctors spent serving in hospitals were essentially retained and the economic misfortunes these physicians had inherited from the late Weimar era would take several years to turn around. It was not until at least 1938 that the situation improved. The Nazi medical administrators, always mindful of the problems of youth and quick to seize a propagandistic opportunity, did what they could to help. Early in 1933, when salaried young doctors in Munich were infringed upon by their employers, the Reich Association of Employed Physicians interceded with Dr. Leonardo Conti, Prussia's commissar of health and the Berlin executive of the National Socialist Physicians' League (NS-Ärztebund). Although his jurisdiction stopped at the Prussian border, Conti assured the Bavarian rabble-rousers of his sympathy.[15] A year later the Reich interior minister, who was responsible for health administration, officially encouraged the hospitals to hire married applicants with children.[16] And as late at 1938 the Nazi-organized medicine sections at the universities (*Reichsfachgruppen Medizin*), which had the explicit support of the Reich physicians' leader (*Reichsärzteführer*), compiled evidence on the economic plight of the young assistants, published it in part, and promised further action with the government.[17]

However gradually, the transition of younger physicians from salaried to independent positions improved to the extent that a growing number of doctors came to be needed in the Reich. The near-closure conditions of the late republic and the regional deployment directives of the authorities after 1933 slowly corrected the supply-and-demand imbalance until an equilibrium was attained. At this point, however, the forces of the marketplace again caused maladjustments resulting from an undersupply of doctors, which led to the chronic shortage at the end of World War II.

As happened at other levels of the German economy, the creation of new functions resulted in new posts to be occupied, a trend that was accelerated when mobilization for war began and the armed forces were reconstituted. In 1933, those seeking jobs still outnumbered the available job postings in the advertising sections of the professional journals.[18] But as the incoming doctors found that if they were patient practices became available, as for example in East Prussia or in the seedier districts of a large city, and salaried positions, perhaps for postdoctoral specialist training, could be had without too much difficulty, those job want ads began to disappear.[19] It would be a safe estimate that the turnaround occurred in 1935, after many Jewish colleagues had been forced out of competition, even though the general concern about a national dearth of doctors did not set in until 1939.[20]

One indication of this new trend was the often advertised availability of new opportunities, some of them with agencies of state, such as consulting physician for the Reich insurance scheme, others with the Nazi party or its affiliates, such as in labor service camps or the SS. Industry, in concert with the German Labor Front (Deutsche Arbeitsfront—DAF), was hiring an increasing number of physicians.[21] In addition, all three branches of the Wehrmacht—the army, the navy, and the Luftwaffe—actively courted young doctors for professional careers as *Sanitätsoffiziere*, especially after the Hossbach Protocol in November 1937, when the planning of aggressive war necessitated an ongoing mobilization.[22]

Yet a third signal of better times for doctors was provided by the career development pattern of civil service physicians, the time-honored *Amtsärzte*. In 1934, the selection process for these moderately well-paid and tenured positions had been rigid, with candidates being required to possess good academic records, a certain amount of private field experience, and the ability to pass additional qualifying tests.[23] But as early as spring 1935, because more attractive options were available elsewhere, certain prerequisites for an *Amtsarzt* career were being lowered by compressing the special training curricula or by partially abolishing the examinations.[24] By 1939 the Reich's health bureaucracy was seeking to employ not only *Amtsärzte* of the first order, full-time, regular officials, but also adjunct physicians and part-time ones, who would enjoy some of the state-sanctioned privileges such as the title *Medizinalrat*, as well as being able to earn money in a private capacity.[25]

With the beginning of the war in September 1939, the occupation of a medical official intermittently became somewhat more popular only because these specialists were less likely to be inducted into the Wehrmacht than were civilian physicians.[26] And indeed, in the war years the civilian health administration fought for retention of every member of its official staff on the home front and often with success.[27] But even though entrance requirements to the *Amtsarzt* office were further lowered and more perquisites were added, the job remained as unattractive to medical neophytes as before the war.[28] In one senior health administrator's opinion, inexperienced as well as seasoned doctors generally avoided this career unless they had "a black spot somewhere."[29] The result was a disastrous understaffing of most German regions with public health officials, among which the Saar Valley, Thuringia, and Prussia fared by far the worst.[30]

For the deployment of physicians on the home front, the history of the *Amtsärzte* during the war reflects the experiences of the entire corps of medical practitioners in that phase of the Third Reich. Because the central health administration had known the war was coming, if not when, far in advance (an assumption that cannot be proved by evidence but seems certain in the known factual context),[31] it had passed the emergency measure of October 15, 1938, empowering it to rule over the Reich's physicians as it saw fit.[32] In the first few weeks of the war many able-bodied doctors, including those serving in various hospitals and medical faculties, received their marching papers. Some had been conscripted in the preceding months, and others were called up early in 1940. By the end of May of that year, 36.7 percent of all hospital staff physicians and 32.4 percent of all self-employed practitioners were serving in the armed forces.[33]

At first the strategy of the Berlin health planners under Reich Health Leader (*Reichsgesundheitsführer*) Dr. Conti, whose only concern was to retain as many male physicians for the treatment of the civilian population as possible, worked fairly well. The shortages of the prewar months were exacerbated, as for example in East Prussia and Silesia, but they could be partially compensated by the readiness of older, retired doctors and married female physicians to step into the breach. In addition, twenty-four hundred senior medical students were consigned to the medical corps after an emergency graduation.[34]

The Reich health officials enacted several special measures to ensure a proper deployment of civilian physicians and the use of all available resources against the far-reaching claims of the Wehrmacht to conscript all physicians in the eligible age groups.[35] On September 2, 1939, the interior minister, as Conti's superior, enabled the Reich Physicians' Chamber to direct resident practitioners toward any work in the interest of public sanitation. Two days later the Reich labor minister pronounced that medical duties should be undertaken, along with the fund insurance doctors, by any physicians with the proper qualifications, be they privately practicing specialists or doctors still waiting for panel certification. All doctors' freedom of horizontal mobility was indefinitely suspended; practitioners were to be completely at the disposal of the regional planning agencies, which could push them around within the confines of the Reich like figures on a chess board.[36]

The government health bureaucracy was always prepared, in principle, to help a doctor avoid active service at the front by attesting to his indispensability within the civilian populace. Hence many a doctor who could show good cause was able, for a while at least, to remain with his practice.[37] When a practice was temporarily vacated by a conscripted doctor, the health bureaucracy co-opted an auxiliary physician (*Hilfskassenarzt*), who could be anyone not eligible for front service (including doctors with Jewish spouses), and temporarily put him in the incumbent's spot. Such a person administered the practice on behalf of his predecessor, and he received a fixed stipend set by the health authorities. This regimentation was aided by yet another provision forbidding German practitioners to close down their premises or sell their medicinal instrumentarium or even their automobiles.[38]

In the next few years a fierce intraregime contest developed between the military and the civilian health administrations, mostly over personnel, in which the ordinary German doctor became an unfortunate pawn. Generally, the Wehrmacht paid no heed to servicing the needs of civilians, which were becoming more serious, especially in rural areas.[39] In 1941, the interior minister was well aware that any male physicians twenty-seven years old or younger would immediately be drafted for war service, usually upon graduation from the university.[40] Since the reservoir of female and older male physicians was slowly being depleted, there were only two ways to countermand the Wehrmacht's ambitions. One was to encourage greater numbers of young men to apply for home reserve status (*uk-Stellung*) with the authorities, and the other was to tighten the logistic controls over all available civilian doctors, including women and fresh university graduates, so as to deploy them instantly, possibly before the army could pursue them.[41] In particular, this purview was to include the nation's hospitals, for if a vestige of professional freedom had still been preserved, it was here, among the assistant and senior staff physicians.[42]

In May 1942 the leaders of the central health administration decided on two further measures to help ease the physician shortage. First, they forbade civilian doctors in Germany to leave the profession unless they received special authorization to do so.[43] And second, they entered into an equilibrium agreement with the Wehrmacht, stipulating that the current deployment ratio of physicians on the home front and in active duty be frozen.[44] The first requirement further restricted the traditional liberties of German doctors; its consequences for the needs of the civilians were at best doubtful. The second afforded only temporary relief. If, as was called for, an older, trench-weary doctor was to be sent home for every young medic conscripted, there would be a time lag of three months during which the newcomer had to undergo basic military and field-sanitation training. To derive maximum benefits from the system, the army turned this time into a waiting period for the health bureaucrats in Berlin by refusing to part with its seasoned veterans before the young medical recruits were ready for combat. Moreover, the army high command was shrewd enough to relieve mainly incapacitated doctors, near casualties, who would be ill-fitted to assume the strenuous medical chores at home.[45] Knowing this, the Reich agencies tended to withhold their candidates for front-line duty.[46] The Wehrmacht, which after the defeat at Stalingrad in February 1943 was in dire need of all categories of officers, strove to continue its recruiting without proper consultation with its civilian partners.[47]

By this time, more Allied bombs were falling on Germany's cities, some of which, like Berlin, had ceded about half of their medical staff to the war theater. Because of a high incidence of injuries to the extremities of air raid victims, specialists like surgeons and ophthalmologists were in particular demand. Internal redeployment difficulties were playing havoc with regional health officials, who had been entrusted with the well-being of massive populations after their transfer, for safety reasons, from one province to another.[48] Partly because of the long-standing tension between the civilian and the military medical sectors, but also because the internal public health direction was in chronic disarray, Hitler had appointed one of his personal physicians, Professor Karl Brandt, to the post of sanitation and health plenipotentiary for both areas of operation in July 1942.[49] This appointment was reconfirmed and strengthened in September 1943, with the object of isolating Dr. Conti, the heretofore dilatory Reich health leader in the interior ministry.[50] But even this reshuffle was without consequence, for the civilian-military relationship remained as acrid as ever, and the internecine battles of Brandt and Conti could not generate more personnel.[51]

In 1944 the allocation problems arising from the notorious scarcity of physicians were compounded. The doctors, who by now constituted the most heavily conscripted professional group in the Reich next to veterinarians, were so susceptible to death and wounding just behind the front lines that the casualties among them could not be replaced by a seemingly inexhaustible university recruitment.[52] The bumbling in the home administration did not help matters. Thus in January the Reich health leader's office failed to secure the records of just-graduated university students and hence lost sight of them. Police Chief Heinrich Himmler, the new and well-briefed minister of the interior, complained in April about serious delays in the assignment of medical personnel to transferred population groups.[53]

Stopgap measures brought no relief. After late March, more experienced hospital assistants were to be distributed among the regions, to be replaced in the clinics by uninitiated medical graduates. Even the Wehrmacht's grudging concession in April that henceforth it would release its older army medics without the three-month waiting period made little difference.[54] The damage had already been done. In the civilian sector the consensus was that "the Wehrmacht is becoming less and less considerate in regard to the medicinal needs of the civilian populace."[55] Ironically, by March 1945 the troops had been decimated to the point that the Wehrmacht had more physicians in its ranks than it could use.[56]

Nevertheless, two more last-minute attempts were undertaken by the Reich authorities. In spring of 1944 female doctors with children were strongly urged to join the health services, even on a part-time basis. By the end of the year, this recommendation was made an order, backed by the emergency legislation passed on the threshold of the war. Even mothers with small children were subject to this dragnet.[57]

And finally, the authorities considered calling on the reserve of alien physicians. These could be roughly divided into a preferred category, citizens of friendly powers or sympathizers from occupied countries, and a less desired category that included citizens of belligerent nations, most of whom were at the Reich's command in prisoner-of-war camps (unless they had become turncoats like some White Russians and Ukrainians). As early as 1942 the Reich health administrators had realized that foreign physicians might have to be employed. But for fear of logistic and political complications, such as with Russian doctors who might be treating Soviet forced laborers, nothing was done. Besides, Hitler himself had voiced strong objections to taking such a step.[58]

This situation changed in the fall of 1943 in the wake of the disaster at Stalingrad. It was then deemed essential to assign alien doctors to hospitals and labor camps, where they could be easily supervised.[59] By the end of the year, physicians of the first category were being phased into the public health system, and by the following spring Italian and other foreign doctors had been provisionally assigned.[60] By the end of 1944, this contingent had been augmented by Czechs and other nationals, and they were deemed to be indispensable in the deteriorating situation at the home front.[61]

At this point, total chaos was at hand. After a long history of personnel shortages, logistic inconsistencies, and tremendous loss of human life, the public health administration was on the brink of collapse. Regional and local conditions were unspeakable, as, for instance, in Münster County, where children in kindergartens had gone without medical care for months and even emergency cases in the villages were neglected.[62] In the last year of the war, for every male civilian doctor under the age of fifty who practiced in the Reich, there were three in the armed forces. It was sadly obvious that the thousand army physicians finally promised by the Wehrmacht under one of Commissar Brandt's emergency schemes would be incapable of staving off disaster.[63]

2. The Nazi Reshaping of the Professional Organization

The corporate reorganization of the medical profession within the National Socialist system followed a mixed pattern of forced and voluntary coordination that has been observed in other pre-1933 German institutions. A certain number of previously loyal Nazi protagonists inside the coveted institutions during the final republican years quietly cleared the path for alignment with the Nazi state after Hitler's coming to power and in the beginning phase of the regime they would be aided by outside pressures generated by agencies of party and state. Professional groups and lobbies of the republican era had to be infiltrated and undermined, and then, if the collusion was not sufficient to facilitate easy surrender, force had to be used. Inevitably, the old groups lost their independence, indeed, their claim to existence, after having been merged with corresponding Nazi agencies that now inarguably enjoyed authority, even though some of them had had humble beginnings as unofficial Nazi party affiliates before the political takeover.[1]

Inside the medical profession, the Nazi fifth column was the National Socialist Physicians' League (NS-Ärztebund), which had been founded, rather inauspiciously, by the Ingolstadt surgeon Dr. Ludwig Liebl and a few like-minded colleagues during the party rally at Nuremberg in summer 1929 to promote the interests of Nazi doctors in the Weimar Republic. Its activities included the careful cultivation of a contentious relationship with the leading physicians' lobby, Verband der Ärzte Deutschlands of Leipzig, also called Hartmannbund (founded in 1900–1901) after its founder Hermann Hartmann. In late 1932, Liebl was replaced by the forty-four-year-old Munich general practitioner Dr. Gerhard Wagner, an old Freikorps fighter and longtime Nazi. Henceforth, friction between NS-Ärztebund and Hartmannbund intensified because the National Socialists were winning over more and more converts from the longer-established lobby, and they could hold dual memberships.[2]

After January 1933, Wagner, now charged with establishing control over the medical sector by the Nazi party, decided to absorb the Hartmannbund into a soon to be created Nazi medical system, with the help of his NS-Ärztebund. This Nazi league, staffed exclusively with physician party members, became the spearhead in the regime's drive to coordinate all medical doctors in the Reich and eventually to use them for its purposes.[3] Characteristically, Wagner, as the plenipotentiary of the party, trod carefully, always preferring suasion over force.[4] Already by late March he could be certain of the unwavering cooperation of the bourgeois physicians' unions. On March 22, on the occasion of the "Day of the Awakening Nation" at Potsdam, both Hartmannbund and Deutscher Ärztevereinsbund, its affiliate, since 1929 under the joint leadership of the fifty-five-year-old Nuremberg gastroenterologist Dr. Alfons Stauder, sent a telegram to Hitler indicating that both organizations were looking forward to serving the "patriotic objectives" of the national government "with pleasure."[5] Thereafter an exploratory meeting between Stauder and Wagner took place in Munich, and as a result both men met with their closest aides in Nuremberg on March 23 and 24. Here Stauder appears voluntarily to have surrendered the headship of both physicians' lobbies at the very time that Wagner was appointed commissar of the physicians' chief organizations (*Kommissar der ärztlichen Spitzenverbände*) by the government.[6] From then on Stauder remained in office solely as a figurehead, at the whim of the Nazi leader.[7] In the following weeks, matters moved swiftly. The members of both bourgeois lobbies convened with the functionaries of the Nazi Physicians' League on April 2 in Leipzig to ratify "unanimously" all the new decisions that had been agreed upon by the leaders. In his plenary speech Stauder declared the need for a new "united-front agency" to complete the "revolution."[8] Three days later, Hitler in an audience with Wagner and Stauder expressed his approval and encouraged both doctors to get on with the total Nazification of the medical establishment. Next, the forced reduction of Stauder's salary and the Nazi functionaries' deliberations on how to acquire the lobbies' considerable assets with a minimum of effort signaled the end of the physicians' organizations as they had existed since the turn of the century.[9] On June 7 Stauder was formally dismissed and his place assumed by Wagner, although, for appearances' sake, Stauder was given a nominal post in the new Nazi physicians' network. The Nazi physician leaders shrewdly used the apparatus of the old institutions when to do so was profitable until a final liquidation was propitious. With the legal basis being provided by the Reich Physicians' Ordinance (*Reichsärzteordnung*) of December 13, 1935, the dissolution of Hartmannbund and Ärztevereinsbund was decreed for the beginning of June 1936.[10]

To this day, leaders of the West German medical establishment are wont to explain the Nazi takeover of the republican physician lobbies as a power struggle between the forces of freedom and democracy on one hand and those of totalitarianism on the other, in which the latter finally won. In marked contrast with this interpretation, East German scholars have tended to stress the same events as consequences of a premeditated conspiracy between an essentially fascist-minded German physicianship and the Nazi political leaders at the dawn of the Third Reich.[11] The truth is believed to be in the middle, albeit much closer to the East than to the West German side. There is no question that many German doctors resented the Nazi dictate of a reorganization of their professional societies. Nevertheless, it would be wrong to exonerate the collaborative functionaries of the Hartmannbund, for instance, as victims of Nazi encroachments. Because their political convictions in the Weimar Republic had been only marginally to the left of dyed-in-the-wool Nazis, someone like Carl Haedenkamp, M.D., the erstwhile editor in chief of the Hartmannbund's major publicity organ and a staunch member of the largely anti-Semitic German National People's Party, found it comparatively easy to adjust to the new rulers, and hence he continued to serve them in an almost unaltered capacity.[12] His example was emulated by professionals with similar backgrounds who crossed over with flying colors and accepted positions of great importance in the new medical administration: Heinrich Grote, the doctor, and Clemens Bewer, the lawyer, to name only the most significant. Such attitudes agreed with the Nazi leaders' philosophy of antagonizing as few people as possible and of making the best of a preexisting condition.[13] In the future, they would be the first to concede the historic importance of the Hartmannbund, and they periodically paid homage to its pre-1933 achievements, always adding, of course, that with the advent of the Third Reich this institution had become forever superfluous.[14]

The annihilation of the two traditional physicians' unions was merely a stepping-stone for the establishment of specifically National Socialist health and medical organizations. According to the unwritten rules of Nazi coordination, the destruction of old and the creation of new forms were to proceed synchronously so that one could take over where the other had left off. But in practice, both processes tended to overlap. Hence in spring of 1936 the property and regional apparatus of Hartmannbund were inherited by a Nazi formation, the German Panel Fund Physicians' Union (Kassenärztliche Vereinigung Deutschlands—KVD), which had sprung to life on August 2, 1933.[15]

The KVD did not represent something entirely new because it, too, had preyed on preexisting republican institutions for its lifeblood. In 1932, to change the acrimonious relationship between the hundreds of sickness insurance funds and thousands of doctors treating patients individually insured with them, privately incorporated, regionally deployed agencies were set up all over Germany by Hartmannbund as neutral bodies, charged with collecting bulk payment amounts from the various funds and apportioning them, according to some lump-sum formula, to all the fund-committed physicians in each region.[16] After January 1933 the Nazis consolidated these approximately six thousand regional boards into a central agency with district subsidiaries and gave the system an official character through public incorporation. The KVD continued as a go-between for sickness funds and panel insurance doctors as before, but it also came to serve as an initial instrument of corporate control over German physicians in the totalitarian spirit. From then on, its main task was to regiment German fund physicians, about 80 percent of all self-employed practitioners, professionally, politically, and even socially.

Headed by the leader of the Nazi Physicians' League, Dr. Wagner, and staffed to a large extent with turncoats from the olden days, the KVD was to oversee the certification and regional deployment of all fund doctors by using the ideal ratio of one physician per six hundred insured patients.[17] Political control of the compulsory fund physician membership was facilitated by the introduction of the fascist leadership principle, with Wagner as the "leader" at the top of a rigid hierarchy. Political affiliations were monitored, and the KVD carried out the purge in Germany of Jewish and Marxist panel physicians.[18] Socially, the KVD's purview extended to an emergency fund and a much needed social insurance scheme for panel doctors and their families, as well as to the invocation of an internal disciplinary court. The latter, it was obvious, could also serve professional and political ends.[19]

As if this were not a sufficient means of controlling doctors, the regime leaders established yet another corporate body in April 1936, the Reich Physicians' Chamber (Reichsärztekammer—RÄK). From Dr. Wagner's perspective, this second organization was necessary for two reasons. Despite its great power, the KVD touched only fund physicians, not privately practicing ones or those employed in hospitals or universities. And Wagner, as head of the KVD, was partially dependent on the Reich labor ministry because its jurisdiction covered matters of public insurance, including medicare. Hence any changes in the structure of the insurance funds dictated by the labor minister could affect not only the modality of fund physicians' remuneration but the disbursing agency itself.[20]

Wagner wanted to solidify his position as the party's overlord of medical and health matters at a time when both NSDAP and government offices in the Third Reich were being built up. In 1932, concordant with his assumption of the NS-Ärztebund leadership, he had been charged with broad responsibilities for health in the party realm within the limits of a new party department, Abteilung Volksgesundheit. In May and June 1934, Wagner's close friend and regular patient, NSDAP staff chief Rudolf Hess, reconstituted this department on an official basis, calling it Main Office for People's Health (Hauptamt für Volksgesundheit). Not only was Wagner reconfirmed at the helm, but he was also granted a new mandate as the regime's putative "health leader," suggesting wide powers in the public and private areas of German medicine.[21]

Wagner used this office to amplify his prerogatives over and above the powers that had resulted from the creation of the KVD some ten months previously. Building on the German physicians' long-standing objective of creating a monopolistic professional union anchored in the public domain and patterned after corporative notions, which meshed with National Socialist ideas of an étatist, fascist state in the early years of the regime, Wagner, now officially Reich physicians' leader, proclaimed the Reich Physicians' Ordinance on December 13, 1935.[22] Its main purpose was to found the publicly incorporated, corporativist Reich Physicians' Chamber with compulsory membership for every graduated physician in the land and to provide a statute containing organizational and ethical rulings pertinent to the entire medical profession.[23]

The Reich Physicians' Chamber was officially in place by April 6, 1936. Its attendant and subsequent statutes, of which there were several in the next few years, reiterated the stipulations of the KVD regulation of three years earlier, but they also issued new ones, with the force of law. For example, mutual social relations among all doctors were once again prescribed. Formerly existing provisions for all manner of professional disciplinary proceedings were enlarged, reflecting the priorities of the developing police state, as did the racial and political screening mechanisms that now were reinforced.[24]

But inasmuch as they were fashioned entirely in the image of the Nazi *Weltanschauung*, some of the new clauses went considerably beyond the expectations of the majority of German doctors, who were ever more tightly regimented. By this statute, sterilization and "race" science became firmly wedded to the medical craft, and the principles of *Gesundheitsführung*, of specifically Nazi dicta regarding public health in the service of the nation, became mandatory for every physician. Medicine lost its former legal categorization as a "trade" (since 1869–71), and its new definition among the classic professions was left open. Thus suspended, doctors were at the mercy of the Nazi manipulators who would redefine their task as called for by the requirements of the totalitarian regime. The formerly egocentric objectives of the German doctors, craftily exploited by Hitler's minions, were gradually twisted and merged with the interests of National Socialist policy.[25]

Wagner played the predominant role in this process. Once again ensconced at the peak of the Physicians' Chamber's pyramid, he was cementing his position as plenipotentiary of medicine and health at party as well as state levels. Supported by Party Secretary Hess, he could hope to rise to the highest plane of government administration, perhaps as minister of health, a post that hitherto had not existed and would not, though he hoped to establish it. To reach this important goal, the temporary supervision over some aspects of the Physicians' Chamber by the Reich interior minister was unavoidable and, in the long run, a small price to pay. Even though this minister had had a hand in his formal appointment as Reich physicians' leader, Wagner knew that he was actually responsible only to Adolf Hitler, who was already listening to him in matters exceeding his comparatively narrow portfolio, namely the ongoing race legislation directed against Jews.[26]

Wagner was not able to enjoy the fruits of his efforts for very long. Beset by his rival Dr. Conti, who had started his Third Reich career as the Nazi Physicians' League deputy for Berlin and then rose in Minister President Göring's favor through the acquisition of several Prussian health offices, Wagner died of an undisclosed but allegedly "vicious" illness at the end of March 1939.[27] Conti succeeded him three weeks later, assuming his various offices and superimposing on all his prior titles that of Reich health leader. The deeper significance of this move was that Conti was charged by his superiors in the party and the state to complete a centralization of the German medical and health systems. This task Wagner had begun but never finished because of the multiplicity of agencies that had to be coordinated, streamlined, and converged and the somewhat disadvantageous location of Wagner's seat of power, in Munich, which rendered him unnecessarily susceptible to Conti's machinations emanating from the capital, Berlin.[28]

As it turned out, the somewhat colorless Conti was to have an even more difficult time than his charismatic predecessor. Contrary to his high-sounding title, Conti was only nominally autonomous as the foremost health functionary in the Reich. It is true that in succeeding Wagner he had outmaneuvered as a possible rival Dr. Arthur Gütt, the former chief of the state-supervised public health system in the interior ministry; the ailing Gütt conveniently retired in summer 1939.[29] But, though the Reich Health Office (Reichsgesundheitsamt) under its president, Professor Hans Reiter, served merely nominal functions (as, for instance, the coordination of learned medical associations like the German Dermatological Society), it lay claim to greater independence than was its due under the Reich health leader.[30] Moreover, Conti's jurisdiction and competency were put in doubt by ranking party greats. Robert Ley, the feisty boss of the German Labor Front, who had a genuine interest in extending social and medical insurance benefits to German workers on a wide populist basis that squarely opposed physicians' interests, nearly managed to wrest partial control over public health out of Conti's hands in 1941.[31]

Conti, who had become secretary of state for health in the Reich interior ministry in August 1939 and thus was firmly lodged in the party and state by the time the war was on, was increasingly incapable of dealing with the problems at hand, as indeed he found it difficult to reconcile such duplicate institutions as KVD and Reich Physicians' Chamber for the sake of greater efficiency.[32] Exploiting this situation, and certainly not to the corporate advantage of a by now fully regimented German physicianship, Hitler's personal doctor Karl Brandt had himself appointed Führer plenipotentiary in all matters of German health in July 1942.[33] From then on he succeeded, with a spate of special Führer directives, in reducing Conti's office to impotence, until some time in 1944 this former Berlin physician fell into a virtual state of apathy, one year before his suicide in a Nuremberg prison cell.[34] This act signified the impending collapse of the already moribund Reich health administration and its medicoprofessional affiliates.

3. Medical Specialization and Income

Within the medical establishment of the Third Reich, a contest was being waged between the exponents of generalist medicine and specialism. This struggle had historic roots in the not so distant past of German physicians, when, during the 1920s, the number of specialists vis-à-vis generalists had been increasing.[1] Specialists had received longer and more sophisticated medical training that warranted the collection of higher fees, they preferred to practice in large cities rather than the countryside, and, until the early 1930s, many of them were Jewish. For these three reasons they were anathema to the Nazi philosophy on health and medicine.

The specialists' vertical rather than horizontal approach to medicine, their preoccupation with human afflictions that fell into their narrow categories of expertise, and their proximity to centers of higher learning conflicted with the National Socialist organicist ideal.[2] The archetypal Nazi held a holistic view toward medicine, tempered with notions of Social Darwinism. Inasmuch as he regarded the individual as an organic part of the racially defined people's community (*Volksgemeinschaft*), this subject was a microcosm that mattered solely through the completeness of the totality of its parts. These parts could be dealt with only in the context of the whole and not singularly, in isolation from the rest of the organism. In principle, this holistic view did not allow for the singling out of any of the body's organs for closer attention, but because it was biologically slanted, a certain positive bias was attributed to the mechanics of reproduction and a negative one to matters of the brain. This tendency was in perfect harmony with the Nazis' constant emphasis on things physical as well as their overall anti-intellectuality.[3]

Hence the original National Socialist ideal of the German doctor was the general practitioner, whose social and professional image had suffered somewhat from the proliferation of specialists at the end of the Weimar Republic. Throughout the Third Reich, one of the battle cries of the Nazi medical functionaries was for the full resurrection of the German all-around practitioner as he was pictured in the past: modest, reliable, and professionally trained to put broad knowledge and experience at the service of his patients. As seen by the Nazi medical leaders, the practitioner's potential ability to transcend the smallest cell of the *Volksgemeinschaft*, the family, while making his house calls, rendered him invaluable as a sort of biological block warden, a biopolitical functionary who could perennially spy on the national health for the party.[4]

In his heart of hearts the Nazi physician was a country doctor. It was in the countryside that the Nazi ideology of "blood and soil" could best be complemented with the holistic, organically oriented practice of medicine. Nazis repudiated urban environments as rational, arid, and inorganic constructions that were cursed with the maladies of modern civilization: materialism, atmospheric pollution, and, of course, Jewry. Reich Physicians' Leader Wagner hated modern hospitals, especially polyclinics.[5] In stark contrast, the rural areas were said to offer open-air activity, closeness to unadulterated nature, and the hardy peasant stock, possessed, as the Nazis fancied, of the qualities of their unspoiled Germanic forebears.[6] In the ideal Nazi scenario, a German country doctor's life was depicted as onerous but honest, and, logically, upon certifying young medical school graduates, the KVD encouraged them to practice in the countryside.[7]

But reality continued to present a different picture. Not least because opportunities for good earnings there were smaller, the national trend among physicians was away from the country and into the cities, as it had been for some decades, so that in January 1934 still only 34 percent of all doctors were country practitioners.[8] As a result, medical services were acutely underrepresented in the provinces.[9]

Perhaps the most important medical skill that the family physician in the country was expected to master was obstetrics, for he had to be at the country women's side when they were giving birth at the rural home.[10] Not surprising for a nation that placed such a premium on propagation and population growth, perfect command of obstetrical techniques turned out to be one of the chief postulates of Nazi medical reform, or what could have passed as such. Once again the rationale was organicist and biological: women who had become used to the easy, comfortable ways of the city, with its specialists and modernly equipped clinics, were to be reintroduced to natural childbirth, without anesthetics, because it could be supervised by every family-minded general practitioner just like in the olden days.

The movement toward natural childbirth in the home was greatly accelerated after Leonardo Conti became Reich health leader in the spring of 1939 because he was under the ideological spell of his practicing midwife mother, Nanna Conti. Under her headship as Reich director of midwifery, the training of young women acquiring requisite skills was stepped up with the object of increasing the number of obstetrical assistants to be employed in the course of natural childbirth, and so to wean even more young mothers away from the hospitals.[11] But progress in this area was slow, and the initial difficulties of the peaceful period were compounded as the war became full-blown. The Nazi idea of childbirth in a country home was endangered because the recruitment of midwives lagged and they were insufficiently taught. Besides, fewer and fewer generalists became available in the rural areas. Peasant wives who were traditionally used to natural childbirth became increasingly susceptible to miscarriages because of heavy work loads in the fields; consequently, they tended to favor adjacent small-town clinics.[12]

Conti, nevertheless, was steadfast. Partially because of his ingrained dislike of clinical medicine, but also because hospital beds were becoming seriously scarce in war, he promulgated ordinances in late 1939 that raised the legal retirement age for midwives from sixty-five to seventy and further encouraged childbirth at the home. He reiterated this objective in early 1942: "To be born in a bad hospital is very bad, but childbirth in an everyday household is good."[13] The midwives, who were still in great demand but inadequately schooled and always at risk of being confused with the presumably lower-ranking nurses, were pressed: it did not help their work morale.[14] But the doctors, too, began to protest. One outspoken report from the Cologne area informs of the distinct reluctance on the part of urban women to suffer childbirth at home amid the chronic danger of air raids. And it mentions the mounting unpopularity of natural childbirth, particularly in the countryside, where sanitary conditions in wartime were said to be dismal and infections prevalent. "Anyone with a stake in this issue," concluded the writer, "agrees that this measure will have to be dropped because of the uncertainties encountered during childbirth and the impossibility of applying hard-and-fast rules."[15]

The author of the report left no doubt that, contrary to Conti's designs, the frequency of home births was actually declining. Information from towns such as Lübeck showed that the growth rate of clinical childbirths had been steadily increasing since 1932 and was expected to continue.[16] Statistics from certain rural regions such as Beckum in Westphalia also indicated reticence by expectant country mothers to deliver themselves to the care of Nazi midwives, preferring instead provincial clinics.[17] Two years before Conti's health administration lay in shambles, this failure marked the bankruptcy of a large and important part of specifically National Socialist medical reform.

At the other end of the professional spectrum, medical specialism in the first few years of the regime was distinctly unwanted. It was the declared objective of the medical functionaries, in conformity with romanticist Nazi thinking on health and medicine, to reduce the absolute numbers of specialists, to redistribute the remaining ones more equitably, away from the cities and across the countryside, and to commit postgraduate students to more rigorous generalist training and field practice so as to make them more appreciative of their lowlier cousins, the general practitioners.[18]

The Nazis succeeded, by the middle 1930s, in reducing the specialist proportion of the physicians' corps to slightly more than a quarter, down from about a third at the end of the republic. Yet this decline occurred less because medical graduates or younger doctors decided to heed Nazi advice than because fund-practice Jewish specialists, who had dominated this branch of the profession, were evicted from the profession in the spring of 1933. After that, despite a second round of Jewish evictions in 1938 and official protestations to the contrary, the percentage of specialists climbed again, to just below 33 percent in 1942.[19]

There was little the Nazi planners could do to redeploy specialists to the rural areas. The right clientele did not exist there. Country folk were used to traveling to the small towns, if not the large cities, for complicated treatments that their regular practitioners could not provide, and those occasions were few enough. Since a considerable number of specialists had opted against the panel insurance system, they were dependent on well-to-do private patients, who usually resided in the urban centers. Hence predominantly agrarian provinces such as East Prussia or Schleswig-Holstein continued to be understaffed with specialists, whereas Berlin, Hamburg, and Leipzig, even when purged of Jews, were oversupplied. In 1937 the capital alone had more than seven times more specialists than the province of Schleswig-Holstein, and Hamburg had almost twice as many as East Prussia. These relationships hardly changed in the course of the war because city specialists rarely were recruited by the KVD for service in the countryside; their generalist expertise still was thought to be wanting.[20]

By the time specialists' training was spelled out in more detail by the follow-up ordinance of November 1937, after the erection of the Reich Physicians' Chamber in 1936, all attempts to include more content oriented toward generalists and rural practice in the candidates' preparation curricula had ceased.[21] But if the Nazis were to have specialties at all, it was clear that they wished to see a hierarchy of them in accordance with their ideological value system. Surgeons were at the top of the list because they had traditionally fitted into patriarchal, male-oriented societies such as Germany and were well equipped to meet the heroic martial standards of a totalitarian regime poised to mobilize for war.[22] "It is no accident," wrote a medical functionary as early as 1933, "that the few natural representatives of the master race usually turn to surgery. Here, if anywhere, strong will and action are evidently still decisive." Complementarily, one year before the war it was averred that "in essential respects, the entire personal make-up of the surgeon has to equal that of the military leader."[23]

Surgery was in that group of disciplines for which a specialist training term of four years became obligatory by November 1937, rather than the usual three years.[24] Always a most favored medical branch in Germany, not least because it was one of two possible prerequisites for the assumption of a hospital directorship (the other being internism), its popularity in the Third Reich was further on the ascendancy. The surgeons' percentage of the total number of specialists in Germany increased from 10.0 percent in 1935 to 15.3 in 1937 and had reached 16.4 percent in 1940. Surgeon certifications for neophytes were up from 22.8 percent of the specialists' total in 1938 to 25.1 percent in 1939.[25] As far as the leaders were concerned, this would be propitious for the war effort.

Internism ranked after surgery. This specialty was popular in part because an internist could become chief of a civilian hospital with relative ease.[26] Moreover, judging merely from the experience of World War I, internists were indispensable in any armed struggle and this, too, augured well for the future.[27]

Gynecology, together with its sister discipline obstetrics, also was near the top of Nazi priorities because of the extraordinary emphasis on fertility and demographic expansion in the Third Reich. It, too, was on the rise after 1933.[28] Yet, because of the ideological issue of natural childbirth, gynecology was potentially tarnished. The Nazi health bureaucracy was concerned over the traditional affiliation of gynecology with obstetrical surgery; it objected to the not infrequent clinical practice of delivering babies "unnaturally" through cesarean sections, claiming that these were usually unwarranted. Ideally, it wanted surgeons who would not dabble in obstetrics and gynecologists who would use scalpels only as a last resort.[29]

Because the regime needed child specialists in the various Nazi crib, school, and Hitler Youth services, there were also fairly good opportunities for pediatricians. Their numbers increased slightly until 1938, when it had become obvious that the party was making undue demands on the time of these doctors, expecting many of them to serve in the Hitler Youth in an honorary capacity.[30] Like surgery and internism, pediatrics and gynecology required four years of postgraduate concentration.[31]

There were other specialties that were of less concern to the health administrators. To this group belonged ophthalmology and otology, dermatology, and organic psychiatry, the latter of which, nonetheless, was needed in insane asylums and later for the "euthanasia" program. ("Jewish" Freudian psychiatry, of course, was virtually banished.) Until 1939, some of those disciplines, which required only three years' preparation, underwent denouements partially because of oversupplies from the days of the republic, as in the case of dermatology.[32]

Only World War II would change basic patterns of this ranking order; the soon-to-be-experienced indispensability of all medical specialties at the home as well as the war front resulted in a fundamental revaluation of that sector of medicine in relation to generalist practice. At the height of the war, one Wehrmacht staff physician insisted that "we now have trouble finding all the specialists we need."[33]

In the course of mobilization and anticipating hostilities in the near future, the Wehrmacht actively sought out all types of specialists as early as 1937, offering instant commissions in its branches.[34] Upon the outbreak of the war in September 1939, leading experts in their fields were appointed to prestigious advisory positions in the armed forces to spot-check hygiene and medical practice at the fronts; those men, often well-known university professors, could justly look forward to quick and steep promotions.[35] Not surprisingly, surgery turned out to be the specialty most in demand right behind the front lines, as well as in army, navy, and air force hospitals situated closer to home; surgeons were requisitioned almost to the end.[36] In time, other specialists were needed, notably internists as well as hygienic pathologists and psychiatrists, but not gynecologists and pediatricians unless they and other experts retrained provisionally.[37]

At home, specialists were needed largely to care for the victims of air raids, which did not present a major problem until 1942.[38] Then surgeons, naturally, attained a new preeminence, along with ophthalmologists, because of the high incidence of eye injuries caused by flying window glass.[39] At the climax of the war, physicians of any calling had become so precious that the home-front authorities would fabricate excuses to retain even the most obscure of specialists.[40] Thus the former arbitrary hierarchy was destroyed, and any doctor who had knowingly built his career on diversification could feel vindicated. However ironic or sad the circumstances, this constituted a belated victory for the entire medical profession.

Except for certain younger groups of physicians, especially during the early phase of the regime,[41] specialists and generalists together consistently belonged to the highest-income social strata and were at the top of all the free professionals, including lawyers. This was so, notwithstanding the hue and cry raised by public relations manipulators in their midst, who would periodically contend, as a precautionary measure, that "the German doctor is not faring well, at least not well enough to be able to endure a deterioration of his present state."[42] And this prosperity obtained for all groups of established physicians: the large majority of the fund-committed doctors, judged to be more than 80 percent of the total, as well as the smaller layer of private practitioners, who were invariably earning more, and also the employed physicians, who sometimes had that opportunity, as did the professors of medicine.

It is true that at the beginning of Hitler's rule the doctors were still suffering from the adverse effects of a combination of ordinances connected, in one way or another, with the emergency legislation of the late-Weimar Brüning cabinet. These had been designed to reduce the deficit in the sickness insurance funds as well as fill the coffers of the Reich treasury, but then massive unemployment kept patients away from the doctors, and that professional group faced economic limbo.[43] Unquestionably, the creation of a centralized KVD after January 1933, which facilitated a smoother transfer of payments from the sickness funds to the physicians, as well as official rhetoric concerning the future safeguarding of doctors' and patients' interests, did a great deal to restore public trust in the health sector, at least for the time being. Certain reforms in the panel fund system, such as the reduction of a mandatory fee patients paid for each visit to a doctor's office from the late republican days, coupled with a quantitative consolidation of the heteromorphous insurance fund structure, further boosted this confidence.[44] The return of patients to doctors' practices as the economic depression was lifting was paralleled by a reduction in the doctors' numbers, relative to the population, in large part because of the disappearance of Jewish physicians. By 1934 the doctors' gross earnings were averaging 10,324 marks, surpassing the bottom values they had reached in 1932–33, and in 1937 physicians were taking home 13,643 marks on average, more than in 1928 and nearly as much as in 1929 (Figure 1).[45]

With the recovery of full employment levels in a harnessed economy and the final removal of Jewish, privately practicing physicians by 1938, the doctors were making even more money in 1939, although exact figures are missing.[46] For 1941, contemporary sources estimated an average income of 20,000 marks, which sounds realistic only if applicable to both fund and private physicians.[47] Two years later, all 356 fund-committed physicians in the South German region of Augsburg, regardless of specialty, drew a gross income from the insurance fund of just under 14,000 marks on average, to which at least a couple of thousand marks could probably be added from private patients. In the city of Augsburg alone, the mean income for 103 panel physicians was nearly 15,000 marks.[48] That year in northern Brunswick, the city's fifty-three general practitioners and seventy-five specialists, all *Kassenärzte*, were grossing over 16,000 marks before counting private side incomes, which, with such a predominance of specialists, could have been substantial.[49] Here in the north, incomes for physicians relocated in the surrounding countryside by the war events tended to be higher, over 17,600 marks, even though in Kreis Wolfenbüttel or the provincial town of Peine opportunities for additional private practice were limited.[50]

From one discipline to another, the differences in earnings were remarkable. In Brunswick city, the generalists were making 12,350 marks compared to 19,300 for the specialists. Among the latter, the ten resident surgeons received the highest fees (RM 24,100), followed closely by nine ophthalmologists (RM 23,200) and thirteen gynecologists (RM 17,300), reflecting the intramedical priorities and attendant peer status of the time. Internists and pediatricians were next in line (RM 14,600 and RM 13,400 respectively), with dermatologists, neurologists, and urologists trailing well behind (RM 12,600; RM 9,250; RM 7,800).[51]

If these incomes appear steep, it must be pointed out, on one hand, that they probably would have been even steeper had the war not taken place. Generally, all doctors lost 10 to 15 percent of net earnings because those fit to fight in the trenches had to be supported communally by the ones left behind to practice, a situation in which all military physicians' salaries as commissioned officers were taken into account.[52] On the other hand, physicians always had substantial overhead costs to defray, approximately 20 to 40 percent of gross earnings, depending on the resident's specialty (such as expensive x-ray equipment for a radiologist, or a sturdy automobile particularly for doctors in the countryside), costs that were apt to rise during the hostilities. Deducted from net earnings after taxes were social and life insurance premiums and payments into a special old-age pension fund to which, even in peacetime, physicians notoriously undercontributed.[53]

In peace as well as war, there were three additional measures by which the physicians' take-home income needed to be qualified to be fully understood: the percentile extremes at either end of the income spectrum, to analyze how these related to the healthy center core; the doctors' pay compared with that of other professional groups; and some indication of how these earnings affected the quality of life for doctors of all types.

In 1934, 63.5 percent of all doctors in the Reich were earning between 5,000 and 16,000 marks, after deduction of overhead costs (Table 1.1). Compared with income statistics for self-employed Germans three years later, showing 21.4 percent in that earnings bracket, the doctors were doing very well, especially considering that in 1937 the overall incomes were higher (Table 1.1). Judged by the values for 1937, the best earners in this middle group of doctors (as of other self-employed persons) would have been subject to a personal income tax rate of approximately 13 percent.[54]

If this was thought to be a more than sufficient emolument to guarantee a comfortable living standard, there were, at the bottom of the physicians' scale, 12.6 percent who made between 3,000 and 5,000 and 8.6 percent who fell below the 3,000 marks-a-year line (they corresponded with 20.5 percent and almost 53 percent in the self-employed sector) (Table 1.1). Indeed, it is possible to make certain inferences regarding the existence of penurious fund doctors after an examination of official KVD support programs that were launched three years after the political takeover. Hence practitioners eking out a living in wayward, economically deficient places in such predominantly rural provinces as East Prussia and Bavaria were guaranteed a minimum annual income by the KVD of 5,000 marks in 1936 and 6,000 marks in 1937. That year 123 such practices were aided at a cost of RM 316,000.[55] Indigent doctors with practices in nonsubsidized areas were helped in a somewhat less generous fashion, as were physicians with large families, who benefited from baby bonuses granted to fund doctors after the birth of a second child.[56] As contemporaries have recorded, a young physician attempting to establish a fund practice in 1936 or so, despite the developing scarcity of medical graduates, was likely to be in this lowest earning group, at least for a few months, until he became reasonably well known.[57]

Such extremes were matched, on the other side, by 11.3 percent who enjoyed between 16,000 and 25,000 marks per annum, and a tiny 4 percent who collected enormous fees above 25,000 marks a year. These still substantial groups of affluent, mostly private-practice physicians, some of whom, in 1936 perhaps, might charge as much as RM 3,500 for a single medical service,[58] contrasted positively with much smaller groupings of self-employed Germans of various trades totaling merely 5.2 percent (Table 1.1).

In the doctors' case, both extremes persisted through the war, even though the exact relations are not certain. Dr. M. in Swabian Amerdingen received only RM 300 from the KVD for the last quarter of 1943, whereas his colleague W. in Lindenberg, some hundred miles to the south, was grossing RM 10,000.[59]

It is possible to place these figures further in perspective, vis-à-vis the earnings of comparable professional groups, only for the incipient phase of the Third Reich, for which statistics on the incomes of doctors, lawyers, and dentists are available. Lawyers, who were earning substantially more money than physicians in 1928, started to fall behind the doctors in 1933 and were trailing them in 1936, when their mean annual income was 10,800 marks compared to the doctors' 12,546 marks.[60] Expressed somewhat differently, the doctors' corporate earnings grew by an annual average of 10.5 percent, judged on a compound basis, compared with the lawyers' income growth rate of only 4.4 percent, between 1933 and 1936.[61]

Additional though somewhat limited comparisons between doctors' and lawyers' incomes may be attempted for the arbitrary dates of 1934 and 1936. In 1934 physicians were pocketing 10,324 marks on average and lawyers 9,784 marks.[62] Table 1.1 highlights this discrepancy by divulging a much larger proletaroid segment of lawyers than of doctors who earned below 3,000 marks that year, 20.3 as opposed to 8.6 percent. This less than happy situation for the lawyers was not compensated, at the other end of the spectrum, by a larger proportion of legal professionals fortunate enough to receive incomes of over 25,000 marks, 6.1 as against 4 percent. (Indeed, the published statistics reveal that not one physician, but 0.2 percent of all lawyers, grossed premium amounts of 100,000 marks and more.)[63] What is significant for this juxtaposition is that in the healthy middling section many more doctors than lawyers were earning the amounts deemed necessary for a high-quality life short of becoming profligate (RM 5,000–16,000): 63.5 against 47.1 percent. More than half the lawyers existed on incomes of less than 7,000 marks.[64] These proportions appear to have been essentially unchanged two years later, when 2,570 physicians but 3,000 lawyers made less than 3,000 marks, and 46 lawyers made over 100,000, 5 more than the physicians who declared that much.[65]

Academically trained dentists, who in present-day West Germany tend to earn as much as, if not more than, physicians, found themselves even behind the lawyers. Their mean income in 1934 was RM 6,361, yet half of them made less than RM 5,500.[66] Almost three times as many as the doctors, 21 percent, resided at the poverty level of 3,000 marks or less, and for every dentist who grossed at least 16,000 marks, there were almost five physicians who did so. In fact, whereas four doctors out of a hundred made 25,000 marks or more, not one dentist could command such fees (Table 1.1). For every six physicians with a comfortable lifestyle (at between 5,000 and 16,000 marks per annum), there were only five dentists who did as well (Table 1.1). Two years later the physicians still earned almost twice as much as their distant cousins in dentistry.[67]

As may be expected, the doctors generally lived well on their generous incomes, even after hefty deductions for overhead. Personal income tax levies, if judged by the figures for 1937, ran to about 31 percent only for the couple of hundred of them who earned over 50,000 marks, and they could well afford the tax.[68] The richest of these men led luxurious lives, such as the surgeon Ferdinand Sauerbruch, who dwelled in mansions, kept expensive horses, and sometimes showered his favorite assistants with miraculous presents such as automobiles.[69] Until 1939, a large number of physicians took their vacations abroad as a matter of course.[70] Most of them could sustain conveniently located and spacious quarters, certainly in peacetime, the exceptions being younger doctors with insufficient means, who lived in such disadvantaged rural areas as Schleswig-Holstein.[71]

Chief among the prized possessions of medical doctors in Germany was the automobile, which many of them were able to justify on occupational grounds. A Mercedes was the preferred make not only of style-conscious figures like Sauerbruch but, judging by advertisements in professional publications, of most of his lesser colleagues as well.[72] In 1936, the five-liter compressor flagship cost RM 22,000, obviously out of reach for any but the truly wealthy, yet a more modest two-liter model had a sticker price of RM 6,000, as much as a fifth or so of the doctors would earn in a year. The cheapest machine of this genre, a four-seater convertible Mercedes, fetched 4,000 marks at the dealer's, and today it would be worth a special effort to determine how many doctors owned this reasonably affordable car in comparison with other professional groups or members of the German social elite, including the new Nazi administrators.[73] Other physicians made do with used cars, even those unaffordable for the average German. For example, one could buy an old Opel P 25, as did Dr. Wilhelm Hagen of Augsburg, for 500 marks in 1935.[74]

During the war, the physicians' automobiles lost their functions as symbols of pleasure and prestige (as, indeed, they did for most other strata of German upper society), for they were often requisitioned by the Wehrmacht or consigned by the KVD to emergency and replacement doctors. It was forbidden to enjoy them in private, and contraventions were sternly prosecuted. In any case, at the height of the conflict, most Mercedes cars had been supplanted with cheaper, unsightlier models converted with wood-burning generators, or by the Fiat Topolino, the gasoline-powered midget on license from fascist Italy, or by the humble bicycle.[75] The change came at a time when most physicians were impelled to reconsider not only the worth of their material possessions but also the very substance of their calling.

4. Practicing Medicine in the Third Reich

In the execution of their professional duties as healers, the entire corps of medical doctors in the Third Reich lost traditional privileges without gaining new ones, while at the same time contracting new obligations without being allowed to shed old ones. The crucial shifts that occurred in this constellation of competencies, which never had been ideally balanced, resulted from the promulgation of measures surrounding the creation of those novel Nazi institutions, the KVD in summer 1933 and the Reichsärztekammer in spring 1936. They were the KVD Regulation of August 1933, the Reich Physicians' Ordinance of December 1935, and its supplement, the Professional Statute (*Berufsordnung*) of November 1937, as well as resultant formal decrees from the late 1930s through the war.

The 1935 ordinance marked a historic precedent by establishing, on a nationwide basis, a fixed body of codes governing the professional conduct of the medical peer group, inside and out of the medical office, and as such it appeared to fulfill the expectations that all its older members had countenanced for decades. But as it turned out, in many remarkable instances the new codification went much further than a voluntarily imposed honor system of the Weimar-republican kind in that it restricted the physicians' freedom by threatening stiff punishment for all infractions. It took the German doctors some time to grasp that the new regulations were not the natural product of their own free will but had been imposed upon them by a small number of Nazi colleagues who claimed to represent their corporate interests without making good their promises in the end.

Consonant with the guidelines of the new ordinances, the German physicians' corps essentially became a microcosm of the larger Nazi sociopolitical system governed by the Nazi leadership principle (*Führerprinzip*). At the helm stood the Reich physicians' leader, and later the Reich health leader, and both would brook neither discussion nor opposition to their corporate dictates. During the process of redefining the medical profession in National Socialist terms, the physicians' conformity and their subsequent control were ensured by a new, two-tiered system of staggered penalties, to be meted out at the disciplinary court level for relatively minor transgressions and at a higher Nazi professional court level for major ones. The lower courts were quick to pronounce warnings, assign demerit points and fines up to a thousand marks, and sometimes suspend physicians from their medical duties. The higher courts invariably considered irrevocable expulsion from the profession and were always prepared to submit the cases before them to the civilian judiciary, if not the secret police.[1]

By the various rulings doctors were compelled to present every private contractual arrangement to the Reich Physicians' Chamber for approval.[2] They had to register with the new Nazi medical agencies and keep them abreast of any changes in their family status or in matters relating to their medical qualification, such as upgrading to a specialty. Details on residence and practice venues were meticulously filed by the KVD and Physicians' Chamber to facilitate logistic deployment of doctors long before the war broke out.[3]

Nor did the doctors' patients escape these intensified controls, and the doctors were chastised for permitting any relaxations. In accordance with Nazi racial tenets, all serious cases of alcoholism and what were deemed incurable hereditary or congenital illnesses such as imbecilism were to be recorded with the authorities, as were highly contagious diseases like venereal disorders. This tight monitoring early in the regime provided the Nazis with a convenient instrumentarium for sterilization, as well as annihilation later on.[4] Moreover, violations of paragraph 218 of the German criminal code, safeguarding the right to life of the unborn child, were sharply indicted by the biopolitically motivated anti-abortionist Nazi leaders. Hence in May 1936 Dr. Heinrich Eckard of Eisenach was jailed for two years for this offense, and Eutin gynecologist Dr. Wolfgang Saalfeldt was repeatedly ordered to appear in court, his loyalty to the Nazi party notwithstanding.[5]

One of the novelties provided for by the Nazi medicopolitical legislation was the imposition of continued training on seasoned doctors, be they general practitioners or specialists.[6] Indeed, it was one of the desired goals of these courses to neutralize further the differences between those two categories of doctors by forcing them both to undergo the training.[7] Under the direction of dermatologist Dr. Kurt Blome, who had been appointed deputy in charge of continuing medical education by Gerhard Wagner in the spring of 1935, the first courses began in the fall of that year. At that time, only country doctors were co-opted, but after some months they were followed by their colleagues from towns and cities.[8] Although it was conceded that any city clinic could host the three-week events, institutions in rural settings were clearly favored. The health functionaries soon developed predilections for special centers in Munich, Berlin, Hamburg (and later Vienna), and Dresden, where, in their own Rudolf Hess Hospital, they endeavored to teach the specifically National Socialist concepts of health and medicine. For every physician under sixty years of age except university lecturers and public health officials, retraining was mandatory every five years so that in 1936 alone more than five thousand doctors attended the sessions.[9] Taught by fanatic Nazi instructors, these courses were anything but popular. It would be advisable for doctors to volunteer more cheerfully for them, wrote one concerned lecturer in 1937, "to avoid the hardships of quota conscription."[10]

German physicians who were naive enough may have thought these indoctrination exercises constituted progress in the formal professionalization of their calling. But if interest in these courses decreased over the years, the doctors could be roused by yet another novel item in the plethora of ordinances that promised to tighten the corporate ranks. By lifting the physicians' vocation out of the context of competitive commercialism where it had resided, along with other gainful occupations, since 1869–71, the Nazi legislators cleared the way for a welcome redefinition of the medical art that would have important legal and social consequences. The curt statement in paragraph 1 of the Reich Physicians' Ordinance, "The medical occupation is not a business," made it possible to exclude from the the doctors' corps anyone who was not properly schooled or licensed in accordance with long-accepted academic standards: the medical quacks.[11]

Along with the large majority of German medical practitioners, the Nazi health functionaries appeared to deplore a situation inherited from the republican, and further back, the Wilhelmine era, in which any person could practice medicine for a fee, without formal training, as long as the medical doctorate was not used. During the republic, the most qualified of these men and women had striven for a certain degree of professionalization by incorporating themselves on a civil-legal basis and by rejecting lesser-qualified and blatantly fraudulent "practitioners." But as late as 1933 the problem was that without more formal distinctions, the German public could not differentiate between certified medical physicians, almost all of whom possessed a medical doctorate, the incorporated natural healers who attempted, with limited means, to help patients to the best of their ability, and felonious quacks whose only interest lay in garnering high fees. In fact, the lower the class a healer belonged to, the greater was his tendency to impersonate those above him, and because the German public had become weary of conventional doctors in the final stages of the republic, this had led to gross abuses to the detriment of the academic physicians whose "crisis of medicine" during the depression it significantly compounded.[12]

After the political takeover, the Nazi health leaders were in a quandary because on one hand, they realized that by outlawing the quacks they could curry favor with the great majority of doctors. On the other hand, however, these leaders were committed to certain planks in the Nazi conception of medicine that favored the lay element over exponents of so-called school medicine.[13] In their reformation of German medicine, they had to find some middle ground, keeping the acceptable lay healers contented while also pacifying the militant professionalists who called for the total extinction of that genus.[14]

By early 1935, when nothing more had been accomplished than prohibiting quacks from calling themselves physicians and interdicting their itinerancy, there existed at least fourteen thousand lay healers, or three for every ten academic doctors.[15] The next feat was accomplished in December of that year with the passing of the Physicians' Ordinance, which, in Reich Physician Leader Wagner's words, removed the medical profession from "alien legal ground."[16] A few months later, the German Natural Healers' Union, to improve its credibility, purged its ranks of unsavory elements, thus reducing the membership by one-third.[17]

After the Professional Statute of November 1937 had once again failed to settle the issue definitively,[18] the aura of compromise was extended into 1939 when finally, in February, the Lay Healers' Law was announced. It called for specific certification for lay healers, who were now to be labeled "healing practitioners" (*Heilpraktiker*), a new title anchored in public law. Compulsory membership in the regime-sanctioned German Natural Healers' Union, whose self-screening was encouraged, bequeathed on these practitioners a semblance of professionalism without making them truly respectable. To solve this long-standing problem, no new recruitment into the occupation was to be permitted. But the other and, for the legitimate physicians, negative side of the issue consisted in dubious concessions to the quacks that unmistakably stemmed from the Nazi health leaders' own empathy with them. Any quack who could demonstrate requisite ability was allowed to graduate to the bona fide group of physicians after adopting the title "physician of natural healing." Moreover, any with extraordinary talent could enter a medical faculty without the usual upper-school qualification and could advance to the licensure stage as a doctor medici. And even those who were not singled out in this manner could continue to engage in old-style quackery as long as they collected no fees.[19]

For the traditional medical establishment, the Nazis added insult to injury when they decreed that regular doctors had to assist registered nature healers at the latter's request.[20] Furthermore, the physicians had no way of ascertaining who in the health bureaucracy would ordain the "good" quacks and who would decide to let them enter the universities. Time was to show that a wrong sense of professionalism and perhaps of social justice on the part of the rulers had augmented the old disorder by leaving the nonstandardized doctors unchecked and in rivalry with the academics, all under the mantle of "reform." Although further regulations against health quacks were on the books in the early phase of the war, nothing was done. One or two years before the war's end, one could have no more illusions about the "dangerous ramifications of quackery" in the Third Reich.[21]

The doctors were abused in yet another manner. The Physicians' Ordinance of 1935 had expressly safeguarded the traditional Hippocratic privilege of confidentiality between doctors and their patients, which was reiterated in the Professional Statute in 1937. Infractions were to be punishable by fines or up to one year in prison.[22] Physicians were allowed to resort to the secrecy oath even when called to the witness stand in judicial proceedings.[23] As late as 1940, when the war was on, RÄK functionary Kurt Blome assured a congregation of doctors, all of whom applauded him loudly, that this hallowed convention would not be disregarded because it formed the "basis of confidence between physician and patient."[24]

But the potential for destruction of this privilege, which protected both doctors and patients, had been built into the first statutory statement, and from then on erosion set in. A medical secret could be laid bare, so the 1935 ordinance said, if the "common sense of the people" demanded it.[25] Not surprisingly, such a rationale would form the premise for the doctors' legal obligation to inform on their eugenically infirm patients to the Nazi health authorities.[26]

The regime's scrutiny over its subjects was tightened during World War II, in consonance with certain programs for ostracizing and liquidating biologically objectionable men, women, and children. This brought on a fundamental change in the functioning of medical ethics in the German context. Thus in March 1942 Reich Health Leader Conti once again publicly repeated the regime's long-standing desire to establish a "health file" on every German, from the cradle to the grave. In the course of assembling this file, he said, it would be necessary to violate the principle of medical confidentiality, even though an effort would be made to keep this violation to a minimum.[27]

The death knell for the time-honored privilege was sounded in January 1943, when Hitler personally decided to suspend medical secrecy in the relationship between the doctors and the supreme official, health plenipotentiary Professor Karl Brandt. As a noted postwar sociologist of medicine has commented, this action signified not only a substantial loss in corporate medical prestige but also the demise of an important function of societal interaction.[28]

At the height of the war many physicians who found it difficult to adjust to the tight regimen imposed by the health bureaucracy between the home and war fronts had every reason to doubt the continued existence of their profession as a free agent of German society after the anticipated "Final Victory." Never had German doctors enjoyed the prize of freedom unto themselves, out of reach of any state controls, as much as during the Weimar Republic, and never had they been more afraid of losing this treasured status as then. Danger had lurked from the egalitarian-minded panel fund administrators who aimed to delete the doctors' free-enterprise privileges (which were guaranteed them because of their commercial business classification since 1869–71) and instead bureaucratize them in such a way as to make them subservient to the administrators' schemes. The result would have been the abrogation of the free contractual relationship between the patient as a client and the physician as an entrepreneur, through a fixed consignment of patients for every doctor controlled solely by the funds. The relentlessness of this socialization drive on the part of the sickness funds made the doctors rally even more strongly to their lobby, the Hartmannbund, and, when it appeared inert, to cross over increasingly to the Nazi camp.[29] In the last stages of Weimar, the medical exponents of the Nazi party proclaimed strong adherence to the idea of a "free" medical profession, with freedom of doctor's choice guaranteed for every patient, and this concept was officially perpetuated after the political takeover. It was essentially enshrined in the Reich physicians' and complementary ordinances and repeatedly paid lip service by men like Gerhard Wagner.[30]

But there were hidden traps. Precisely because the legal classification of physicians was newly defined in December 1935, this profession could be said by some to have been forced onto the mercy of the state. For if the doctors were removed from their commercial base, this could be read to mean that their liberties so insistingly flaunted in pluralistic Weimar were also gone. In that sense, then, the Reich Physicians' Ordinance was a true product of the totalitarian regime. The Nazi leaders never precisely said so, but Wagner surely knew what he meant when, by various means, he forced commitments from the doctors to the specifically Nazi program of public health and when he intimated that in future the freedom of patients to change their practitioners would have to be curtailed.[31]

At the beginning of the war, when Wagner's successor Conti embarked on extraordinary measures to procure the supply of doctors necessary for civilian and military use, some physicians verbalized their fear that the emergency situation might lead to a permanent state of socialization for them after the victory. From then on Conti and his underlings found themselves periodically challenged to deny that this might happen.[32] Although at heart the Reich health leader understood his colleagues well and even rescued them successfully from bureaucratization attempts made by DAF leader Ley, he, too, could not escape the need to solve ever-recurring supply-and-demand impasses through stringent regulation.[33] The doctors' fears regarding socialization would have been substantiated by certain plans in the Reich health administration calling for a permanent implementation of the martial contingency deployments even in peacetime, after the Final Victory, rather than a return to the moderate control exercised over certification regionally by the KVD. This would have meant the institutionalization of those barriers to horizontal mobility which the large majority of physicians had come to dislike after fall 1939.[34]

But those antiprofessional tendencies caused by a regime bent on rigid discipline in the service of the *Volksgemeinschaft* did not go away, and there was widespread fear in the medical profession after the defeat at Stalingrad, when even more resources were harnessed for the war effort. In August 1944 Himmler, by then Conti's superior, said that doctors should be put on fixed salaries and made financially accountable for every day their patients were sick. At that time, with Conti veritably out of commission, the bureaucratization of physicians was again seriously considered by the authorities and most likely would have been established along with other, no less total, reforms of German society intended for the postwar period.[35] In the end, German doctors owed it to the Nazi defeat, not to any victory, that the blanket suspension of their professional liberties never did come to pass.

Bureaucratization would only have hindered the doctors' fight against diseases. For the health casualty index in the Third Reich shows that physicians had to contend with a higher rate of illnesses and accidents than observed at that time in England and the United States; moreover, it is probably safe to assume as well that in the purely German context the incidence of sickness increased from 1933 to 1939 over the preceding period.[36] As the effects of the Great Depression subsided slowly after 1932, the general living standard, including nutrition, did not improve sufficiently to lead to better comprehensive health for the people of Germany, even though there was progress in certain sectors until the war broke out. After that, the situation deteriorated dramatically up to the final catastrophe. Air raids after 1940 augmented ordinary health and sanitation hazards by the dangers arising from surface impact and firebomb devastation, with a resultant climb in civilian mortality.

After 1933, the doctors were kept busy by a gradual but certain worsening of the general health situation. From 1933 to 1935, the rate of increased sickness among health-insured persons (approximately 90 percent of all Germans) was 20 percent. From 1935 to 1938, this increase amounted to nearly 30 percent. The post-1935 increment may be explained by a return of more and more members of the work force, still weakened from the depression, including older people and invalids, to jobs that required greater application because of the forced policy goals of autarky and mobilization for war.[37]

Certain illnesses, like tuberculosis and venereal disease, were on the downswing at first, with physicians taking well-earned credit.[38] Because of the Nazis' inordinate preoccupation with human fertility, doctors also tried successfully to hold down the number of miscarriages, baby deaths, and cases of maternal mortality to a respectable minimum, hence keeping the birth rate high.[39] There was, however, an alarming increase in diphtheria and scarlet fever among children of more than 100 percent between 1933 and 1939. In the twelve months from 1938 to 1939 alone, scarlet fever shot up from 114,000 to 154,000 cases and diphtheria from 150,000 to 175,000 cases. As often happens with epidemics, the gravity of these cases differed from region to region and was unpredictable; diphtheria struck particularly hard in the Palatian town of Speyer, where it was lethal, and in Westphalian Herne scarlet fever was more than four times as widespread in 1939 than it had been in 1933.[40]

Another dark spot in the health record of the regime during the prewar period was the mounting incidence of industrial accidents among clerical employees and especially blue-collar workers, who were driven to the limits of their capacity.[41] The more menial the tasks to be performed, the more critical the calamities that occurred. Laborers at new autobahn or aqueduct construction sites had to suffer the merciless regimen of brutal foremen who pushed them on the job, at the risk of accident or death. In the quarry of Silesian Striegau in autumn 1935, in only one week a laborer's chest was crushed, another's head was pelted by stones, and a third was burned to death during dynamite blasting. At some work sites, as in the Mansfeld coal mines, the total fatality increase from 1933 to 1939 may not have been as noticeable as at others, but at the national level the accident growth rate appears to have surpassed that of the entire work force.[42]

Original documents in West German archives prove that the Nazi health administrators knew full well where the events were taking them.[43] Nevertheless, in official publications and communications to the press they minimized the problem and displayed optimism when they should have been giving stern warnings. After Conti had succeeded Wagner in the national health leadership and with a war in the offing, this peacetime practice was perfected to a fine art. Diphtheria, for example, said Conti in spring of 1940, was on the way out, and so were other pediatric ills, as well as tuberculosis; in general, according to Conti, there was no reason to panic despite the false rumors "malicious Jewish emigrants" had spread abroad.[44]

The blunt fact was not only that all those ailments continued to multiply, but also that the accident rate rose precipitously after 1939 and that new, sometimes exotic diseases were poised to strike the German populace. The influx of conscripted Polish laborers in 1939–40 and the Wehrmacht's sojourn into eastern Europe brought dysentery into certain areas, for instance Bavaria, although it could be extinguished before posing a national threat, and a recurrence in 1942 was controlled.[45] Spotted fever and typhoid followed a similar pattern in the incipient war phase, but they remained latently virulent until the end.[46] Better-known and justly feared disorders such as cancer were on the rise throughout, and seasonally, as in spring 1942, there was a high frequency of afflictions triggered by the conditions of war, like scabies, bacterial food poisoning, and intestinal ulcers.[47]

Because of nutritional deficiencies, scarlet fever and diphtheria were difficult to control, and, encouraged by the extremely cold winters of 1940 and 1941 and thereafter by the bombings and forced evacuations, infant mortality was approaching a frightful proportion by the end of the war.[48] Tuberculosis, too, was reaching crisis proportions. After the start of the war, this scourge spread virtually unchecked, from over 70,000 lung and throat afflictions in 1939 to over 100,000 in 1942 in prewar Reich territory alone, not counting skin and other types of tuberculosis. In Herne, 2,579 cases of all manner of tuberculosis were registered in 1943; in this location the disease had grown fourteen times as fast from 1939 onward as it had from 1933 to 1939.[49] At the end of 1941, for every 100,000 inhabitants of a large German city, 67 people were dying of tuberculosis, whereas one year later, there were 73.[50] Because of a conflict of interest between the desire to inhibit lethal contagion and the need for man-hours for war production, patients were kept in civilian work programs and exposed to other civilians to the point that an open tubercular condition made institutionalization unavoidable; but often the removal occurred much too late and more damage had been done, both to the patients and to their work colleagues. It was characteristic of the Nazi medical leaders' view of hospitalization and severe human suffering alike that they procrastinated in making more beds available to chronic tuberculosis patients but thought nothing of interning terminal cases behind bars.[51]

Industrial accidents, which increased significantly over the span of the war, were intimately tied to both overexertion and work absenteeism, a disastrous combination that wrecked the people and cut down on production efficiency. In the Mansfeld mines serious accidents causing work layoffs of more than eight weeks grew from 1.3 to 1.9 percent between 1940 and 1944, and lighter ones from 26.3 to 29.6 percent. And in the Penzberg mines of Upper Bavaria the number of mishaps rose from about seven per ten thousand shifts in 1939 to twice that in 1943.[52] If more and more hardworking Germans were calling in sick as the war progressed, it was the women, mostly between twenty and forty years of age, who were particularly susceptible to exhaustion and disease, so that by the middle of 1942 their absentee rate stood at four to five times that of the men's, already at a record.[53] There was no doubt in the last few years of the Nazi regime that the health administration, and with it the many overtaxed physicians, were waging a losing battle against consumption, illness, and death, in the best of conditions at the toll-exacting worksites or in the underprovided schools, homes, or hospitals, and in the worst during and after air raids. How hollow rang the public reassurances of Reich Health Leader Conti, who desisted neither from making flattering comparisons with the World War I situation nor from lying outright to conceal the unpleasant truth.[54]

The German physicians' life in the Third Reich was not made any easier by complications arising from the national hospital network. To a large extent, these conditions were, in one way or another, connected first to war mobilization and then to the war itself.[55] But admittedly, they were also a partial consequence of the health administrators' aversion to the concept of institutionalized patient care, which kept the German hospital tradition in disrespect and discouraged the enlargement of any existing clinical facilities. Such views were consonant with the Nazi suspicion of city environments in which rationally organized hospital operations, with their high concentration of specialists and their cooperation with university medical faculties, flourished best.[56]

Because fewer and fewer hospitals for inpatients had been built since the beginning of the regime, the safety occupancy margin was dwindling from 1932 to 1938. In the last year of the Weimar Republic, at the end of a steady growth of hospitals for the nation's sick, only 62 percent of all beds in the Reich had been occupied. In 1935 this figure rose to 64.6 percent, and it was at 69.3 percent in 1938. In this entire six-year period, the number of hospital patients grew at an average annual compound rate of more than 3 percent, twice as fast as the number of available sickbeds.[57] In one Lübeck hospital alone, the annual patient growth rate was more than 9 percent.[58] In the years before the war, hospital directors and medicine professors alike negotiated strenuously with the authorities for additions to existing clinics or for the construction of new ones, usually without success.[59] By the time the war was on, the number of beds in the Reich for civilian use had fallen by approximately one-quarter since the end of 1938, even though the facilities of newly annexed territories had been added.[60]

War mobilization influenced the regime's planning as early as July 1935, four months after general conscription had been announced. At that time the health authorities were asked to file a comprehensive list of all the Reich's hospitals with the government.[61] The purpose of this measure became more explicit in August 1937, in the context of the Four-Year Plan and in anticipation of territorial annexations in the following year. It was then that a specific inquiry was held as to the number of hospital beds that would remain after a necessary consignment to the armed forces. As this redeployment was taking place and it was revealed that not enough space would be left for civilian purposes, more beds in auxiliary hospitals were procured, for the time being still without difficulty. By the beginning of the war, even with Wehrmacht hospitals established, Germany had somewhat more beds than in 1938, enough, at any rate, to satisfy the expanding population's needs for adequate hospital servicing.[62]

For the duration of the Polish and the western campaigns, the Wehrmacht's additional demands for civilian hospital beds came close to endangering this basic capacity, even though civilian hospitals experienced a certain relief after the "mercy killing" of about one hundred thousand genetic misfits, whose beds were a welcome increment.[63] Still, in the early war years, there was no real hospital crisis even if beds for inpatients remained in somewhat short supply and bombing raids damaged the wings of some institutions, as in the case of the Düsseldorf university clinic. Fund insurance subscribers were often treated in outpatient wards and then sent home, and for the affluent, private clinics or parts thereof were still open, some in very plush settings.[64]

Nonetheless, although relatively few casualties among patients were occurring as a result of British bombings, the development of a total conflict that did not exempt civilians was becoming clear. In the concept of *Blitzkrieg*, the Nazi leaders thought nothing of harming innocent civilians who were nationals of enemy countries, while considering their own population to be immune from outside attacks. This was a hubris which, in the case of air warfare, was individually reflected in venal Reich Marshal Hermann Göring's overestimation of his own abilities as the nation's air warden. As late as 1938 the leaders responsible for the health sector downplayed the likelihood of severe air damage on civilian installations, including hospitals, although the potential for a higher frequency of injuries of a more conventional type, other than those resulting from enemy bombs, was conceded.[65] Hence air defense was neglected. But in 1940–41, to the disbelieving scorn of Göring, more and more British bomber planes were making inroads over Germany, and Joseph Goebbels noted in his diary that "if really heavy air raids occur, things in Berlin will look pretty nasty. Our new shelters are nowhere near sufficient."[66] It was becoming painfully obvious to clinic directors like the Berlin gynecologist Professor Walter Stoeckel that their establishments, in the middle of large cities and sometimes close to military compounds, were vulnerable.[67]

The doctors' already overworked nerves were strained further as the British raids gained momentum in 1942. In late May Cologne was subjected to a serious air attack, and Göring's fortunes at headquarters declined visibly.[68] By the fall of that year a twofold problem emerged regarding the hospitalization of civilians. The hospitals still available were filling up, to 82.2 percent of their capacity in the entire Reich and as high as 86.6 percent in the densely built-up capital.[69] More important, those critical reserves were useless as long as hospitals remained prime targets in the city centers. Hence it was imperative either to establish proper shielding or to construct new, adequately protected buildings in safer areas. The Nazi authorities had little luck with either of those makeshift solutions. Karl Brandt may have been appointed as Hitler's emergency envoy in July to take charge of such important matters, but any measures would come much too late and would have run aground in the heavily tangled bureaucracy of old, established institutions such as the Charité Hospital in Berlin, where corruption was rampant and little opportunity for structural modifications existed.[70]

Early in 1943 no more than 150 hospital patients had been killed in the Reich. This was about to change, however, as the British intensified their nightly air strikes and the Americans joined them in the daytime.[71] In March Berlin was hit, sustaining heavy losses, including damage to the still unfortified Charité.[72] Meanwhile, several replacement hospitals had been started but, because of the constant disruptions, were nowhere near completion, so that the previously existing reserves had to be further tapped. By now the Reich health authorities were readily conceding an acute scarcity of beds.[73] At no time was the seriousness of the situation more glaring than during the firebombing of Hamburg in July to August, when up to fifty thousand inhabitants perished and 60 percent of the university clinical complex was destroyed. Before this disaster was visited on Germany's second largest city, Hamburg had merely 630 provisional auxiliary beds in sheltered surroundings, with over 3,000 projected; twelve main hospitals and fourteen replacement institutions within city limits were fully exposed to attack. After the calamity, Hamburg's air-sheltered reserve for new casualties had shrunk to 3,000 beds, and 4,000 more beds were said to be wanting.[74]

In the last two years of the war, the dearth of sickbeds was compounded by other material shortcomings and human failures that greatly hindered the physicians' work. Some of these were caused locally, as in Leipzig, where the ambulances did not function, or in Kassel, where the mobility of health officials was hampered by a lack of staff cars.[75] As the eastern front moved westward, the Wehrmacht further encroached on the civilian health authorities with its unrelenting claims to civic hospitals.[76] And, despite the urging of knowledgeable clinicians, the Charité in Berlin was insufficiently evacuated. Many patients and personnel remained in the ancient structure, and it was only a miracle that even after heavy bombing, which jeopardized two-thirds of the buildings, no appreciable number of lives were lost.[77]

In the end there was virtual chaos, after destruction had struck repeatedly, in the final, desperate phases of the war. The near total extermination of such noted institutions as the university clinics in Leipzig, Münster, and Düsseldorf, or the municipal hospital system in Stuttgart, was accompanied by a degree of human misery afflicting innocent patients and desperate doctors that defies any attempt at recounting, even from the sobering distance of today.[78] The Allies found few hospitals intact in the spring of 1945. Most were reduced to rubble, the result of Conti's and Brandt's many miscalculations, but also, in a more tragically profound sense, the ramifications of a vengeful Nazi policy against humanity that rebounded against the German people.[79]

Nevertheless, despite the many professional and institutional strictures that the Nazi health administrators imposed on German physicians in the period after the political takeover of 1933, the quality of medical service did not suffer inordinately in comparison with the republican era until the start of World War II. In the mid-1930s, most doctors still had been schooled in the universities of the republic, and they adhered to a professional standard that was, by and large, universally accepted. But in the late 1930s, a new crop of specifically Nazi-trained young doctors entered medical practice, and their standards came to leave much to be desired, even though many of them were still under the supervision of older, monarchy- or republican-educated colleagues, even while serving at the military fronts.[80]

Previously unforeseen factors arising from a planned economy and the circumstances of the war itself came to have an increasingly serious impact on the quality of medical work after 1939, and in some cases even before. For instance, as labor was seen to be in short supply after the restoration of full employment, it was becoming difficult to hire physicians' helpers because qualified nursing staff was requisitioned by the Wehrmacht.[81] Because of restrictions against the importation of foreign raw materials, certain drugs and medical implements were running low and doctors had to make do with inferior or replacement materials, as in the case of surgical gauze.[82] In a situation of overemployment, many patients who felt that they were unduly pushed to their physical limits in plants and factories asked their family physicians for certificates of ill health, claiming faked ailments. Staying at home for a few days would not cost them too much money because the panel funds still paid a half-wage. Perhaps out of sympathy, perhaps to avoid losing their clientele, the doctors tended to comply, much to the chagrin of the economic planners who attempted to curb this practice.[83] Not least because of these repetitive visits by laborers and white-collar employees alike, and being faced with more and more patients as their own number in the civilian sector decreased, doctors were tiring more easily and becoming prematurely old as well. The Reich health leadership had determined that in 1939 male physicians' life expectancy was nine years less than the average for all males in the Reich, and that did not bode well for the war phase.[84]

The war exacerbated these problems and created a few novel ones. The shortage of matériel continued to be bothersome even though one could be inventive and get around it, if one tried. Early in the war, the health bureaucrats issued directives on how to avoid using imported drugs and how to save on bandages. Insulin was to be employed very sparingly; the same applied to morphine, for which no synthetics had been developed. Rhubarb from Central Asia was to be produced at home. Much more currency was to be placed on home-grown herbs than on the expensive imports such as cough medicine, a guideline that sprang directly from the back-to-nature ideals of the Nazi health politicians.[85] These instructions proved useful for some time to come, but by early 1943 new challenges arose. Because glass was at a premium, medicinal containers, thermometers, and syringes were extremely hard to obtain by 1942. Around the time of Stalingrad, morphine, insulin, and chloroform were well-nigh non-existent on the home front because the military hospitals were running out of them.[86]

As the lack of medical support staff proved unrelenting,[87] the burden imposed on the practitioners by would-be work shirkers was turning into a nightmare for most of them. Late in 1939 the authorities decreed that henceforth doctors were to judge the patients' condition but not their capacity to withstand work routines. Somehow this order failed to have any effect on absenteeism, which was daily getting worse, particularly in the war production plants and among masses of women there who felt they could not take the pressure. Soon the KVD was initiating sterner measures by threatening permissive doctors who would, in any case, much rather attend to genuine afflictions, although it was debatable even then where exactly to draw the line. Unfortunately for the physicians, a new dimension was put on this contentious issue when in June 1942 it was ordained, at least for certain regions, that annual vacations for workers be made contingent on a medical certificate.[88]

Physicians received plenty of opportunity during this war to test their sense of altruism in accordance with the Hippocratic Oath. At the height of the conflict, some of them were seeing eighty or more patients a day. These patients were increasingly testy, overly nervous, hypochondriac, and also ready to blame their doctors for their having to wait hours on end, sometimes in the company of "dirty Poles." Regardless of office hours and beyond the already onerous chores during patients' visits, it proved a trying experience for physicians to administer emergency aid to air raid victims whose eyes had been injured or who were in shock, let alone those whose limbs had been torn off or whose skulls had been crushed. Indeed, the health of the doctors themselves was at stake, especially of those past normal retirement age who had been recalled to help out. In the hospitals, too, the medical men and some women performed superhuman feats. In the Berlin Charité, for example, surgeons were operating for up to eighteen hours daily, with such bad food to eat in between that all of them suffered drastic weight loss. And their mortality rate was staggering: between the beginning of the war and

January 1943, 3,883 physicians at the home front had died, more than four times the number of those who fell in the trenches. Small wonder that by July 1941 the morale among doctors was worn thin and their animosity to the Reich health leader and his subalterns was critical.[89]

Ordinary medical practice in Germany was a veritable trial after the defeat at Stalingrad in early February 1943 and with the Allied bombers poised to strike ever more forcefully against city-dwelling civilians. To the equipment and material wants now were added, in the last year of the war, virtual supply stoppages for such essential items as insulin for the nation's diabetics and gasoline for the physicians' cars.[90] More doctors had to put up with sloppy and unconscionable assistants, for such staff had become so precious that many nurses imagined they could take any liberties they wished.[91] And the physicians were still beset by the Nazi functionaries, who suspected them of favoring absentee workers by issuing them certificates of ill health. This problem had become so unmanageable that in March 1944 Reich Mobilization Minister Albert Speer contemplated a term in concentration camp as a proper deterrent against medically certified slackers.[92]

A new harassment for medical practitioners in 1943 was the devastation of their office premises, notably those located in the insufficiently protected cities, from air raids. Often expensive medical gear and equipment were lost, and even if replacements sometimes were available, they did little to bolster the doctors' self-confidence. A certain measure of relief in this situation was provided by mobile emergency units in some towns, all the more so because they made service assignments after air raids very practical. Some doctors, like the bombed-out Berlin internist Theodor Brugsch, were able to continue provisionally, seeing patients at the offices of cooperative colleagues, but always the question was, how long? The damage inflicted on the Reich's health system by this devastation for the average German physician was psychologically as demoralizing as it was physically crippling, even though under the scrutiny of the authorities all pessimistic impulses had to be repressed. After a series of raids on Stuttgart's inner city in September 1944, 52 medical offices were entirely wiped out, with 118 still in operation, as the town council recorded in its minutes, scarcely concealing its desperation.[93]

Doctors toiled and labored as best they could. With every month the health of these exhausted men and women deteriorated further, and especially because of the high number of older physicians in the Reich, their death rate continued to be excessive.[94] The daily regimen of these healers, before some of them broke down completely, was grueling by any recognized standards. The following case histories of a few of them were believed to be representative of the great majority by the authorities who collected them in September 1943. One seventy-six-year-old specialist, an orthopedist, was tending the practice of his conscripted son. Although he was impeded by rectal cancer, he was seeing about one hundred patients per day. Another, a forty-nine-year-old general practitioner, collaborated with his physician wife, who also looked after their child. Their consultations would start at 7:30 in the morning and end, with hardly an hour's break, at 8:00 in the evening. After that, in the absence of a medical secretary, the paperwork had to be done. The telephone could ring all night long, and nocturnal visits occurred no less than three times a week. Since 1939, this man had lost thirty-three pounds and had developed an abdominal ulcer. Yet a third, a sixty-six-year-old internist, suffering from coronary sclerosis and chronic bronchitis, worked ten hours in an office far from his home without interruptions or meals, treating up to sixty patients a day. And a woman internist aged thirty-four had lost fifteen pounds in only nine months; her subsequent sterility was no doubt traceable to a workday of sixteen hours, including the care of two toddlers.[95]

The doctors were compelled to witness scenes of human drama they would hardly have imagined in peacetime. Urologist Werner Forssmann, stationed in Berlin in 1943, was pressed into service at the Brandenburg-Görden penitentiary, where scores of political prisoners were beheaded by the guillotine. Among the macabre details he recorded was that not two minutes elapsed from one execution to the next. Forssmann was rebuffed by the wardens when he invoked professional ethos and asked to sedate the delinquents. His own special ration of cognac and cigarettes he found utterly revolting.[96] Werner Catel, a pediatrician, was exposed to even starker realities when he survived the bombardment of Leipzig. During the night of December 3, 1943, the city center, containing his clinic, was set aflame. Those children, his patients, who were able to reach the street, were rolling on the frozen pavement, moaning and bleeding from open wounds. There was no water, no food, no bandages. With bombs raining down incessantly, doctors and some staff were risking their lives to save children, carrying them piggyback over the rubble. It was an inferno. "As I was running toward the burning tuberculosis station, I suddenly saw the head of a nurse, one of our best, protruding from the ruins, her facial expression frozen in fear of death and despair."[97] And in the final throes of the Nazi Reich one young Dr. Brandt happened upon a throng of country people led by a political functionary about to lynch a British pilot, just descended. It took great power of persuasion on Brandt's part to keep the angry Germans at bay and eventually arrange hospitalization for the injured airman.[98]

Physicians posted in cities by the Reich health leadership were not allowed to evacuate themselves or sometimes even their families to safer places in the provinces, as many other civilians did at that time. Hence personal tragedies transpired that might have been avoidable, had doctors not been doctors. No sooner had dermatologist Edmund Hofmann, fifty-three years old and with a brilliant academic career still ahead of him, returned from the Balkan front at the end of 1943 than he was surprised by an air raid in his Kassel residence. He perished with three of his children.[99] Young Dr. Gustav Heinrich Hahn, who had married into one of Hamburg's patrician families, took his calling so seriously that the human misery he viewed depressed him. Drifting closer and closer to suicide, he died of pneumonia combined with heart failure in June 1944.[100] Berlin gynecologist Stoeckel's two assistants, Drs. Caffier and Breipohl, were shot in the back of the head by marauding Red Army soldiers over a simple misunderstanding, in the very end. As a further cruelty of war, Stoeckel's grandson Goswin was felled by a stray grenade, just as he wanted to discard it, only a few months later.[101]

However chilling, these final months of the war in Germany were not only times of heroism for the doctors. Human as they were themselves, many of them were cracking under the strain and slipping into danger of moral corruption. It was understandable that with hundreds of patients upon them, some started to mete out preferential treatment.[102] Potentially more perilous was the increasing consumption of alcohol and morphine to help these doctors through the day; partially as a result, wrong diagnoses and inappropriate therapies were not infrequent. As well, incidents of sexual misdemeanor in the company of female patients, a fairly common professional problem even under normal conditions, appear to have been on the ascendancy.[103] Principles of professional conduct were flagrantly violated when physicians failed to appear for duty or, unable to face their responsibility as committed regime servants, hurried from the scene of catastrophe during the finale, leaving their sick charges to an unknown fate.[104] Clearly, not just this colossal war itself but also the moral depravity of the political forces that had unleashed it brought out the worst in those physicians to whom the concern for their fellows' lives had become a calculated game with death.

Against the hardships suffered by their civilian colleagues, the opprobrium of those doctors conscripted for service in the war should not go unnoticed. The main medical business in wartime was surgery, and the men with the scalpels became the most sought-after specialists for emergency work just behind the trenches and in the stationary field hospitals further off, where they and their patients were relatively secure. In the course of the entire conflict, the casualties included up to 60,000 Germans wounded during the Polish campaign, 220,000 in the western one, and well over 650,000 at the Russian front. In more than half those cases, the men's limbs were injured; only about five of every hundred suffered from head, lung, neck, or abdominal wounds.[105] All these conditions called for surgeons of various specializations, excepting circumstances in which soldiers were afflicted with plagues such as dysentery, typhoid, spotted fever, or, in the Crimean region or North Africa, malaria. In these areas pathologists, hygienists, and internists were needed most.[106]

All military doctors, yet especially surgeons and notably those at the eastern front, performed unbelievable feats, often against seemingly insurmountable odds.[107] Those surgeons are legion who worked for days and nights on end, with hardly a few hours' sleep in between and constantly under the influence of coffee, nicotine, or other drugs, assisted rudimentarily by a few undertrained orderlies.[108] Their emergency operations took place with only a modicum of protection from the enemy, sometimes under the hail of bullets or grenades or in the pall of winter, when the soldiers' heavy clothing made it difficult to obtain proper access to injuries. Grenades exploding nearby could unsteady the hand that was guiding the scalpel, and ever so often lice and flies would infect the wounds and spoil the bandages, as well as causing skin disorders among the medics themselves. The West German best-selling author Peter Bamm, who experienced the war as a conscripted surgeon, tells of mice that not only devoured cigarette paper and personal letters but also jumped across the injured during operations.[109]

The military doctors' working conditions were complicated by peculiarities that were a function of the severity with which this war was being fought, particularly in the Soviet Union. One of these was a comparatively high incidence of frostbite and hypothermia, which often necessitated amputations. This became a major problem not only in the combat theater but also during air transport of the wounded behind the lines because in unheated planes toes would often freeze even if heavily wrapped. For every two soldiers who became terminal victims of enemy fire, German army staffers had concluded by 1944, one died from the extreme Russian cold. Repeatedly the doctors faced the difficult decision of exposing a wounded man to the perils of hypothermia during transport or retaining him behind the lines. The lesser evil was frequently apparent only after a patient's death.[110]

Yet more serious cases in which doctors had a direct influence over life and death involved self-inflicted wounds by men who had broken down under the tribulations of war and gone to any lengths to be sent home. Unfortunately, these soldiers paid no heed to martial law, which in severe cases stipulated capital punishment if such self-mutilation could be proved. It was a challenge to the German doctors' sense of medical ethics to attempt to circumvent these rulings by not only saving their unfortunate charges' health but also avoiding their deliverance to the SS or into the hands of the merciless war judges. This was by no means an easy task. For not only did they have to remove the culprit from the authorities' attention during the recuperative period, but the cause of the injury had to be concealed in the logbooks so as to stifle all suspicions. It is not known how many field doctors accepted the considerable personal risk of shielding such malingerers, but those who did and lived to tell about it have erected fine monuments to the art of medical practice in war.[111]

For the physicians, this was a time of professional and personal decisions at many levels, decisions neither more nor less important than during the civilian practice, but made more onerous because of the urgency of the front and a potential conflict with the military code. Much was left to the individual doctor's judgment when medical textbooks, the advice of colleagues, and even the guidelines of military superiors were not immediately at hand. When should the wounded be marked for transport? Was it safe to risk an operation in the face of another possible attack?[112] Doctors could be subjected to court-martial after having sent certain abdominal cases back to the hospital and the lightly wounded to inactive troops. Triage was practiced: soldiers seriously hit during a Russian snowstorm sometimes had to be abandoned to save others. And how close to the active-combat lines should one venture to retrieve the casualties to be expected?[113] What to do with prisoners of war who badly needed attention?[114] The question of whether one should help against one's better medical knowledge was one that many combat doctors often asked themselves. One colleague, beleaguered in the ruins of Stalingrad, routinely moved from one dying soldier to the next, applying iodine and faithfully dressing every wound—an utterly futile act and still a very humane one.[115] "Once again I know why I am here and what it means to be a doctor," wrote twenty-six-year-old Dr. Gottfried Gruner from the shores of the Black Sea, just a week before he fell in October 1943.[116]

Such details suggest that the Nazi military leadership did not do all it could have to ensure a good working environment for those physicians and to safeguard against so high a number of casualties. Even though this problem cannot be definitively solved here, there is sufficient evidence to demonstrate that the Nazis were lacking in medical concern as early as the Polish campaign in autumn 1939. The medical network for World War II, which was very closely patterned on that for the preceding war,[117] was outmoded in several respects before it even began to function. The land transportation system employing both automobiles and trains was cumbersome and detrimental to the wounded, even though the increasing use of aircraft alleviated these problems later on; the field hospitals were largely immobile.[118] Shortages of instruments and sanitary equipment combined with faulty assignment routines and inadequate hygiene haunted doctors and patients alike. Auxiliary personnel were in short supply and improperly schooled; sometimes scissors had to serve as scalpels.[119] All medicines were scarce, but some, like antibiotics, were not tried or their development was neglected. Nutrition was generally poor because of a dearth of suitable foodstuffs, if not for the fighting troops, certainly for their wounded comrades.[120]

In the everyday rush of emergencies, the older physicians were losing their finely honed skills, while the younger ones, carelessly trained in the medical faculties, never acquired the touch but tended to resort to shortcuts bordering on unprofessionalism, all the exceptions notwithstanding.[121] Occasional breakthroughs in some areas were more than canceled out by failures in others. For example, even though the Germans succeeded in establishing a special clinic for the brain-injured, they were slow until the end properly to use blood transfusions and lost many lives for that reason.[122] But whether they amputated excessively, as has recently been claimed, must remain disputed as long as the opposite can be charged as well.[123] There is, indeed, a need to examine much more closely the assumption that it was the "relative backwardness of Nazi medicine" that made the Third Reich lose more human lives at the military fronts than absolutely necessary and aided in the gradual dehumanizing of the medical art until the catastrophe in 1945.[124]

Chapter 2

The Challenge of the Nazi Movement

1. Doctors in the Nazi Party

At the outset of the Third Reich, the popular German author Peter Bamm was still practicing surgery in Hamburg under his real name Dr. Curt Emmrich. He was residing in a city that had a reputation for reticence toward the National Socialist movement. Its burghers were said to be less sympathetic to the Nazi phenomenon than those of other places. Nevertheless, Bamm does recollect that during 1933, in the casino of the hospital in which he was employed, "one after the other of the colleagues, rather occasionally and always somewhat sheepish at first, arrived in a brown or black uniform."[1] The strongly anti-Nazi Dr. Otto Buchinger, a Quaker and famous even then for having found a patent health formula for overweight patients, joined former naval physicians at a reunion ceremony, somewhere else in Germany, in September of that year. A minority, he notes in his memoirs, were nonparty comrades.[2]

Such evidence infers that German physicians, whatever their monarchical and republican party leanings in the past, were overrepresented in the Nazi party as well as its adjunct organizations as early as 1933. For the NSDAP, statistical data prove this assumption with graphic clarity. Just before the National Socialists came to power, less than 7 percent of all the physicians appear to have been attracted to the NSDAP.[3] But along with other social and professional groups, the doctors joined the party when it seemed like the right thing to do, in 1933 and 1937, when the membership rolls were open to every eligible German over age seventeen. They were also inclined to sign up in 1940–41, after the party leadership had lifted a temporary entry barrier in 1939 (Table 2.1). In 1934–36, 1938, and 1942–45 party entrance was closed to all but the youngest applicants and a few favored groups; hence doctors, who usually were over twenty-six, did not join at these times. Although membership was open in summer 1939, few physicians joined, possibly because the signals of mobilization, a planned economy, and imminence of war, already had bruised the reputation of the party.[4]

Physicians were academically trained professionals; they were members of the social elite, which, of course, constituted the highest and smallest stratum in the hierarchically structured neophyte Nazi membership between 1933 and 1945, as depicted in Table 2.1.[5] As a whole, the joining pattern of the physicians, the academic professionals, and the social elite was the same as that of the membership at large, with a few significant exceptions. Overall, the party received a strong boost from very young members between 1942 and 1945 (17.7 percent of total membership), during a stretch when closure affected most older Germans. Accomplished, more mature members of the social elite hence were barred from entering the party in its final phase, but university students and a few privileged persons belonging to the older generation were not. This situation is reflected in the low 2.6 percent for the physicians (Table 2.1). Further, if 1937 rather than 1933 was the prime year for all Germans to enter the Nazi party, this probably was related to the political success of the Nazi regime in having beaten the depression and brought about nearly full employment. But members of the social elite, including most academic professionals, were motivated by special interest, occupational, or psychological considerations. Hence they saw this matter differently, joining the party in greater numbers during 1933 and dropping off somewhat in 1937.[6] The doctors within the larger social subgroup of the academics proved the exception. Hesitating in 1933 (32.9 percent), they reached their new membership peak in 1937 (43.4 percent), in this instance paralleling the collective membership pattern (from 22.0 to 27.2 percent).[7]

Unlike the remaining upper-class members, there were three chief reasons for the doctors' behavior. First, at the beginning of the Third Reich most physicians were suspicious, waiting to see how the Nazis would solve their own socioeconomic dilemma, which, in recent times, had been compounded by the pressing needs of the young recruits to the profession. But as was indicated in the previous chapter, by 1937 the regime could be credited with having improved the employment and deployment picture; doctors' average earnings that year were higher than ever. Till then, these developments had already been aided, second, by a partial Nazi solution of the "Jewish problem," in that by 1934 many Jewish practitioners had been removed from participation in the panel practice system, and Jewish medical employees had been dismissed from universities and clinics.[8] And third, by 1937 the Nazi physician leaders had accomplished most of the promised reorganization of the profession, notably by restructuring the mode of allocating fund payments and creating a comprehensive professional code (*Reichsärzteordnung*) with a complementary association (Reichsärztekammer). A welcome side effect had been the neutralization of the hated fund insurance bureaucracy. Before that, German doctors had not been certain how the new Nazi measures might affect them professionally. The novel changes purported to interfere little or not at all with traditional privileges and to bode well for the future of physicians vis-à-vis, for example, the medical quacks, and thus encouraged a closer affiliation with the Nazi regime via membership in its monopolist party.

In 1939, however, even before the inception of World War II in the fall, doctors were constrained and set upon by the regime in ways that threatened their mobility and hence their earnings. Other disappointments were also making themselves felt, such as inertia in the legislation regarding lay healers and overly harsh applications of RÄK and KVD regimens, and, as will be shown below, the party and its affiliates made increasing demands on the physicians' precious time. It is significant that at this stage the doctors came to contribute much less to the new Nazi membership than the academic professionals and the social elite as a whole did; among physicians, the party was half as popular as among all new joiners. As the vagaries of war affected the doctors on the home as well as the war front, their percentages as new party members until the end of the conflict, measured against previous periods when they joined the party, remained consistently below those for the other three groups whose membership in the NSDAP is charted in Table 2.1. But interpreting this behavior as a sign of hard times must not be taken too far, for it is valid only in a comparison of joiner periods, in the nexus with other newcomer groups. By a different count, as will be seen below, it can be demonstrated that the actual proportions of physicians who continued to approach the NSDAP remained formidable.

The relationship between physicians, academic professionals, and the social elite within the framework of new party membership is clarified in Table 2.2. In 1933, the second highest point of concentration for physicians as new members in the party, the doctors constituted not quite one-quarter of all academic professionals and about one-fifteenth of the social elite to join the party. In 1937, the apogee for physician joiners, these shares changed to about one-third of the academic professionals and one-tenth of the elite. Two years later, not even one-fifth of all university-schooled professionals who joined the NSDAP were physicians, amounting to one-twentieth of all upper-class newcomers. For the last phase of the regime the absolute figure of merely two new physician joiners for a full three years appears somewhat low to venture any judgments regarding the doctors' trend in comparison with that of the academic professionals and the elite.[9]

On the basis of the values shown in Tables 2.1 and 2.2, which stem from a randomly drawn sample of 18,255 new Nazi party members (1925–45) on file in the Berlin Document Center, as well as on the basis of figures published from the 1933 Reich census, listing a total of 27,047,899 socially classifiable persons, it is possible to conclude that from 1933 to the end of the Third Reich the physicians were overrepresented in the party by a ratio of three to one.[10] Yet another randomly drawn sample from the Document Center of 4,177 physicians, recorded to have been members of the Reichsärztekammer between the time of its founding in 1936 and the Reich's capitulation in 1945 indicates that Protestant physicians were more prone to join the party than their Catholic colleagues (Table 2.3, column A). This is in keeping with older and more current findings that Catholics in the Third Reich were less susceptible to the National Socialist lure than Protestants.[11]

Further proof of the strong connection between National Socialism and physicianship is contained in Table 2.4, facilitated by the RÄK sample. It demonstrates that 44.8 percent of all physicians in the Reich, that is, of those who were compelled to register with the Reich Physicians' Chamber from 1936 to 1945, followed the Nazi party either before or after 1933.[12] Among those, the professionals who had been licensed between 1925 and 1932 exhibited the strongest tendency to join, at 53.1 percent, and those licensed from 1919 to 1932 were the next strongest, at 50.8 percent. In contrast, the category of Nazi doctors inaugurated between 1878 (the earliest date mentioned in this sample) and 1918 was significantly weaker, at 39.1 percent, as was that of those licensed after 1932. This is a clear indication that the primary movers among Nazi physicians were rather recent medical school graduates before Hitler's political takeover, who, particularly in the years of the Great Depression, were suffering from professional closure imposed upon them by their older, established resident colleagues, and all manner of attendant hardships.[13] They had been socialized in an era of ideological acerbity and had been exposed to an increasing Nazi presence in the body politic. Up to and including 1933, they approached the Nazi camp out of resentment for past and present conditions and in hope of a brighter future at the hands of the predestined leaders. It is very probable that those formerly junior doctors as mature men were in the group of professionals who contributed to the membership surge of 1937 because they were satisfied with the visible changes during the early years of the regime. Nor did university graduates between 1933 and 1938 shrink from fixing their star to the Nazi wagon, for at that time the Third Reich appeared as a firm guarantor of professional security—their proportion was in the 43 percent range (Table 2.4, column E). That this rate remained virtually constant through the war (1939–45) is less a sign of the Nazi party exerting pressure on upper-school and university students to join after compulsory membership in the Hitler Youth had expired than an expression on their part, if not exactly of contentment with the ways of the rulers in war, yet still one of trust in a bright future after the expected Final Victory.[14]

Tables 2.5 and 2.6 further show that throughout all Nazi party recruitment periods, physician candidates tended to be mature men and women well advanced in their profession, the only exception being 1938, when the entering doctors' mean age was twenty-seven. This happened to be the age at which they normally received their medical licenses. Hence they did not share in the infusion of younger blood that the Nazi membership at large experienced, especially toward the end of the regime. In this doctors resembled other cohort peers among the social elite, the academic professionals, and the corps of higher civil servants, whose entrance into professional life was often governed by factors similar to those affecting physicians such as long periods of university schooling and apprenticeships (Table 2.5).

Moreover, Table 2.6 (columns A and C) shows that in 1937, the heyday of new Nazi membership for RÄK-registered German doctors, those between thirty-one and forty years of age were overrepresented in the NSDAP, opposite the corresponding age cohort among all the doctors in the land. Also overrepresented were colleagues in the lowest age group, thirty years and under. The cohort between forty-one and fifty was proportionally represented, and the age groups over fifty years clearly showed less interest in the NSDAP.[15] The projected image of Nazi-prone physicians as stable but reasonably youthful people is also supported, even though statistically much less surely, by the values for the thirty-three new NSDAP joiners in that year (Table 2.6, column B). Here the first three age cohorts appear as overrepresented, with the two middling ones as substantially so.[16] A juxtaposition of these figures with those for established Nazi members and medium-level functionaries, the Kreisleiter, of late 1934, would suggest that the bulk of the Nazi physicians were older than the general membership. Moreover, the Nazi RÄK physicians of 1937 could not match the Kreisleiter corps of three years before, which consisted primarily of men in their thirties, an age that the reigning hierarchy deemed ideal for assuming political leadership.[17] At the beginning of the age spectrum, Nazi RÄK physicians were neither as immature as the party membership at large, nor did they monopolize the thirty-one-to-forty-year bracket as did the functionaries, in fact occupying a position between both those extremes. This last comparison once again underlines that in age the National Socialist doctors more closely matched the rest of the German physicians in the Reich than the typical Nazi stooges and vanguard leaders.[18]

This sociogram held true for physicians in the entire Reich, which is not necessarily to say that similar conditions obtained for individual regions or localities. Variations undoubtedly existed, but the details regarding them are sparse. In 1933, in Rhenish Stolberg, a town of some thirty thousand inhabitants, probably because of intense peer-group pressure, eleven out of thirteen doctors joined the party, or nearly 85 percent.[19] By 1945, almost 80 percent of the self-employed doctors in Thuringia were in the party.[20] Half of the thirty-two physicians in the Bavarian county of Laufen-Berchtesgaden in February 1935 were registered party members.[21] In all of Bavaria, for our key year of 1937, a majority of doctors (51 percent) was in the NSDAP, of whom 80 percent were between thirty and sixty-one years old.[22] But the established benchmark of approximately 45 percent for Nazi doctors was much lower in other Reich locales. Traditionally liberal-minded Baden had only 30 percent on record, Hesse-Nassau had 33 percent, and Württemberg 36 percent.[23] Presumably counts such as these excluded Jewish physicians because they generally could not be bona fide members of the KVD and RÄK, the agencies that punctiliously compiled such statistics. A published note about Berlin, distinguishing between Jewish and "Aryan" physicians, indicates that less than 26 percent of its doctors were NSDAP adherents in 1937. This might be surprising in view of the capital's record number of Jewish physicians but makes some sense if one remembers that Berlin's snootily sophisticated population was long notorious for giving the Nazis more trouble than that of any other German city.[24]

How do these Nazi membership figures measure up alongside those for other, socially compatible subgroups? Even though research into the social history of National Socialism and the Third Reich has progressed appreciably over the last few years, little is as yet known about the sociopsychology of Hitler's most dedicated followers in the various professions. In party membership the physicians were, without a doubt, at the very top of any list including other academic occupations. They were ahead of the lawyers, who, according to a recent educated estimate, never exceeded 25 percent.[25] Other groups also fell below the doctors' level, such as the teachers (including upper school ones), every fourth one of whom was in the party. Trailing even the teachers were all the other civil servants, notwithstanding both groups' still recognizable overrepresentation in the NSDAP.[26] The engineers were remarkably immune to the Nazis' beckoning for reasons not yet obvious—contrary to what Hermann Rauschning noted about them at the height of World War II. Thus far, the insufficiently informed critical literature on engineers infers a high degree of underrepresentation in the party in spite of the grossly atypical example of Albert Speer and the much-touted Third Reich craze for technology and technocracy.[27] Ironically, academically trained pharmacists, who collaborated closely with doctors of medicine, also retreated into the background when prompted to join the ranks of the Reich's only party; the causes have yet to be divulged.[28]

To be a member of the Nazi party was one thing, but to be a leader, subaltern, intermediate, or superior, was still another for lawyers, apothecaries, or physicians. Not surprisingly, there were legions of jurists among the Nazi functionaries, of whom Hans Frank, Roland Freisler, and Werner Best may have been the most prolific. Until December 1932 a strong-willed pharmacist had put his stamp on the hierarchy, in the person of Gregor Strasser. There were a few exposed engineers such as Fritz Todt, Gottfried Feder, and Speer, and dozens of diversely qualified teachers. With one undistinguished exception, however, one searches in vain for a doctor of medicine serving the National Socialist cause in high places.[29] The *Führerlexikon* of 1935, that veritable *Who Is Who* of the early National Socialist dictatorship, lists only sixty-three physicians as prominent leaders of party, government, economic, or cultural institutions of the Third Reich in late 1934, and their biographies are approximately 3.7 percent of all those in the book. Compared to delegates from the other professions, in particular the jurists, who are hugely overrepresented in the tome, doctors are distinctly underrepresented. Forty of those sixty-three were professors of medicine, who were apt to be included simply by virtue of their university office, leaving only twenty-three ordinary doctors licensed to practice medicine. Their average age at that time was forty-four, with a range from twenty-eight to sixty-five. All but two had seen active duty in World War I, and not quite half had been engrossed in postwar Freikorps or similar vigilante-style ventures. Twenty expressly emphasized some affiliation with the Nazi regime.[30]

Before the details are filled in to provide a somewhat fuller portrait of these men and others like them not listed in the Nazi handbook, a preliminary reflection on the discrepancy between the doctors' overrepresentation in the party and underrepresentation in agencies of government and state is necessary. One might speculate that physicians, who from earlier decades had a reputation for being apolitical in the sense of joining political parties, so much identified with their profession, which involved dealing with people in a person-to-person relationship, that other, wider social contexts did not matter to them, unless, of course, basic professional needs were at stake, in which case political party attachment might serve a lobbyistic purpose. It may be presumed that this is what happened to the German doctors before and after the year of National Socialist takeover. Their much talked about "crisis of medicine," with its economic, social, and ethical ramifications, was either very real, or imagined, or, indeed, thought to be threatening a majority to the extent that they used the influential Nazi party as a pressure group, perhaps in lieu of the Hartmannbund, which many viewed as inert during the last years of the republic. Yet they hesitated to assume offices that would place them into multifarious social frameworks, unlike person-to-person relationships between physicians and their patients. Unlike a lawyer, who upon assuming some public office could still apply the skills of his calling to the business at hand, a doctor had to stop practicing medicine. A second factor, but no less important, may have been the expected loss of income that some, if by no means all, party or government offices might entail. Physicians were the highest-earning professionals in the Third Reich and, understandably, loath to surrender that privilege. The intelligence branch of the SS complained in 1938 that physicians were exerting themselves less and less for the party, which in large part was blamed on their "materialistic attitude."[31]

The politically active doctors may be divided roughly into three subgroups: those taking an interest in the administration of their profession to the extent that it had been politicized, those participating in the bureaucracy of the NSDAP in the widest sense, and those who controlled some facets of government.

Most of the men who worked on behalf of the Nazi medical bureaucracy like the KVD or RÄK had active World War I and Freikorps records and, as Old Fighters of the Nazi movement, had entered the NSDAP before 1933.[32] They had filled key functions in the founding and evolution of the Nazi Physicians' League after 1929 and had tended, particularly in the final phase of the republic and ever since Hitler came to power, to sacrifice medical practice and professional upgrading to the goals of the movement at large. If ever there were fanatical believers in the aims of National Socialism, especially as they might pertain to the medical sector, these were the ones. Today one may fault them for upholding false ideals and for narrowness of vision, but it is impossible not to take their dedication and, within Nazi party terms, their sense of duty seriously. These men may have been politically very ambitious, as was blatantly obvious in the early career of Leonardo Conti, but they were not opportunists in the conventional sense of the word and certainly not, so far as one can make out, interested in material riches. In the vanguard of this group, besides Conti, were Gerhard Wagner, the first Reich physicians' leader, Friedrich Bartels, his deputy until 1939, and, as Bartels's successor till the end of the war, Kurt Blome.[33]

Of the same ilk but functionally less significant were such men as the Stuttgart neurologist Eugen Stähle, born in 1890, military staff physician (*Stabsarzt*) in World War I and thereafter a member of Freikorps Epp, which in early 1919 quashed the Munich-based Bavarian Soviet Republic. Stähle joined the party in 1927, became the Nazi Physicians' League deputy for Württemberg in 1930, and on April 30, 1933, took charge of that province's KVD chapter, thus facilitating its Nazification.[34] Stähle's Breslau colleague Karl Peschke, eight years older and a generalist, had a very similar career with the exception of Freikorps service; in 1934 he directed the KVD in Silesia.[35] Another such functionary was general practitioner Carl Heinz Behrens, born in 1889 in Celle and a Hitler follower since 1924; in Gau Hesse he worked as the party's deputy for "people's health" (*Gauamtsleiter für Volksgesundheit*).[36] Country doctor Heinrich Grote has already been mentioned as a functionary of the Hartmannbund who had no trouble crossing over to the Nazi camp after January 1933. The former World War I *Stabsarzt* was an early Nazi party member, destined to win the confidence of Gerhard Wagner, who, after 1933, would put him at the helm of the KVD, first in Berlin and then in all of Germany.[37] To round off this group profile one might mention Kurt Klare, forty-nine years old in 1934, who in 1941 would describe himself as a "German Christian" (formerly a Roman Catholic) and, racially, a "Nordic." Klare, whose military World War I career was thwarted because of ill health, became a NSDAP member in 1927; in 1929, he helped to found the Nazi Physicians' League, whose membership number two he acquired. A committed anti-Semite who propagated his views in print early in the regime, this respirologist became the head censor of medical publications under Wagner, for which he was rewarded with the honorific title of "professor."[38]

Several medical doctors were or became Nazi party officials after the change of power in 1933, but their total number, for reasons indicated above, must be assumed to have been much smaller than the group of medicopolitical functionaries. These men tended to serve the party at local or regional but seldom at Reich levels. More or less typical of this cohort were the local party bosses (Ortsgruppenleiter) Friedrich Mennecke of Eichberg, Wolfgang Saalfeldt of Eutin, and Walter Krauss of Eichstätt.[39] The first-mentioned was an incompetent schemer who made no effort to conceal his party over medical priorities; the latter two were venal, given to excesses in private life such as heavy drinking and women-chasing, obviously using their social and political station for pleasure and personal aggrandizement.[40] But not many medical doctors were content to stick with this comparatively lowly party position, preferring instead somewhat elevated posts, if any at all. Characteristically, the internist Karl Kötschau, who was born in Thuringian Apolda in 1892 and who served both in the imperial army and an

East Prussian Freikorps, led the NSDAP's Beelitz chapter between early 1933 and June of that year. Kötschau also assisted in the formulation of Nazi medical dogma, and thus he aspired to a university chair; minor political chores likely to confine him to provincial backwaters impeded his pursuit of greater things. Fittingly, he won a full professorship at Jena in 1935.[41]

The talented Kötschau could have been at least a regional party representative, a Kreisleiter, as were some of his more astute colleagues. One such man was the generalist Anton Endrös, too young to have served in the war yet a veteran not only of the Freikorps Möhl but also of Hitler's 1923 Beer Hall Putsch. Endrös was adept at public speaking, and he adroitly represented the party's interest in independent regional broadsheets earmarked for Nazi usurpation.[42] Dr. Helmut Otto, born in 1892 and with a sterling World War I and Freikorps past, was an expert in medicine as well as in law and agronomy, and in 1933 he was the Nazi Kreisleiter of Solingen.[43] Because he could not adhere to the standards of that post and could not, in the end, put out for his party, Dr. Theo Rehm, a physical ruffian and Old Fighter four years Otto's junior, was ingloriously dismissed from his Kreis leader's post at Emmendingen, in 1936.[44]

Ancillary, no less worthy party offices could accrue as a consequence of social status, talent, and proven political experience. Onetime surgeon Erasmus Pauly, born in 1888, married into a wealthy family business, joined the party in 1931, and became a functionary in the regional administration of the NSDAP at Giessen.[45] Dr. Heinrich Haselmayer, some eighteen years younger and a Hitler man of the first hour, in March 1933 was put in charge of continuing education (*Volkshochschule*) sponsored by the NSDAP in Gau Hamburg.[46] Both physicians were accorded the rare distinction of being listed, as paragons of the movement, in the Nazi *Who Is Who* of 1935.

Finally, doctors could avail themselves of opportunities nominally in government but in actual fact on the borderline between party and state that fetched a very respectable salary and sometimes a measure of tangible influence. By 1936, six physicians were Reichstag members, doubtless a reward for loyalty to the Nazi movement, if not a sign of greater things to come for these incumbents.[47] In March 1933 Dr. Erhardt Hamann was summoned to the Saxon Landtag, and for a few months hence he served in the municipal administration of Halle.[48] In tandem with party appointments, a few medical doctors became city mayors and councilmen.[49] With NSDAP backing, some doctors obtained career postings with the state police, which in the war ahead could lead to powerful positions in the administrative network of occupied territories, such as in Poland, as well as to more critical assignments, as were those within the SS.[50]

2. The Nazi Physicians' League and Other Party Affiliates

The second major Nazi organization inviting medical doctors in the Third Reich was the National Socialist Physicians' League, or NS-Ärztebund. Tables 2.3 and 2.4 illustrate that of all the doctors registered with the RÄK between 1936 and 1945, (i.e., all doctors in the Reich), 31 percent entered this league, or one-third of all the Protestants and one-quarter of all Catholics, considerably fewer than were attracted to the NSDAP.[1] But the pattern of entering the NS-Ärztebund by age cohort vaguely coincides with that for the party, with the age group licensed before the Weimar Republic being less interested in the league than the republican medical graduates.[2] And as in the case of the party, the 1933–38 license cohort appears to have displayed less enthusiasm for the doctors' league, suggesting a relative preponderance in its membership of the more mature doctors, many of them undoubtedly Old Fighters of the movement. The real surprise, however, comes after examining the figure for 1939–45: only 7.4 percent of all doctors who registered with the RÄK just before and during the war joined the league, and they were from the throng of freshly inaugurated medical neophytes.[3] In absolute numbers the league is said to have had 2,786 members in January 1933, about 14,500 in 1935, and 30,000 in 1938. If these figures seem high it is because veterinarians, dentists, and even pharmacists, who were all entitled to membership, most certainly were included in the count.[4]

Table 2.4 further shows that nearly 28 percent of all RÄK physicians between 1936 and 1945 were members both of the NSDAP and the NS-Ärztebund and that the same people tended to join both organizations. The Nazi Physicians' League was a specialized branch of the party; technically, no Nazi doctor could be in it without prior membership in the NSDAP.[5] But this rule was not strictly enforced, for the league was always eager to strengthen its membership and tended to admit candidates who belonged to Nazi organizations other than the party, such as the SA or SS. It also welcomed doctors who were barred from entering the party when the NSDAP was closed in 1934–36 and 1938 on the tacit understanding that they would apply for NSDAP membership. Because the NS-Ärztebund was one of the more socially elitist institutions of the Nazi movement and its ranks thinned after the first five years or so of the regime, a ban against membership of certain former Freemasons was lifted in the case of doctors in May 1938 by the league's dictatorial leader Gerhard Wagner.[6]

The NS-Ärztebund's notable loss of popularity after 1935 and particularly during the war was the result of a credibility gap that dated from the earliest history of that institution, harking back to the Nuremberg Nazi party rally of August 1929. This had been a period in the Nazi party's history when the founding of specifically National Socialist formations by social or economic pressure groups within the bourgeoisie was becoming more common. In February 1926 the Nazi Students' League had sprung to life, and it was followed in October

1928 by the similarly oriented Nazi Lawyers' League and in April 1929 by the Teachers' League.[7] The Nazi leadership in Munich used these self-motivated lobbies to broaden its party base in the lower and particularly in the upper middle classes. To follow up on those efforts, Alfred Rosenberg created the Society for German Culture in 1927 that tended to stress spiritual and nationalist bonds between the professional groups and Hitler's movement, rather than just economic chimeras.[8]

Against this background Dr. Ludwig Liebl and his fellow founding fathers of the NS-Ärztebund in August 1929 made a point of declaring in their statute that the new league was "not an economic or professional organization of physicians, but part of the fighting organization of the NSDAP." They promised to fulfill the functions of health and race-biological advisers to the party and to serve it whenever the need arose. Furthermore, they pledged to permeate their profession with a specifically National Socialist vocational ethos and to support their younger colleagues in true Nazi spirit, as well as wield a positive influence on the current crop of university students.[9]

These goals were altruistic rather than self-interested, and they represent a unique page in the chronicle of the early Nazi movement, if one regards it primarily as a social protest phenomenon in a time of socioeconomic turbulence. At least rhetorically, these founders created a legacy of altruism that was to be perpetuated well into the Third Reich: virtually unaltered statements of noble intent form the nucleus of additional pronouncements by the NS-Ärztebund hierarchy up to January 1933 and as late as 1943.[10]

Yet they did not express the true sentiments of the bulk of Nazi supporters among the physicians, who before 1933 were young rather than old, insecure rather than established, desperately casting about for chances of gainful self-employment and economic stability rather than opportunities for self-sacrifice to augment the fortunes of some political party.[11] In the various pre-1933 statutes of the league one comes across references, in at least one document, to "racial disintegration" (an allusion to the competition of unwanted Jews), or to "socialization of the general health system" (hinting at the dreaded expansion of the republican public health delivery scheme).[12] But though the author of those lines in 1931 was Leonardo Conti, then a thirty-one-year-old physician, who could easily identify with the disillusionment of his peers in professional limbo, his was a lone voice of the younger generation generally suppressed in the management phalanx of the early physicians' league. All five original NS-Ärztebund founders mentioned in one key source were older, established doctors, of the sort that were in evidence in the pre-1918 licensure group joining the NSDAP and physicians' league before 1936.[13] It is significant that Dr. Fritz Lejeune had not been invited to cofound this physicians' league. Since 1925 he had led the Weimar republican *Jungärzte*, younger doctors pushed to the end of the waiting queue, and was well known for his National Socialist proclivities. Born in 1892, he had one of the lowest party membership numbers.[14]

The forces of youth might have won the upper hand in autumn 1932. At that time Conti, then the league's deputy in Berlin, precipitated a leadership crisis by remonstrating against Liebl's Munich guidance as not being forceful and belligerent enough. Yet at the close of that year, it was not Conti but Wagner who finally succeeded the ailing Liebl; the Munich generalist, though more youthful, was on no account a spokesman of the young. By a hair's breadth Conti was expelled from the league, and the incident would exacerbate the already extant friction between himself and Wagner for years to come.[15]

In essence, then, the NS-Ärztebund's purpose was conceived by a respectable plurality of late Weimar republican physicians who eyed and eventually joined it, those who were progressively disillusioned with the professional policies of the Hartmannbund, as that of an economic combat union, a role that none other than Gregor Strasser, then the prominent Nazi party organization chief, saw cut out for it as early as 1930. The league would take charge of "important professional status interests of physicians," wrote Strasser in September of that year, after he had been prompted by a cautious inquiry on the part of the watchful Hartmannbund.[16]

After the political takeover in 1933 Wagner, at the behest of Hitler and Hess, used the NS-Ärztebund primarily as a political weapon against the still existing bourgeois physicians' associations. Indeed, through their liquidation as well as the establishment of novel Nazi institutions such as the Reich KVD and Physicians' Chamber the professional and economic interests of all German doctors, including the former Young Turks, were seen to be served. Hence the relatively stable frequency of Nazi Physicians' League joiners until 1939.[17] But already the league was suffering from a serious identity problem. In day-to-day affairs the Nazi physicians' professional interests, tallying, as they did, with those of almost all the German doctors at that time, were being looked after by the KVD and RÄK on one hand, and by the Nazi party on the other. As members of all three of those institutions, many physicians of the Third Reich thought the NS-Ärztebund superfluous. They may also have resented that theirs was not an exclusive professional association, as were the sometimes bothersome KVD and RÄK, but that instead they had to rub shoulders in the league's ranks with medical personnel of lower qualification, dentists, veterinarians, and even untitled pharmacists.[18] And as if they were not already sufficiently regimented by the honor courts and professional practice stipulations of the KVD, RÄK, and, for many, NSDAP, the NS-Ärztebund added yet another set of codes that was apt to constrain the doctors in professional forums.[19]

Nevertheless, vis-à-vis its membership and the movement, the NS-Ärztebund tried hard to justify its existence after 1933 by acting as a political mobilization cadre for medical doctors behind the front of a cultural center. For appearances' sake, physicians were socialized in the sophisticated setting to which the upper bourgeoisie, men and women with expensive tastes and a superb education, was conventionally accustomed. Ambitious art exhibitions were scheduled, such as the show "Old and New Romanticism in Germany," enhanced by the expert remarks of art historian Juliane Harms, in early October 1934 in Wiesbaden.[20] There were special university-style lectures, for instance on German Culture in Hesse-Nassau, and appropriate book exchanges.[21] Such cultural pretensions were rendered more creditable when early in 1935 the physicians' league concluded an agreement with Rosenberg's party-officious Nazi Cultural Community (NS-Kulturgemeinde) to facilitate the mutual crossover of talents: Rosenberg would help in the areas of theater, music concerts, and film, and the Nazi doctors would reciprocate by sending medically knowledgeable speakers.[22]

These ties with yet another NSDAP agency accentuated the squarely political intentions of the Nazi physicians' leadership, for these regular social events were ultimately designed to initiate the doctors to mandatory extracurricular routines that could become iron regimens in a period of emergency. Political onuses were always built in, and ideological insinuations abounded. Hence one week after Harms had spoken about art, the Nazi physicians of Wiesbaden were impelled to listen to a race-biological lecture titled "The General Practitioner and Hereditary Diseases." And in Berlin at about this time, Richard Lepsius, a business executive with highest regime connections, enlightened the local doctors regarding the impact of national autarky on the supply of raw materials, warning his audience about the current shortage of imported medicinal aids in a planned economy.[23]

Other subjects that came up were more political, and some related to the professional well-being of the members. The physicians' league disseminated biographical information on Jewish colleagues still practicing medicine and sought to steer all loyal party folks away not only from their offices but also from the practices of "Aryan" doctors who were oblivious to the Nazi regime.[24] Members were marched off, in mufti or in uniform, to significant political events, but just as often merely to drills and flag ceremonies and similar trifles.[25] Invariably, the local chapters of the NS-Ärztebund served as sounding boards for labored political addresses as well as clearinghouses for the recruitment of Nazi doctors to parallel organizations such as the Hitler Youth.[26]

By far the most important political objective of the physicians' league was to fashion the German doctor, insofar as he was malleable, after its own conception of the ideologically inspired soldier and leader. Such an ideal was well aligned with the Nazi movement, whose overriding principle was to level off traditional social differences by bringing the classes closer together. For the onetime elite this meant forsaking privileges of long standing and adopting the customs, predilections, and mannerisms of ordinary people. These desired sociocultural metamorphoses would not come overnight, and they would be resisted by the designated changelings unless the path to humility was paved with rewards and the conversion process sweetened with commendations.

In the case of the doctors, who for decades had been pillars of German society, such mutations had to be effected through carefully planned training courses, in amiable, tasteful environs, and with a calculated admixture of work and relaxation, sports, study, games, and restful contemplation. The proper doses of outdoor activity, cleverly administered, would reduce the doctors' penchant for academic preoccupation that was the fulcrum of their elitism. Moreover, if their professional discipline was to be married to political acumen, then medical content and National Socialist conditioning would have to balance each other perfectly. The process would begin with the trusty colleagues already in the movement's league, as those most likely to comply, set a good example, and return to professional life as even better Nazis than they had been before.

The experiment was attempted at a so-called Leadership School of German Physicians at Alt-Rehse, a breathtakingly beautiful spot on Lake Tollense in Mecklenburg.[27] Billed in the Nazi literature as the "character school of the German doctor" and based on the model of continuing medical education for all physicians by Kurt Blome, the training camp was to feature lectures on Nazi *Weltanschauung*, public health administration, holistic medicine, and professional politics by high-ranking functionaries such as Wagner, Conti, and Haedenkamp, as well as Nazi celebrities like Rosenberg and Hess.[28] The two-week course, for batches of about a hundred participants each, commenced early in June 1935, under Blome's resident director, Hans Deuschl.[29] In an atmosphere of forced camaraderie the vitalistic instincts of the participating doctors, who as members of the NS-Ärztebund were conscripted to attend, were appealed to through physical exercise and folksongs to the point that medical shoptalk outside the classrooms was frowned upon. The course's anti-intellectual stance sometimes included beer-induced vulgarities.[30] But it was considered suitable in reducing even those German doctors with sincere Nazi leanings, who could not help being products of the cultured homes and haughty universities, to their essential manliness. Command jargon, pep talks, and roll calls would sharpen their National Socialist awareness and ready them for martial prowess. By early 1936, nearly a thousand physicians, mostly committed functionaries, had been treated, and the program was now to be aimed at junior doctors considered prime material for future political leadership.[31]

Today it is difficult to gauge the popularity of this scheme even among loyal NS-Ärztebund members. The outbreak of the war interrupted the Alt-Rehse activities, rededicating its facilities to military purposes. Thereafter, physicians from the recently conquered "Germanic" countries and resettled German nationals—Dutchmen, Alsacians, and Lorrainers—were trained there in accordance with Nazi geopolitical tenets.[32] But for insiders, the declining fortunes of Alt-

Rehse were a telling symptom of the denouement of the physicians' league over the past few years. Since 1933 the NS-Ärztebund, sandwiched between the party on the one side and the KVD and RÄK on the other, had become a nuisance to many Nazi doctors. Its activities were an unwanted burden, and, since its financing was never too stable, the various "voluntary" membership contributions to pay for them were resented.[33] The league's regional functionaries lost interest in their work; some either became sloppy administrators or withdrew from their posts.[34]

Between 1939 and 1945 only 7.4 percent of all physicians then graduating joined the doctors' league, down from 32 percent before the war (Table 2.4). As the war relocated entire groups of physicians on the military fronts and the KVD stepped in to control almost all functions of their life in Germany, the social and cryptomilitary uses of NS-Ärztebund became fully redundant. The planning for a national German physicians' convention was halted, and regional meetings were canceled.[35] Officially, the league continued to exist as a branch of the party's Hauptamt für Volksgesundheit, and it was occasionally employed for the reconvening of Nazi doctors home on furlough, its rallies peppered by functionaries' speeches full of propaganda but also exhibiting resignation.[36] By the time the party chancellery declared the league a dormant organization till the Final Victory because of the exigencies of "total war" in early 1943, thus forcing it to share the fate of such other institutions as the Nazi Teachers' League, it was clear even to its most avid supporters in Conti's hierarchy that its end was long overdue.[37]

According to Table 2.4, the Storm Troopers or Brown Shirts (SA) and Black Shirts (SS) ranked third and fourth in the physicians' choice of Nazi groups to join; 26 percent of all the doctors inaugurated before 1945 and registered by the RÄK after 1935 were SA members, before or after 1933. This compares with a mere 11 percent for lower- and upper-school teachers.[38] A surprisingly low 17 percent of the doctors belonged to SA as well as NSDAP, for as in the case of the doctors' league Nazi party adherence was said to be a precondition for membership in adjunct organizations.[39] The SA was less popular with those Weimar republican graduates who were prone to overrun the NSDAP and NS-Ärztebund; physicians licensed between 1933 and the outbreak of World War II, however, favored it most. There was a drop in SA membership for doctors arriving on the scene after 1938; less than 22 percent of the total sample joined then as compared with almost 37 percent in the peaceful regime phase. But this decline was not as precipitous as the physicians' league's; one obvious reason was that the SA, though not exactly in vogue after 1934, never was temporarily suspended (Table 2.4).

The percentage of Weimar medical graduates in the SA (28.5) given in Table 2.4 is low enough to suggest a significant difference between it and the corresponding figure for the NSDAP (50.8 percent), even if figures for female NSDAP members are discounted.[40] One inference one can draw from this is that among the Old Fighters in the Nazi physicians' camp, the SA had not been an obvious first choice. As research over the last few years has revealed, the pre-1933 Storm Troopers in their rank and file were preeminently a proletarian and lower-middle-class phenomenon, attracting very few members of the social elite.[41] Upper bourgeois men were much more likely to consider the SA's leadership echelons. Without a doubt, physicians would automatically be assigned to leadership posts, for the Weimar republican Brown Shirts were chronically short of medics, who, as tradition prescribed, would wear officers' insignia.[42] A number of Nazi doctors in the vanguard of the movement, among them Conti, Blome, Saalfeldt, and Otto, served actively as SA physicians, tending the wounded after skirmishes in the depression period with the communists.[43] Because of such onerous chores, it is fair to say that few opportunists among the doctors approached the SA before 1933; those who took that step were part of the die-hard core, willing "to put their bodies on the line."[44]

But after the seizure of power in January 1933, this was to change. As the Storm Troopers, under the vigorous leadership of Captain Ernst Röhm, increased their formations by leaps and bounds, they needed many more physicians. Hence an SA rank became much more attractive to German doctors, including those who were testing the waters before an honest, long-lasting commitment to this new Third Reich.[45] On one hand, Röhm's attempt to duplicate the apparatus of the Reichswehr meant the institutionalization of medical services on a regular military pattern. This appealed to many physicians who wanted to but could not join the Reichswehr because of its chronic closure.[46] Such SA medical service, however, in a period of peace and in the absence of interparty strife along republican lines, entailed none of the risks of the Time of Struggle (1919–33). Minor demands were made on SA doctors, such as occasional donations of money for SA welfare purposes and the free dispensation of medicare in SA camps, as well, of course, as participation in some rallies and marches.[47] Young physicians who had joined the SA before January 30, 1933, now learned that they were eligible for immediate placement in panel practice and may have been envied by previously noncommitted colleagues.[48] On the whole, then, the doctors benefited from a situation in which Röhm had resolved to lure them early in 1933, in exchange for sybaritic privileges.[49] When the veterans' organization Stahlhelm was forcibly inducted into the SA in early 1934, hundreds of doctors, to the obvious delight of Röhm, augmented the existing medical units, with scarcely any objections from the men involved.[50] Physicians were able, within a relatively short time, to attain high SA officer ranks, which they could never have earned in the Reichswehr had they been allowed to join it.[51]

Hitler's purge of the SA in June–July 1934 presented a problem to these physicians, who did not want to be compromised, especially because few of them had taken SA service seriously. Committed Nazis or the circumspectly career-minded characteristically were apt to switch to the SS.[52] If new doctors now and during the war continued to frequent the Storm Troopers, they may have done so because the SA had been so severely emasculated (Table 2.4, column F). This state, often rendering SA membership merely honorific or nominal, afforded the best of two worlds: the bonus of a Nazi shield in return for a modicum of political input.[53] In contrast, the SS was an altogether different organization, particularly after summer 1934. Because it aspired to be an elitist corps, it always restricted its membership intake. About 7 percent of German male doctors who registered with the RÄK after 1935 were counted as SS recruits (Table 2.4). About 9 percent of all male physicians licensed between 1933 and 1939 joined the SS, and the percentage may have increased for the 1939–45 cohort.[54] These figures may appear small, but they must be appreciated from the perspective of other professional cohort memberships in the SS. Only 0.4 percent of teachers were Black Shirts, for instance, in the period from 1925 to 1945, far behind the physicians.[55] The two groups may also be compared in proportional SS representation. Almost 1.3 percent of all SS men and leaders at the end of 1937 were physicians, including veterinarians but not dentists. By conservative reckoning, doctors were overrepresented in the SS by a factor of seven, whereas the teachers' representation was only slightly above their proportion of the population.[56] The one profession that was even more heavily overrepresented in the SS than the physicians was the lawyers, at a ratio of twenty-five to one.[57]

It is well to speculate briefly about the causes of this remarkable attraction between doctors and SS, and, for that matter, between lawyers and SS. As in the case of the SA, the SS offered responsible leadership posts to members of the upper bourgeoisie, but consonant with its enigma and large measure of real power, much more prestige was attached to SS than to any SA posts. Physicians and lawyers considered themselves pillars of a more traditional society, not quite at ease initially with the changes promised by the Third Reich. Hence they craved permanent professional and social security and continued recognition even in a "revolutionized" polity; besides the army, the SS was most likely to provide that. Moreover, in the SS there reigned an aura of technical perfection and, at least on the surface, intellectual brilliance, which fascinated these high achievers.[58]

More important, however, the SS dealt with matters close to the everyday business of their profession and in a manner that was of profound concern to them. It was preoccupied with a redefinition of legal concept and practice, and "law" could come to have a different meaning from the one law students had been taught in the universities. Many lawyers may have been wary of the perversion of the law but were intrigued enough by the potential for legalistic tampering to wish to witness this process and perhaps even to participate in it, to feed their sense of importance by destroying the law's former independence and raising themselves above it.[59]

"Doctors," observes Robert Jay Lifton, "regularly function at the border of life and death."[60] Hence doctors were doubtless conscious of the SS's seemingly absolute control over life and death, a situation not unlike their own. For centuries the physician's charisma, indeed his very real powers, had derived from the manipulation of a patient's health, sometimes at the brink of death, impelling the patient to place his fate in the doctor's hands. Similarly, the black-uniformed SS leader was a persona whose decision-making prerogative put others at his mercy. For a physician in the Black Shirts' ranks, death took on a somewhat different hue than it had in the civilian career and even in the military, whose norms followed accepted codes of behavior. The factor of death loomed large in the SS, which brandished a skull as its symbol. Death assumed a versatile quality in that it might be used in a threatening pose. Patients had traditionally seen doctors as professionals who would try to avert death; respect for doctors was based on this attribute. In a society whose leaders were in the business not only of saving from the process of dying but also of inflicting it at will, doctors could receive even more respect. This motivation helps explain why doctors were visibly overrepresented in Himmler's elite guard units.

There were commonly two avenues of success for physicians in the SS. Much as in the SA, they could elect part-time membership in the General SS (Allgemeine SS) that would not detract unduly from their professional activities. The majority of black-shirted doctors chose this option, putting in weekend service and donning their SS uniforms only on special occasions. A typical case is that of Dr. Gregor Ebner, who since 1931 served a regional SS network out of Munich while devoting full-time energies to his general practice in Upper Bavarian Kirchseeon; only in 1937 would he become a regular employee of the SS-Lebensborn.[61] But even with part-time status, and unlike their colleagues in the SA, these men could be mobilized expeditiously and suddenly. The SS was systematically developed to fulfill narrowly defined functions during wartime. After the creation of the armed SS squadrons (1940: Waffen-SS) as early as 1933, but especially after 1938, his reserve status made every part-time member of the General SS subject to the draft in the Waffen-SS sector. He could then be delegated to shock-troop front-line duty or to specific tasks such as partisan combat and concentration camp service. By such deployment a formerly "normal" doctor might become fatally tainted by war crimes.[62]

Individual cases had tragic results, as the example of Percival Treite shows. This native of Berlin was twenty-two years old when, still a student, he joined the Allgemeine SS in 1933. After his medical state examination in 1936 he took additional training in gynecology with Professor Walter Stoeckel of the Charité Hospital. After being certified in his specialty in 1938, he stayed on as Stoeckel's highly regarded assistant.[63] In World War II, he was requisitioned for military service, apparently against his own and Stoeckel's will; the master almost managed to reclaim him for the hospital. But by April 1943 the armed SS finally inducted Treite.[64] In September of that year, the young gynecologist was appointed staff doctor in the Ravensbrück concentration camp for women. Here, to the later disbelief of his teacher, he engaged in cruel experiments on inmates.[65] Treite's end was ignominious. After deserting Ravensbrück on April 30, 1945, he was arrested by the British on May 11. Charged with war crimes and sentenced to be hanged on February 3, 1947, the doctor took his own life in a Hamburg jail a few weeks later.[66]

The careers of other SS physicians were more obviously shaped for the instant and dynamic success that a full-time commitment to the elite guards was noted for. The prescient Himmler and his lieutenants had created the proper channels to facilitate such success. Government-salaried medical units outside the party-financed General SS existed as early as 1936.[67] By spring 1939 permanent Waffen-SS physicians were guaranteed credit for any specialist training they had undergone as civilians.[68] As the war proceeded, the Waffen-SS had a complex structure for military physicians, and it was constantly updated.[69] There was a *Reichsarzt-SS*, comparable to a surgeon-general in the army, who oversaw all facets of medical and health care in the shock troops. His position was strengthened when Himmler, in August 1943, united the medical branches of all the wings of the SS under this doctor's command.[70] This move was a result of the police chief's own elevation to the post of Reich interior minister, in which capacity he obtained nominal jurisdiction over all the civilian doctors.[71] There even was an SS medical academy, at first in Berlin and after 1940 in Graz, loosely conjoined to that city's university, where aspiring SS physicians received specific schooling.[72]

Until the time of martial adversity surrounding Stalingrad, Waffen-SS careers were fairly attractive to physicians who were militarily inclined and liked opportunities for quick promotion coupled with a respectable measure of power and good pay.[73] Typically, one might have aimed for a responsible position with the militarily deployed police detachments so as to qualify automatically for the armed SS. Dr. Hans-Jochen Boye of Dresden was licensed in February 1939, at the age of twenty-six. After working in a Berlin police clinic and as a Luftwaffe doctor in occupied Warsaw, he applied for a police physician's posting certain to procure for him the emoluments and privileges of a higher civil servant. Boye's transfer from the air force to the SS became fully effective in October 1941, even though his subsequent progress at the police hospital was temporarily interrupted by additional service on the eastern front in a combined police and SS formation.[74] In another corner of the Reich, police physician Dr. Josef Fischer had a reputation as an "agreeable young colleague of diminutive size but wiry and of good posture." Already on record as very ambitious and enjoying the fruits of uncommonly early promotion, the thirty-four-year-old SS leader and partisan combat specialist became a senior staff physician (*Oberstabsarzt*) of the police in 1942.[75] Somewhat older doctors could also fare well in the joint SS and police forces. In late 1938, forty-seven-year-old Dr. Ernst Wenzel, a pre-1933 career policeman, was proposed for the rank of *Obersturmbannführer* in the SS as well as physician-colonel in the police. At the same time, he was singled out for a directorship in the state police hospital, a section of which he had successfully administered.[76]

And then there were doctors who fanatically went every inch of the way with the SS and hardly knew anything else. Friedrich Entress was born in 1914 in the Polish-Prussian province of Posen and graduated from that city's medical faculty in June 1939 when it was once more under Polish rule. As the member of a local ethnic German vigilante group supported by illegal SS, he had, at the termination of the Polish campaign, naturally drifted into the SS Death Head's Squads by November. Serving first in an SS intelligence unit, he eventually became the garrison doctor of Gross-Rosen concentration camp. From there he moved to Auschwitz, then to Mauthausen camp near Linz in 1943, acting as its senior physician at only thirty years of age. Entress, who was said to have a "Nordic" profile, with gray eyes and dark blond hair, was a surgeon with an SS tank division when in May 1945 the Allies captured him—at the pinnacle of his career.[77]

Entress's colleague Josef Mengele, three years older, hailed from a family of well-to-do Swabian machine manufacturers. After acquiring a Ph.D. from Munich University in 1935, he became a doctor of medicine in Frankfurt three years later. He had early been influenced by race research in Munich and Frankfurt and married a young woman who was vouched to be a "dependable fighter for the National Socialist idea." Mengele joined the party in summer 1937 and the SS one year later. After active trench service in the Waffen-SS from 1941 on, he arrived at Auschwitz concentration camp in May 1943, already impressively decorated and with a war injury. His superiors credited him in August 1944 not just with having served in his regular capacity as camp physician but also for efforts beyond the call of duty. SS Captain Mengele had sought to continue his Frankfurt research in hereditary race science and was highly vaunted as an anthropologist. His professional opportunities were practically limitless: "He assuredly appears suitable for any other kind of application, not excluding one at higher levels."[78]

Almost every tenth German doctor in the Third Reich had some association with the Hitler Youth (Table 2.4, column G), which, in the early years of the regime, was built up by Baldur von Schirach as the Nazi monopolist youth organization until it reached some 8 million members at the outbreak of the war.[79] Among the Hitler Youth (HJ) physicians, who were led by Karl-Walter Kondeyne, yet another early fighter for the Führer's movement, the generation licensed between 1933 and 1945 was more heavily represented than those inaugurated in monarchical and republican times, reflecting the comparatively youthful makeup of the HJ-accredited doctors.[80] Within the HJ, physicians were to control epidemics and drug abuse, as well as undertake general health supervisory chores.[81] HJ service apparently was not as popular with the physicians as Schirach had hoped because there were so many other, more convenient and promising options for political engagement. "Securing doctors exclusively for service with the Hitler Youth," wrote a Hessian NS-Ärztebund functionary in October 1934, "might meet with considerable difficulty around here, for among the younger colleagues I hardly know anyone who is not already active in the SA, the SS or with aviators, gas protection squads, or medical and technical emergency patrols."[82] Nonetheless, in November 1935 Schirach, who could never lure enough physicians into his ranks, had managed to integrate former SA doctors rendered redundant after the Röhm purge fifteen months before, thus adding to the staff of six thousand medics already at his beck and call.[83]

As Schirach was reminded by that Hessian physicians' leader, there were still other Nazi institutions to which Third Reich doctors could belong or be affiliated with, however loosely. Some of these held a special attraction for doctors either because of the latter's lifestyle or their occupation. The National Socialist Motor Corps (Nationalsozialistisches Kraftfahrkorps—NSKK), for example, was fairly popular because it needed members who owned automobiles, and the doctors equipped with them found the NSKK's rallies an enjoyable if politically innocuous way to participate in the Nazi movement.[84] Of all the physicians, male and female, 1.6 percent belonged to Nazi People's Welfare (Nationalsozialistische Volkswohlfahrt—NSV), for which they had to furnish assessments or act in some other advisory capacity.[85] Doctors patronized Nazi aviator clubs, SS solidarity groups, and women's leagues. With over two-thirds of all physicians in Germany admitting to some connection with the NSDAP or its derivatives, the medical profession surely emerges as one of the most highly Nazi-oriented occupational strata in the Third Reich.[86]

3. Forms of Resistance

The heavy participation of doctors in various sectors of the Nazi movement during the Third Reich suggests that their antiregime activity was inversely related to National Socialist association. The evidence to be presented below will prove this to be so. It dismisses an earlier claim by Georg Bittner that German physicians from 1933 to 1945 suffered "quiet, unpolitical heroism" by retiring to what he calls "inner emigration," and it further exposes the spuriousness of Hans Schadewaldt's assertion that overall, the medical profession was wronged by wanton Nazi rule.[1] Few doctors would oppose the Nazis on political, ideological (including religious), or medicoethical grounds. A handful risked their lives; a somewhat greater proportion merely issued queries or aired discontent, often ingenuously unaware of the consequences. After all, the scale of negative reactions to the Nazi regimen, between political indifference on one side and tyrannicide on the other, was finely calibrated, ranging from verbal disagreement to demonstrative protest, and from there to political conspiracy and murder. It is moot today, as certain British and West German historians have done, to label these expressions of dissatisfaction for the purpose of marking gradations. The activities in question were subjectively experienced and thus are hardly measurable by hindsight criteria masquerading as objective; the present ascriptive categories are nominal, not interval, and frequently blurred by the inconsistencies of language. One would do better to explain perceived differences of degree by attempting, as in the case of all historical actions, to get inside the minds of the actors and circumscribe their motives within some generally comprehensible terms of reference, leaving, as in statistical analysis, sufficient leeway for potential errors of judgment and subsequent correction by those better qualified to judge, not excluding the actors themselves.[2]

Such a qualifying search must, of course, be undertaken after the application of a commonly accepted yardstick with which to measure recognizable extremes at either end: altruistic self-sacrifice for the cause of freedom on one side and contemporary or post-1945 distortions or deceptions on the other. As regards the former, documented death sentences and executions speak for themselves. Regarding the latter, however, the historian of doctors under Hitler must be wary. Given the official Nazi desiderate that every German doctor practice his profession "in the spirit of National Socialist physicianship," which had been legalistically secured by a plethora of ordinances,[3] it was easy for them to fall under the suspicion of recalcitrance on the slightest pretext, as easy as it was for the Nazi bureaucrats to construe a pretext for allegations. Thus Dr. Werner Schmidt of Reichenbach in 1935 was accused of performing abortions, a serious enough felony under the new legislation, but to defame the man entirely the KVD saw fit to call him an "unsavory Marxist and Communist."[4] Dr. med. et dent. Fritz Baerwolf of Gotha, who in 1934 had failed to receive authoritative recognition as an oral specialist, openly charged that he had been libeled by jealous colleagues as a communist.[5] And during the war, hospital physician Dr. Sch. in Wolfsburg was repeatedly reprimanded for irregularities of all sorts, resulting in the doctor's claim that someone wanted to see him in a concentration camp.[6] Twenty-five-year-old Dr. Kurt Herlitschka was condemned to a five-year penitentiary term in autumn 1943 for having plotted a surreptitious retreat to France. But he had committed this infraction during his incarceration in an SS camp, after having caused the death of a comrade while himself in Himmler's order.[7] Was he a hero, then? It appears that in all these cases National Socialist accusation, specious or not, could after 1945 without difficulty have been stretched by those misfortuned men to simulate political opposition when in reality there had been only professional friction or common unruliness.

Nonetheless, the most committed group of politically motivated resisters among the German doctors were the Marxists, almost all of them uncompromising communists, in the company of a few Social Democrats and left-of-center sympathizers. But even they were inconspicuous. Among one known group of 485 dedicated communists who became victims in the fight against Nazism from

1933 to 1945 there were five physicians, one of whom was Jewish. Similarly, sixty-year-old Eutin Dr. Ernst Wittern, detained in a hastily improvised concentration camp in Holstein in 1933, was one of 283 inmates there, for having derided the regime and its official symbols. The inclusion of these professionals in the ranks of other victims from all walks of life appears to push the representation of physicians in the resistance considerably above that in the population at large, but these instances were isolated and not necessarily typical. Physicians were not usually found among Marxists.[8]

To some extent, the opposition of Marxist physicians to the Third Reich was triggered by the regime's proscription of such doctors in the spring of 1933, by the Law for the Reconstitution of the Civil Service. Along with their Jewish colleagues, "Aryan" physicians who had a proved record of Marxist activity in republican times were dismissed from hospital, *Amtsarzt*, or other employment situations and ostracized from panel insurance practice.[9] In preparing such action against individuals, the physician functionaries of the KVD habitually were much more radical and unforgiving than the legislation had provided for, doubtless because of the notorious hatred among German establishment doctors for anything resembling socialized medicine. Hence of 338 bans pronounced by the KVD against Marxist colleagues by summer of 1933, 231 subsequently had to be rescinded by the Reich labor ministry, which, in rendering the final decision, employed a far more conservative, if not humanitarian, standard.[10] KVD officials who wished to uproot as many unwanted rivals as possible aimed for an excessively broad interpretation of the new law, expecting to be able to circumvent the more accommodating rulings of the civil servants. They hoped that their own preemptive judgments would withstand any future revisions so as to avoid civil lawsuits for financial compensation, which several defiant doctors attempted. The question was of considerable significance for the new Nazi medical hierarchy, wrote Dr. Grote in October 1934, because of the possibility that "an appreciable number of excluded doctors, whose exclusions had been canceled, would demand retroactive payment for fund-insurance services," resumed after the initial injunction.[11]

The problem was complicated by the potential inclusion within the group of Marxist doctors of Jewish physicians, who were subject to curtailment by yet another clause of the same decree. Realizing this, the labor ministry lost no time in commenting that no precise definition of Marxist-active physicians was feasible, implying that it was better to err in favor of the suspects.[12] This consideration is important not least in today's efforts to assess the case of Marxist doctors fairly. For inasmuch as the large majority of socialist physicians was Jewish, it would be difficult to trace their persecution at Nazi hands solely to an ideological conviction, when in fact the racist argument took precedence. Unhappily, in trying to present an analysis of the circumstances leading to the deplorable fate of blacklisted doctors at that time, certain of today's West German scholars have paid little heed to this complexity: virtually all of the leftist physicians they mention are identifiable as members of the Jewish minority.[13]

There were two additional sources of annoyance for communist and Social Democratic physicians early in the regime: the dissolution of Marxist physicians' unions and the forced disruption of ambulatory services. The principal lobbies, present since the days of the republic, were the League of Socialist Physicians (Verein sozialistischer Ärzte), originally founded in 1913 and reactivated after the Great War, and the Workshop of Social Democratic Physicians (Arbeitsgemeinschaft sozialdemokratischer Ärzte), harking back to 1926. In both organizations Jews proliferated. Hence for Saxony it was announced in June 1933 that the state's Reich commissar had dissolved the socialist physicians' league: "As is generally known, the league consisted of a horde of mostly communist physicians."[14] Furthermore, socialist-committed doctors who had been employed by the SPD fund–supported ambulatory networks dealing out medicare to the needy largely in big city centers after spring 1933 found themselves on the street, their contracts annulled without due legal process and being owed thousands of marks in back pay and pension premiums.[15]

Within the group of Marxist-oriented physicians whose opposition to the Third Reich is documented it is wise to differentiate between the full-time conspirators and the more incidental activists. Foremost among the former were Karl Gelbke, Elfriede Paul, Fritz Gietzelt, Rainer Fetscher, and Johannes Kreiselmaier.[16] Their life histories and the circumstances under which they became sworn enemies of Hitler in the communist camp were not identical but remarkably similar. A few of them had always sympathized with the KPD and considered themselves friends of the Soviet Union. Dr. Gelbke was a suspect for the republican police even in Weimar days when, from 1930 to 1933, he served as contract physician at the Soviet trade mission in Leipzig. After Hitler's political takeover, Gelbke and his wife, Dina, were instructed by the soon to be illegal KPD to employ their medical practice as a cover with a view to assisting communist *agents provocateurs*. Astonishingly, the doctor was able to sustain his large Leipzig practice against all odds, treating patients as well as running an intelligence network for the underground. Gelbke defied Nazi stool pigeons and house searches, and he remained unbroken during Gestapo questioning. In fact, his medical reputation was so high that he was invited to treat the sick child of one of his interrogators. Many German communists, conscripted foreign workers, and prisoners of war owed their health and their lives to Gelbke, who miraculously survived the Third Reich.[17]

Equally committed to the communist cause was Dr. Elfriede Paul, who practiced generalist medicine near the Kurfürstendamm in Berlin from 1936 to 1942. Together with her paramour Walter Küchenmeister she belonged to the communist resistance organization Red Chapel, directed by Harro Schulze-Boysen and Arvid Harnack, for whom she wrote and distributed handbills and posters with anti-Nazi slogans, maintained clandestine radio contact with Soviet cadres, and encouraged the infiltration of German workers. Among other feats, she helped to create escape channels to Switzerland later once used by Kurt Schumacher, the postwar founder of the SPD.[18] Although it is not known how much time and effort she invested in her medical practice then, she was able to apply her professional skills, albeit to a limited extent, to help fellow prisoners after her capture and incarceration in September 1942. Küchenmeister died on the executioner's block in 1943, but Dr. Paul was liberated from the Leipzig penitentiary in April 1945.[19]

Unlike Drs. Gelbke and Paul, Dr. Rainer Fetscher was drawn to communism by patients during office hours, after he had been dismissed from his chair in social hygienics at the Technical University of Dresden in autumn 1933. Until the end he claimed that he did not wish to be pigeonholed as a card-carrying communist; he was simply a "bourgeois democrat." By 1936 he had organized his medical office so it could function as a support center for illegal communists. Fetscher developed an ingenious system of treating affluent Nazi leaders and then using the money they paid him in the anti-Hitler struggle. Comrades visited him not only for medical but for moral and material assistance. He never once interrupted his liaison with the Dresden communist cadre led by Hermann Eckhardt. In early 1945 Fetscher was convinced of the imminent victory of the Red Army over fascist Germany; he was making plans for a reorganization of the German health administration along Soviet lines. Already he had successfully undermined a local Dresden police station and, backed by his contacts, was endeavoring to save strategic bridges and buildings from destruction by the SS. But then Himmler's elite corps struck, and he was murdered on May 8, on the very day the capitulation of the Third Reich was written in stone in the fallen capital.[20]

The Leipzig internist Fritz Gietzelt was not originally a communist, but he was agonizing over the Nazi politicization of German medicine just commencing in 1933, when he received his license. An attempt to emigrate to Sweden foundered on the obstacle of Swedish certification—a common problem for most would-be physician émigrés. Thereupon Gietzelt specialized in internism and in 1939 established a radiology practice that soon made him one of the wealthiest doctors in Germany. Like Fetscher, he counted a sizable number of Nazi notables among his patients. It is a testimonial to his political shrewdness no less than to his medical proficiency that his expert assessments were valued by Wehrmacht offices and Gestapo headquarters alike. Gietzelt, who carefully revealed his criticisms of the regime to some of his acquaintances, was finally recruited for communist undercover work by a leading local cadre, the artist Karl Krause. Consequently, this doctor used his offices in much the same fashion as did Fetscher and Gelbke. In 1943 Gelbke acquainted Gietzelt more closely with the antifascist platform of the Leipzig KPD. Even though he never became one of the movers among the Leipzig communists, Gietzelt lent them his support in a variety of ways, communicating cryptic radio messages and collaborating with Russian officers, who were interned in the nearby prisoner-of-war camp at Taucha. Trusted by the Leipzig Nazi brass, he frequently forged health certificates for conscripted foreign workers to free them from their arduous chores. These laborers then engaged in the sabotage of Germany's munitions industry. His ruses enabled Dutch, French, and Belgian forced workers to return to their home countries and saved German resistance fighters from transport to the military front. On June 30, 1944, however, Gietzelt was arrested, subsequently tried, and condemned to death. Luckily for him, his execution was postponed until February of the following year, and in the confusion following an air raid, Gietzelt fled from his Dresden jail. Hiding out in nearby Meissen, he was truly safe only after the arrival of the Soviet troops.[21]

The last exemplar of communist opposition, Johannes Kreiselmaier, was not so fortunate. He was decapitated by his Nazi tormentors in Berlin-Plötzensee on November 27, 1944, after a prolific career in the orthodox Marxist resistance. Kreiselmaier was a relative latecomer to the resistance scene. This pious son of a Lutheran clergyman had actively sympathized with the SS since 1936 and had joined the Nazi party one year later. At the height of his career in the Nazi Wehrmacht, after his promotion to *Oberstabsarzt* in November 1940, he was confident of Germany's Final Victory. But the calamitous loss at Stalingrad in February 1943 changed his thinking. Like many Germans, Kreiselmaier experienced this disaster as the turning point of the war, if not the regime, whose criminal nature he had begun to comprehend. Back in the Reich in 1943, the doctor was introduced to the resistance group of Anton Saefkow and Franz Jacob. Kreiselmaier began to act out his anti-Nazi convictions by offering free medical care to communist cadres, sometimes using as shelter the military hospital he was in charge of. Cadres were also convened on the premises of his practice in Berlin-Zehlendorf. He, too, kept German men from being marched off to the fronts, and he collected valuable information from his influential Nazi patients. He is credited with having supplied to the underground details about the ominous V-2 rockets so that much of this nefarious hardware could be destroyed before it did any damage. And he, like Fetscher, was instrumental in the planning for a restructured German health system, with particular attention to the prevention of mass epidemics, to be implemented after the fascist reign. But Kreiselmaier was arrested by the Gestapo in July 1944. He betrayed none of his conspiratorial friends despite the usual threats and torture.[22]

Other Marxist physicians may have been less effective in their actions, and some may have risked far less to begin with; nevertheless, in their moral fortitude, they still were many cuts above their Nazi professional peers and hence deserve mention here. In Berlin, Dr. Wolfgang Kühn worked closely with Saefkow and Jacob, and he in turn was assisted by Drs. Gerhard Pagel and Helmut

Müller. As far as is known, all survived.[23] Dr. Margarete Blank, a communist activist since the late republic, valiantly used her practice in Saxon Panitzsch much like her colleagues Fetscher and Gietzelt, listening to anti-German radio news and aiding Soviet prisoners of war. Her life was snuffed out by the guillotine in February 1945.[24] Dr. Theodor Brugsch, an eminent Berlin internist, who like Fetscher had been forced out of a professorship, helped colleagues implicated in the July 1944 plot.[25] Nor ought the twenty-one medical doctors be forgotten who early in the Nazi regime decided to demonstrate their aversion to fascism by signing up with anti-Franco forces in the Spanish Civil War. Among them at least one woman distinguished herself.[26] Not included in those twenty-one heroes was Dr. Karl Schnell, who had first emigrated to France, then directed a field hospital for the Spanish republican forces. When the hospital was liquidated by Nazi interventionists, Schnell lost his life.[27] Social Democratic physicians who have gone on record for their anti-Nazi stance include a Dr. Braun of Coburg in Franconia, who was arrested in spring 1933, and Julius Nördlinger, once a dedicated Augsburg proletariat doctor, who in 1934 lent a helping hand to persecuted local SPD officials.[28]

The best of the non-Marxist opponents of the Nazi regime among the doctors were motivated by ethical considerations that sprang directly from the Hippocratic Oath and by more general humanitarian factors consonant with an upper-bourgeois German lifestyle and mentality, which was anathema to the lower-middle-class *Spiessbürger* sordidity of Hitler's rule. This attitude could have translated into a rejection of overt and even covert racism and hence the persecution of Gypsies and Jews or a basic skepticism regarding nationalist megalomania, or the party's oppression of the Christian churches. Last but not least, etiquette, comportment, and aesthetics contributed to the elitist professionals' revulsion against boorish Nazi manners and the profligate lack of tact of these would-be revolutionaries.[29]

Paragons of medical resistance on ethical grounds have become known mainly in the area of what the Nazis called "euthanasia," the killing of demented or crippled civilians just before the war, many of whom actually were fit to live. This, at least, was the professional opinion of some of the physicians involved in the various processes of selective liquidation, all of them within the geographical boundaries of the Reich.[30] Doctors with great moral qualms about murdering innocent victims of Nazi racist ideology found it next to impossible to refuse to cooperate in the scheme or openly to sabotage the killings. Decoys had to be used such as falsifying documents or finding a pretext for delaying the "treatment" of certain patients. Hence Dr. Roemer, the director of a mental institution in Württemberg, sidetracked the evacuation of many of his wards to a killing station after constant wrangling with Dr. Eugen Stähle, now the leading health official in that state and as staunch a Nazi as ever. Other patients were released into the care of their relatives, as was successfully done by Dr. Conrad, a woman physician at the

Eichberg institution, who managed to dupe her director.[31] Although it was very difficult, some doctors even retreated forever from the ignoble sites, either by voluntary enlistment for front-line duty or by insisting on premature retirement.[32]

Still, a very few outstanding cases of defiance have been chronicled. Dr. Martin Hohl, the director of Bayreuth's mental institution Wendelhöfen, after laborious subterfuges, told his suspicious Berlin supervisors outright that he would never play a part in the murder of innocent people.[33] Similarly, Dr. F. Hölzel was brave enough to inform his superior at the infamous Upper Bavarian asylum of Eglfing-Haar in writing during summer 1940 that he thought the state-decreed "euthanasia" measures were "convincing" in their objectives. Nonetheless, to affirm the importance of official provisions and personally to live up to them were two different things. "Thus with all my rational insight and goodwill, I cannot help but feel that by nature I am simply not equal to the task."[34]

Medical ethos was invoked during other Nazi ventures involving human lives. After the Reichstag fire in late February 1933, when the hooligan SA capriciously beat up well-known German communists, brave civilian doctors tried to prevent the worst by offering aid, at great risk of being manhandled by the Brown Shirts.[35] In May 1934 a Düsseldorf *Amtsarzt* may knowingly have jettisoned officially sanctioned sterilization procedures by refusing to ordain surgery for a local Indochinese-German half-breed.[36] During the war, the occasions for such professional trepidation were multiplied many times. Occupied Warsaw's health officer Dr. Wilhelm Hagen in December 1942 deemed it a weight on his conscience when he learned that seventy thousand Poles, old people and children under ten, were to be killed, "just like the Jews," and he protested to the Führer.[37] Some eight months later, certain of the local Würzburg physicians lodged vocal complaints with the authorities when it was rumored that the ball-bearing plants of Schweinfurt, lately the targets of American bomber pilots, were to be relocated to their town, critically close to hospitals and clinics.[38]

If some German physicians came to resist the increasingly evident anti-Jewish measures, Hippocratic ethics tempered with general humanitarian sentiments were the most likely cause. Casting all precautions to the wind, several "Aryan" doctors ignored the requisite Nazi rulings and continued to be sociable with their Jewish neighbors. At Professor Ernst Rüdin's Kaiser Wilhelm Institute for Psychiatry in Munich, some German physicians protested against the removal of "Jewish art," paintings by the Russian expatriate Leonid Pasternak, in the face of the fulminations of their Nazi colleagues.[39] German doctors secretly went on treating their Jewish patients after the promulgation of the discriminative race laws of September 1935, some far into the war.[40] During that conflict, German doctors who honored personal ties with Jews or were related to them by marriage exposed themselves knowingly to the regime's defamatory campaigns; the SS and concentration camps were menacingly close. Professionals who put themselves at risk to help the "U-boats," German Jews who had gone into hiding after the fateful evacuations started, were especially vulnerable. Although there were few such physicians, their names have been preserved in the annals of history: Josef Schunk, Walter Seitz, Theodor Brugsch, and M. Helmy, all of Berlin, virtually the only place in the Nazi Reich where Jews might successfully be hidden.[41] But Bruno Schulz and Leo Mager worked out of Rüdin's famous institute in Munich, and we know of at least two German "Aryan" physicians who ended up in Auschwitz for having aided Jews.[42]

There were physicians who still held high the ideals of freedom and democracy and who deplored the authoritarian strictures imposed by the ruthless Hitlerites. They showed it by facilitating employment opportunities to regime pariahs or, later, by brushing aside the ordinance forbidding "Aryan" Germans from offering commensal privileges to Polish domestics.[43] One doctor demonstratively ripped apart his ballot in the polling station during the referendum of August 1934, while another denounced the SA in a public place.[44] During the war, there were Anglophile young doctors in Hamburg who met with like-minded intellectuals in surreptitious surroundings, discussing banned books, "degenerate" art, and, ever again, the hubris of Hitler's campaigns. They danced the nights away with equally defiant young actresses, to the music of American swing.[45] In the capital, meanwhile, Dr. Vera Gaupp was providing shelter for runaway conspirators of the July 1944 plot.[46] One could never be careful enough, however. Erika Mann tells of a Munich doctor at the start of the regime who habitually passed "derogatory remarks"; his wife, visiting with Mann in Switzerland, showed herself perilously contemptuous of the potential consequences. Before too long, the doctor ended up in Dachau, with his wife imprisoned and their young son tucked away in a party home.[47] Political criticism was most safely voiced in the guise of parabole and metaphor, as did the noted Berlin physician Dr. Munk in summer 1941, when he compared the state of freedom under Friedrich Schiller's Duke Karl Eugen of Württemberg with the present tyranny.[48]

If it is sometimes said that German physicians were essentially unpolitical, and if by that is meant that they showed naiveté rather than coolheaded balance, then indeed some expressed this behavior during the dictatorship. In September 1934 the country doctor Theodor Ensinger in Haltingen near Konstanz was reported to the authorities because he had rambled on about how he, who had once been imprisoned by the "Commies," still preferred them to the Nazis, that Göring had set the Reichstag on fire, and what with the Röhm putsch and the horrors of the concentration camps, "I cannot see the slightest sign of progress brought on by National Socialism . . . no one may speak his mind!" This man, possibly under the influence of alcohol, was spontaneously voicing his dissatisfaction with the current political system as did so many of his fellow Germans, whether they were physicians, streetcar conductors, or candlestick makers.[49] But Dr. Carlo Pietz of Berlin, a gynecologist intermittently pressed into war service, nearly lost his life because of denunciatory remarks made by his former governess. Visiting the old lady in his hometown of Darmstadt in spring 1943, he was confronted by the ruins of his father's house. Enraged, this member of the Nazi party and Physicians' League (1940; 1942) hurled invective at the Führer, who had caused the death of millions in his desire to conquer the world: "One must do away with him!" It was only because Pietz's Wehrmacht superior was sympathetic and destroyed his court file that he remained among the living. A personal sense of material loss was hardly the proper motive for political reaction, expressed with volatility and without perspicacity.[50]

Among some doctors, pro-Jewish and anti-Nazi sentiments sprang from a genuine Christian conviction that had shaped their view of medicine for years and sometimes decades. Municipal staff doctors of Bayreuth were imprisoned by the SS in 1938 after being accused as obstinate Christians and Jew-lovers.[51] Dr. Otto Buchinger of Witzenhausen, a fervent Quaker, was repeatedly bothered by the party because he was suspiciously religious and deemed to be a crypto-Semite; at the height of the war, a jealous younger Nazi colleague plotted to take over the lucrative practice until, luckily for Buchinger, this man was found to be insane.[52] The Catholic doctor with three degrees Albert Niedermeyer, an Austrian gynecologist and strong defender of prenatal life, showed fortitude when he pronounced against the Nazi eugenic policy while still a practicing physician in Lusatian Görlitz. First, the local KVD revoked his medical license, then the Gestapo apprehended him. In 1938 he suffered a term in Sachsenhausen concentration camp; upon his release, he resumed his practice in Vienna, closely watched and constantly harassed.[53]

Many German doctors serving in the Wehrmacht were moved by the Hippocratic Oath, as well as by principles of religion and common decency, as if the stark horrors of the trenches were necessary to remind them once again of the essence of their calling.[54] The example of army physicians mending the self-inflicted wounds of would-be war shirkers and covering up for them later must be regarded as a form of political resistance against the dictatorship, inspired by the noblest of medical considerations.[55] Army medics, especially toward the end of the conflict in which many were losing faith, are known to have provided affidavits helping draftees to escape from the service or to prevent them from entering it.[56] The deeply religious Freiburg pathologist Franz Büchner influenced young military doctors home on furlough who craved his words of wisdom on the evils of "euthanasia," and, in so doing, openly took sides with the professor and against the regime.[57] Dr. Alois Hauer, an Austrian physician serving with the German occupation forces in Norway in 1942–43, was a prison inspector in charge of captured Norwegian patriots. He did what he could to rescue them from the SS physicians, inventing diseases such as diphtheria that would deliver them from the dreaded evacuation to Germany. He also supported his Norwegian captive colleagues in their bid to help their wretched fellows. "He saved the life and health of many" is the postwar verdict of Dr. Astrid Lange Ahlson, who knew him then, "and redeemed them from torture, suffering, and death—not without endangering himself."[58] And finally, overcome by compassion for the burghers of Regensburg, two Wehrmacht *Oberstabsärzte* on their own authority declared that city neutral territory for the approaching U.S. forces in early May 1945, lest any house-to-house combat would harm the population. But no sooner had they issued their courageous orders than they were strung up on flagpoles by fanatical Nazis who made them pay with their lives for such humanity.[59]

4. The Problem of Motivation Reconsidered

Against the background of such impressive evidence of physicians' anti-Nazi attitudes, why did the majority of German doctors array themselves politically with the Third Reich? Before probing more deeply the issue of motivations, it must be stressed once more that hardly ever was a single moral action or the lack thereof black or white but that, instead, various shades of gray predominated. If some human motives were completely altruistic, others were crassly self-interested, and others were a mixture of both, with the proportions often changing. This qualifying rule would appear to apply not only in the case of supporters of the regime, but also in that of the saboteurs, or those medical professionals who may have passed as such. Who was to know then and who is to utter final judgment now upon what actually went on in the minds of people at that time? As one observant contemporary poignantly remarked at the end of 1943, when the war was considered by many to be all but lost, physicians in the Third Reich may have had more freedom of movement and expression than other citizens because even the tyrants were clinging to them for dear life.[1] Hence any concern or unrest doctors may have expressed must today be evaluated with more scrutiny than the valor, for example, of schoolteachers, who, as salaried state servants and invested models of authority for younger generations, would have chanced a great deal more in the event of open tumult.[2] Nor must it be forgotten that much the German doctors said and did may look like acts of political resistance in our time when in reality, given their unique position, matters of professional status and peer privilege could have been at stake. If it is true that Dr. Fritz Gietzelt's 1944 execution was delayed because prominent Leipzig physicians protested as a group, they may have done so for humanitarian reasons as much as for the sake of a collective egotism: to safeguard their professional pride and sense of corporate solidarity.[3]

A corollary would hold true for those physicians who served or joined the Nazi movement in any conceivable capacity. Certainly, not a small number of them did so for idealistic, politically motivated reasons: Dr. Kurt Klare, the Hitler disciple of long standing who soon was on Gerhard Wagner's payroll, or that anonymous young physician who in fall 1933 found occasion to propagandize "Hitler and his tremendous movement" to colleagues in open letters of the party press.[4] Some listened to the regime's clarion call that doctors *must* be National Socialists and "leaders of their people" that was issued to them incessantly.[5] But for many, plain necessity was the mainspring for political action. Young doctors hoping to start out with a panel fund practice appeared to have little choice: in the wake of the novel KVD controls in 1933, they were driven to what may be termed an involuntary form of opportunism. For the KVD *required* every medical professional on its certification waiting lists to produce a spotless National Socialist record; registrants with Old Fighter laurels were to be given preference.[6]

Thus the cases of Dr. Herbert Volkmar and Dr. Hanna Donnerberg may stand for many others. Volkmar's candidacy for KVD installment was already filed with the Wiesbaden KVD chapter in November 1934 when an ailing older physician petitioned that Volkmar assume his fund practice. It was in Volkmar's favor that he had been an SA man since 1933 as well as a regular member of the NS-Ärztebund.[7] And a pristine Nazi reference was called for as late as 1938, when physicians were becoming scarce and were already being courted by the regime. Because the KVD divined that the forty-two-year-old Dr. Donnerberg of Rhenish Neuwied, previously a privately practicing professional, had shown insufficient commitment while attached to the Hitler Youth and had failed to make her mark "in any other affiliate of the party," she was rated politically unreliable and her KVD certification was withheld. Donnerberg appealed the decision claiming that she had been libeled, pointing to her excellent service record in the Nazi Women's League and the Labor Front, among other organizations. Her appeal was judged valid at higher KVD levels, after evidence showed the doctor to have been a faithful Nazi activist who had not, as charged, patronized Jewish stores as late as 1935. She was promptly instated.[8]

Moreover, in the early years of the regime, when many young doctors still were desperate for work, established Nazi practitioners would advertise full-time takeovers or part-time deputyships only for colleagues with a demonstrable party association.[9] The political factor was even more instrumental in the case of institutions such as municipal or private clinics seeking junior and senior staff.[10] Small wonder, then, if realistic job-hunters became expert at emphasizing their Nazi titles when they went soliciting for opportunities.[11] He wished to become a factory physician (*Betriebsarzt*), for the pay was not bad, wrote a neophyte doctor in November 1936. But would he be accepted, he wondered, because he lacked the preferred status of an Old Fighter of the movement.[12]

Doctors slated for employment by publicly administered institutions or by the government always had to endure an assiduous political screening that could take considerable time. Typical is the case of Dr. Hans Joachim Sewering, who was mentioned in the Introduction. Before he was to assume his posting as tuberculosis specialist in Schönbrunn in summer 1942, the Nazi Gauleitung, in accordance with requirements, was asked for a political bill of health. It responded that Sewering had joined the SS in 1933 and the NSDAP in 1934 and that he was currently on front-line duty. Still, the verdict was equivocal. "Nothing detrimental is known," it said in neat letter type, "objections exist neither on political nor on social grounds." The final comment was penciled in and potentially damaging: "Until now he has shown no interest in the local party chapter and hence in the Nazi movement." As we have seen, this doctor's career progress was not impeded.[13]

Ways were known of using personal connections beyond nominal memberships and token affidavits that smacked of careerism bordering on ruthlessness, and these were in keeping with the scarcely hidden system of spoils and corruption that was a major dynamic of Nazi rule.[14] Thus a gynecologist in Upper Bavarian Murnau did not hesitate to ask the local mayor for a lucrative hospital position because he was "a party comrade of many years."[15] But in another sense, these routines were reminiscent of channels of protection and influence characteristic of social structures more properly associated with pre-Nazi conventions, in particular the old-boy fraternity networks. This once again points up the curious marriage between reactionary interest-peddling and new political ambition, which bound, however tenuously, the traditional social elites to the new power brokers for the temporary expediency of both. Was Hans Pfundtner, secretary of state in the interior ministry and a confidant of Conti and Frick, not aware of this when he used his offices to curry favor on behalf of junior fraternity alumni, all physicians who were keen on quick advancement and promotion?[16]

There may, in fact, have existed several more dimensions to the political compromise of Third Reich physicians not easily interpreted today, for the pressures exerted by the Nazi movement were manifold, subtle, and complex, to the point of appearing not only confusing but paradoxical at times.[17] Amid general exhortations early in the regime for doctors to align themselves with the movement, what was one to make, for instance, of the public derision of Thuringian physicians by one of Wagner's functionaries, who exclaimed: "In the world of politics, it is easy to coordinate yourself. All you have to do is to exchange your black tuxedo for a brown shirt and the matter is settled!"[18] If patients in the party were broadly encouraged to patronize the doctors of their regional NS-Ärztebund chapter and if many doctors admittedly joined the NSDAP because "it meant good business," why were the movement's physicians still discriminated against at certain of the nation's clinics?[19] What of the post–World War II assurances of some that they approached the party "because all the others were joining, without inner commitment," and that of others that physicians were tricked into the movement with the bait of a party uniform but never the tenets of Nazism?[20] Was it not an anomaly that a known critic of the regime, upon attempting to leave the medical bureaucracy, was implored to enter the party as a guarantee of continuing employment, while another doctor, eager for NSDAP service and eventually in the pay of the police, was banned from the party's ranks because of his father's SPD past?[21] And did it fit together if some Nazi block warden pressured a doctor to sign up for the NSDAP when at the same time it was stressed that party members, after malpractice suits, would be more harshly dealt with than political abstainers?[22]

Even if the confusing pieces of this puzzle cannot be put together on these pages, a final, residual possibility must be considered. It would be that physicians entered the Nazi movement for the purpose of resisting the system from within: the classic "Trojan Horse" theme said to have been enacted several times in the course of the Third Reich, as it was by Wolfram Sievers and Kurt Gerstein in the SS. But Sievers was a liar, and Gerstein very probably was deluding himself; the potential for such premeditated spying-cum-sabotage in any regime apparatus after 1933 was always diminutive.[23] Not one doctor is known to have joined a Nazi organization for the express purpose of countermanding the dictatorship,[24] or even of exerting a moderating influence, notwithstanding any assertions to the contrary.[25] The case of chief Auschwitz physician Eduard Wirths, described so eloquently by Lifton, convincingly bears this out.[26]

Such legends have recently received new nourishment, at the risk of further distortions, by a widely publicized story of altruistic anti-Nazi acts at the hands of a nominal collaborator of the Hitler regime. Valentin Senger, a Jew who survived the Hitler era in his native Frankfurt, has told touchingly of Dr. Kurt Hanf-Dressler, the gastroenterologist practicing medicine while clad in his Storm Trooper uniform on Blittersdorfplatz, and how he overlooked the Jew's circumcision and helped him against abdominal cramps some months before the war.[27] Years later Senger claims to have discovered that the good doctor had used his rank in the "mounted SA" to help "any number of Jews," even assisting them in secret hideaways.[28] Hanf-Dressler may well have been a hero and aided Jews, and thus he must be counted among the intrepid men and women credited with having been what the Israelis call "righteous gentiles," but the part about the SA is patently fictitious: Hanf-Dressler's RÄK records show that he never joined any Nazi organization.[29]

Still the case of Hanf-Dressler demonstrates the plausibility that some physicians became wary after entry into the Nazi system and then did their best to wreck it. Again, however, the chaff must be separated from the wheat. Dr. L., for example, was a Rostock radiologist with a Jewish brother-in-law and preregime SPD connections. Joining the party in 1940, he constantly made derogatory remarks about the Third Reich, such as publicly criticizing the Führer's radio addresses. As a National Socialist, his peers judged him "cosmopolitan" as well as "unreliable."[30] Yet did the party see this man as a wolf in sheep's clothing? An unconventional Nazi pedigree and periodic bickering could hardly have placed him in a class with systematic, or even occasional, opponents of the regime.

Such resisters working from within the ranks did indeed exist, but it is impossible to ascertain whether they were intermittently entrapped by pangs of compassion or whether they fulfilled the function of double agents. The former is more likely. High-ranking health officials in Würzburg and in Hamburg refrained from reporting pro-Jewish colleagues and looked out for Social Democrats after their release from concentration camp captivity.[31] The physicians Kurt Gauger and Curt Thomalla carved out careers for themselves in propaganda media such as films, all the while remaining genuinely sympathetic to more critical colleagues; Gauger is said to have helped many of the persecuted.[32] Psychiatrist Dr. Karsten Jaspersen, a Nazi party member since 1931, developed moral qualms over "euthanasia" he was involved with and in 1940 intervened with Münster's bishop Graf von Galen and even Martin Bormann—to no avail.[33]

Some attempted even more, and at greater risk to their safety. The chronicle of their noble deeds spans virtually the entire course of the Third Reich. In 1933, when the Bavarian aristocrat Erwein von Aretin was detained in a Munich prison cell, Dr. Meixner, a young SS physician, copiously examined him and, with an appropriate certificate of illness, preserved him from the Dachau camp.[34] In August of that year a Nazi doctor complained about the ill treatment administered to a regime victim in the streets of Wuppertal, whereupon he himself was put away.[35] Dr. Werner Kirchert, adjutant to chief SS physician Ernst Robert Grawitz, removed himself from any potential implication in the "mercy-killing" programs that began in autumn 1939, after strongly stating his objections.[36] In the Flossenbürg concentration camp, Dr. Baader was known as the solitary humanitarian among the resident SS physicians because he evaded orders and prevented torture and murder until he managed to exchange his garrison duties for front-line service in summer 1940.[37] Lifton has told the incredible story of SS "Dr. B." (his real name was Wilhelm Münch, the only death camp doctor to be acquitted in postwar trials), who never participated in Auschwitz ramp selections for the gas chamber and tried to help the inmates as best he could.[38]

The tragic fate of a Pomeranian physicians' leader, details of which have recently surfaced, may attest to the decency of other regime-conformist German doctors who may have acted likewise but never lived to tell about it. The man in question had refused to dismiss a Jewish colleague from his hospital. This Nazi doctor was charged in a party court and subsequently lost his position, and the Jew committed suicide to thwart his impending deportation. Later, during the war, the benefactor perished in an air raid.[39]

Chapter 3

The Dilemma of Women Physicians

1. Demographic Trends and Tendencies

From 1933 to 1945 the proportion of women among German physicians grew remarkably, continuing a trend that had started before the Weimar Republic, as soon as women were allowed to become certified medical doctors.[1] In 1907, just over 0.5 percent of all German doctors were women; they had graduated in countries other than Germany, which opened medical examinations to women only a year later. This percentage rose to over 5 by 1925, and because male doctors despised as well as feared competition from women, their professional lobbies introduced a 5 percent limit for women seeking licensure by the end of the republic.[2] But this closure affected only the early years of medical school, and so the cumulative percentage of female physicians increased from 6.5 in 1932 to 7.9 in 1937. That figure climbed to 9.8 percent in 1939 and 12.4 percent in 1942.[3] It is still not certain what the percentage of women doctors was in 1944–45, but among all doctors registered with the Reich Physicians' Chamber from 1936 until the end of the regime, women made up about 17 percent.[4]

Toward the end of the war, a leading Physicians' Chamber functionary estimated that with very few exceptions, "every certified female doctor" was tied into the national health delivery system.[5] This had not always been so because, as will be seen in greater detail later, many of the women doctors did not choose to practice medicine until they were urgently required to do so during the war. Thus of the 17 percent mentioned above, not all may have been active. And if only 17.4 percent of all women doctors who registered after 1935 enjoyed the security of a panel practice (as opposed to 45.1 percent of all male doctors so registered), the remaining 82.6 percent of the women were either professionally engaged or idle. The unique position of female doctors is further highlighted if one considers that none of the 44.9 percent of male doctors who were not in panel practice can be presumed to have been idle.[6]

Table 3.1, constructed on the basis of one of the two extant RÄK samples, shows that among the female physicians registered with the Reich Physicians' Chamber between 1936 and 1945 those who had been licensed before or during 1918 constituted almost 5 percent of the doctors inaugurated at that time. Although the frequency of licensures for women relative to those for the men increased during the Weimar Republic, it is clear that a high proportion of the women did not actually practice medicine but instead remained at home, usually as the wife of a breadwinner, most likely a medical one. This holds true for the first half of the Third Reich as well, but not for the second half, when more than one-quarter of all young doctors who were then licensed were female. In the early 1940s, because of the exigencies of war, for every twenty-six women who graduated there were seventy-four men who did so and almost certainly joined the work force immediately.[7]

In 1939, a leading woman physician wrote: "For most female doctors the accessibility of panel practice is, for reasons of economics, of decisive importance."[8] But significantly, those female medical graduates who did enter the profession were always given less of a chance than the men to establish themselves on their own. Having been on an almost equal footing before the Weimar Republic (because in that phase they were still a curiosity, and their male colleagues needed time to develop effective arguments against them), the women fresh out of medical school faced heavy obstacles during the 1920s. This tendency continued on into the Third Reich, when, as Table 3.2 makes clear, a young male colleague had almost twice the chance to establish himself in panel practice as did his female counterpart.[9] Typical is the case of general practitioner Dr. Margot Gressler, involuntarily co-opted by the KVD just before the war, who in March 1939 wanted to found her own practice in Thuringian Ohrdruf. Her claim that this town of some eight thousand was badly in need of a female generalist because there already were three male practitioners was rejected by the panel admission boards, thus perpetuating Dr. Gressler's employee status.[10]

This antifeminist discrimination can be illuminated for the entire Nazi period with the help of absolute figures. If 21.8 percent of all women physicians had been in some dependent employment by 1932, that figure rose to 24.1 percent in 1935 and to 41.4 percent in 1939. By 1942 54.6 percent of all women doctors were salaried.[11] In that year, 5,146 such women doctors were counted. Of those, 3,453 worked in hospitals and clinics, and about 700 were auxiliary panel doctors deployed by the KVD.[12] The rest might have held jobs in industry (pharmaceutics), in party agencies such as the NSV, or be contracted as shop physicians (*Betriebsärztinnen*) in factories.[13] Self-reliant female practitioners with their own offices could consider themselves fortunate in that a September 1941 plan to exchange them for male assistant physicians from the nation's hospitals was never implemented.[14]

As women doctors were obviously disadvantaged in their quest for professional (and economic) independence, they were also hampered in their attempts at specialism. But to the extent that female physicians collectively were becoming more acceptable over time, the degree to which specialization hindered a woman's career was getting smaller. Of the female physicians registered as specialists in 1936 and after, the group that graduated before 1918 had constituted 5 percent vis-à-vis 95 percent for the men. That percentage rose steadily during republican times, until in the first six years of the Third Reich 19 percent of all specialists were women (Table 3.3).[15] By contrast, female generalists proliferated much more visibly: their percentages compared to those of men increased from 4.6 to over 27 in the same time span and by the same terms of accounting (Table 3.4).[16] But because women physicians abrogated their profession after licensure much more frequently than did men, the number of female doctors actually practicing was much lower. Hence women specialists with a money-earning job constituted merely 5.5 percent of all specialists in January 1937 and 5.6 percent a year later.[17]

Moreover, even though the ratio between generalists and specialists among the women doctors, as among the male ones, was about two to one,[18] the women still were largely relegated to sex-specific areas of endeavor. But here, too, a gradual change was discernible. Pediatrics, which was by far the most popular specialty with women doctors and was expressly conceded to women by Nazi propaganda,[19] was being displaced after 1932 by some less "feminine" areas: its frequency index declined from 45.7 percent in 1930 to 44.1 in 1932, 43.3 in 1935, and 42.4 in 1937. Throughout 1938 only twenty-six women, 37.1 percent of the total of female novice specialists, became pediatricians. Of course, they still made up 42.6 percent of all the pediatricians.[20]

After pediatrics, gynecology, another sex-specific specialty, was very popular with women doctors, even though their proportion in it, too, declined from 14.5 percent in 1930 to 14.0 percent in 1937.[21] Gynecology had been popularized for German women by Dr. Agnes Bluhm, who was among the first three female physicians to establish an office in Berlin, in 1890, after graduating with a medical degree from Zurich. Early in her career Bluhm turned to eugenic dogma as it was being preached at the time by Alfred Ploetz and later by his student Fritz Lenz. She tied gynecological and obstetrical issues to a vulgarized Social Darwinism, which, to the Nazis, legitimized gynecology as a "natural" specialty for women.[22]

Women doctors participated in other specialties to a noticeably larger extent than they had before the Third Reich—internism, otology, ophthalmology, and dermatology. This and the emergence for the first time in 1937 of female experts in orthopedics and particularly in urology conveyed the impression that women doctors had successfully infiltrated formerly traditional preserves of male doctors.[23] There were even a few aspiring female university lecturers before the war who excelled in one specialty or another.[24] Yet though this pattern may have signified slight progress for female medical professionals in the ten-year period from 1930 to 1939, it was overshadowed by the decline in the proportion of women in men's most hallowed specialty, surgery, from 2.0 percent in 1930 to 1.6 in 1937.[25]

This decline reflected the peculiarly *völkisch* assumption that surgery called for and represented the essential qualities of German masculinity,[26] and it served as the final criterion in an overall judgment of female physicians in Nazi Germany. Women could no more be surgeons than physicians in chief, wrote Dr.

Roderich von Ungern-Sternberg, and such was the consensus in the medical faculties.[27] Women physicians, even those who in principle would recommend a female doctor to a female patient, appeared to agree, as did the otherwise contrary Mathilde Kelchner.[28] In the Third Reich, women may have elected branches of surgery requiring little or no physical strength, such as plastic restorative work, but how many women went into that as opposed to men is still in need of further exploration.[29]

The careers of female specialists would differ, typically, according to the period in which they were licensed. Because of the growing trend toward third-party employment, it was generally easier to found a specialist's practice, supported by membership in the panel fund system, before the outbreak of World War II than after. Bertha Essig, who was born in 1894, established herself as a generalist in 1932 and as a pediatrician three and a half years later. Her colleague Charlotte Geisler, however, sixteen years her junior and certified as a pediatrician in 1943, never had a chance for independent practice or for panel insurance status: upon licensure in Munich she was retained as an "auxiliary assistant" (*Aushilfs-Assistenzarzt*) at the Schwabinger Krankenhaus.[30] Similar to the case of Essig was that of Susanne Bergk, born in 1904 and set up as a general practitioner in 1937. After 1935, she was also a neurologist. The careers of Edith Wermter and Gertrud Daniel, a respirologist and internist, were more like Geisler's. Wermter was born in 1909, received approbation to treat lung disorders in 1940, and thereafter was assistant physician in an East Prussian institution for tubercular children. Daniel, who was a year older, was licensed in internism only in 1944 and subsequently could do no more than deputize as *Oberärztin* in a Munich private clinic.[31] Neither Wermter nor Daniel served as a model for female doctors who looked to the ultimate in professional emancipation.

2. Marriage, Motherhood, and Militancy

From its very beginnings, *völkisch* dogma, later elevated to official National Socialist ideology, had always taught that, rather than attend university and establish themselves in some academic profession, German women should marry, stay at home, and have children. Double-earner status (*Doppelverdienertum*) among married couples, with both the professional husband and his occupation-bound wife leaving the home to make a daily living, was particularly frowned upon.[1]

To the extent that the Nazi health administration ever systematically discouraged women from practicing medicine, it was the married ones who would be targeted first. In the first year of the regime, whenever young doctors were wanted for positions in a hospital, it was made clear that male ones were preferred and that unmarried ones would have priority. Such a policy discriminated heavily against married female physicians.[2] From 1930 to 1937 the proportion of nonpracticing female doctors climbed from 4.8 percent of all women doctors to 17 percent, and in 1939 to 25.7 percent, and almost all of these were married women.[3] Yet two important considerations qualify these statistics. The pre-1936 percentage figures were higher than printed in the sources, for before the establishment of Reichsärztekammer in that year nonpracticing women physicians were not required to register with any agency. The percentage values published for 1933–35 also reflect Jewish physicians who, contemporaneously, were forced to retire from their jobs.[4] In 1939, just before the war, of all the married female doctors in the Reich, just over half were not working gainfully.[5] But as early as 1938, when even unmarried female doctors had difficulty finding a panel practice, especially in competition with married male colleagues,[6] this trend was beginning to reverse. The combination of an ongoing rejection of Jews and a war-bound economy that was responsible for an increasing shortage of doctors in the Reich caused even married women physicians to be recalled to clinics and medical offices, albeit in positions subordinate to men.[7] From 1939 to 1942 the proportion of female physicians intermittently or permanently out of work decreased from 25.7 to 22.0 percent.[8]

Before this trend took root, however, married female doctors had to endure the humiliation of being, at least formally, struck from the roster of established panel physicians in the Reich. This occurred in the course of a precipitate campaign against women inaugurated by Nazi physicians' leader Gerhard Wagner, who in December 1933 publicly declared the NSDAP's intention to rid the nation gradually of all female doctors by curtailing university (medical) training for women, and then, in January of the following year, barred those married women doctors from the panel registries who did not depend on a separate income to safeguard the economic well-being of their families.[9] Yet for various reasons, including a strong protest by the women physicians' spokesperson Dr. Lea Thimm and a decline in the oversaturation of the medical profession, few married women doctors actually suffered in the end. Altogether only about 115 of them were excluded by Wagner's order, and by 1939 the ban, though officially still on the books, was merely theoretical.[10]

One of the chief arguments employed by the misogynist male physicians against their female colleagues was that professional work would prevent married doctors from fulfilling the ultimate National Socialist goal of bearing and raising an appropriate number of children. Dr. Friedrich Bartels, the former ruffian Freikorps warrior who eventually was to become Wagner's deputy as Reich physicians' leader, in 1933 argued that though he might concede that practicing female physicians performed a social service function, it was imperative to "reintegrate the married woman, the working mother, into the family."[11] His compatriot Carl Haedenkamp, equally male-centered, held a year later that conjugally committed female physicians should "devote themselves to their duties as women and mothers and should leave the battle for survival to their men."[12] And in 1938–39 Dr. Gerd Hegemann of the University of Münster demonstrated that female physicians tended to marry much later in life than other women, hence shortening their period of fertility, and that, consequently, the number of children to be expected from them on average was "unsatisfactory." Hegemann was emphatically seconded by gynecologist Professor Ernst Bach, the highest medical official in the Reich education ministry.[13] But in their eagerness to push their women colleagues against the wall, the male doctors argued unfairly. In 1933 Dr. Charlotte Graetz-Menzel of the Hygienics Institute at Munich University had shown, in a scholarly disquisition, that in a scientific sample of Weimar republican women physicians 41.2 percent of the married ones had remained childless.[14] Some two years later, Dr. Julius Hadrich, of Gerhard Wagner's staff, turned this figure against female doctors by stating that Dr. "Grisetz-Menzel" had proved that a large number of them were not mothers.[15] Had Hadrich intended to support the married women doctors, he could have cited a statistic of 1933, according to which 46.4 percent of all married Berlin women then in the work force were without children, a considerably higher proportion than of the female doctors.[16] Indeed, figures published in early 1936 by the German women's journal *Die Frau* indicated that 70 percent of all married female doctors were mothers.[17] During the war, when female doctors knew they were needed, those who were married made a special point of publicly announcing the birth of each new child.[18]

Using reason, women physicians, whether married or not and regardless of the number of children they tended, further defended the existence of women professionals in medicine against the encumbrance of the male-dominated medical establishment in several ways. In literary polemics, three lines of argument were pursued with varying degrees of consistency: (1) the submissive motherhood argument, (2) the neutral sexual parity argument, and (3) the militant antimasculine argument. The advocates of these positions were women doctors who were, at the same time, subordinate functionaries in various Nazi welfare and social service organizations, including of course medical ones.

The motherhood line of reasoning capitalized on the specifically Nazi axiom that maternity was the quintessence of womanhood in German society.[19] Thus Erna Orlopp-Pleick, a married gynecologist born in 1894 who served as an advisory physician in the League of German Girls (BDM), explained in 1936 that as director of the League of German Women Physicians in East Prussia she had made certain, as early as November 1933, to delegate a number of female doctors to the Reich Mothers' Service of the German Women's Front (Deutsches Frauenwerk), for it was here "that we realized special needs for women doctors to look after."[20] Erna Röpke, who was not a physician but section leader in the Reich Mothers' Service, applauded her by reminding a Berlin assembly of female doctors in the same year that the training and schooling of mothers in the Third Reich was the specific task of *married* medical women.[21] Not twelve months later, those sentiments were echoed by Ursula Romann, a Berlin student of medicine who held a post in the Reich student leadership and was soon to marry.[22] Edith von Lölhöffel, a sports physician who had given birth to four children, summed it up in 1939: "Among all academic professions for women that of the female physician is the most feminine and the most motherlike. These tasks, which any woman has to solve in the midst of her family at home, are the very same ones a woman doctor must deal with in the great people's community."[23] Because the issue had become of secondary importance by then, representatives of the women physicians in the Reich maintained this stance somewhat less enthusiastically during the war.[24]

The sexual parity idea was somewhat more audacious than the motherhood argument. It fed on the notion that if, according to Nazi ideology, women were indeed different from men, then their special disposition called for sex-specific medical care. Hence, if women were more emotional, intuitive, and spiritual than men, only the intuitive female doctor could understand and treat them. Dr. Mathilde Kelchner, a staunch protagonist of women's causes who had joined the party as a sixty-year-old matron in 1932, in a meticulous treatise of 1934 was careful to draw a fine line between male and female physicians, with each of the two groups attending to its own clientele, naturally delimited by gender. Her attitude was nurtured by a strong emancipationist ambition. The female physician is not "a copy of the male physician," wrote Kelchner brashly, "but rather, she is able to put her own particular imprint on medical practice." Women patients would prefer women doctors in many situations, especially gynecological ones, in which they felt uncomfortable in the presence of a man; this, then, would serve to define the work sphere of the woman doctor.[25]

In 1934, Kelchner's views formed the basis for further musings in the circle of women physicians bent on equity with their male colleagues.[26] Two years later, in 1936, Kelchner summarized her thesis in the pages of *Die Ärztin*, the publicity organ of the female physicians and to a large extent a forum of emancipatory thought.[27] By that time, too, Agnes Bluhm, that venerated senior figure among Germany's medical women, expounded on this theme, albeit strictly within a *völkisch* framework, so that the leaders of the medical establishment could not help but notice that a potentially dangerous movement was afoot. In October 1936 the KVD, in what was probably intended as a Solomonic decision, established that male patients were no more entitled to treatment by male doctors than were female patients by female doctors.[28] Although this dictum could be interpreted to read that women physicians were free to treat patients of both sexes just like their men colleagues, it was not the privilege these sex-consciously determined women professionals were seeking.

In a phase when other female professionals in the Third Reich were being squarely put in their places by the male rulers,[29] this directive ended one variant of liberationism from the women doctors' camp. A decidedly radical belief was that male "exemplars" counted for nothing and should be ignored. Women doctors who subscribed to such militancy rejected the traditional male tenet that because women were physically inferior to men (and their brains were smaller and lighter), they were not fit to be elevated to the same professional levels as the males.[30] This point was seized upon by Dr. Lizzie Hoffa, a functionary of the German Women Physicians' League, who insisted in 1933 that because women mastered both child education and housework they were the equals of men in coping physically with a doctor's chores.[31] In 1934 Dr. Lea Thimm, who was fighting Wagner's obstinate misogyny in restricting panel practice, denounced the spiteful envy of young male doctors who had been seen to be the favorites of the older colleagues who dominated the panel admission boards. According to Clifford Kirkpatrick, that shrewd foreign contemporary observer of women under Hitler, Thimm complained openly that a jealous man doctor "once threatened a woman doctor with a concentration camp if she did not give up her practice."[32]

By 1936, young aspiring sister professionals had moved even further, although for female emancipationists of any age time was running short. For a woman to attempt to adapt to a male's way of thinking and work was a mistake often committed in the past, spokeswomen of female medical students from all over the Reich proclaimed. It would have been far better for a woman to expose the essence of her differences from males and render it productive. At the same time, all that talk about a woman's mission toward "spiritual motherhood" was gibberish. Medical women should marry if they wished and then mobilize on behalf of the German people in multiple capacities, with a natural emphasis on preventive, curative, and social services.[33]

But all these considerations, important as they were for the fate of individual women doctors since the beginning of the Third Reich, were rendered meaningless before the war because the health administration became ever more dependent on qualified physicians regardless of gender. After the decrees of the Reich ministers of the interior and labor in early September 1939,[34] female doctors, who might not have wished to practice medicine unless they had their own offices, were ever more frequently requisitioned by the agencies of the Reich health leader.[35] Hence in January 1941 Leonardo Conti was pleased to acknowledge "the performance of women who had jumped into the brink despite family obligations."[36]

In the following months the problems with female labor in the Reich were becoming more acute. In particular, it was noticed that women of the more well-off classes hesitated to integrate themselves into the war economy, so that Goebbels, who favored compulsory female labor conscription over the Führer's scruples, exclaimed in frustration, "Our fine ladies will not come voluntarily."[37] In the medical sector this meant that since young male medical graduates were immediately being sent to the military fronts, the health administration came to rely almost exclusively on young, inexperienced female physicians to staff its hospitals and auxiliary practice positions at home.[38] Family status now had largely ceased to be an issue. Anne-Liese Schwang from Danzig-Oliva, for example, was twenty-four years old and single when she was licensed in March 1940. She was immediately drafted to serve as an assistant doctor at Gotenhafen's municipal hospital. Her colleague Gertrud Wohlfeil was twenty-eight and married upon licensure in 1941. She was co-opted for duty in a private sanatorium on the fringe of the Black Forest.[39]

During 1942, incentives and all manner of coercion were intensified to ensure that not merely the neophyte female doctors but also previously retired ones entered the medical network. On one hand, the Reich health leadership removed certain formal impediments to coax a larger number of female physicians into state-supported *Amtsarzt* careers. On the other, public opinion was beginning to exert pressure on the authorities to force more women, not excluding the married ones, back into the health care system.[40] But even in 1943 the situation of women physicians in the Reich still was sadly paradoxical in that they were in great demand and moved about the German landscape by Conti's administrators at will, while at the same time being despised by the bigoted party troglodytes because they could not stand the women's urbanity, as manifested in their "painted faces and their colored fingernails."[41]

In 1944, finally, the Reich health leadership went after senior medical students as well as mothers with children. An ordinance of April stipulated that women physicians who had children could not be compelled but should be encouraged to accept medical employment of some form, even if it was part time. But two months later this was qualified to read that only mothers with children under the age of fifteen could be exempt from service, pending further notice, and that those mothers who had managed some modus vivendi even with younger children should be conscripted.[42] This was the time that Dr. Jacoba Hahn, wife of Hamburg general practitioner Dr. Gustav Heinrich Hahn, who had just died of despondency, and the mother of a preteenage son, felt prevailed upon to resume her profession, as an assistant physician in the state hospital of Neustadt in Holstein.[43] By the fall, as young girls about to graduate as physicians were being allocated for medical service by Conti's men, it was suggested in Bavarian medical circles that women physicians with children, no matter what their age, should be seriously considered for public health care deployment. "It is self-evident that from now on those women physicians must come forth and serve whose domestic burden is a light one. That which women in the armaments industry and in the rest of the work force are called upon to do, namely to entrust the care of their household and their children to others, today may also be expected of medical women with children. Nor will it always be possible to allow those women to become professionally active in their place of residence. A separation from the family simply cannot be avoided in each and every case."[44] Indeed, some four months before the Hitler regime came to its ignominious end, women physicians with very small children were made subject to conscription anywhere in the Reich, provided the toddlers were looked after in some fashion.[45] Whatever gratification some female doctors may have derived from this regulation, it turned out to be a strange compromise between the apodictic notions of early unbending Nazis on womanhood and the liberationist ideals of the most formidable female doctors.

3. University Students

The fluctuations in the enrollment of female medical students from 1933 to 1945 to a large extent reflect the variations of National Socialist doctrine and practice on the role of German women in general and that of women doctors in particular, but they also contributed to them. Even though closure against new women medical students had been introduced in 1930, the cumulative percentage of women of all semesters registered in medicine vis-à-vis men had reached an unprecedented high of just over 20 percent in the summer of 1933. It was only then that the incessant propaganda against women students by pre–Third Reich misogynists, now carried over into the new regime by the Nazis, was taking hold, for after 1933, when some professors made a point of ignoring their presence, the number of female medical students steadily declined, reaching a nadir of 15.9 percent in the spring semester of 1939.[1] Naturally, those percentage figures varied according to locale. At the Reich level, during summer 1937, 17.9 percent of all medical students were women, yet in Würzburg University, in a small town and therefore more susceptible to Nazi controls, this figure reached only 17.1 percent.[2]

But this phenomenon, seemingly a deterioration in the state of women medical students over time, has to be carefully qualified. In the first place, it does not appear to bear out Gerhard Wagner's intention of December 1933 to eliminate medical studies for women altogether.[3] For if from summer 1933 to summer 1934 the percentage of female medical students decreased from 20.2 to 19.1, possibly signaling a short-term effect of Wagner's militant announcement, it was up to 19.3 in the following summer.[4] Indeed, the officially positive attitude toward women physicians by 1938 or so was already being foreshadowed in university circles in 1935, as student self-government leaders were prepared to subscribe to the principle of financial support for young medical women in training, who were said to be just as indispensable in the future as women teachers.[5] Second, because medicine, as a curative and service-oriented discipline, was considered to be more "feminine" than others such as law or physics, the pre–Third Reich trend among girls graduating from high school to favor medical studies at the university rather than something else continued forcefully for the time being. As a matter of fact, under Hitler medicine augmented its share of women students compared to other disciplines by 12.4 percent until 1939, and medical studies became the most popular course for women, surpassing the humanities, traditionally in first place.[6]

In the total of university enrollment, the rate of overrepresentation of women in medicine increased by half a percentage point between summer 1928 and summer 1938, whereas in the same decade women's underrepresentation in law expanded by 2.3 percentage points.[7]

Several new factors regarding the proportions of female medical students came into play during the war, mirroring conditions in the medical profession but also influencing them. The required presence of male students at the fronts translated into almost a tripling of the corresponding percentage of female students at institutions of higher learning, from 11.5 percent in summer 1938 to 27.0 percent in spring of 1941.[8] Although an increase of women medical students vis-à-vis male ones was embedded in this general process, female medical students, though obviously important, lost their subjective exclusivity because of the recent Nazi administration policy to admit a greater number of women to disciplines from which they had formerly been discouraged. Physics and law were cases in point; both were expressly mentioned even before the war as areas of fruitful activity for the academically trained German woman.[9] And although medicine, along with teaching, still had not lost its place on the Nazi roster of most desirable occupations for academic women, the new emphasis on law, for instance,[10] probably caused many a bright, emancipation-bound young German woman to seize this opportunity for self-realization and professional advancement, at the expense of medicine.

Hence a paradoxical situation developed in that Conti and his bureaucrats were beckoning girls to enter the medical faculties and urging them to become doctors, at the same time that conflicting economic and professional needs resulting from the overall war effort were reducing the previous monopoly of medicine on women.[11] It is true that in the winter semester of 1943–44 the percentage of women medical students compared to males had climbed to 33.8, up from 16.6 some five years before, but simultaneously the ratio of these women to those enrolled in other disciplines such as law had changed to render medicine somewhat less significant. At the end of the regime women medical students were underrepresented in the total of disciplines in which women enrolled at German universities by a rate of 18.5 percent.[12]

Because these young medical women were in such great demand at the height of the national struggle, the quality of their instruction came to suffer just as much as their actual performance on the job. Insofar as the same was true for the whole of the medical student body,[13] it is possible that the standard for women students sank even lower than the one for men, chiefly for two reasons. One was contingent on the new National Socialist practice of depriving girls of Latin instruction in the upper schools. But since Latin was still required as part of the medical curriculum, female students in the medical faculties had to study this classical language on the side if they were to pass the qualifying examination. This not only led to a much higher dropout rate for female medicine students than for male ones before final examinations, but it also meant that those women students who managed to pass the Latin and the medical tests were likely to do poorly in both, making their expertise questionable later on.[14]

Yet another decline in quality is suggested by the statistical datum that during the war women medical students at graduation averaged twenty-six years of age, one year younger than their male cohorts.[15] Whereas for the men this marks no change from the 1933–38 period, the women had, in that same period, been twenty-seven as well, leaving them one year of medical instruction short in wartime.[16] One may infer that in the war years the men received a comparatively better medical education simply by default because many of them, dreading active service at the fronts, sought to stay in the medical schools as long as possible, using ruses such as dodging examinations, until inescapable deadlines were prescribed by the Reich education ministry in summer 1943.[17] Conversely, women may always have been under pressure to finish their studies quickly and join the work force—until at the end of 1944 they were provisionally deployed as doctors even before having taken their final examination.[18] What all this amounts to is that if a certain latitude was granted to male students but withheld from female ones, to the professional detriment of the latter, this would serve as yet another example of unequal treatment of the sexes in the vocation of medicine, inspired by the utilitarian cynicism of the Reich health administration in its reluctant tolerance of women colleagues.

But the female medical students of the Third Reich differed from their male cohorts in other respects. One was social origin and, interdependently, economic status. Unfortunately, accurate records regarding the social makeup of medical students under Hitler, divided by gender, are not known to exist. With the exception of a special sample, we have recourse only to statistics for female students on one side, or medical students on the other, but not to a combination of both. The special sample is one of needy students who sought out financial assistance in the form of loans from the authorities; its usefulness for sociohistorical purposes is more fully discussed in Chapter 5. But it can briefly be stated here that the sample is heavily skewed toward the lower middle and lower classes, at the expense of the social elite. Inferences to be drawn from it, including those regarding the relationship between sex and class of medical students, therefore have to be treated with the greatest caution.

As incomplete as the available data are, the following conservative judgments may, after careful analysis, be rendered: (1) In the Weimar Republic, a rising number of university students tended to hail from the lower middle class, at the expense of the upper middle class or social elite (upper middle class increasingly including the old aristocracy) that had formerly monopolized higher education.[19] (2) This trend continued into the Third Reich (Table 3.5).[20] (3) Since the early days of the republic, female students tended to be upper middle class rather than lower middle class because during years of general financial uncertainty university studies were considered a luxury for girls that could best be afforded by the well-endowed members of society. This held true particularly during the Great Depression, whose tail end coincided with Hitler's ascension to power. In the Third Reich, not least because of the lingering opposition to education for women that characterized its beginning phase, the tendency for women students to be upper middle class persisted.[21] (4) Although in the Weimar Republic medical studies were becoming much more of a vehicle for upward mobility for male and female members of the lower middle class than was any other discipline, upper-middle-class women were more likely to be found in medicine than were upper-middle-class men. This phenomenon extended into the Third Reich.[22] And finally (5), at least in the case of the students seeking loans for which we have data, there are interesting differences in the treatment by parents with certain lower- and upper-middle-class occupations of their sons and daughters. White-collar worker fathers, perhaps for reasons of social mobility, were inclined to send daughters rather than sons to medical school, as did fathers belonging to the nonacademic professions (or perhaps those daughters went on their own accord?). Within the elite social class, higher civil servants seem to have been the most eager to follow this pattern, whereas farmers, in the lower middle class, appear to have had the least use for a daughter in medical school, as opposed to a son.[23]

In the absence of better records and within its given limits, the loan-student sample is useful for gaining insights into yet another set of differences between male and female medical students: attitudes toward Nazi politics. Even granting that loan students were under greater pressure than other students to join any of the extant Nazi organizations because they needed money from the regime,[24] it seems remarkable that some students still thought it possible to abstain from politics altogether, which would indicate less than rigorous controls for the entire student population (Table 3.6, column A). In any event, the data suggest that female medical students were three times more likely than male ones to remain aloof from Nazi politics, but also that they were somewhat more likely to abstain politically than were young women enrolled in the sum total of the disciplines.[25] Moreover, it is clear that university women studying medicine were rather less active in Nazi political organizations than men.[26] But there was no difference between female and male medical students with regard to the age at which they customarily joined a Nazi group: the members of both genders were twenty-two on average.[27]

Female and male medical students also differed in the type of Nazi organization they felt attracted to. In this case choice could have been restricted by sex-specific factors, and, as befitted a male-oriented dictatorship, women would have been more restricted than men. Hence only males could join the SA, the SS, or the National Socialist Motor Corps (NSKK). And while 35.6 percent of all politically active male medical students opted for the Brown Shirts, which was the most popular Nazi unit for them, the medical women chose membership in the

Nazi Student League (in their particular case it was ANSt, the female branch of the NSDStB) as their preferred organization (Table 3.7). In joining the NSDStB, the women were ahead of the men by a factor of three to one, but they were still below the total of female university students, of whom approximately half joined the Student League.[28] As in the case of graduated female physicians, who will be discussed below, female doctors in training were much less likely to swell the ranks of the NSDAP than were their male cohorts, who flocked to the Nazi party proper at a rate almost double that of the women. Yet female medical students who joined the NSDAP appear to have liked it better than did female students from all the disciplines combined.[29] Not surprisingly, female medical students tended to be drawn to service-oriented organizations like Hitler Youth and the Nazi women's groups; in the former they outnumbered the men by three to one in total political affiliation, and in the latter they were unto themselves.[30]

Indeed, the ANSt branch of the Nazi Student League, the League of German Girls (BDM) in the Hitler Youth (HJ), and the various women's organizations were all charity, care, and service-related. ANSt funneled medical students into *Kliniker-Fachschaften* or medical training units that were quasi-extracurricular and commonly led to voluntary health care work outside the medical faculties, as well as to optional training camps or lecture courses.[31] The BDM was eternally in need of medical students to instruct the younger girls in hygiene and general health care, to act as orderlies in youth camps, and to assist female physicians in physical checkups. It, too, channeled prospective women doctors into adult organizations such as the Nazi welfare institution NSV, short of recruiting its very own neophyte BDM physicians.[32] As early as summer 1939, in the course of intensified mobilization, the Reich authorities recognized this need by making unpaid service in the health units of the Hitler Youth (BDM) obligatory for every female medical student, unless she wished to work at Red Cross facilities. Despite their busy schedules in wartime, this order for women medical students remained on the books until the very end of the global conflict.[33] Membership in adult women's organizations such as NSV or NS-Frauenschaft (NSF) for female doctors in training entailed after-hours chores such as assisting mothers and their small children, dispensing free dietetic advice, and making oneself useful in recreational institutions of the National Socialist welfare network.[34]

Female medical students, like their male counterparts, were concentrated in *Medizinische Fachschaften*, or medical work units that were organized by the Nazi-dominated student self-governments and superimposed on the regular medical faculty structures. *Fachschaften*, originally extracurricular yet not extrauniversity, were activated in all the university departments "for the spread of National Socialist propaganda" and "to put a Nazi slant on scholarship," but they also possessed purely social functions, if only to attract a modicum of students.[35] Work in these medical study units was once again sex-specific. For the women, it was designed to condition them for welfare and service applications, as well as for properly defined tasks in mobilization and war, so as to discourage them from any conception of leadership such as heroic young male doctors were supposed to embrace.

The most common service within the *Fachschaften* was nursing and caring for the sick in hospitals, either during the semesters or on holidays.[36] Other activities included welfare service, as in Heidelberg, and pregnant women's or young mothers' training, as in Würzburg.[37] Ever and again, the women doctors in training were summoned to special camps organized by the *Fachschaften*, often in conjunction with ANSt and other Nazi women's groups, to safeguard their development as National Socialist health care cadres.[38] Mobilization demands were fulfilled as early as 1935 when special air raid schooling for women physicians was devised.[39]

Reportedly, the women students tried to escape from tasks they viewed as useless and time-consuming, keeping them from essential work in the laboratories and lecture halls for which they would receive proper academic credit. Nonpolitically minded medicine instructors, too, were becoming worried about their students' scholastic progress. In time, the young women were dodging *Fachschaft* obligations in Freiburg no less than in Cologne, and in Würzburg, where not even half of all the enrolled young female clinicians showed interest in *Fachschaft* activity in winter 1937–38, the number of events initially scheduled had to be scaled down.[40]

The original designation of *Fachschaft* work as "voluntary," holding out few rewards for any but the most craven devotees,[41] soon resulted in such an embarrassment to the regime that its leaders were impelled to make parts of the program compulsory. Significantly, it was the paramilitary portion dealing with training to protect against air raids, later extended to the treatment of disorders inflicted by combat chemicals (*Kampfstoffe*), which introduced partial *Fachschaft* membership obligation by making eligibility for medical examinations dependent on attendance in study-unit courses.[42] Somewhat more popular were hospital training courses because such experience was valuable by traditional standards and it counted toward academic credit in university examinations.[43] But on the brink of war, as the Reich student leadership had left no doubt about the primary ideological purpose of the medical *Fachschaften*—they were to be platforms for later incorporation in the Nazi Physicians' League—the young medical women were found grumbling. From the University of Breslau the Security Service of the SS alleged in November 1939 that *Fachschaft* leaders were considering expelling female medical students who, through irreverent behavior, had disgraced themselves in public.[44]

By that time, other, additional obligations had further complicated the life of these students. ANSt and *Fachschaften* imposed on them to ensure their entrance into race-political schooling camps, and some of them actually held unpaid part-time jobs in the party's Rassenpolitisches Amt, directed by Nazi fanatic Dr.

Walter Gross.[45] In the annual Reich vocational contests, female medical students were called upon to be represented with strenuously composed entries, and in the 1937–38 competition, one of their teams, from Würzburg, actually emerged victorious, after handing in a report on the physical condition of babies and toddlers in the mountainous Rhön region.[46]

As soon as the war was on, the regime was able to draw distinct benefits from such peacetime regimentation, for now the mobilization of female medical students began on a hitherto unprecedented scale, while *Fachschaft* and ANSt work receded into the background. A complicated system of mandatory services now forced female students to devote even less time to classroom studies and more to extracurricular tasks. Hospital service recruited every one of them for a period of three months per year, from 1940 on.[47] After summer 1941, upper-school graduates wishing to study medicine had to perform orderly duties in a hospital for six months before being allowed into medical school.[48] Also from early 1940 on, there was an obligatory "field service," usually at harvest time, pressing the girls into physical labor, or a "factory service," placing them alongside blue-collar workers on industrial assembly lines.[49] At the height of the war, only the older students with children, whose husbands had fallen at the front, were declared exempt from those regulations, and only after individual dispensation.[50]

After a change of venue to the wide plains of the conquered East, medical application by these young women to the multifarious problems of eastern European, ethnic German settlers constituted the apex of such war-related mobilization. Here the young women were truly unique because they were isolated from their male cohorts. Usually, their work centered on the prevention of the Asian eye affliction trachoma or the teaching to Polish-German mothers of proper baby care and good dietary habits, but it also entailed race-hygienic, eugenic tasks. This work was always performed under the jurisdiction of the SS. The preeminent duty was "to instill 'master race' (*Herrenvolk*) notions into the settlers." In such a capacity, the future German female doctor seemed fated, upon full graduation, to play a contributory part in the new Nazi order, determined as it was by the priorities of blood and soil.[51]

4. Medica Politica

An account of the female physicians' involvement in politics during the Third Reich largely amounts to the attempt of professional women to maintain an individualistic form of organization, separate from the men's. Initially, it was within such a framework that emancipationist sentiments were vented, with the varying degrees of militancy described above. Participation in actual Nazi party politics was secondary, at least until the coming of World War II.

In 1933, most German female physicians were incorporated in the League of

German Women Doctors (Bund Deutscher Ärztinnen—BDÄ), a thoroughly bourgeois group that had been founded in Berlin by three hundred independent-minded women to look after group-specific interests, headed by one Dr. Schröder-Jakowski, in October 1924. Regional chapters had been quickly established, some of them led by resolute women physicians who later managed an easy transition into the Nazi era, as did Dr. Clara Soergel, the original BDÄ steward for Saxony-Thuringia.[1] By 1928, the league had more than doubled its membership.[2] To a certain extent, this meant an antisocialist and pro-*völkisch* bias, twin attitudes that would explain typical social establishment positions such as the stand of the BDÄ's right wing against the decriminalization of abortion, which was one of the most hotly contested issues during the troubled times of the Great Depression, when jobless families simply could not afford more children.[3]

After the political changeover in 1933, the BDÄ, like similar bourgeois groups, was not immediately dissolved but "coordinated" through affiliation with specially created control institutions of the Third Reich. Hence, like the Reich League of German Female Academics, it became a subgroup of that huge umbrella organization, the German Women's Front (DFW).[4] It received as its new leader a dyed-in-the-wool Nazi in the person of Berlin physician Dr. Lea Thimm, who had an unsullied party record as far back as April 1926; regionally, too, the leadership was ostensibly Nazified where it had not already been.[5] In East Prussia, for instance, Erna Orlopp-Pleick, a thirty-nine-year-old doctor who was a member of the party as well as the Nazi Physicians' League and a contractual adviser for the Hitler Youth, had assumed the BDÄ area directorship in Königsberg by autumn of 1933.[6]

Nonetheless, although women physicians were now set, to all intents and purposes, to be properly inducted into Nazism, the BDÄ became, ironically, the very instrument to fight for female doctors' privileges, under the tutelage of the headstrong Hitlerite Lea Thimm. In January 1936, at a plenary session of the BDÄ in Berlin, Thimm acidly remarked that no sooner had the party invested her with the old league's leadership than her energies "had immediately been consumed by the struggle for recognition and preservation of the women doctors' status."[7] She was of course referring to her quarrel of two years earlier with Reich Physicians' Leader Wagner regarding the right of women to study medicine and the then impending suspension of female panel physicians.[8] It is more than likely that Wagner had to recoil in 1934–35 in front of the intrepid Thimm, an event upon which she loved to reflect during her years in power—and because preparations for a tight Nazi regulation of physicians in the Reich were still not finalized.[9]

For the time being, then, the Bund Deutscher Ärztinnen was granted a stay of execution. Under the continued presidency of Thimm, and with equally resolute National Socialist doctors acting as her aides, the BDÄ strove to provide the organizational underpinning for the battles of principle these women physicians were waging against their Nazi male cohorts. Dr. Helene Sauer, a general practitioner from Wuppertal, acted as Thimm's treasurer, and Dr. Auguste Hoffmann, who officiated in Berlin, scheduled training courses for sports physicians; both women were accredited with the party's Main Office of People's Health.[10] Dr. Edith von Lölhöffel, a party member since 1933, became editor of the BDÄ's journal, *Die Ärztin*, in February 1936.[11] But Thimm was brazen enough to delegate for office women colleagues who enjoyed no Nazi affiliation whatsoever: Margarete Schubert was put in charge of a detail assisting medical novices who were seeking to establish themselves professionally, and Elisabeth Geilen was appointed as the BDÄ's executive secretary in December 1936.[12]

For the fifty-year-old Lea Thimm the ax fell at the end of 1936, in a phase when other outspoken intellectual Nazi "feminists" were also silenced in the Reich.[13] Coincidentally, the monopolistic character of the new Reich Physicians' Ordinance from 1935 on obviated other, preexisting organizations that would have rivaled the KVD and RÄK.[14] In October Thimm still was able to reassure herself and others that the "tendency gradually to obliterate women physicians, because they were redundant and bothersome, by throttling them economically," had finally been "liquidated," even though one would always have to be watchful. In November, she made sure to assume the secretarial duties for the BDÄ, perhaps because she had a sense of foreboding.[15] A few weeks later, Wagner dissolved the League of Women Physicians, on the characteristic pretext that the "seclusion of the female doctor" would have led to the establishment of a special university for women.[16] In 1937 Dr. Ursula Kuhlo, a twenty-eight-year-old party member dating from February 1932 and therefore, presumably, trustworthy in the eyes of Wagner, tried to prevail on the Reich physicians' leader to resuscitate a self-contained women physicians' group. But this was not to be. One of Wagner's last acts as head of all the German doctors was to constitute a new chapter for women physicians, directly subordinate to his authority, in the fall of 1938. Because Kuhlo, as a professional newcomer, was considered relatively untouched by the wiles of Thimm, she was named to the chapter's directorship.[17] The institutional annihilation of the female physicians as a self-expressive entity was completed in May 1939, when Wagner's successor Conti appointed Kuhlo to the governing board of the Reich Physicians' Chamber; a solitary woman, she was outnumbered by thirteen men.[18] In 1942 the journal *Die Ärztin* became an official organ of the RÄK.[19] Under pressure from Conti's programmatic centralization of medicine in the Reich, Kuhlo demurely toed the men physicians' party line until the end of the war.[20] In such circumstances, timid attempts by a few women physicians to reactivate the unique esprit de corps of their older colleagues of yore never got off the ground.[21]

To the extent that gender-specific organizational politics was diminishing in importance for the women doctors, Nazi party affiliation was gaining. Table 3.8 shows that even though more than half of all the women physicians maintained connections with Nazi cadres from 1933 to 1945, they were underrepresented compared to the males.[22] Nevertheless, according to Table 3.9, in the period from 1939 to 1945 the underrepresentation of women was decreasing, from index figure 1.56 to 1.31, vis-à-vis the prewar period.[23] This came as a natural consequence of the increase in formal recognition, leading to greater nominal parity with men, which all women were experiencing after 1939, especially the job-skilled ones, because of the demands of war.[24]

Table 3.8 illuminates the curative and welfare-related character of women physicians' Nazi recruitment in the Third Reich. The women doctors' presence was stronger proportionately in the service-oriented cadres of the Nazi Student League and the Hitler Youth (appropriately, the BDM), while their representation in the strongly male-centered formations of the party and of the Nazi Physicians' League was down. To be sure, if the party was disinterested in the services only women doctors were reputed to be good for, the NS-Ärztebund was known to the women as the source of much of their trouble in maintaining independent status and as the home territory of the unpopular Gerhard Wagner. References to it by female physicians were never more than perfunctory.[25] Hardly surprisingly, women, by dint of gender, monopolized the Nazi women's organizations, the German Women's Front and the more tightly structured NS-Frauenschaft (Nazi Women's Organization—NSF), to the same degree that their male colleagues dominated the SA and SS.[26]

The value of Nazi party membership for female physicians has already been demonstrated in terms of the history of their professional organization: such membership was ideal for documenting political loyalty while at the same time allowing greater leverage in maneuvering against the medical establishment. And without question, it helped in obtaining the tokens of more mundane, everyday career progress. Since political reliability was a factor in gaining employment or improving one's station in any event,[27] but doubly so in the face of the unrestrained animosity of their male colleagues, straight party membership was by far the best ploy for women doctors. Proof of affiliation somewhere else in the movement counted for less. Thus already in the early years, when *Jungärzte* were competing against their established colleagues for panel practice, female physicians shrewdly mentioned party affiliation in their job advertisements; as doctors became scarcer after the mid-1930s, this habit subsided.[28]

Biographical details regarding five women doctors, Hanna Donnerberg, Margot Gressler, Hildegard Schönberg, Herta Russ, and Hilde Tries, appropriately conclude this account. I have already cited the case of Dr. Donnerberg, who in 1938 was seeking a generalist's practice in Neuwied. At first she was not allowed one by the KVD admission board on the charge that she had never been actively involved in any National Socialist organization, least of all the party itself, even though she had been doing free consulting work for the BDM since September 1934. It was only after Donnerberg, who was also accused of having shopped "in a Jewish store" as late as 1935, filed a strong protest with the aid of the local NSF leader and emphasized her service as a staff physician in the BDM that a higher-level review board attested to her dependability in "party organizations" and permitted her to open a practice.[29] Margot Gressler, however, was unsuccessful in setting up her own office in Ohrdruf two years later, mainly because she had to contend against male colleagues; but it certainly did not help her cause that evidently she was completely devoid of party ties.[30]

Hildegard Schönberg, in contrast, fared much better. At age twenty-nine this gifted pathologist had joined the party in 1931, and by 1938 at the latest, Schönberg was also a member of the Nazi Aviation Corps (NSFK). Doubtless, this aided her career. First an assistant physician at Berlin's Auguste-Viktoria Hospital, she became a section leader at a children's clinic in 1936, and by the time of her death in 1939 she was working in three Berlin institutions at once. Still finding the time to publish the results of her original research, Schönberg was on her way to a promising academic career when she contracted a fatal case of diphtheria.[31]

During the war, such Nazi connections had by no means lost their power. Vienna-born physician Herta Russ reminded the Reich health leadership in November 1940 that she had suffered, as an illegal National Socialist, for her "Nazi orientation" before the Anschluss, thereupon proceeding to lay claim to her own private practice. Indeed, it was on record that she had joined the Nazi party openly in 1938 right after Hitler had marched across the Austro-Bavarian frontier.[32] Dr. Hilde Tries could show no such credentials when she became the candidate for a position as shop physician in Hessian Kelkheim in summer 1942. A practicing Catholic, whose immediate family was already under suspicion for its strong church ties, this twenty-six-year-old doctor was said by the party to be "in no way positively disposed" toward the new regime because she was "neither in an ancillary branch of the movement nor in the NSV," to say nothing of the NSDAP itself. The party assessor neglected to credit Dr. Tries with her membership in the BDM, but, possibly, her religious background forever ruined her chances for professional advancement.[33]

Of all the Nazi affiliates holding out professional opportunities for women doctors, the BDM was the most popular. It contained no men, and work in its ranks was considered to be the most gratifying, even if, like virtually all other such jobs in the movement, it brought no financial rewards.[34] But presumably, it was useful as a springboard for attractive, remunerative careers in the future, such as in the nation's school system, the *Arbeitsdienst*, or as a sports or factory physician,[35] apart from providing the necessary political covering that was almost obligatory in the Nazi system. It was not until 1937 that the BDM started employing women doctors on a full-time basis, yet as the regional network of the Hitler Youth expanded during the war, the number of gainfully employed higher-echelon BDM women physicians went up accordingly.[36] Full time or in a voluntary, advisory capacity, there were thirteen hundred female physicians in the BDM by 1939 and fifteen hundred two years later.[37] Until the beginning of hostilities, special training courses schooled these BDM physicians at the RÄK camp of Alt-Rehse every September from 1936 on; the first course was attended by an enthusiastic 130 women.[38] In daily practice the BDM doctors supervised hygiene in the female Hitler Youth, performed health tests, stood by in emergency and accident situations, offered all manner of advice in matters of sickness and health as well as more formal instruction, and during the war even directed the first aid services of BDM teenagers after air raids.[39] One of their specifically assigned tasks was to collaborate with civil service *Amtsärzte* in the routine health care of schoolchildren.[40]

Work in the NSV, which, like the medical BDM chores, was organizationally under the purview of the Hauptamt für Volksgesundheit headed by the Reich physicians' leader, usually revolved around care of mothers and babies, a particularly important mandate within the official program of the Reich's health preservation planning (*Gesundheitsvorsorge*).[41] To the women physicians, it seems to have been less attractive than BDM service only because men proliferated and tended to be in charge (Table 3.8). Nevertheless, the curative work in the NSV was frequently coupled with identical schemes originating in the two major Nazi women organizations, the DFW and, most notably, the NSF.[42] On the whole, then, this work was rewarding to the female doctors. Pregnant women and young mothers with their babies had to be sent to spas and specially established homes in the country, where they were to benefit from extended rest periods in clean air, recuperative exercises, and strengthening diets. As well, there were courses to be taught in proper mothering.[43] As stands to reason, a racist philosophy underlay these efforts: only biologically fit German women, no matter of what social class, were to be looked after, so that they would produce even fitter offspring.[44] Finally, in the ranks of the NSV, female physicians might assume an important role through counseling in the psychiatry of youth, often in conjunction with legal agencies.[45]

Apart from these major areas, there were other services female doctors could render to the Nazi movement, of which only the most extreme might be mentioned here, to project the limits to which the most fanatical National Socialist women professionals were prepared to go to salvage their vocational identity at any price. A certain Dr. Bahr was an employee of the Rassenpolitisches Amt, where at the height of the war she checked for Jewish ancestors in the pedigrees of ordinary citizens, with disastrous consequences for those who were found positive.[46] Opportunities existed for women physicians in the SS institution Lebensborn that cared for racially promising children born out of wedlock and their mothers, certain of whom had entered into sexual congress with physically impeccable SS men.[47]

In this respect, Dr. Herta Oberheuser surpassed them all. This pediatrician, who was born in 1911 and joined the party as a twenty-six-year-old intern, eventually got on the medical staff of Ravensbrück, the only concentration camp just for female captives. Ironically, as a woman among women, she participated in cruel experiments and helped cause the death of many a victim.[48] To this day she remains as the epitome of the ideologically perverted but nevertheless ambitious female professional of those unique twelve years. To the extent that she may initially have been a victim of the politics of the Third Reich, she ended up bearing a major share of responsibility for its crimes.

Chapter 4

Medical Faculties in Crisis

1. Infection of Medical Science with Nazi Ideology

In the Third Reich, the faculties of medicine collectively became the preeminent academic discipline in all the colleges and universities. This was the case in absolute as well as in relative terms. Not only did medicine become the strongest discipline, with about 30 percent of all university faculty being medical teachers by 1935 and more after that, but it also came to exceed by far the other faculties in university power politics. Having grown after the middle of the nineteenth century, the German medical faculties became the most prominent of all university schools in the Weimar Republic; during this period, medicine scholars notoriously dominated the university administrations as rectors. From 1923 to 1932 almost 36 percent of all the rectors were medical men. In the Third Reich this trend continued, for in the 1933–45 period the 36 percent figure jumped to nearly 59 percent, overrepresenting medicine as a discipline in the rector's office by a factor of two to one, if judged by all the disciplines together. The medical sector's influence was heightened because after January 1933 the rector of every university was appointed by the Nazi state and endowed with Führer prerogatives. Therefore, he emerged with absolute powers at the top of the university hierarchy, responsible only to the Reich ministry of education, albeit under some influence of the party's academic representative.[1]

Any events occurring in a medical faculty were apt to set precedents for developments in other faculties or could signify changes or indicate changes to come for the university community as a whole. In that sense, medical faculties may be said to have become, over time, role models.[2]

In keeping with the increased significance of medical schools in the Third Reich, one may point to the establishment of new pseudo-disciplines in the medical faculties as portentous for a novel trend in higher education. The quintessential novelty as a pseudo-discipline permeating the medical schools after January 1933 (and subsequently affecting other faculties as well) was *Rassenkunde*, or race hygiene, also often referred to as "eugenics," the main ingredient of which was, of course, the premise of the National Socialist doctrine.[3] Indeed, it is fair to say that the ideas of *Rassenkunde* or *Rassenhygiene*, to the extent that they were conceived by scholars of medicine, represented a truly medical content within the body of Nazi dogma as it evolved since the beginnings of the *völkisch* movement. This meant that important portions of the National Socialist program were medicalized during the Nazi Time of Struggle and that certain medical scholars had a hand in this medicalization. Ultimately, one can perceive an organic link between distinct tendencies in German medicine predating the 1920s on one side and the race-hygienically inspired horrors of Auschwitz on the other, a link that went largely unnoticed in the critical literature on National Socialism and the Third Reich until the publication of George Mosse's and Robert Jay Lifton's seminal studies.[4]

According to its original *völkisch* criteria the "science" of *Rassenkunde/Rassenhygiene* possessed three equal components: an anthropological, a sociopolitical, and a purely medical one. The anthropological property of *Rassenkunde* predicated the performance and recording of measurements of human bodily characteristics as a basis for comparisons and, finally, value judgments imputing inequality which, nonetheless, always remained totally arbitrary. These value judgments were inspired by sociopolitical, that is, expansionist or imperialist, assumptions which, for the faithful, attained an axiomatic quality. They would subsequently provide the intellectual framework for the manipulation of the human species, either as individuals or in a group, by the medical techniques of "selection" or "counterselection." The aim was to improve and augment one discreetly defined "race" deemed to be superior (*Aufzucht*), while impeding and extinguishing another, thought to be inferior (*Ausmerze*).[5]

The scientific atmosphere in which *Rassenkunde* was allowed to take root in academic medicine and thereafter to influence other scholarly disciplines was that of the last quarter of the nineteenth century. It was the immediate post-Darwinian era, which in the Second Reich ruled by Kaiser Wilhelm II witnessed the rise of a new, racially motivated form of anti-Semitism, intellectually presided over by the zoologist and onetime physician Ernst Haeckel.[6] In a sense, Dr. Alfred Ploetz, though not an anti-Semite, can take credit for having been the spiritual father of *Rassenkunde*, through his elaboration of vulgarized Social Darwinian theories. He was a medical practitioner, lecturer, and author born in 1860, who lived long enough to receive an honorary doctorate from Munich University's faculty of philosophy in 1930 and a professorial appointment at that university from Hitler personally six years later.[7] Ploetz had adopted a very crude Darwinian scheme when he suggested that the white ("Westaryan") race was superior to the other races: Jews still were tolerated as almost "Aryan" and anti-Semitism was eschewed. In any case, the Germanic peoples were reputed to be "at the very top."[8]

According to Ploetz, such views were subject to the dictates of racial hygiene. During a war only inferior members of a race should be sent to the front lines to serve as "cannon fodder." Ploetz even divined that to keep a superior race healthy, a caucus of physicians should decide at the birth of each new child whether it should be allowed to live. As Mosse has aptly noted, "The ruthlessness inherent in this method of racial hygiene was due to the exaltation of human power, inevitable as long as it was maintained that human survival depended upon the cultivation of an elite and the eradication of the weak."[9]

The 1930 Munich University festivities for Ploetz bespeak the importance to which *Rassenkunde* in Germany had risen by that time. Ploetz himself no less than his loyal disciples was responsible for this. That doctor of general medicine served as a pioneer in several capacities. In 1895 he published what was regarded as a fundamental volume on the superiority of the Germanic race, and nine years later he founded a pace-setting journal for all *völkisch*-inclined scholars, the soon to be famous *Archiv für Rassen- und Gesellschaftsbiologie*. (One of the first physicians to collaborate in this venture was the gynecologist Dr. Agnes Bluhm.) Along with Bluhm, Ernst Rüdin, and others Ploetz also established, in 1905 at Berlin, a "scientific" society, the Deutsche Gesellschaft für Rassenhygiene, which soon attained status for white racist scholars beyond the confines of the Reich.[10]

One of the cofounders of this society was Philalethes Kuhn, Ploetz's junior by ten years, who began his professional career as a physician in the German colony of Southwest Africa. He participated in the Kaiser's ruthless campaigns against disobedient native tribes and in particular joined in the genocidal warfare against the proud Hereroes in 1904. From this experience he derived his notions about German superiority as a master race, which initially was predicated, in the *völkisch* manner, on an assumed inferiority of blacks, thought to be interchangeable with Jews.[11] In 1920 Kuhn obtained a full professorship in clinical hygienics at the Technical University of Dresden, and in 1924 he was the new local chapter leader of the Gesellschaft für Rassenhygiene and an enthusiastic if surreptitious supporter of Adolf Hitler, then in captivity at Landsberg. By 1926 Kuhn had moved to Giessen, and here, as formerly in Dresden, he took care to infuse his medical hygienics seminars with specifically racial messages.[12] Kuhn's example soon was followed by Professor Hans Reiter, born in 1891, who since 1919 taught hygienics, with a similar racist tinge, as an adjunct professor in Rostock. Also an avid disciple of Hitler, Reiter would in 1932 claim a deputy's seat for the NSDAP in the Mecklenburg Landtag.[13] Throughout the 1920s, Kuhn and Reiter were in league with yet a third physician vitally concerned about the "race question," Dr. Fritz Lenz. A former student of Ploetz's, he at age thirty-six occupied the first chair dedicated to race hygienics, established in 1923 at Munich, albeit only as an associate professor.[14] Through Kuhn, Reiter, Lenz, and lesser medical teachers with an anthropological inclination race hygiene eventually was being taught at several universities in the 1920s and early 1930s, though in no way systematically.[15] Yet despite an aura conducive to a modicum of racial studies in the medical faculties some years before the inception of the Third Reich, hardly any of its later theorists on race were able to earn their degrees in *Rassenkunde* in the republic. As an example *Dozent* Siegfried Koller, who was to play a remarkable role in eugenic planning years later, received the first of his two doctorates not in medicine but from the philosophical faculty at Göttingen, on the uses of statistics in blood group research, in the year 1930.[16]

The established medical schools were reluctant to accept *Rassenkunde* as a serious discipline. But after Hitler's ascension to power this situation was to change, if not overnight. It is certain that Hitler had been influenced by Lenz's medicalized ideas on race as early as 1924, when he had read the professor's first important book in Landsberg prison. It is equally well known that Lenz had hailed the imminence of the Führer's racial program, insofar as it had been publicized by the early 1930s, even though the scholar noted that Hitler had perhaps radicalized his own original concepts somewhat unduly, especially in regard to Jews.[17] At any rate, today there is no doubt that after January 1933 Hitler, supported by Rudolf Hess and Hess's protégé Dr. Gerhard Wagner, unequivocally endorsed the institutionalization not only of racist-eugenic organizations of various provenance, to be logistically supported by party or state, but also, and especially, teaching positions in *Rassenkunde* in the medical faculties.

This government support is borne out as much by the new chancellor's open acknowledgment of Kuhn's work[18] as by his ostentatious appointment of Fritz Lenz to the first regular full chair of race hygienics ever in a German medical faculty in 1933, at the prestigious and highly visible University of Berlin.[19] At about this time, Kuhn and his colleagues issued calls for the erection of many more race-scientific posts in the medical faculties, preferably at the full professor level.[20] The contemporaneous appearance of myriads of racist-inspired agencies of an official or semiofficial nature all over the country augured well for the future of *Rassenkunde* as an academic field.[21]

This development was in keeping with the new tasks that were constantly announced as preconditions for the survival of the German "Aryan" race, however that was defined, unmistakably in the ideological tracts of Ploetz, Lenz, and Kuhn. Thus Professor Walter Schultze, a physician and Bavaria's new state commissar for health, held publicly that "the significance of questions of race" now was paramount to the extent that the old practice of caring for the weak would have to be abandoned "in favor of the racially intact and the congenitally sound." Psychopaths were said to resemble imbeciles, from whom the race would have to be shielded in the future. Since sterilization was an insufficient measure, annihilation (*Ausmerze*) would become necessary. The chaff would have to be separated from the wheat. "In part," said Professor Schultze, "this policy has already begun in our present concentration camps."[22] Professor Reiner Müller, who had taught in the medical school of Cologne since 1914, wrote in a 1935 hygienics textbook under the caption *Rassenhygiene* that races suffered different degrees of susceptibility to disease, thus suggesting that they could be identified and kept from social or sexual congress with each other, which, after all, was the purpose of properly executed "race hygienics." Diabetes was more frequent among Jews and Hindus than among any other people, declared Müller in this context. The professor made a point of not singling out German-"Aryans" as specifically disease-ridden. Rather, their superiority was posited by dint of the Nordics' well-known talent for survival of environmental hardships, which had, in the course of time, produced the present German type: "productive, intelligent people, who excel through a combination of inventor's initiative, logical lucidity and a strong will."[23] In the same year the Dessau physician Böttcher even went so far as to recommend the application of race science toward the practical goal of "making the blood of the Jew visible in a test-tube," although this would not be possible as long as Jewish scientists at German universities were allowed to boycott such nationally vital research.[24]

Between 1933 and 1939 positions in *Rassenkunde* were launched in most medical faculties, and if there were no chairs, courses in this subject were assigned to faculty members who had an abiding interest in the issue. Berlin, Greifswald, Munich, Halle, and Leipzig had their own chairs or university institutes in 1933. Frankfurt received one in 1935 (Otmar Freiherr von Verschuer) and Giessen in 1938 (Heinrich Wilhelm Kranz). In Tübingen, faculty members Wilhelm Gieseler, Heinrich Hoffmann, and Otto Stickl, every one a staunch National Socialist, looked after the needs of *Rassenkunde*, even though no chair had been established.[25]

Indeed, one of the problems to be surmounted was the dearth of qualified candidates for such posts, for no tradition of training in *Rassenkunde* existed. Except for the conventional subject of anatomy, the unique combination of anthropology and medicine had not yet become part of the accepted curriculum; a logical sequence of instruction had still to be worked out. As a result, most, if not all, "specialists" in *Rassenkunde* hurriedly invested with teaching duties turned out to be pathetically incompetent. One outstanding example was the Czech gynecologist Lothar Gottlieb Tirala, who succeeded Lenz in Munich in November 1933 after eight years as a private practitioner in Brünn. In spite of two doctorates, Tirala lacked basic knowledge even about current theories of heredity such as Mendel's; instead, he concentrated his efforts on curing all manner of diseases through breathing exercises. In public speeches as well as in continuing education courses for practicing physicians he would accuse Albert Einstein of plagiarism and begrudge Paul Ehrlich his epochal discoveries toward the control of syphilis. No wonder that for his students Tirala soon became a source of levity and laughter.[26] But even one of the more respected personalities in this new field, Eugen Fischer in Berlin, who enjoyed an international reputation both as an anthropologist and as a medical scholar, became fanatically bound to the hodgepodge of ideas that constituted *Rassenkunde*, as much as he was in awe of "the great Führer," so that questioning students found it difficult to establish an intelligent dialogue with him.[27]

Over the years a paradox developed in that the quality of university instruction in *Rassenkunde* and its status at the higher schools of learning remained extremely dubious, while its practical uses, especially in wartime, increased to the point that medico-ethical limits were strained and surpassed. In March 1936 *Rassenkunde* became a proper subject for academic examinations as part of a physician's prescribed course of studies.[28] At bulwarks of *Rassenkunde* such as Giessen, doctoral dissertations in the subject soon proliferated.[29] But by 1938 critics within the universities and state ministries were once again calling attention to the problem at hand. In January Professor Reiter published a reminder that university courses in race hygienics were still not sufficient either in quantity or in quality. One month later Dr. Herbert Linden of Conti's health department in the Reich interior ministry echoed this complaint, combining his critique with a proposal for improvement.[30] Little more than a year later, however, this deficiency still had not been redressed. Since qualified university teachers for *Rassenkunde* were not available, courses of instruction had to be held in improvised workshops or be delivered by external personnel. "Expert circles are doubting the success of this method," commented the Security Service of the SS curtly.[31]

Toward the end of the war the Reich ministry of education still had no choice but to concede failure in the area of *Rassenkunde* instruction; certified faculty did not exist and the students' grasp of the subject matter was found to be wanting.[32] Such failure became manifest in daily practice when "Aryans" with Nordic features were identified, who after passing the test with flying colors would turn out to be Jews.[33] And yet, the other side of this was the vicarious advice administered by the leading race hygienicists to the manipulators of the racial-eugenic machinery. This machinery had long been put in place to implement the mutations thought indispensable for upgrading the German race: sterilization, castration, "euthanasia," and subracial annihilation. After June 1933 Professor Lenz vigorously applauded the proposed sterilization of habitual alcoholics.[34] And in summer 1942 Professors Fischer, Verschuer, and Lenz sanctioned Leonardo Conti's plans for a tighter race-hygienic orientation of German health policy—the same Conti who had already implicated himself in the "euthanasia" killings backed by the tenets of those professors' *Rassenkunde*.[35]

By far the worst of the intellectual troglodytes who occupied chairs in *Rassenkunde* during the Third Reich was Heinrich Wilhelm Kranz. His career may be detailed here at some length because it conformed closely to the stereotype of the fanatical Nazi Old Fighter physician from the early 1920s on, who was to reap the harvest in the regime phase.[36] Kranz was born in 1897 in Göttingen, the son of a local postal official. His early life was marked by the sort of violence that characterized many original devotees of Hitler. He entered the Gymnasium, but before he could attend the university he joined the imperial troops, at age seventeen, to fight in the Great War. Having survived the war with the rank of lieutenant, he enrolled in the University of Marburg's medical school.[37] Here, in spring 1920, he was a member of the notorious student Freikorps unit that in cold blood shot to death fifteen unarmed leftist workers in the forests near Thuringian Mechterstedt. Although charged before a military tribunal, the students were all acquitted of murder, and the incident caused a months-long national scandal.[38] Now a hero on the nationalist extremist fringe, Kranz moved on to Freiburg, where he received his medical doctorate in 1921. This was followed by ophthalmological specialization in Frankfurt and Giessen, so that in 1926 Kranz passed the *Habilitation*, the obligatory qualifying examination for prospective German university teachers. Thereupon he opened for business as an eye doctor in Giessen.[39]

Presumably under the influence of Professor Kuhn, who was teaching in Giessen by that year, Kranz intensified his interest in *Rassenkunde*, which he intimately tied to population planning, while at the same time honing his relationship with Hitler's *völkisch* movement. A member of the Nazi Physicians' League and of the party proper in the early 1930s, Kranz scheduled race-hygienic training on behalf of the NSÄB in 1931.[40]

After January 1933 Kranz's political as well as his professional progress began to take shape. First he became Dr. Wagner's deputy in Upper Hesse and the highest KVD delegate in that region. Thereafter he was accorded a variety of party and Nazi physician organization offices related to race hygienics, notably its application in special law courts facilitated by several edicts of race and "hereditary health" legislation in the early regime years. Still essentially an ophthalmologist and without even the rudiments of formal anthropological schooling, Kranz was on his way to becoming one of the most powerful ideologues of race and population politics in the Third Reich.[41]

Kranz took great care in preparing for his entrance into the hallowed halls of higher learning, and his success was impressive. As early as January 1934 he had acquired official permission to conduct continuing education courses in race hygienics for nurses as well as for physicians on the premises of Giessen University. He was joined by sympathetic faculty members such as Professor Rudolf Edler von Jaschke, director of the university's gynecological clinic, but also by well-known outside experts in the field, like the Frankfurt professor Otmar von Verschuer.[42] For winter semester 1934–35 Kranz was given a mandate to lecture in race hygienics, and early in 1937 he was appointed a tenured associate professor responsible for this subject at the university.[43] The Institute for Hereditary Health and Race Preservation (Institut für Erbgesundheits- und Rassenpflege), which Kranz had established as a party-sponsored organization in autumn 1933, had been partially transferred to the university, with the help of Professor Kuhn, by January 1936. Two years later it became a full-fledged university department, financed by the state. In 1939 Kranz advanced to the position of leader of the Nazi Lecturers' League (NSD-Dozentenbund), Giessen chapter, and, after a brief stint in the Wehrmacht that took him to vanquished Czechoslovakia, was chosen rector of the university in 1940. He continued his spectacular career as a full professor, successor to Otmar von Verschuer in Frankfurt, after that stellar race scholar had assumed Eugen Fischer's coveted position in Berlin in 1942.[44]

Kranz is said by some to have taken his own life in May 1945, presumably on the run from the Allies, who had added his name to their list of war criminals.[45] His suicide would be proof of his own acknowledgment that his past work as a race hygienicist would not meet with universal scientific approval because it had transcended the outer boundaries of Hippocratic ethics. To be sure, if Kranz through any of his deeds had become criminally responsible by 1945, a question that was never tested in a court of law, he would have had to be classified as a planner, a theoretical perpetrator of evil, what the West Germans have fittingly termed "desk murderer" (*Schreibtischtäter*). Legal prosecutors and scholars alike have largely passed Kranz by not only because he died in 1945 without leaving great tomes of scholarship, but also because much of the evil he and his followers wrought was evil only potentially, for many of Kranz's brainchildren never matured. Nonetheless, Kranz's example is important in the development of German medicine under a racist aegis, for, next to the already familiar scenarios from Auschwitz and other concentration camps, his institutes in Giessen and Frankfurt document the lengths to which a criminalized medical profession under Hitler was able to go. Kranz's career highlights not only the vacuity of *Rassenkunde* as an academic discipline bereft of any contextual locus in the tradition of international science, but, and more important, it illustrates the infestation of German scholarship with Nazi ideas and, after their conversion from theory into practice, the complicity of *Rassenkunde* scholars, draped in the white uniforms of medicine, in the eventual death of millions.

The danger of Kranz's academic work to human species that did not make this doctor's predefined grade lay in his individual control over them collectively, once he had recorded and classified their characteristics and, based on his learned value judgment, pronounced on their ultimate future. Kranz commenced such tasks in the institute he had set up with the aid of the NSDAP in 1933. In the interest of the "race improvement process" (*Aufartungsprozess*)[46] Kranz was collecting and filing away for constant reference health and other personal details on hundreds of thousands of Hessian residents, including inmates of insane and tuberculosis asylums, but also "racial aliens" and "mongrels," among whom would be included Jews, Gypsies, and persons of mixed ethnic origin. As well by 1939 a separate "hereditary-statistical" (*erbstatistische*) card file was extant listing eighteen hundred sets of twins from Giessen's hinterland. Yet another section of the institute dealt with the biological specifications of prospective marriage partners; this unit was always ready to assess the merits of a marriage loan, but also of possible sterilization to be subsequently decreed by the hereditary courts. One of the more sinister activities engaged in by the institute's staff was rendering binding opinions in paternity issues, not just for settling alimony cases but for preventing further offspring by sterilization on congenital or racial grounds. The records of the institute contained virtually complete information on Hessians deemed to be "asocial" by Kranz and his assistants: prostitutes, vagrants, beggars, petty criminals, and drunkards.[47]

What to do with this miscellaneous inventory? In 1937 Kranz's assistant Dr. Otto Finger elaborated the antisocial properties of 136 persons who belonged to two large Gypsy clans. In the conclusion of his fastidious study on such "racially alien parasites" Finger expressed the need for their physical containment—a measure that was implemented forthwith through the consignment of German Gypsies to concentration camps, where they awaited sterilization or transport to liquidation sites.[48]

In 1934 aspiring race hygienicist Dr. Siegfried Koller arrived at Kranz's institute. Eleven years younger than the ophthalmologist, this blood-group expert had joined the NSDAP in 1933. He now proceeded to work toward his second, a medical, degree under Kranz's direction, which he had accomplished by 1938; a year later he was a nontenured university lecturer (*Dozent*). Turning increasingly to the application of statistical methods to population macroanalysis, Koller recommended before the war that the circle of people who ought to be sterilized, castrated, or physically removed from society should be many times greater than could presently be justified by valid National Socialist race legislation.[49] Such views were radicalized in subsequent publications by Kranz and Koller with potentially disastrous consequences for millions of ordinary Germans, whose "asocial" qualities were judged to be hereditary rather than the result of an inclement environment. The two physicians received a mandate from the regime to design a new biopolitical law. It would create the apparatus for removing the "inalienable *völkisch* rights"—a category invented by these scholars—including the right to undisturbed life amid the *Volksgemeinschaft*, from 1.6 million designated unfortunate persons. Only the reversal of the Wehrmacht's successes at the eastern front in 1942, which necessitated the deployment of Koller as a martial medicine (*Wehrmedizin*) statistician in the army's service, obviated this gruesome plan.[50]

Kranz probably had a decisive influence on the killing of disabled persons at the beginning of the war in Hadamar, some fifty miles from Giessen. Alice Platen-Hallermund, who surmised his role, was one of the earliest German chroniclers of Nazi medical abuse. She has called Kranz "one of the few university professors of race science, whose will to destruction was so blatantly obvious."[51]

If *Rassenkunde* admittedly was the most precarious, it was certainly not the only questionable innovation in the landscape of academic medicine after January 1933. To a certain extent, the entire discipline was permeated with typically *völkisch* notions, many of which had been around long before Hitler came to power. These notions embodied what in the late 1920s had constituted grounds for a critique of and correctional proposals for a deep-felt "crisis of medicine" in the entire profession in Germany, mostly emanating from rightist political quarters.[52]

At the core of the revisionist medicine was the *völkisch* conception of organicism.[53] Building on the ideas of the irascible Danzig surgeon Erwin Liek, a baroque, charismatic figure who exerted a tremendous influence on German medicine in the latter half of the Weimar Republic,[54] Nazi doctors rejected what they contemptuously called modern "mechanistic" medicine. In conformity with totalitarianism, they demanded that in the new medical cosmology the human body be viewed holistically, as a natural entity within which all parts were physiologically related to each other. Hence it was wrong to search for the seat of a specific disease in individual organs of the body; rather, the entire organism had to be considered for treatment. An analysis of these biological precepts helps to explain the disdain of Nazi medicine for the specialist and, conversely, the predilection for generalist practice.[55] The *völkisch* physicians strove for a return, medically speaking, to a preindustrial state, where the forces of nature such as sun rays or fresh air or herbs, rather than synthetic pharmacological products and the technology of a laboratory or operating room, were enlisted to aid the human body in maintaining or recovering its balance. It was their conviction that healing was a craft, to be carefully executed in a directly personal doctor-to-patient relationship, more on the basis of intuition than of reason.[56]

In such a setting, applied medicine based on hunches tempered by experience was rated far more highly than theoretical medical science, which was known to reside in the universities.[57] The conventional medical faculties were therefore attacked in a double capacity: as pinnacles of intellectual aloofness that sponsored the theoretical exercises of scholars devoid of any ties with the organic *Volksgemeinschaft*, and, more specifically in the medical context, as bastions of "objective" specialist research unrelated to the real needs of ordinary patients.[58]

Imbued with such ideas, Nazi physicians' leader Wagner, who early in the regime succeeded in obtaining a certain degree of influence in the universities as a whole,[59] embarked on a raucous propaganda campaign against the medical schools. Ideally, his strategy was to institutionalize Nazi medicine, but in his day-to-day treatment of the medical faculties he used a two-pronged tactic. Because this pragmatist realized the value of the traditional university structure with its proven apparatus for Nazi medical purposes, he would not go along with the most radical Nazi revolutionaries who wished to throw the baby out with the bathwater by demolishing the medical faculties altogether. Claiming that he aimed for a synthesis between Nazi naturopathy—what was called "New German Healing"[60]—and what he referred to as "academic medicine" (*Schulmedizin*), he envisaged the infiltration and gradual conversion of the traditional teaching body through the appointment of his own people but also by making use of the residual prestige of established scholars, insofar as they would acquiesce in changes they at first were bound to regard as radical.[61]

In addition, Wagner was planning, with as much help from state and party agencies as possible, the erection of counterinstitutions to check any untoward development of the medical schools in the future because he suspected that unreconstructible, "reactionary" scholars would resist him after all. As a first step, Wagner chose to collaborate with his close ally in the party, the Bavarian state commissioner for health Dr. Walter ("Bubi") Schultze, in the establishment of a new state academy for public health officials in 1933, as well as a Bavarian Academy for Continuing Education one year later, both in Munich, at Wagner's seat of power.[62] Next came the inauguration of a new teaching hospital specifically devoted to the dissemination of New German Healing in Dresden in June 1934, which was suitably named Rudolf-Hess-Krankenhaus, after Wagner's influential patron and patient, who himself was beholden to herbal cures.[63] The founding of the NSÄB-sponsored continuous-training course of studies for Nazi physicians in Alt-Rehse one year later was marked by distinctly antiacademic invective on the part of Wagner and his aide Kurt Blome that had to be interpreted as an immediate threat by perspicacious university administrators.[64] Also in Dresden by 1938, a Nazi academy for continuing medical education on the Bavarian model had been superimposed on an already existing conventional institution; it was to complement the teaching hospital.[65]

It is a measure of the spinelessness of certain of the established medical scholars that they not only did not resist Gerhard Wagner's incursions into the realm of medical education but went out of their way to meet him on his own terms. Presumably for opportunistic reasons, these men adjusted to the changed situation without a struggle. Thus when the Bavarian academy for continuing education organized a race-hygienic course of studies in September 1934, three members of the Munich medical faculty appeared in person for the National Socialist closing ceremony.[66] In Alt-Rehse, too, almost all the deans of Germany's medical schools and many of their faculty colleagues were gathered in June 1935 to listen to the antiprofessorial insults of the party's medical functionaries.[67] Still before the war, glaring concessions on the part of the academic establishment were to go beyond the realm of mere formality, for they came to affect the curriculum. In autumn 1937 Heidelberg's medical school organized a prize contest for candidates who could elaborate on "people's health," a specifically Nazi formula, and Breslau's followed suit a few months later with an essay topic on the new heredity legislation.[68] Of course this matched the ideological perversion that had by now tainted so much of the medical faculties' formal teaching, what with the introduction of courses such as "Race and Hereditary Biology as Tasks of the National Socialist State," offered by Professor Theodor Pakheiser, or "Race and Race Hygienics," taught by Professor Carl Schneider, both at Heidelberg.[69] Even long-established medical scholars such as the surgeon Ernst Heinrich Seifert, a professor at Würzburg since 1923 and the university's rector in 1938, now paid lip service to Hitler's proclaimed aims and conjured up the peculiarly Germanic phenomenon of "an inner coherence between physicianship and leadership."[70] The internationally respected Munich pathologist Max Borst spoke publicly about the necessity for science and scholarship to serve "the people" in a time of need and repeated the Nazi physicians' demands for an organicist application of medicine.[71] And the Berlin medical historian Paul Robert Diepgen amplified such views when he wrote in his popular textbook of 1938 that "it depends how *völkisch* science is defined. Certainly science, in serving all mankind, has to be cosmopolitan. But this does not contradict the fact that each people will understand and support science from its own particular vantage point." Diepgen concluded: "We as Germans could not have a better ideological fundament for our medical practice and course of studies than the National Socialist fundament in the spirit of Hitler."[72]

This is not to say that all of medical science at the universities was adulterated after 1933. There were islands of prodigious scholarship and, as we shall see later, there was downright resistance to the regime in a few cases. In the final analysis, the question must at least be posed whether those good examples were indicative of the state of academic medicine under the Nazis or whether the compromised and sullied ones were. If at all, a balanced judgment can be rendered only after a review of the entire spectrum.

Several mature medicine scholars, especially those with international reputations, were able to continue teaching exactly what they had taught before Hitler came to power, without making the slightest concessions. They saw no reason to change their proven ways. They could easily brush aside a charge by the Nazi racist Dr. Walter Gross as early as April 1933 that the developments in *Rassenkunde* had passed them by.[73] Wagner and his cronies would not have dared to molest them, for fear of risking the vestiges of Germany's traditionally awesome medical prestige.[74] The memoirs of unspoiled medicine professors such as the book by the pathologist Franz Büchner demonstrate this convincingly. Büchner, a pious Catholic, writes about the thoroughly scientific atmosphere he encountered first in Berlin and then in Freiburg, and he is equally laudatory about his senior colleagues and younger peers.[75] Ludwig Aschoff, that great Freiburg pathologist whose chair Büchner was later to inherit, in 1934 openly declared in contradistinction to what the Nazis thought that there was no such thing as a "nationally delimited medicine," for diseases were "not contingent on individual cultural or political circles," and medicine was, like no other discipline, dependent on "the cooperation of peoples."[76]

There is no denying that even then the coryphaei of German medicine were still capable of internationally important feats, as was proven by the pathologist Gerhard Domagk, who in the 1920s had interrupted a promising university career to join the IG Farben trust. In 1936 Domagk explained to a university gathering how he had experimented with the health of his own daughter in the ultimately successful development of sulfa drugs for the treatment of bacterial infections.[77]

Domagk was awarded the Nobel Prize in 1939, but the Nazi government forbade his accepting it. And also in 1936, the internist Theodor Brugsch analyzed aspects of organicism in medicine, without being slavishly committed to the Nazi preconceptions.[78] It was to the credit of famous Heidelberg internist Ludolf von Krehl that in 1937 at the age of seventy-eight he published a small booklet entitled *The Physician* in which he ruminated on the ideal qualifications of a doctor without a trace of Nazi ideology, although it had been written at the behest of Wagner's aide Kurt Klare.[79]

Even during the war such overtly decent attitudes to medicine as a Hippocratic trust did not change for those scholars of medicine who did not want it to. In 1940 the surgeons Emil Karl Frey, Erwin Payr, and von Seemen publicly held forth on the latest improvements in their field; what they had to say was impressive by the international standards of the period.[80] And the internist Ferdinand Hoff, who like Büchner survived the Third Reich to write his memoirs, tells of a paper he gave before the Medical Society during summer 1943 in Berlin, on which occasion such luminaries as the surgeon Ferdinand Sauerbruch, the gynecologist Walter Stoeckel, and the internist Gustav von Bergmann joined him in discussion, accompanied by most members of the Berlin faculty.[81]

But on the other side there were unconscionable physicians who used the National Socialist climate to further their scholarly careers in any way possible, acting on the old assumption that if formal progress in their professional development could be shown to have taken place, they would enjoy the customary tokens of advancement resulting from such labors. The problem with these medical pseudo-scholars was that they were aware of their innate mediocrity and that to bridge over whatever difficulties they experienced, they were prepared to violate their fundamental integrity, take shortcuts in their science, and collect easy rewards. In the course of doing so, they became criminally responsible. For exemplary purposes five men will be dealt with here, but this list is by no means exhaustive: Ernst Günther Schenck, Kurt Heissmeyer, Johann Kremer, Sigmund Rascher, and Josef Mengele. All of them ultimately aspired to be full professors of medicine.[82]

Schenck was born in 1904; he received a doctorate in natural science in 1927 and another one in medicine in 1929.[83] He joined the SA in 1933 and the NSÄB and NSDAP in 1937.[84] By that time he already was an executive physician in one of Munich's municipal hospitals and a lecturer in internism and physiology at Munich's medical faculty. In the summer of 1942 Schenck became an adjunct professor.[85] Initially on Wagner's Munich staff and a champion of biologized New German Healing, he had no difficulty changing over to Conti's Berlin office after Wagner's death in 1939. Soon he was one of Conti's closest advisers on national health policy.[86] In April 1940, Schenck had joined the Waffen-SS as a lieutenant, second class, and by fall 1944, he had reached the rank of lieutenant colonel (*Obersturmbannführer*).[87] By 1942 Schenck had become inspector general of nutrition for the Waffen-SS, personally responsible to the head of the concentration camp system, SS General Oswald Pohl (who was later hanged at Nuremberg).[88] He was charged with improving the diet of SS troops fighting at the fronts, for instance by finding new and portable natural staples with a high protein content for them. Late in December 1943 Pohl and Schenck conspired to test one such new product, derived from chemical waste that was said by Himmler to kill freshwater fish, in the camps of Dachau, Buchenwald, and Sachsenhausen, involving 100,000 prisoners as guinea pigs.[89] For unknown reasons, only 100 prisoners were fed the "protein sausage," but Schenck did perform nutrition, or rather hunger, experiments on 370 inmates of Mauthausen camp in 1943–44, in the course of which all of them suffered discomfort and pain and many became so emaciated that eventually they died.[90] It is obvious from the extant documents that as an SS officer, Schenck was eager to please Himmler and Pohl, but beyond that, there is little doubt that he wanted to use the sum total of his "research" to obtain for himself a full chair in physiology as soon as he was able to leave active SS service.[91]

Kurt Heissmeyer, though not incorporated in the SS, nevertheless was a member of the party since 1937. He was a year younger than Schenck and the nephew of influential SS general August Heissmeyer. After being licensed in 1933, Kurt Heissmeyer became a specialist in the treatment of tuberculosis. Since 1934 he had been associated with Himmler's boyhood friend, the SS surgeon Karl Gebhardt, and in early 1944 he was an *Oberarzt* in the employ of Gebhardt's SS sanatorium at Hohenlychen. Academically ambitious but without real scholarly merits, Heissmeyer, too, dreamed of becoming a medicine professor. To qualify himself for university teaching (*Habilitation*), he conceived a plan for curing tuberculosis. He would conduct experiments, not on animals as had been the previous practice, but on humans; with the help of his friend Oswald Pohl and the backing of Himmler he would find such an opportunity in Neuengamme concentration camp near Hamburg.[92]

The idea was to infect living organisms with tuberculosis bacilli, going on the outlandish, homeopathically inspired theory that the disease could be checked with a dose of its own germs. Heissmeyer's theory had long been disproved by the experts, and it serves as testimony to Heissmeyer's severe deficiency as a scientist that he was not aware of that.[93] In June 1944 the doctor started his experiments, injecting the tuberculosis bacilli into Russian and Polish inmates of Neuengamme, some of whom already had the disease. Under minimal hygienic conditions and lacking any proper medical care, many of the men died. The East German authorities who tried Heissmeyer twenty years later judged that this would-be professor had rendered his experiments "devoid of any scientific quality."[94] Indeed, Heissmeyer himself realized the futility of his work by fall 1944, but he still wanted to push on so he could write his *Habilitation* thesis.[95] So he topped off this ghastly series by injecting twenty Polish-Jewish children, aged four to twelve and all delivered from Auschwitz, with the bacilli. In April 1945, however, when time was running out and the murderous evidence had to be destroyed in a hurry, he had them all killed by poison or hanging.[96]

Johann Paul Kremer already was a professor of medicine in Münster when he came to Auschwitz to function as a camp physician in August 1942. He had been an SS member since 1932. His problem was an inferiority complex; for although in 1942 he was close to sixty years old and possessed two doctorates, he had still not been promoted beyond the rank of adjunct professor of anatomy. That did not sit well with this scientist, who thought the regime owed him something because he had been the first Nazi party member of the entire teaching body of his university in 1932.[97] In Auschwitz Kremer participated in selections for the gas chamber, but he also sampled "live-fresh material from human liver, spleen and pancreas" for hunger research, excised from specially chosen prisoners after they had been killed just for that purpose.[98] Back in Münster in early 1943, Kremer was hoping to be rewarded for his efforts with a regular chair in hereditary biology, only to be sorely disappointed. Increasingly, he regarded himself as the victim of intrigues at the university. As he saw it, he was "gradually getting on the nerves of the gentlemen at the university because of my scientific record and my years-long activities in the party. They have a very bad conscience." He wanted to use his "Auschwitz material" to force his colleagues into a full recognition of his worth as a scholar, perhaps by authoring a book under the title "Histological Regression."[99]

Sigmund Rascher, a doctor's son, was thirty years old in spring 1939 when he toiled in the comparably humble job of assistant physician at Munich's famous Schwabinger Krankenhaus. In April he met Himmler, who took an interest in his cancer research to the extent of allowing him to use Dachau concentration camp facilities in an effort to switch from animal to human experiments. The doctor's oncological work was intermittently hampered by his conscription to the Luftwaffe just before the war, but Rascher maintained contact with the SS. By early February 1942 he had been conveniently stationed in Munich and was beginning terminal experiments on men in special pressure chambers to help develop the wherewithal for combating the usual difficulties pilots experienced at great heights. This research, which lasted until May and caused the deaths of upward of one hundred Dachau inmates, many pursuant to vivisection, was jointly sponsored by the Luftwaffe and SS. By August Rascher was involved in freezing tests that caused death to about ninety prisoners and terrible pain to some two hundred others. The point of it all was that Rascher, who meanwhile had been transferred to the Waffen-SS, was once again extremely eager to obtain his academic credentials for a high university position, and in this he was actively supported, for reasons of his own, by Himmler with his SS apparatus. A *Habilitation* to be based on Rascher's arcane "research" failed, however, first at Munich and then at Marburg and in Frankfurt, mostly because of the formal requirement that results be exposed to public scrutiny. When Rascher finally was set to join the SS professor August Hirt in Strassburg in early 1944, he was arrested (and later shot) by Himmler's men for having abducted babies.[100]

Dr. phil., Dr. med. Josef Mengele arrived in Auschwitz in May 1943, where he continued research he had begun as an assistant to Professor Otmar von Verschuer in Frankfurt in the late 1930s. While his mentor now held the prestigious chair at the Kaiser-Wilhelm-Institut in Berlin, Mengele collected organs from prisoners, often twins or dwarfs, such as heterochromatic eyeballs or unborn fetuses that he carved from his victims in the same manner as Kremer, to be sent on to Verschuer in Berlin. There is circumstantial proof that Professor Verschuer had commissioned Mengele to perform these acts and would reciprocate by facilitating the assistant's entry into the world of academe.[101] Mengele's scholarly goals were no secret to anyone who knew him at this time. He had an "overweening desire to become recognized as a great scientist," and his *Habilitation* was already on its way.[102]

2. The Mechanics and Essence of Faculty Politicization

Gerhard Wagner's first attempt at influencing medical faculties consisted of establishing platforms outside of the universities. But his second was to enter the universities. He had legally been enabled to do so early after Rudolf Hess's edict of September 6, 1933, prescribing that all medical faculties in the Reich consult Wagner in his capacity as head of German physicians. Wagner subsequently set up a network of stooges in each faculty coordinated by the Munich professor of dermatology Franz Wirz.[1] This caucus met for the first time in January 1934 to construct a long-term agenda. Those resolutions were implemented later, by an extension of this caucus, the party's own Commission on Higher Education (Hochschulkommission der NSDAP). It was established in July 1934 under Hess and included, among others, Alfred Rosenberg and Wagner, who quickly monopolized it. Its immediate purpose was to check on Bernhard Rust's Reich Education Ministry (REM), newly constituted on May 1. But although the commission's mandate was to control all university faculties, Wagner himself remained primarily interested in the medical schools—to effect the appointment of the party's own candidates. Thus still in 1934 thirty-four medical positions were filled at several of the Reich's medical faculties as a direct consequence of the commission's meddling, and to the obvious chagrin of the Berlin ministerial officials.[2]

One of the first university appointments Wagner managed with the aid of the more amenable Bavarian authorities was that of his Munich colleague and friend Dr. Walter Schultze, born in 1894, whose claim to party fame was that, as surgeon and first SA staff physician, he had treated Hitler's wrenched shoulder during the putsch of November 1923. In September 1934 Schultze, just anointed as Bavaria's health commissar, became adjunct professor of people's health at

Munich University. To underline the programmatic significance of this appointment, Wagner himself spoke, during Schultze's inauguration, of a precedent at Munich that would soon be followed at other medical faculties.[3]

Until now Wagner, with Walter Schultze at his side, had maneuvered himself into a commanding position to exercise more power in medical faculty investments by launching candidates of his own as referees in the education ministry. Under Rust and his section leader in Amt Wissenschaft, responsible for all academic appointments,[4] the first head of the medical unit in 1934 was a certain Dr. Fricke, but because he stayed only a few months it is doubtful whether Wagner had sufficient opportunity to bring his weight to bear on him. Later in 1934, Fricke was replaced by Dr. Werner Jansen, a physician and author of light fiction with a *völkisch* flavor, who remained in the ministry till June 1937. That Jansen was a kindred spirit of Wagner is suggested by his preoccupation with ideas of New German Healing, such as hydrotherapy, "houses of health," and prophylactic methods, in proximity with "nature." Though never formally qualified, Jansen had been made a professor on the occasion of his nomination, which in itself serves as a comment on the ongoing politicization of the academic medical establishment.[5]

A genuine chance for Wagner to gain a foothold in the REM arrived in the summer of 1937, when a replacement for the ailing Jansen was sought. The choice of both the Reich physicians' leader and Schultze was Dr. Ernst Bach, a Munich gynecologist and another man after Wagner's own heart. Born in 1899, he had joined the imperial army in 1917 and emerged from the war with the rank of reserve lieutenant. In 1919–20 he was an active member of at least two Freikorps. Having founded one of Munich's early Nazi party chapters in 1922–23, Bach naturally took part in Hitler's Beer Hall Putsch. In 1925 he was licensed as a physician, and by 1930 he had completed his specialty training. In July 1933 this successful gynecological practitioner accepted Wagner's offer to become Bavarian representative of the Nazi Physicians' League. Two years later he had his *Habilitation* in place and was a *Dozent* at Munich's medical faculty. It is virtually certain that both Wagner and Schultze were responsible for that appointment, for by publicly rhapsodizing about naturopathic medicine Bach had made sure to please Wagner, and Schultze in accord with Wagner suggested his friend's name for the Berlin post.[6] But Wagner, too, intervened heavily with the ministerial officials on Bach's behalf.[7] Henceforth Bach could justly regard himself as the physician leader's "confidant in matters of the university."[8]

Bach assumed his Berlin duties in the spring of 1938, and although there was consensus that his academic qualifications were no better than "average," he, too, through Schultze's special prompting, was elevated to a titular professorship.[9] After some strenuous manipulation that posting was changed to a full chair in gynecology at Marburg, replete with university clinic directorship, in autumn 1939.[10] Wagner, who in November 1937 had frankly admitted to Rust's deputy

Otto Wacker that he had a stake in "the training of medical students and in continuing medical education,"[11] had little opportunity to avail himself of Bach's services because he died in spring 1939. Nonetheless, as will be shown below, political appointments in the medical faculties were made consistently throughout Wagner's tenure as Nazi head of the German doctors—whether under Wirz or through the Hochschulkommission, Schultze's additional office as Reich lecturers' leader (since July 1935),[12] or through Jansen or Bach directly. One of the last and potentially most far-reaching actions Wagner undertook in medical school affairs was to channel into the regular student body promising natural lay healers, some of them on special scholarships, who would be sure to safeguard the ideals of New German Healing in a formal academic setting.[13]

Under Leonardo Conti and still before World War II, a new era in the regime's health policy was ushered in, one of whose telling features was, much unlike the case of Wagner, the relative absence of party prerogatives and the proximity of the health administration, now formally an integral part of the Reich interior ministry, to Himmler's SS.[14] Also important in this new constellation was moving the Reich physician leadership offices from Munich to Berlin, which decreased the influence of someone like Schultze in academic medical planning, for he was a creature more of the party and SA than the Black Shirts.[15] And although it was Himmler's wont to disclaim any interest in the Reich's universities and specifically in the affairs of the medical faculties, he is known to have cared a great deal about what transpired in seminars and classrooms and what sort of scholar should be appointed to a teaching position.[16]

Thus, although the exact circumstances of Bach's departure from the Berlin ministry are not known, it is at least likely that the termination of his ministerial duties was connected with the death of Wagner. For in early 1940 the gynecologist was replaced by Dr. Max de Crinis, professor of psychiatry at Berlin University's teaching hospital Charité and a man not only acceptable to Reich Health Leader Conti but also tied to the SS. Moreover, as successor in Karl Bonhoeffer's chair de Crinis was a nationally respected scholar, quite the opposite of Ernst Bach.[17]

De Crinis, born in 1889 in Austrian Steiermark into a doctor's family, had undertaken his early medical as well as his specialty training in Graz; by 1924 he was an associate professor of neurology there. Ten years later he received an offer for a full chair in Cologne. This offer must have been very welcome because this physician, too, had exposed himself for years on the extreme rightist political fringe, in this case on the side of the pan-German Schönerer movement that clamored for union with Germany. As such, like so many early Austrian followers of Hitler, de Crinis was persecuted by Vienna's clerico-fascist regime, possibly for having participated in the futile July 1934 Nazi coup that killed Chancellor Engelbert Dollfuss. The psychiatrist moved to Berlin in early 1939.[18]

An entry in his personnel records attests that de Crinis had been "a well-known pioneer in the anti-Semitic realm," and indeed, beyond the apex of the war this doctor, whom contemporaries have described as firm but charmingly sociable,[19] remained ferociously committed to the fight against Jews, especially in medicine.[20] This may explain his early links with the SS, whose ranks he joined in 1936. More precisely, he became a member of the Security Service of the SS, the SD (Sicherheitsdienst), whose chief for extranational affairs, the younger Walter Schellenberg, he soon befriended like a father.[21] No doubt it was Schellenberg, well liked by Himmler, who facilitated repeated meetings with the Reichsführer-SS, for since the beginning of his service in the REM in spring 1940 de Crinis was thought of as having a special value for the SD.[22] By the end of 1943, at least, the SS Security Main Office (RSHA) was convinced that the psychiatrist had discreetly worked for the SD "with optimal success."[23]

Until the end of the war, de Crinis virtually single-handedly pulled the strings behind any medical appointments in the nation's university faculties. He did so craftily with a blend of uncanny instinct and disarming logic. First he used his personal prestige as a scholar to insist on appointments of his own choice, dictating to the deans of faculties if no agreement with them could be reached.[24] Yet ideally he always sought to satisfy those faculties; that was his second virtue.[25] Third, he quickly put to work whatever information came his way, and for years he maintained a close relationship with his predecessor and friend, Ernst Bach.[26] And fourth, to benefit the regime this fanatical Nazi truly believed in, he loyally served its ends, shrinking from nothing, and that included placing politics before science. Thus de Crinis contributed, in his own peculiar way, to the ongoing deterioration of academic medical standards in the universities that became a major theme of the period.[27]

Leonardo Conti's own input into this machinery was limited not because there were insurmountable differences between himself and de Crinis (in fact, there may not have been any), but because his administration could not coordinate the various facets of public health until the very end. Formally, Conti's position was in the interior ministry, not the ministry of education. Hence Werner Forssmann's claim that Conti offered him prospects for *Habilitation* as early as 1939 is probably spurious.[28] Timid efforts by Conti to obtain a stronger say in medical faculty appointments early in 1943 led nowhere.[29] By the time Conti had been effectively surpassed as chief health officer by Professor Karl Brandt around the summer of 1943, Conti's political edge had been blunted beyond repair. If on anyone, it now would be incumbent on whoever Brandt chose as his delegate to take an interest in these matters. And indeed, there was such a person: the surgeon Professor Paul Rostock of the Berlin faculty, but he got along well with de Crinis.[30]

Himmler's determination to exert some influence on academic medical appointments was nurtured by a twofold interest in medicine: he sympathized with naturopathic methods and hence was close to the ideals of Wagner's New German

Healing, but beyond that he saw the potential of applied medicine through experiments for his SS, especially after the beginning of the war, and increasingly by way of the "human material" that his own camps could provide. Because he knew the traditional medical professoriate to have scruples in this area, he would best be served by implanting within the faculties men of the Black Order whom he could totally trust.[31]

The Reichsführer's manipulative touch in academic medicine proved to be a deft one. He closely watched the process during which Ernst Bach was appointed as Jansen's successor in the REM, giving his own approval only after the ministry's bureaucrats had seen fit to report to him.[32] Through his SS apparatus he patronized the eminent internist Professor Alfred Schittenhelm, who had moved from Kiel to Munich in 1934 and became a Black Shirt one year later.[33] Similarly, Wilhelm Pfannenstiel, a professor of hygiene in Marburg who had once studied at Oxford and joined the SS at age forty-four in 1934, was turned into a stool pigeon of Himmler's. In his case, the SS's intentions are perfectly clear from a letter penned in December 1936 by Josias Erbprinz zu Waldeck-Pyrmont, Himmler's deputy for the Fulda-Werra jurisdiction, which urged that the REM be asked once more "what the state of Dr. Pfannenstiel's investiture as rector of Marburg University is."[34] By early 1939 Pfannenstiel had fulfilled some of Himmler's scientific expectations by having tested a method for the preservation of bread, to be tried in the field by regular SS units.[35] During the war Pfannenstiel officiated as a hygienics adviser in the Waffen-SS, and such consulting work even took him to the annihilation camp of Belzec, where he witnessed the gassing of Jews.[36] It was Schittenhelm in Munich and Pfannenstiel in Marburg who were to push through Dr. Rascher's *Habilitation* so that this ambitious experimenter could be widely supported by the SS "by being instated into a lectureship or even a professorship."[37] In 1942 Himmler was also very interested in launching the Frankfurt radiologist, Professor Hans Holfelder, who had x-rayed hundreds of his SS men for the detection of tuberculosis, into an appropriate chair at the new university of Posen.[38]

Moreover, Himmler most certainly obtained access to some medical faculty politics through such regional Nazi Lecturers' League representatives as anatomy professor and SS leader Enno Freerksen of Kiel University, who were coterminously informers for the SD; for the Lecturers' League still had a modest say in appointments.[39] As late as January 1945 Himmler wanted to ensure that his favorite candidate, *Dozent* Dr. Bernward J. Gottlieb of his own SS medical academy in Graz, receive the soon to be vacated, prestigious chair in the history of medicine at Berlin, protesting all the while that he had no intention of meddling in the affairs of Reich Education Minister Rust.[40]

This example and those of Rascher and perhaps Mengele show that Himmler was not merely dependent on university insiders who could be drafted into his SS, but that he also could reverse that process by turning his own men into university academics. Indeed, beneficial to Himmler's interests, the three chief medical officers of the SS were, at one point or another in their political careers, named to professorships, although their actual university obligations remained little more than perfunctory.

The internist Ernst Robert Grawitz, born in 1899, son of the noted Berlin hematologist Professor Ernst Grawitz,[41] and, according to Göring, once a student activist on behalf of the incipient Nazi movement, became Himmler's chief SS physician in May 1935. In December 1941 he was created, presumably at Himmler's behest, an honorary professor at the University of Graz. Himmler may have regretted this appointment, for he often found Grawitz, who not only coordinated experiments on humans but also messed about with them himself, wanting as a scientist, even by his own weird standards.[42] Further, Joachim Mrugowsky, once an undernourished, struggling student[43] and Grawitz's chief hygienist during the war, first became a *Dozent* in 1941 and then, in September 1944, an adjunct professor at Berlin University.[44]

Neither Grawitz nor Mrugowsky appears to have bothered to secure a certificate of *Habilitation*,[45] but that was not so with the last member of this trio, Dr. Karl Gebhardt. Besides the SS sanatorium that he directed at Hohenlychen, he became Grawitz's uppermost SS surgeon and in 1943 SS chief clinician. Ironically, though he probably was the most qualified physician of the three, he also, through odious and totally unnecessary bone transplants and other experiments on camp inmates, became the most notorious.[46] Born in 1897, this school chum of Himmler for a while trained with Sauerbruch in Munich and had his *Habilitation* as a surgeon in hand in 1932. He became a prominent expert in sports and accident medicine, treating, among others, the king of Belgium in 1937. In that year he already was a full professor in the medical faculty of Berlin, after he had sworn himself to the SS in 1935, at the initial unusually high rank of major.[47]

Knowing that ordination by the SS was perhaps the shrewdest method to ensure professional success, several aspiring medical scholars took care to enroll not only in the party but also, and especially, with the Black Shirts. A case in point is the surgeon Friedrich ("Fritz") Hartmann, born in 1900, who had a less than perfect academic vita but a polished political record. Like de Crinis, Hartmann was an Austrian with a formidable (illegal) Nazi past, for he belonged to the radical fringe of the right-wing, pro-Hitler Steirischer Heimatschutz. While studying medicine in Graz he began to worry about "the preservation of the German and Aryan character of the student body and the universities in the face of undue Catholic and Jewish influence in Austria." After graduation in 1923, Hartmann went to Tübingen as an assistant to Professor Wilhelm Trendelenburg. He joined Sauerbruch's team at Munich University in 1926 and was taken to Berlin by him in 1928.[48] In 1936 Hartmann, with Sauerbruch's help, received his *Habilitation* and a *Dozentur* there.[49] But arguably more important, by that time Hartmann had already spent three years in the SS. The Black Shirts greatly valued him "because he is in constant close contact with the National Socialists in Austria." In 1935 the surgeon had completed the obligatory political training for university lecturers as "probably the best man of the course, ideologically speaking." His party membership was secure by 1938.[50] The combination of unwavering support by his superior Sauerbruch and flawless SS connections produced for Hartmann, predictably, a Berlin adjunct professorship in July 1941, forced through prematurely against more qualified competitors. His unfair advantage is implied in the carefully worded opinions of two medical authorities, who judged Hartmann's tangible academic achievements little more than mediocre.[51] Such verdicts notwithstanding, Hartmann remained Professor Sauerbruch's protégé until the end of the war.[52]

Several more examples could be cited, demonstrating that in the Third Reich academic dullness was no impediment to career progress if skillfully paired with Himmler's political power. With the SS looming in the background, success could be counted on, as experienced by yet another assistant to Sauerbruch, Max Madlener, two years older than Hartmann, party member in 1933, SS trooper in 1934, and adjunct professor of surgery in Düsseldorf in 1940.[53]

The crassest but also the most ironic case in this category, however, is that of the surgeon Kurt Strauss. For it shows that if the political factor was grossly exaggerated, then by the Nazi physicians' own criteria of the survival of the fittest, literally, the unfit had to go under, not, unfortunately, without having done mountains of damage. Strauss, too, could look back on a long personal history of political violence in the ranks of the Nazi movement, and by that movement's honor code he was entitled to compensation for the sacrifices he had endured.[54] As early as 1932 Strauss was good friends with Conti and Robert Ley; somewhere along the way, he also had found his place in the SS. On the basis of a pitiful slate of publications yet with a plethora of tricks, this physician managed to get his *Habilitation*. It was a dubious feat for a man whom Nobel prize winner Werner Forssmann, his erstwhile assistant, has recently described as a butcher always skirting litigation, a habitué of parties, and a woman-chaser.[55] Early in the war Strauss was provisionally entrenched in a full chair at Prague University, but in addition he directed an institute of his friend Ley for the reconstitution of wounded and disabled men. Here he fell into trouble by misappropriating resources, exploiting his wards, and suspicion of marriage fraud. Back home in the education ministry, de Crinis, beset by personnel problems, was still searching for an elegant way to relocate this generally disliked surgeon, whom he credited with some ability, possibly to Münster.[56] Then, in the fall of 1944, disaster struck. As Strauss was awaiting court-martial for his various malefactions, Himmler first had him demoted and then expelled from his order. Shortly thereafter, Strauss's life ended in a jail cell, expunged by his own hand.[57]

Membership in the SS was the most reliable means of achieving a teaching job in the universities, with much better than average prospects for an eventual full chair. Conversely, previous or existing ties with organizations not aligned to National Socialism, be they of a political or religious nature, could result in a candidate's being overlooked for an appointment or, perhaps worse, in summary dismissal, if the position predated Hitler's coming to power. Although there were not many of them, non-Jewish teachers of medicine were known to have fallen victim to the so-called Law for the Reconstitution of the German Civil Service of April 7, 1933, or subsequent, related legislation.[58] Hence realists with strong ambitions had to make overtures to the regime to avoid even the slightest suspicion of political disloyalty. After all, competition had been fierce since the days of the republic; in 1932 it had been well publicized that statistically, only one of seven medical lecturers could expect an offer for a full-time, tenured post.[59]

In those circumstances, pressures to conform and court the powers that be naturally affected the younger academics more than the older and established ones. At teaching clinics and university medical departments, assistant physicians and lecturers with an eye on a regular chair after January 30, 1933, would therefore suddenly be seen to flaunt formal Nazi affiliations that might have much embarrassed them in prior years.[60] Others were quick to learn that the Nazi Lecturers' League, in which physicians tended to proliferate,[61] was soon exerting its routine influence on even the most junior of academic appointments and adjusted themselves accordingly.

Examples of pronounced Nazi behavior by young academic hopefuls eager to rival and perhaps supplant their older, more experienced teachers abounded early in the regime, especially if those teachers were Jewish. Thus in Tübingen, the entire corps of medical faculty assistants joined the SA in May 1933. In Berlin the NSDAP was favored for membership along with the SA, and at year's end the overenthusiastic among the assistant doctors compared Hitler to the ancient god Wotan in a Christmas celebration. At Bonn University some assistants commenced to intrigue against their superior, the (non-Jewish) dermatologist Erich Hoffmann, in the hope of ousting him. For those assistant physicians, collaboration with fanatical students often proved to be just as efficacious as backing from the Nazi Lecturers' League. Hence in Leipzig assistants and medical students in unison insisted on the execution of the Hitler greeting on all occasions, and in Freiburg medical students and assistants alike gathered around Nazi *Dozent* Otto Bickenbach, who in wartime would acquire infamy through concentration camp experiments on humans.[62]

Throughout the medical ranks, from the lowest to the highest, appointments now tended to be made on the basis of political criteria, and of obviously younger men, so much so that the West German historian Hans Schadewaldt's verdict that new faculty continued to be chosen "solely for objective reasons" borders on distortion.[63] The preeminent case of Heinrich Wilhelm Kranz has already been dealt with.[64] Others in that category were Heinz Kürten, Willy Usadel, Johannes Stein, and Heinrich Hoffmann. Kürten, born in 1891, began his scholarly career in Halle, where he was a *Dozent* for internism in 1925. Engulfed, like Kranz, in *Rassenkunde*, he organized continuing education courses in race hygienics and assisted in the purge of Jewish colleagues from the Halle faculty. Not surprisingly, Kürten became a tenured professor at Munich University one year later.[65] The surgeon Usadel, three years younger than Kürten, had been a *Dozent* in Tübingen in 1928 and in 1933 was a hospital chief in Berlin. Usadel was fortunate to have an influential brother in the party hierarchy, was himself a party member since 1931, and had publicly supported Hitler just before the precarious Reichstag elections of November 1932. Therefore he was appointed full professor in Tübingen in 1934, over the heads of two better-qualified colleagues and despite the cautious judgment of his peers that he did not enjoy the measure of collegial "confidence" necessary for such a chair.[66] Johannes Stein has been described by Karl Jaspers, psychiatrist and philosophy professor in Heidelberg, as a "fanatical National Socialist." At Ludolf von Krehl's funeral on June 18, 1937, SS and party member Stein, who had a solid reputation as an anti-Semite, roundly condemned the enemies of Nazism and intoned a hymn in honor of race science. These remarks were designed to assure the National Socialist authorities of his own continued loyalty. For in March 1934 Stein, an associate professor since 1931, had inherited Krehl's chair and had become the university's vice-rector in 1935—a decidedly political appointment.[67] Similarly, psychiatrist Heinrich Hoffmann harvested the fruits of early anti-Semitism and timely party entrance when he was called from Giessen to Tübingen to serve as its leader-rector in fall 1937.[68]

A sensitive issue even by contemporary criteria, but nevertheless indicative of the high degree of Nazi infiltration suffered by the medical schools at that time, was the *ad hominem* investiture with professorial honors of party men without any formal postgraduate qualifications whatsoever. Such appointments, amounting to sinecures, were given on the strength of the candidates' Old-Fighter status and Hitler's prerogative as the nation's leader-president, usually on the recommendation of Wagner and his entourage. Doctors Wilhelm Holzmann, Kurt Klare, and Hermann Boehm are examples.

General practitioner Wilhelm Holzmann, who had established the Nazi Physicians' League in Hamburg late in the republic, was rewarded with a professorship in 1933.[69] Kurt Klare, the *völkisch* lung specialist and cofounder of the NSÄB and an aide to Wagner, became an adjunct professor first in Munich in 1935 and in 1940 accepted a similar offer from Münster.[70] Retired *Amtsarzt* Hermann Boehm's merits extended even farther. A veteran of the 1923 Munich Beer Hall Putsch, he too became instrumental in the early Nazi Doctors' League. After having been named a staff member of the naturopathic Rudolf Hess Hospital in Dresden in 1934, Boehm became a professor of *Rassenkunde* in neighboring Leipzig a year later. Active in the Nazi training camp Alt-Rehse, this Old Fighter thereupon was thought to be sufficiently well-rounded to advise in the nomination of new chair holders and was himself on a short list for a chair in Strassburg during World War II.[71]

Clearly, the regime leaders expected medical faculty to enter into some relationship with party and state if they wanted to sustain a career, even though they could be thoroughly despised for doing so. Near the end of the war the SD observed sarcastically that the most prolific of the medical teachers "had learned only one thing from National Socialist problems, namely to be in the party, in order to show to outsiders that they know how to go with the times."[72]

After proper identification, the above-mentioned cases of obviously compromised medical scholarship for political-careerist reasons all lend themselves to easy classification. Invariably, the men in question distinguished themselves through a smaller or greater mark of incompetence in their chosen field. It may even be possible to posit a negative correlation between competence and political involvement: the worse the man was as a scholar, the more likely his Nazi contamination.

But where does one draw the line between true pro-Nazi conviction and mere lip service to the regime, which could have manifested itself in some nominal Nazi affiliation? Mixed types are conceivable in cases in which a scholar of integrity outdid himself in demonstrations of pro-Nazi loyalty to protect his professionalism but at the same time sincerely accepted at least some of the precepts of National Socialism. Such behavior was typical for many of the ordinary physicians as, indeed, it was for the educated elite and even the other layers of German society, especially before the war.[73] In attempting to grasp the essence of this problem, the historian is hampered by the appearance of conflicting evidence pertaining to prominent professors in their personal reminiscences and their official dossiers.

One may take Professor Oswald Bumke, for instance. In his postwar memoirs, this retired Munich psychiatrist expends a great deal of energy on the exorcism of the Nazi ghost. Those passages culminate in the contemptuous characterization of a polyclinician who, in a university lecture, confronts his students with a picture of Hitler, to be employed as a last source of inspiration after all other diagnostic tools have failed. Yet, tucked away in some obscure publication, there is a remarkably different statement by Bumke. When this same internationally renowned scholar presided at the convention of the Society of German Neurologists on September 27, 1934, after reviewing the years of the republic just gone by, he spoke the following sentences: "Gentlemen, today we have gathered in quite another Germany. Today once again each German heart is filled with hope. But this time around it is not the last onset of a people slowly tiring, but an uprising that has definitively lifted the whole of Germany out of the timidity of the postwar years, an uprising that will fortify us once more, after earnest application, internally as well as externally."[74] This was not reticence, neutrality, or naive lip service—it was a heartfelt homily to the new regime. In fact, those remarks suspiciously approximate the officious loyalty declarations of reliable Nazi rectors put in place for that very purpose, for example that of oral clinician Johannes Reinmöller, who greeted his colleagues in November 1933 in Erlangen, invoking the Führer in every other sentence.[75] Upon closer examination of Bumke's career one finds that his brand of psychiatry was not out of joint with Nazi conceptions justifying criminal eugenic manipulation and that this professor actually endorsed the law of July 14, 1933, for the prevention of hereditarily diseased offspring.[76] Indeed, younger West German critics have described Bumke, once an objective scientist, as a "champion of fascist psychiatry."[77]

In their recognition of at least a partial commitment to the Nazi cause, it is evident that for the sake of survival in a new democratic Germany after 1945, or merely for saving face, some medical academics have suppressed or misrepresented their former allegiance, making it difficult for the modern historian to sort out the truth. In his memoirs, Bonn emeritus Erich Hoffmann goes to great lengths to detail machinations against him by invidious younger faculty and, like Bumke, to deplore the Hitler regime.[78] But according to several passages at the beginning of his book he appears to have taken many facets of the "revolution" in the "fatherland" seriously, until it allegedly got out of hand, without informing the reader how extensive his initial empathy for the Nazis really was and how exactly he was converted.[79] Hoffmann lightly brushes over the fact that along with three hundred colleagues he had lent fatal credibility to the dictatorship in March 1933 by affixing his signature to a document putting trust in Hitler's new government and pledging energetic support, a document made nationally public in the *Völkischer Beobachter*.[80] But the reader has no way of knowing if Hoffmann did not seriously believe in his action, which implied a strong commitment to anti-Semitism and anti-Marxism, at the time.

Also deleting essential facts or withholding proper explanations are the West German senior scholars Werner Forssmann, the urologist and Nobel laureate, Hans Bürger-Prinz, the Hamburg psychiatrist, and Ferdinand Hoff, the internist. Forssmann obfuscates the issue of his pro-Nazi loyalties by emphasizing the Nazi implications of others, such as his former superior Kurt Strauss, and, correspondingly, by making light of his own party involvement. The circumstances of his party entry purposely remain shrouded in darkness. In the original German version of his memoirs Forssmann never alludes to them—instead the reader is suddenly confronted with the physician's NSDAP membership as a given by autumn 1933. In the English-language version, which was published two years later, there are totally new sections, intimating among other things that Forssmann may have joined the Nazis before 1934, but this particular passage is marked by a distinct lack of clarity. The truth is that Forssmann joined Hitler's party in August 1932, when no one was compelled to do so, but after auspicious

Nazi electoral victories in July. As both versions of the book move on, the party is belittled as an unavoidable nuisance but nevertheless something that did not come to be a bother, and Forssmann's SA obligations, too, are played down.[81] Forssmann chooses to say nothing at all about his membership in the Nazi Physicians' League, which today is evident from his Physicians' Chamber card.[82]

In instructive episodes from his rich and varied life as one of Germany's foremost psychiatrists Bürger-Prinz ruminates on all manner of psychosomatic disorders but neglects to explain why he commented favorably on "hereditary psychoses" in 1935, in the spirit of the hereditary legislation just passed.[83] Moreover, the psychiatrist recalls the circumstances of his installation as full professor in Hamburg in 1936–37 but studiously avoids the question of whether that appointment was not, perhaps, the consequence of his having joined the NSDAP in May 1933, as well as the SA—seeming biographical trifles that are self-servingly omitted from his volume.[84] As well, Bürger-Prinz conveniently deletes that part in his vita which proves knowledge of psychiatric killings and connivance at the escalation of penal servitude for "asocial" juveniles, who could be assigned to interminable incarceration. "Euthanasia" murderer Werner Heyde (whose illegal "Dr. Sawade" existence Bürger-Prinz would shield after 1945) and Hans Heinze, the Brandenburg penitentiary psychiatrist, were privy to this scheme, and members of the Swing Youth, jazz fans in Bürger-Prinz's hometown of Hamburg, were potential victims.[85] Neither does this psychiatrist disclose his inglorious role in the Degkwitz affair. When Bürger-Prinz's pediatric colleague Rudolf Degkwitz was indicted for "defeatism" in late 1943, the psychiatrist, then dean of his medical faculty, instead of attempting to intervene on Degkwitz's behalf, wrote demurely to Commissar Brandt's deputy: "Prof. Degkwitz has indeed been arrested by the Gestapo because of defeatist writings or talk. As far as I have been able to ascertain, he will be put on a regular trial. We are certainly not counting on seeing him in the faculty again." Instantly, Bürger-Prinz began looking for Degkwitz's replacement.[86] By the strength of the formula that in Third Reich academia politics was somehow inversely related to science Bürger-Prinz's own political background suddenly is struck in stark relief, for during that period there was no clear consensus on his scholarly merits. At least in one expert opinion as late as 1944, Bürger-Prinz was thought to be "a very nice man" but "not significant as a scholar."[87]

Ferdinand Hoff, too, produces an impressive record as a medical scientist, who, well qualified from republican days, after 1934 advanced quickly from one university to the next, always bettering himself, and all on the strength of objective contributions.[88] His personal file substantiates that he was unflaggingly respected by his peers and a perennial favorite with the Berlin ministry.[89] Still, nowhere in his book is there the slightest suggestion that such progress could have been linked, however tenuously, to Hoff's own good standing in the Nazi movement. When those political ties are mentioned, they are rendered almost threadbare. Hoff convincingly stresses that there was a need for some political shielding because of his former, documented, membership in the German Democratic Party, but he defuses his own role in making contact with the Nazis. According to his published story, a colleague in 1933 suggested that Hoff join the SA in a perfunctory capacity, without having to assume any leadership duties. Later, in 1937, it was to have been this SA which filed a Nazi membership application on his behalf that turned out to be successful.[90] Evidence proves, however, that Hoff joined the Brown Shirts at the comparatively high rank of captain (*Hauptsturmführer*) in 1933 and that, judging from the party's files, he was active in his formation. When he exchanged SA incorporation for membership in the NSDAP, he received an "honorary discharge." Early on in Königsberg Hoff's wife was a local official in the NSV, which he himself had joined as well, and their two daughters were members of the BDM. Later, in Würzburg, Hoff willingly collaborated with the political study units (*Fachschaften*) by contributing lectures on New German Healing. Moreover, Hoff also belonged to the Nazi Teachers' League (many professors did for opportunistic reasons) and to the NS-Ärztebund. The Hoff family contributed generously to the frequent party collections—all of these symptoms of a much better than nominal Nazi status and neatly blanked out in Hoff's postwar memory.[91] Moreover, Hoff joined the party only after having "submitted an application for entry into the NSDAP," as is felicitously written in his papers, and not on the SA's suggestion. He was trusted as someone who "will, without reservation, act in the best interests of the National Socialist state at all times."[92] That was hardly the typical profile of a fellow traveler.

In this respect, perhaps the greatest enigma of all was the celebrated surgeon Ferdinand Sauerbruch, for though his physicianship was weighty, his pro-Nazi convictions appear to have been much stronger than has commonly been held. It is true that Sauerbruch made only three formal concessions to the new regime, which brought him benefits and much intraregime prestige: he accepted the title of state counselor (*Staatsrat*), allowed himself to be honored, along with Professor August Bier, a much more overt Nazi sympathizer, by accepting the Nazi substitute of the Nobel Prize, and officiated as surgeon-general for the Wehrmacht in wartime.[93] Never a party member, let alone an adept of the SA or the SS, Sauerbruch, a profoundly conservative monarchist at heart, ostentatiously forbade SA troopers to hoist a Nazi flag on the roof of his clinic. He also bore the brunt of vicious attacks by the party's expert on *Rassenkunde* Dr. Walter Gross for having upheld the ideals of the Great War and the traditional universities as a model for youth in the Third Reich.[94] In his teaching and as the innovative researcher that he was, Sauerbruch remained beyond reproach, despite idiosyncratic and, in interpersonal relations, frequently offensive mannerisms.[95]

It is also true, however, that even though the surgeon may privately have disliked Hitler and have gotten into arguments with pronouncedly National Socialist scholars,[96] he supported many of the political objectives of the new regime, including its aggressive anti-Western stance, the ideology behind the new official anti-Semitism (although he rejected its radical mode of execution), and some of the stereotypical views about organicist medicine.[97] Sauerbruch made clarion appeals to Germans and foreigners alike, attempting to explain to them the new Nazi policies and asking for sympathy and understanding, and thereafter he knowingly allowed his international prestige to be shabbily abused by Nazi propaganda.[98] He supported acolytes like Fritz Hartmann not least because his father was a pan-German in opposition to the Dollfuss regime, and Hartmann himself received pristine approval as a "long-standing" Nazi, "honest and politically true to the Führer and his state."[99] Despite what some modern historians have insinuated, Sauerbruch's contact with the representatives of the classic resistance to Hitler such as General Ludwig Beck and Colonel Claus Graf von Stauffenberg was also fleeting, even though it is likely that he was urged to make a much stronger commitment to the anti-Hitler cause.[100] The point, of course, is that he chose not to do so. On balance, then, the final verdict on Ferdinand Sauerbruch might well be one that could apply to a whole phalanx of lesser colleagues in the medical faculties: in the eyes of two recent West German analysts of the available evidence, he lived "in qualified agreement" with the Nazi state, "albeit vacillating."[101] Thus on several counts, for all its enigmatic characteristics, the figure of the master surgeon may aptly serve as a symbol for the ultimate dilemma of German medical scholars under Hitler, in the best and the worst of times.

3. Anti-Semitism, Resistance, and the Future of Medical Academia

For ideological reasons and because of the shortage of academic vacancies at the beginning of the Nazi regime, aspiring National Socialist teachers of medicine sought ways to rid themselves of Jewish colleagues who would be rivals for a university post. If this was generally in keeping with attitudes in other academic disciplines, the medical faculty, along perhaps with that of law and certain natural science departments such as physics, was singled out for especially severe treatment because here the proportion of Jewish instructors was particularly large. Exactly how large is still not known, but it was assuredly greater than the figure of approximately 17 percent for physicians as a whole.[1] As early as March 23, 1933, the Nazis were charging that "Jewish lecturers are dominating the chairs in medicine," and in his speech at the Reich Party Rally of September 1934 Dr. Wagner still maintained, probably in exaggeration, that half of the Berlin medical faculty was Jewish.[2]

The expulsion of Jewish assistants, lecturers, and professors of medicine from the universities began with the promulgation of the Law for the Reconstitution of the German Civil Service of April 7, 1933, on which subsequent ordinances were based. Jewish civil servants, including all university teachers of medicine, now were subject to immediate dismissal unless they had been in office before 1914, had fought in World War I, or had lost a father or son in that war. Medical teachers received the extra benefit of exemption if they had risked their lives in a quarantine camp for an epidemic. Salaries and pensions were to be paid only after a certain length of service and were, in any case, considerably scaled down, whenever they came due.[3] Compounding this body of legislation were other statutes, such as the Editor's Law of October 4, 1933, which forbade German-Jewish medical scholars to publish the results of their research in German books or journals.[4]

The speed with which the Jewish medicine instructors were let go could vary from state to state, as could the individual circumstances, for each state was to announce its own version of the April 7 edict and was free to interpret it in any way it saw fit, as were most universities.[5] Yet most expulsions had occurred by early 1934. Some professors were viciously treated before being dismissed, as happened to the internist Hermann Zondek, an associate professor at Berlin, who officially lost his right to lecture on September 5, 1933, after he had been harassed and his Jewish assistants beaten by the SA as early as March.[6] Internal medicine *Dozent* Hans Krebs, too, was immediately suspended in Freiburg (Baden) in mid-April and legally terminated by early July.[7] The gynecologist Egon Pribram, a *Dozent* since 1923, met with the same sudden fate at Giessen.[8]

Because in the Third Reich anti-Semitism in practice was always both a function of official state control and the result of nonmanipulated, populist spontaneity,[9] the purge of Jewish medical teachers was invariably accompanied by the insidiousness and expressions of private hatred on the part of "Aryans" who now stood to benefit. Weeks before the law of April 7 took effect, Dr. A. Nückel, a gynecologist once employed by Berlin's Frauenklinik Cecilienhaus, charged that the clinic's director, Jewish Professor Wilhelm Liepmann, who had dismissed him in 1932, was a notorious Marxist and intriguer, openly blaming the Nazis for the burning of the Reichstag a fortnight before.[10] Rudolf Nissen, Sauerbruch's favorite assistant and on his way out of Berlin in May 1933, on top of the decreed injury had to suffer insults from a former friend whom he had frequently helped out—significantly—in preparation for the *Habilitation*.[11] Sometimes professors who might have been suspect politically, or were disliked for any reason, were taken as Jewish by their colleagues and accosted.[12] Dr. Wagner's organized Nazi doctors approved of and shared in such detestable behavior. Professor Otto Lubarsch was a distinguished pathology professor in Berlin who out of a misguided sense of patriotism had turned to anti-Semitism and Hitler early, although he was a Jew himself. After the confused old man had died on April 1, 1933, thus avoiding a possibly ugly future, his memory was gratuitously smeared by the editors of *Ziel und Weg*, the National Socialist professional journal.[13]

For a few Jewish faculty physicians, legalized persecution at Nazi hands was deferred but not aborted. The Nuremberg Race Laws of September 1935 revoked the privileges of those formerly exempted because of veteran status.[14] Thereafter, the Anschluss of Austria in spring 1938 extended the injustices to an additional 28 professors and 120 lecturers.[15] By the time new *Habilitation* regulations had been announced on February 17, 1939, no person of Mosaic faith or Jewish ethnicity was entitled to certification as a university medical teacher.[16]

Just before World War II, then, a second, smaller group of proscribed Jewish medical scholars included the Heidelberg psychiatrist Willy Mayer-Gross, an associate professor, and the young assistant in psychiatry Karl Stern. Unique among his peers, Stern had enjoyed an American Rockefeller grant (and hence special protection) allotted to the Munich Kaiser Wilhelm Institute under the directorate of Nazi professor Ernst Rüdin.[17] In Halle, the neurologist Alfred Hauptmann, a full professor who had earned the Iron Cross and other medals in World War I and still was a military reserve physician, was ejected from the university in December 1935, after Hartmannbund and the KVD both insisted to the rector that he be discharged.[18] In Berlin the famous gynecologist Robert Meyer and in Frankfurt the equally noted dermatologist Karl Herxheimer, a fellow of several international learned societies, were acutely at risk.[19]

Paradoxically, as repercussions against the Nazi regime increased abroad because of its unfair treatment of the Jewish medical scholars, some of them of world renown,[20] foreign countries for reasons of their own were making it more and more difficult for those scholars to continue work at their medical colleges. There were virtually no faculty positions for medicine professors in Palestine, then under British administration.[21] England was one of the more generous nations in trying to accommodate younger and older medical researchers. Hans Krebs thus was welcomed first in Cambridge, then in Sheffield, and finally at Oxford; he became a British citizen in 1939, and for his discovery of the citric acid cycle (still in Nazi Germany) and seminal studies in nutrition he was awarded the Nobel Prize in 1953 and a knighthood five years later.[22] Mayer-Gross, too, succeeded in establishing himself in Britain, where he coauthored an important psychiatry text and pioneered the pace-setting psychiatric day-and-night clinics system.[23]

As Krebs has emphasized, the more theoretical a researcher's approach to medicine was, the better were his chances for a university position, at least in the favored Anglo-Saxon realm. For the United States, which was not as magnanimous as Britain, the surgeon Rudolf Nissen has corroborated this maxim.[24] In America, only the most distinguished Jewish personages could be certain of an uninterrupted university career; younger instructors, particularly those with a more practical inclination such as internists, became dependent on private practice, the establishment of which met difficulties because of licensure restrictions.[25] Among those who were to succeed at American universities eventually were Siegfried Thannhauser, the Freiburg internist, no doubt because he, too, had been supported by a Rockefeller grant for some time; by spring 1935 he was at

Tufts University in Boston.[26] The physiologist Rudolf Höber of Kiel, author of a respected textbook in the field but dismissed in April 1933, found a haven at the University of Pennsylvania Medical School when in his fifties.[27] That same faculty also received Heidelberg Professor Otto Meyerhof, yet another physiologist and Nobel laureate (1922), who before the Third Reich had supported the much younger Krebs.[28] Berlin Professor Robert Meyer was seventy-five when he was offered a faculty position in Minneapolis in 1939.[29]

Nissen started practicing surgery in New York in 1941, after years of tenure as a professor in Istanbul, where he and several other German-Jewish scholars, among them the gynecologist Wilhelm Liepmann and the ophthalmologist Joseph Igersheimer, had helped to restructure that Turkish university in the modern spirit of Kemal Pasha.[30] A few Jewish medical teachers were able to immigrate to Switzerland or some Balkan country, though none of them had realistic prospects for a university chair.[31]

In the end, only a handful of not wholly Jewish medical scholars or Jews married to "Aryan" German women were allowed to stay in the Reich, but if they worked in universities at all, it was in humiliating circumstances. Friedrich Löning, whose faith was Lutheran but whose paternal grandfather had been Mosaic and who himself had served in the Great War as a staff physician, was pensioned off as an associate professor of internal medicine while still in his fifties, and he even stopped keeping office hours in Bavarian Schongau.[32] Robert Oppolzer, one-quarter Jew and a decorated veteran of World War I, was needed as a surgeon at the University of Vienna early in 1940, when his colleagues were being drafted for the front. "All the physicians of the clinic, who are, without exception, members of the party, the SS or the SA, have petitioned to retain Dr. Oppolzer."[33]

Even if the inadvertent irony of this official statement today is vexing, it assuredly did more for this assistant physician and his family of four than any order for compulsory labor in the armaments industry could have done. Other German physicians incorporated within Nazi formations, not excluding academic ones, probably were pleased that those fully Jewish medical teachers who had remained in the Reich till the height of the war now were either in concentration camps or in the process of being "evacuated" to the East, destined for liquidation. The exact number of Jewish instructors of medicine who were ultimately murdered is not known. At least two teachers of the Berlin faculty were in that group, the dermatologist Abraham Buschke and the internist Hermann Strauss, and possibly a third one, the pathologist Ludwig Pick.[34] Frankfurt's Karl Herxheimer, who had refused to accept exile abroad, also became a victim, as did Giessen's Professor Soetbeer, who after arrest by the Gestapo killed himself in his cell in March 1943.[35] In the end, Germany may have lost as many as 40 percent of its medical faculty to racist fanaticism; the harm to science and education was unfathomable.[36]

Nevertheless, however disturbing this piece of medical history is for the modern reader, it must also be emphasized that not all German-"Aryan" professors of medicine agreed with the anti-Semitic policy of the Third Reich and that some expressed disapproval or even opposition. Most effectively, this would be done collectively, as is alleged to have happened in Marburg, where the pediatrician Professor Ernst Freudenberg was to be dismissed because of his Jewish wife. The entire medical faculty intervened with the Reich education ministry, though to no avail.[37] In Heidelberg, Dean of Medicine Richard Siebeck sent a submission to that ministry as early as April 1933, in which he maintained that even though it was necessary for academic teachers to be "of German stock and German spirit," it was self-evident that "German Jews take part in advances of science and that great medical personalities have emerged from their midst." A few months later Siebeck was removed as dean by the new Führer-rector and nothing more was heard of this petition.[38] Similar attempts were made at Düsseldorf, with similarly pathetic results.[39]

Political protest was not, of course, confined to the Jewish issue. In Bonn the medical faculty desired to entrust the psychiatrist Hans Walther Gruhle, already an associate professor, with a full chair. Gruhle, known as an opponent of the sterilization laws, was rejected by the Berlin ministry, reportedly after Ernst Rüdin of Munich had wielded his influence in summer of 1934. In October the Bonn faculty tried again, citing Gruhle's popularity with students. But the Nazis wanted Kurt Pohlisch, who appeared to be much more malleable in sterilization matters. Gruhle was barred from university teaching until 1946.[40]

This raises, once again, the fundamental question of resistance on the part of doctors, this time those ensconced in academe. Munich's Oswald Bumke, a doubtful figure in any event, thought he had definitively dealt with it when he asserted, in reference to his own case, that anybody who dared to resist was dispatched to a concentration camp. "Certainly, one could have gone there, if anyone would have been served by that. But this was out of the question. If I, for instance, had disappeared—because of dismissal, consignment to a camp or an 'accident'—then someone else would have come along. The nurses would have been at large, the patients gassed, and the students would not have been educated to become what I would call physicians. I for one have never cared for Don Quixote and his pranks—except for those in the novel."[41]

Bumke illustrates his cynical argument with an example from his own career. He attempted to resign his chair some two weeks before the Röhm affair in June 1934 because of the appointment of the Czech charlatan Tirala to the Munich faculty.[42] Yet even if this were true, it would only prove that some teachers of medicine were insulted in their professional sensibilities by changes, some of them merely procedural, wrought by the new regime, rather than disturbed by ideological or ethical problems. That the former was indeed so is shown by the comportment of several of Bumke's colleagues. The Leipzig pediatrician

Werner Catel, who was a party member and collaborated in the "mercy-killing" of retarded children, quarreled with his dean, who was an inordinately fanatical Nazi and a friend of Gauleiter Martin Mutschmann, and Catel claims to have suffered endless party intrigues thereafter.[43] Psychiatrist Ernst Kretschmer at Marburg, too, complained about perpetual friction with his Gauleiter and lesser Nazi cadres whom he deemed to interfere in purely academic affairs, and though he was no friend of the regime, he applauded its "annihilative sterilization procedures," enjoyed a collegial relationship with arch-Nazi Rüdin, and, for some time at least, maintained institutional ties with the academically and politically ambiguous psychotherapy institute of Martin Göring.[44] Yet another member of that institute, Professor Johannes Heinrich Schultz, got into trouble with his Nazi boss Göring toward the end of the regime by being branded a "defeatist," but in itself this was no suitable political alibi for the culprit, who was, indeed, a member of the Nazi Motor Corps and had applied for membership in the party at least once.[45] One also has to examine with great care the motives of Münster radiologist Paul Krause, who demonstratively shot himself on May 7, 1934, for his "fatherland," on account of "the terrible terrorist pressure, the persecution, which is both unjust and superfluous."[46] If these words in Krause's suicide note sound passionately altruistic, it must be remembered that Krause had been a right-wing nationalist, a declared enemy of Marxism and Social Democracy, who had hailed the coming of fascism in Germany as a "deliverance." On the day Krause became an opponent of Nazism, "he was not motivated by an antifascist, democratic or ideological principle," writes one of his more perceptive biographers. Perhaps he was, after all, even to a high degree, but there also had been obnoxious machinations engendered by his immediate subordinate who wished to inherit his post, and Krause had remonstrated against some of Dr. Wagner's organizational measures as intolerably unprofessional.[47]

Humanly understandable, the powerful element of fear for one's safety or position closed the mouth of many a would-be opponent in the academics' ranks. The Viennese internist Professor Julius Bauer recollects how, after a scathing attack on Nazi "scientific" racism he had published in a prominent Swiss journal in 1935, he was excluded from the German Society of Internal Medicine and viciously smeared by Gerhard Wagner. Thereupon he did receive some sympathetic letters, transmitted secretly, from German university colleagues. But on the whole, Bauer writes, "no one could dare to stand up in public and declare his support for me, unless he wanted to lose his office, his freedom, or even his life."[48]

There were, however, teachers of medicine who risked not only their careers but also their lives for ethics, religion, or ideology. These were not scholars who would mention in their publications approvingly the feats of Jewish pioneers because even dyed-in-the-wool Nazis might still do so if it suited them.[49] Rather, this list would once again be topped by Marxists who unwaveringly acted out the precepts of their creed, although it was Russian-linked, which placed these scholars under the shadow of high treason.

Georg Groscurth was a *Dozent* for internal medicine at Berlin University and a friend of the noted chemist Robert Havemann. Through a resistance group named European Union he monitored information for the illegal KPD that he secured from patients in high places such as Rudolf Hess, but he also protected potential victims from Nazi encroachments. Groscurth was beheaded at forty years of age on May 8, 1944, after a show trial orchestrated by Roland Freisler's infamous People's Court.[50] The same fate befell Dr. John Rittmeister, two years older than Groscurth and, intermittently, a brilliant employee of Martin Göring's institute. Though he was not technically a full-fledged instructor of medicine, research for him was paramount, and he influenced a wide circle of Berlin students. Rittmeister, after having signed on with the communist organization Red Chapel, was found out by the Gestapo at the end of 1942 and executed in May of the following year.[51]

Other venerable men prevailed, albeit not of the communist persuasion. At Munich University in 1933, Max Lebsche worked as professor of surgery, much appreciated by senior colleagues such as Sauerbruch, who would have liked to take him to Berlin when he himself moved there in 1927. Lebsche was such a pious Catholic that he came to condemn the 1933 Concordat between the Vatican and Hitler, and when he was forced to make even nominal concessions he resigned from his post in protest.[52] Religious conviction also was the mainspring for the courageous actions of Freiburg pathologist Franz Büchner. In a continuing education lecture in 1941 he openly criticized the Third Reich's "euthanasia."[53] When in October 1942 Büchner attended a closed experts' meeting on human survival in extreme weather conditions, the villainous Dr. Rascher revealed details about his freezing experiments on humans. Büchner is reputed to have protested to his military superior in Berlin (Büchner was a consulting pathologist for the Wehrmacht), luckily with no apparent consequences for himself.[54]

Also apparently in this category of political opposition is Berlin pharmacologist Wolfgang Heubner, who grieved in a letter of December 1938 to the secretary of the Göttingen Academy of Sciences about the expulsion from that body of those members "who are Jewish or related to Jews by marriage" and asked to be removed from the membership himself. The sixty-one-year-old Heubner's specific mention of his own teacher, the Jewish Richard Willstätter, as being among the intended victims, made him truly stand out from among the large crowd of opportunists and pro-Nazi followers of the period.[55] Not surprisingly, Heubner later sought to snatch Dr. Groscurth from the fangs of the executioner.[56]

Equally intrepid, though expressing their anti-Nazi sentiment in different ways, were Professors Paul Schürmann, Emil Krückmann, and Rudolf Degkwitz. Berlin pathologist Schürmann taught his students constant adherence to the Hippocratic catechism. He practiced this philosophy when he was asked by the party to camouflage the exitus of Oranienburg (later Sachsenhausen) concentration camp inmates by issuing false death certificates. Schürmann instead indicated the real cause of death and consequently fell out of grace with the regime. He surrendered his university career and joined the Wehrmacht. In July 1941 he fell during action on the eastern front.[57] Berlin ophthalmology professor Krückmann, retired since 1934, during the persecution of the Jews kept on treating his non-"Aryan" patients, without charging them a fee and in the face of possible Nazi recriminations; he even visited some of them in prison.[58] Hamburg pediatrician Degkwitz, despite his early Nazi sympathies, came to loathe the Third Reich so overwhelmingly that he constantly risked critical remarks in the presence of his students until he, too, was tried by Freisler's court in February 1944. His life was spared only because his earlier research toward the prevention of measles was deemed epochal by his judges. Degkwitz survived the Third Reich in the penitentiary.[59]

Last to be counted among the opponents of the Hitler regime were those medical scholars who resisted sterilization and "euthanasia." The question of whether there were relatively few or many of them still is a matter of dispute, as may be the nature of the resistance rendered, at least in the eyes of some authors. Whereas Alice Platen-Hallermund, that early chronicler of Nazi medical abuses, in 1948 maintained that most full professors of psychiatry had "stayed away from 'euthanasia,' several even actively opposing it, though without success," Dirk Blasius, a more current expert, believes that the corps of psychiatric notables "emphatically backed the National Socialist legislation."[60] This paradox may be the result of irreconcilable assessments, yet it also seems to assume shape in the personality of Professor Karl Bonhoeffer, the nestor of German psychiatrists, who condemned medical killing but does not appear to have opposed sterilization with any consistency, if at all.[61] It is reasonably certain that in 1938 Frankfurt psychiatrist Professor Karl Kleist pronounced fearlessly on the deplorable physical and nutritional state of insane asylum inmates after having inspected them and later denounced "euthanasia" to his students.[62] Neither can it be discounted that Freiburg psychiatrist Kurt Beringer as late as November 1944 prevented his mentally deranged charges from being evacuated for purposes of annihilation, for this testimony comes from the redoubtable Franz Büchner.[63] Similar resistance, we are reliably informed, had been displayed by his Kiel colleague, Professor Hans Gerhard Creutzfeldt.[64]

The doubts and contradictions inherent in men of the caliber of Krause and, less so, Bonhoeffer, appear in others also and, if properly recognized, may help in preventing hasty judgments. Hence they illustrate how difficult a fair evaluation of the phenomenon of resistance, without consideration of all the motives and the entire prehistory of the persons involved, was and continues to be. Professor Gottfried Ewald has recently been mentioned as a psychiatric worthy who may, indeed, have been of two minds when he withdrew from the "euthanasia" project in August 1940 and, against express orders to do so, voiced his scorn for it. Customarily referred to as the resister par excellence of the medical profession,[65] Ewald has been found to have had an active World War I and Freikorps past and was originally a trusty National Socialist who applied for party membership, unsuccessful only because of the amputation of an arm in the war. He joined the SA reserve so as not to miss military maneuvers altogether and was rated in 1939 as "completely sympathetic to the aspirations of the NSDAP." Ewald may have been entirely selfish in his motives because he must have been painfully aware of his crippling condition. According to his wife, Ewald was afraid of concentration camp punishment at the time of his brave deed, but in 1944 he again stood in line for a chair in Strassburg, the SS-protected university. After the Nazi experience Ewald appeared to side with those erstwhile colleagues who were not indicted, and he may have destroyed self-incriminating records.[66] Whatever else the personal history of Gottfried Ewald might illuminate, it once again demonstrates the dangers inherent in painting the characters on the stage of Nazi medical academe either black or white.

In August 1940, when Ewald took his courageous stand, the future of the medical faculties already was very much in jeopardy. As with some other university disciplines, the problem harked back to the mid-1930s, when the vacancies created by the dismissal of so many able Jewish teachers had been filled with non-Jewish recruits, who were generally of lesser quality. By 1938 there existed a shortage of certified candidates for prestigious chairs in medicine demanding the greatest talent, but also at the lowest assistant levels, a shortage that had been aggravated because the rewards of an academic career seemed puny measured against onerous and expensive training and in comparison with what now was offered in private industry or in the various armed services. It was significant that in this year of 1938 the great Charité gynecologist Walter Stoeckel, sixty-seven years old, was asked by the Berlin ministry of education to carry on for another twenty-four months, for lack of a suitable successor.[67]

For the academic discipline of medicine the difficulties were further compounded by a relatively heavy acceleration in student enrollment even before the beginning of the war. Early in 1939 it became clear that certain subjects, such as race hygiene and history of medicine, could hardly be sustained with the staff available; in both fields officers of public health and specialists such as gynecologists, as well as a few bona fide professors, were doing all the teaching.[68] Additional signs of acute understaffing appeared when in the fall of that year, because of the war, the universities were threatened by the specter of closure, and some were temporarily shut down. By that time several medical deans, perhaps against better knowledge, scrambled to assure the Berlin education ministry that despite higher student numbers they still had enough instructors on hand to avoid the cancellation.[69] And yet, younger and older faculty were being conscripted at such an alarming rate and in such an uncoordinated fashion that the rector of the

University of Würzburg asked the Berlin authorities whether the planning needs of the universities could not be heeded more assiduously.[70]

Yet another complication arose regarding new medical faculties and academies that were the direct result of National Socialist imperialism in that they were being conceived in connection with newly to be founded institutions of higher learning in the conquered territories. Foremost among these were the Reich Universities in Strassburg and in Posen, to be opened under Nazi auspices in 1941.[71] Here the putative institutionalization of medical chairs, but even lesser posts, seriously countermanded the already strenuous attempts to keep positions in the core Reich filled.[72] To attract eligible staff for Strassburg, for instance, higher than average salaries were earmarked; but these, it was feared, would unnecessarily arouse greed in medical instructors everywhere.[73] In Posen, which was not generally popular with any but the politically most ambitious, it was anticipated as late as fall 1943 that for lack of qualified incumbents the chief physicians of the local hospitals might have to be appointed to full chairs—a horrifying vision for the conservative Berlin medical administrators.[74] Because it was nonsensical to entertain them in all seriousness, designs for extra medical schools in Cracow, Dresden, Klagenfurt, and Linz never left the drawing boards, for the Berlin ministry also had to accommodate the needs of the newly acquired faculty at Prague.[75]

Hence it did not require much shrewdness to observe, as Professor Rostock of Berlin did in July 1942, that in future years it would become ever more difficult to find personnel for the existing medical chairs, "unless we are prepared to lower the standard for our professors."[76] Already the standards had deteriorated, as had been roundly asserted in a widely circulated memorandum authored by Berlin's Professor Wilhelm Guertler, a prominent metallurgist, with specific inferences to be drawn for medicine.[77] Medical teachers continued to be drafted, and the casualties of dead or wounded at the fronts were making themselves felt. The medical schools were bartering for every staff member they could get. Not surprisingly, therefore, Professor Stoeckel needed little coaxing to agree to a further, indefinite stay.[78] Meanwhile, the end of 1942 had produced openings for almost every medical field, five in physiology alone.[79]

The year 1942 also marked the beginning of risky stopgap measures. At first it was decreed that university medical assistants at the fronts be allotted more time off so they could look after the requirements of their faculties.[80] Next it was considered to appoint foreigners to existing chairs, with "political reliability" as a natural precondition.[81] (Nationals of which Nazi satellites should have applied, one wonders. Belgians, Danes, or Bulgarians? Their countries also had problems.) As the military conscriptions of indispensable teaching personnel did not abate and many men appeared to be gone for good,[82] more and more professors long past their prime were being prevailed upon to remain at their posts, despite the potential consequences of such senescence.[83]

But the Berlin planners knew the other side of this shortage as well. In the capital in February 1944, at a time when resourceful academic recruits were scarce as never before, the physical and mental health of Wilhelm Trendelenburg, professor of physiology, was said to be critical. Sixty-seven years old and still not an emeritus, Trendelenburg was in such a state that he could not be approached; he was interested only in going for walks and playing his cello.[84] In Vienna at this time, the sixty-nine-year-old ophthalmologist Josef Meller was said to have passed his peak long ago and to be physically in bad form, and his equally old colleague, the internist Nikolaus Jagic, was judged "no longer capable of classroom instruction, what with his light-weight scholarship!"[85] For Meller, reported to have "neglected the direction of the clinic," a "more active" replacement was scheduled in the Vienna Academy of Sciences in the person of internist Professor Hans Eppinger, who had just turned sixty-five.[86] Indeed, by July 1944 one-third of all the medical instructors in the Reich had reached the conventional age limit of sixty-five.[87]

In the final twelve months of the Nazi regime many medicine professors died of old age or overexertion and suffered from hardship, self-ingested drugs, or air raids, and medical teaching was constantly hampered by the interruptions of war on the home front.[88] Not the least result of these conditions was that Germany fell fatally behind in basic research. One of the most devastating testimonies of this consequence of years of neglect was a document near the end of the war detailing the most urgent research needs. Of twenty-three essential items, penicillin was mentioned in third place.[89] Without straining anyone's credulity, it can be easily maintained that German mass production of this drug, which was available in the Reich in tiny quantities by 1944, would have delayed the Allied victory. Instead, penicillin and its application to war-related casualties had been invented and developed in Britain and the United States. One of the three men responsible for this historic feat was the Jewish doctor Ernst Boris Chain.[90] As a twenty-seven-year-old assistant, Chain had been expelled by the National Socialists from the Berlin Charité Hospital in 1933.[91]

Chapter 5

Students of Medicine at the Crossroads

1. The Development of the Medical Discipline in Peace and in War

Since the middle of the Weimar Republic, medicine, for reasons outlined elsewhere, had been a very crowded profession. Consequently, measures short of establishing a university quota were taken in the final half of the republican regime to discourage Gymnasium graduates from entering the medical faculties. But even though these measures resulted in a decline in the absolute number of medical students in the last months of the Weimar era, they could do nothing to prevent the continued rise in the proportion of medical students vis-à-vis students enrolled in other university disciplines. From summer 1926 to the winter of 1932–33, there was an increment of medical students within the entire student universe from 13.0 to 26.2 percent.[1] Thereafter, from the end of 1932 to winter of 1938–39, the absolute number of medical students declined steadily, but in total university enrollment, their proportion went up, from 26.2 to 38.6 percent. From then on into the war, because of military needs and official encouragement of physicians, even the absolute numbers shot up, so that the negative annual growth rate (in absolute numbers) of the prewar phase was visibly reversed. For the entire Third Reich, then, medical enrollment in absolute figures experienced a positive average annual (compound) growth rate of 4.40 percent, compared to a loss of 4.74 percent for the total of university disciplines. In this period, measured against the development of all university subjects taken as a unit, medicine alone grew at an average annual rate of 9.61 percent (Table 5.1).

In this respect, medicine compared favorably with its traditional rival discipline of law, but also with its lowly cousin, dentistry. Unlike medicine, law had started on a decline relative to all university fields of study in the summer of 1925, and this decline, from an impressive 30.1 percent of total enrollment, continued through the Third Reich, until in winter of 1943–44 a mere 6.7 percent of university students were in law, compared to a whopping 71.9 percent in medicine.[2] Dentistry, too, between 1933 and 1945 plunged in absolute as well as in relative numbers, with only 2.5 percent of all university students left there in the end. Perhaps even more startling, however, is that enrollment in pragmatic engineering subjects at the technical universities (*Technische Hochschulen*) collapsed from 1932 on: absolutely as well as relatively, that is, in terms of university disciplines, especially medicine. Against medicine's absolute (compound) annual growth rate of nearly 5 percent, the engineering faculties registered a decrease of

7.65 percent (Table 5.1). As will be seen later, the significance of this disturbing trend was not to be lost on those martial planners of the Third Reich who were technocratically minded.

In the early years of the Nazi regime, the relative ascendancy of medical students still precipitated much alarm because vacancies to be created by the removal of Jewish colleagues had not yet fully materialized and future mobilization needs could not yet be anticipated with any degree of accuracy. In 1934, for instance, the authorities warned that although no more than 2,000 new physicians could be absorbed by the work force annually, at the most (for the overflow of doctors licensed at the end of the republic, now waiting to be certified for panel practice, was still strong), the annual numbers of medical school graduates would far exceed this benchmark figure until about 1939, when some equilibrium would be reached. In 1936 it was pointed out that in 1934 as many as 2,930 medical dissertations had been approved, and 3,600 a year later, signifying an increase of nearly 23 percent. Of course, in the same time span the absolute number of medical students had actually declined by 13.3 percent.[3]

Indeed, the demographic problem of a surplus of physicians had been largely solved by 1938. But the beginning of the war in fall 1939 brought on new concerns. For reasons that will be discussed below, there was a run on applications for medical school in the autumn trimester of 1939, with absolute figures for enrolled candidates rising to 16,565, from 15,905 less than a year before (Table 5.1). In Greifswald, for example, there was room for only 380 freshmen, but 492 were enrolled. Similar conditions obtained for other universities; but Marburg had to close registration in October because its introductory courses had tripled.[4] The officials estimated that at the ten medical faculties that were still open (several universities had been closed at the war's beginning), 35 percent more first-semester students were now studying than at the twenty-six institutions available a year before.[5] Early in 1940, at most universities more than 50 percent of all the freshmen were medical students, with 75 percent at Tübingen.[6]

To facilitate effective planning, the Nazi administrators decided to resort to polls. Hence over the years it became clear to them that medicine was likely to maintain its preferred status among potential students of higher learning, at least until a change in the structures dictated by the war rearranged the entire rank order of national priorities. Although it is true that within the various groups thus sampled technical subjects were finally starting to become more popular, with engineering usually ranking even before a military career (which still failed to be reflected in the actual figures for technical students as shown in Table 5.1), medicine easily kept its strength, as was borne out by continually high proportions of students in the medical faculties.[7] In contrast, law was observed to fare badly in the projections of secondary school pupils until the end. After an inquiry conducted among southern German Napola students in early 1944, for instance, it was found that over 22 percent of the prospective graduates wished to study for an engineering degree, 18 percent for a military career, over 11 percent for the medical doctorate, and merely 1.8 percent for the legal profession.[8] The neglect of law in large measure was a direct consequence not only of war, during which legal procedures as matters of civilian concern tended to be obviated, but also, and increasingly, of the lawlessness that was an unavoidable by-product of the Hitlerian, totalitarian system of governance.[9] This was the case even if it must be conceded that the Napola students were not typical of the bulk of German upper-school pupils because their institutions were administered by the SS.

Those dry statistics may signal but cannot explicate certain policy decisions in high places that influenced the development of medicine as a university discipline in the Third Reich. This discipline came to suffer structural permutations that were the direct consequence first of mobilization for war and then of the war itself. Hitler's introduction of mandatory conscription for the newly constituted Wehrmacht in 1935 meant that male personnel of eligible age who might usually be lingering at the universities had to be diverted, for a while at least, to the armed forces. To some extent, this had been paralleled by the contemporaneously valid induction into the Labor Service (Reichsarbeitsdienst), and both obligations affected all students of higher learning, not just medical ones.[10] But regarding those, the Wehrmacht soon was in a quandary, for though its leaders appreciated having the prospective medics in their companies as fighting men like everybody else, they also realized that in the event of war as many qualified physicians as possible would be needed and therefore undue impediments in the course of medical studies ought to be avoided as ultimately counterproductive. Hence in 1938 the Wehrmacht made provisions that conscripted medical students would spend a portion of the two-year training service in a medical capacity, perhaps as orderlies, which would also count as part of the university's required curriculum. Yet another measure in 1938 permitted the army general staff to shorten the conscription term only for students of medicine.[11]

The early demands of the Wehrmacht lent added weight to the argument of higher education planners that courses of academic study, including medical ones, be shortened for economic as well as biological reasons: to allow students to enter the labor force and get married sooner, thus contributing both to the gross national product and to the celebrated cause of procreation. With this in mind, an upper-school reform lopped off one year from the traditional thirteen-year curriculum by Easter 1937, and similar cuts were planned for university studies, interestingly enough over the protests of race hygienicist Fritz Lenz, who was afraid of deterioration in quality.[12]

A first step in this direction was the introduction of trimesters in the fall of 1939, meaning that by the outbreak of the war three shortened "semesters" were to be fitted into the old academic year replacing the former two, as well as the customary semester holidays. This system remained in place until spring of

1941.[13] Indeed, several more male medical students could be graduated this way quickly than would have been possible otherwise, and many of them, often after provisional final examinations or sometimes none at all, were hurried to the fronts.[14]

Yet realizing that military medics ought to be fully accomplished physicians, the Wehrmacht general staff soon decided to exempt university students from active service altogether as long as they stayed enrolled in medical studies. Moreover, it provided military postings for already conscripted medical students at a university site, to enable them to complete their studies before returning to the war theater.[15] From 1941 on, special Wehrmacht platoons were organized, self-contained medical *Studentenkompanien*, whose members were assigned to individual universities where they observed military protocol and undertook their studies in uniform.[16] These became very popular with male secondary school graduates. A survey conducted in 1942 produced evidence not only that parents would encourage their sons to choose this path, but also that, given the present hard times, the young men all agreed on the benefits of such a course of action. To the question why they were now studying medicine, they would typically answer, "Because this is a guaranteed method for me to play hooky from the war, and especially from front action, without any cost to myself and with the full support of the army."[17]

It is therefore not surprising that other male students resolved, in time, to transfer to the medical faculty after they had finished courses in the humanities or law. The latter is documented in a letter written by an unidentified official early in the war, in which he complains about falsely motivated medical students. "If doctors of law and theologians during armed hostilities discover their liking for medicine only when they are past the age of thirty, then one can believe them just in the rarest of cases. . . . We therefore will have to apply much tougher standards to this group than to the others."[18]

The suspicions of this writer—probably de Crinis—were well founded. Given the hitherto undisputed fact that Hitler's war was unpopular with the large majority of young men who stood to be drafted, medical studies seemed to provide an easy way out of immediate conscription for front service. This implied, however, a lack of proper motivation for a medical career as called for by Hippocratic tenets, and it did not require much perception on the part of the experienced medicine professors to notice it. The medical faculty had been chosen by many young students "who earlier on would never have thought of becoming a doctor," lamented the dean of medicine at Marburg as early as October 1939.[19] Other experts, including Conti, concurred that the present policies would only result in a negative selection of future physicians.[20] The highest charges in government and party were fulminating; Goebbels demanded the instant suspension of the preferential system.[21] Himmler may already have been briefed by his SD that in Königsberg alone, more than half of the Gymnasium graduates had changed their minds suddenly, choosing medicine—the Reichsführer wanted such "cowards" shot.[22]

By the fall of 1940 it was slowly dawning on the administrators that the solution to this problem lay in tighter control over final medical examinations because students would try to procrastinate as long as possible to remain at the universities.[23] In February 1942 Conti, who held formal responsibility for these matters on behalf of the interior ministry, decreed that all medical examinations be enforced within the shortest possible time span, not excluding holidays or furlough, but he still did not threaten sanctions.[24] And so male medical students continued to take weeks off from their studies or to occupy themselves for months with the finalizing of a dissertation, even though the medical state examination, once passed, would enable them to be licensed and subsequently practice. A July 1943 ordinance stipulated maximum examination periods and recommended sharp action by the regional manpower offices, should medical candidates still prove to be obstinate. In the worst cases such attitudes were to result in the loss of the privileged medical student status.[25]

These regulations notwithstanding, upper-school graduates continued to flood the medical faculties. Thus in August 1943 some spokesmen for the University of Berlin were considering closure, despite the partial shutdown of bombed-out facilities in western German medical schools by that time.[26] Representatives of the University of Greifswald were contemplating similar measures one year later.[27]

By summer 1944, important developments affecting the nature of medical studies already were well under way. The medical curriculum had been changed since 1933 to compress courses offered, delete or dilute conventional subject material through the imposition of Nazi-specific disciplines, and to introduce stringent regimens for medical students of both sexes.

The trimester system introduced at the beginning of the war, which was obviously designed to cater to the demands of the military, was only one of several measures intended to shorten the medical studies program over time. The official medical studies regulation (*Studienordnung*) in effect at the beginning of the Nazi regime was still based on schedule and examination guidelines instituted in 1927 and reinforced in 1932. It called for a total of eleven semesters of medical teaching, divided into a preclinical section (from five to six semesters), a qualifying test midway (*Physikum*), and a fully clinical section, again of five or six semesters. During semester breaks students would customarily engage in voluntary practical training under the supervision of a hospital chief physician, mostly unpaid (*Famulatur*), to gather valuable experience. After that a lengthy final examination period was provided for, generally from six months to a year, depending on the candidate's own pace. The maximum duration was two years, which could include repeat time if a test had been failed. After the medical state examination (administered by the executive ministries of the individual states that were subservient to the Reich interior ministry) the candidate had to undergo a *Medizinalpraktikum*, a year of internship, which was to be spent, usually for little or no pay, at a recognized teaching institution such as a university clinic. During this period, the doctoral dissertation, usually well under a hundred pages, could be written for a university medical faculty, which then conferred the actual degree. With the *Medizinalpraktikum* behind them the young physicians were licensed by the state in which they had passed the final examination and were free to strike out on their own, either seeking employment or entering independent (panel) practice, unless they sought courses of specialization.[28] All these provisions were incorporated in the licensure decree (*Bestallungsordnung*) of March 25, 1936, which sought to conform with the spirit of the National Socialist Reich Physicians' Order passed in December 1935, without disturbing the traditional system unduly.[29]

On April 1, 1939, certainly in expectation of an armed conflict but in line with new requirements dictated by a labor-shortage economy, significant cuts were made in the medical curriculum. The final examination was clipped to about six weeks, one of the preclinical semesters was abolished, and the practical year between final examination and licensure was halved and tucked inside the new, streamlined course of studies, with the first three months of internship (now officially called *Famulatur*) to be served after the seventh semester and the last three months after the ninth. Two years were saved, but students had less time to spend on their studies and, in particular, the summer holidays after the seventh and ninth semesters were sacrificed so students could experience training.[30] Yet at least in peacetime a two-year practical term after licensure was obligatory, six months of which could be served as part of the mandatory draft. With the beginning of the war the term changed to one year and it became redundant, as the Wehrmacht pulled in doctors who were scarcely graduated.[31] This compression of the medical course left little time for composing the perfunctory dissertation; it had to be done in the second, clinical half or right after the final state examination. This chore happened to be a favorite for artificial extension by the men to help them avoid active service at the fronts.[32]

The trimester system from fall 1939 to spring 1941 deflated the medical curriculum by yet another few months, but only for students who had the bad fortune to be caught in that time stretch. Certainly, problems arose for those of them who wanted to attend to their internships but could not do so because of a lack of the required free time between trimesters. Hence to a certain extent trimesters proved to have a deleterious effect, as was patently evident when special regulations had to be enacted regarding the resumption of internship after the final medical examination.[33]

Because it became necessary to facilitate medical studies further (with a view to sending a maximum number of graduates into combat zones), by May

1943 some disciplines such as botany and zoology encompassed in the first examination scheme (*Vorprüfung*) for premedical candidates were moved forward in time.[34] At the beginning of 1944 students no longer had to bother learning topographical anatomy and pathological physiology because these had been struck from the roster of examinable subjects.[35] Finally, a fifth preclinical semester could be substituted for one of the clinical ones by November 1944, when the entire course of studies had already been badly thinned out.[36]

These time-saving modifications were complemented by basic changes in the subject matter. The new, important criteria of an applied science turned out to be practicability, racial-eugenic potential, and martial philosophy. Adjustments were made to accommodate each one of these goals. In the spirit of New German Healing, whose tenets Gerhard Wagner had been carrying into the university forums via devious faculty conduits, ever greater emphasis was placed on hospital on-site training, and students were encouraged, specifically in the preclinical semesters, to toil as orderlies and nurses.[37] Nazi administrators aimed to make *Rassenkunde* an integral part of the prescribed course of studies; at the same time chairs in race science were established at various universities. As *Rassenkunde* gained momentum, in spite of the chronic dearth of personnel to teach it, it tended to overshadow or squeeze out the more conventional subjects.[38] *Wehrmedizin*, or military medicine, increasingly found its way into the curriculum, with special attention paid to the requirements of the Luftwaffe.[39]

Bit by bit, medical students were being regimented. In 1937 the Reich education ministry decreed that the first three semesters had to be attended at the same university, curtailing the students' customary privilege of changing from campus to campus at will.[40] After spring 1939, the students were forced to complete six weeks of ordinary factory or agrarian field service some time in the course of their studies, usually right after secondary school. At first three months, later six months of hospital nursing or orderly service were declared obligatory as of 1940, to be pursued after secondary school or inserted between semesters. These requirements applied both to young women and those men incapable of active service; in the case of the able-bodied and normally eligible, they were regularly waived in favor of military substitutions.[41] And as if this were not enough, during the war the ratio between preclinical and clinical semesters also became inalterably fixed, in a four-to-six formula, as opposed to the flexibility that had still been permitted by the order of March 1936.[42]

2. Implications of Politics and Social Class

Programmatically, the politicization of German medicine under Nazi aegis was to begin among students in the universities, as a function of the Nazification of all of academe in the Third Reich.[1] For students, this meant the establishment of suitable mechanisms of everyday political and ideological control. As proclaimed by Dr. Gustav Adolf Scheel, a physician and leader of the combined Nazi student organizations by November 1936, students, after having been conditioned to National Socialist dogma, were to become instrumental in reshaping the entire university system. Like others before and after him, Scheel invoked the proximity between race science, medical responsibility, and National Socialist ideology as the premise for the German people's survival, when at a Heidelberg rally in June 1938 he addressed the German student body: "The mainspring of our science is the struggle for existence and the life of our people. From these, science derives its value and significance. From the life of the German people's community and the race doctrine of the national Socialist movement German science receives fresh impetus and new objectives." Further: "German students recognize the need for a new German university, but their actions are exclusively determined by the National Socialist movement. Only their spirit is capable of reviving the university."[2]

German medical students no less than other university students were expected by the regime to be committed to National Socialism, and the *Medizinische Fachschaft*, the medical study unit, was to organize these students politically and subsequently to monitor their attitude toward the regime from one semester to the next. These quasi-extracurricular *Fachschaften*, one type for the preclinicians, the other for the more advanced finalists, were institutionally tied to the Nazi system of student self-government, and they coexisted with and were plugged into the network of those party institutions the students were expected to belong to as well.[3] As the prominent Berlin historian of medicine Professor Paul Robert Diepgen phrased it in his introductory textbook, work in the *Fachschaft* was designed to impart to every student "knowledge about the tasks and specific application of physicians in the National Socialist state."[4] Diepgen neglected to mention, as everybody knew, that incorporation in the *Medizinische Fachschaft* was compulsory.[5]

The role of the *Fachschaften* in the medical schools was multifarious. Typically, they would organize lectures at various levels of comprehension, to be delivered by ideologically firm faculty members outside of the formal curriculum, on subjects usually touching on the desired intersection between medicine and *völkische Weltanschauung*. Preeminent Nazi physicians such as Dr. Curt Thomalla would speak about such topics as "Population Policy and Race Care as a Question of Fate for the German People," as he did in early 1934 in Würzburg.[6] Balneological excursions were staged, directed by compliant faculty, as well as special work camps such as the one organized by the Heidelberg *Fachschaft* in winter 1935–36, at which anatomist August Hirt spoke on "race issues" (during the war this scientist would kill to set up a Jewish skeleton collection for Himmler).[7] A similar purpose was served through study groups (*Arbeitsgemeinschaften*), in which faculty members dispensed gratuitous advice; these served the career advancement of students and instructors both. Hence in 1937 in Würzburg

"Population Policy" was covered just as thoroughly as "Hereditary-Biological Examinations of Slow-Learner Student Families" or, very prosaically, "Situation and Attitudes of the Physician in the *Volksgemeinschaft*."[8] Race hygiene, of course, was paramount. Other, related subjects to be treated included Nazi public health policy, political Catholicism, Freemasonry, and Jewry.[9] Inasmuch as practical hospital experience was desired of freshman medical students either before the formal course of studies or during semester breaks, the study units administered those, too.[10] The *Fachschaften*, however, also had a social side in that they organized student festivities such as pre-Christmas dances.[11]

Even though the leaders of the *Fachschaften* claimed that attendance at most of their events was voluntary, medical students often had no choice because the study units customarily assigned candidates to the important *Famulatur* training slots. Until the new study regulation of April 1939 much was to be gained professionally through the experience of the optional *Famulatur* between semesters. Therefore at medical schools such as Würzburg, Leipzig, Hamburg, Düsseldorf, and Heidelberg, where excellent working relationships existed between the Nazi student leadership and the Nazified professoriate, only loyal *Fachschaft* members could acquire such training, some of it sweetened by financial incentives.[12] Internally, political patronage was unabashedly admitted: "Above all, the proven and worthy candidates and collaborators must be given the plum positions."[13] *Fachschaft* control over internships (until 1939 *Medizinalpraktika*) was also attempted but does not seem to have been as prevalent because here the clinic chiefs reserved for themselves the right to select junior physicians who would, after all, be given considerable responsibility. These, then, were significant operational barriers to political pork-barreling. According to the records, only the Munich hospitals appear to have succumbed to the *Fachschaft* bosses.[14]

Nonetheless, the study unit leaders exercised powerful blanket controls over their co-opted members in a number of situations, for instance whenever the more senior medical students wanted to change universities. Routine *Fachschaft* reports on costudents soon became just as vital as academic evaluations after examinations and could have a bearing on such mundane matters as the granting of a bursary, but also on entry to all manner of political organizations, viewed by the majority as indispensable for career progress.[15]

Although the medical *Fachschaften* originally fell within the purview of the Nazified student administration, they were also, gradually, locked into Dr. Gerhard Wagner's expanding network. It was clear that Wagner recognized in the study units a tremendous potential for recruiting National Socialist physician cadres. By January 1934 the *Fachschaften* had become cogs in Wagner's machinery of university control, when he reached an agreement with one of the student leaders that future heads of study units be appointed only after consultation with Wagner's caucus of regional faculty stooges. In future, *Fachschaft* leaders and those medical scholars who reported to Wagner's confidant, Professor Wirz, were to observe close mutual council.[16]

A few years later interns were invited to courses at Wagner's training camp in Alt-Rehse; some of this work was to count toward academic credit.[17] In March 1937 the *Fachschaft* leaders were themselves convened there, in an all-out effort to anchor them firmly in Wagner's own ground. One of the crucial points discussed at this meeting was the construction of closer ties between study units and the Nazi Physicians' League.[18] On June 10 Wagner promulgated an ordinance that stipulated the appointment of NSÄB representatives on the *Fachschaft* boards.[19] A second gathering was arranged for the summer semester, attended by Dr. Blome, Wagner's deputy for continuing medical education, Dr. Dingeldey, the Reich physicians' leader's specialist for *Jungärzte*, and Wagner himself. This highlighted an even closer alignment between medical student functionaries and Wagner's apparatus. By that time, too, the national director of the *Fachschaft* system, Dr. F. Gauwerky, had moved his office into Wagner's own Munich headquarters.[20]

Such cross-connections afforded Wagner considerable input into medical students' affairs, as in regard to their participation in the annual Reich Vocational Contest.[21] By 1937, Wagner's guidance was firmly entrenched. In March 1938, the Reich physicians' leader summoned the medical assessment committee to his Munich premises and lectured its members on the relationship between "biological thinking" and "political and scientific leadership recruits." Predictably, the victorious competition entries for that year were in keeping with Wagner's catechism of Nazi public health leadership.[22] Wagner's unceasing attention to the medical students[23] prematurely led to their involvement at levels of party health administration, such as the Race-Political Office of Dr. Gross, that might have helped their careers but surely detracted from their quality as physicians.[24]

Long before World War II, then, the *Medizinische Fachschaften*, with Dr. Wagner's connivance, secured all-pervasive powers, not the least of which was taking a stand in university politics in the hiring and promotion of instructors.[25] But their most dangerous aspect was their ideological influence over the minds of their rank and file. This is starkly illustrated by the case of a third-semester Freiburg student named Vollmann, who early in 1934 underwent orderly's *Famulatur* in the famous Bethel asylum for the handicapped. Here he witnessed and empathized with the Christian, humanistic care extended by deeply religious wardens to epileptic children (Bethel's director, Friedrich von Bodelschwingh, was an exposed member of the Confessional church). Profoundly moved, Vollmann sent a report to his *Fachschaft* leader in which he appeared to support the Bethel philosophy of dedication to such patients because they were "God's dearest children." His letter caused an uproar in the study unit that reverberated through the highest leadership, for such a concept was "absolutely un-National

Socialist," according to the already valid tenets of *Rassenkunde*. Even though the Nazi student leaders distanced themselves from the thought of what later was to become Nazi-style "euthanasia," there are eerie forebodings of this in the correspondence—five years before those crimes actually were perpetrated.[26]

After the death of Wagner and some months into the war, the *Fachschaften* receded in importance, giving way to "comradeships" or *Kameradschaften* that fulfilled essentially the same functions but were totally subservient to martial requirements.[27] As has already been said about female medical students in war, *Kameradschaften* deployed the would-be physicians in special-task units in the conquered East. As part of their internship now stuffed into the regular curriculum, male students, like the female ones but apart from them, were sent to work among ethnic Germans, but also, unlike the young women, in concentration camps and "euthanasia" wards. If anything, such application was even more political than in peacetime.[28]

Membership in the study units always was closely linked to the medical students' incorporation in regular Nazi cadres and especially the Nazi party. More often than not, this was a function of social and even professional circumstances. Therefore, before the frequencies of medical students' membership in those political formations are examined, it would be wise to scrutinize their socioeconomic background.

As has proved practicable before, this may best be done in the context of other disciplines, especially in juxtaposition with the operationally related subject of dentistry and the socially related one of law. At the end of the Weimar Republic, medicine was the outstanding academic discipline to be studied by Germany's social elite, followed very closely by law, which had been in leading position at the turn of the century.[29] But until 1935, the lower-middle-class as well as the working-class representation among medical students was growing somewhat, as were those of law and all the other students, at the expense of the elite (Table 3.5). Hence the universities continued to lose their traditional character as bastions of social privilege, a trend that had started well back in the republic.[30] Until 1941, however, and probably beyond, this trend seems to have reversed itself; one cannot say for certain because wholly conclusive data are still beyond reach.[31]

The available records for the mid-1930s point to a process of medicine continuing, slowly, to outdo law as the most socially acceptable discipline, with dentistry trailing far behind. The percentage of elite-class students in medicine and law was noticeably above the average for universities and Technische Hochschulen (THs), whereas dentistry's was well below. Conversely, the lower middle class was underrepresented in medicine and law and overrepresented in dentistry, compared to the overall student enrollment (Table 3.5). If anything, this social cleavage between medicine and law on one hand, and dentistry on the other, probably widened during the war years, for which data are unreliable.[32]

Did medical students, with a stronger social-elite consciousness than students of any other discipline save law, exhibit a particular propensity for the Nazi party and its affiliates? This important question cannot be answered on the basis of the extant census material because information on student Nazi affiliation was never sought on a large scale. But an answer may be arrived at circuitously if the surviving personal files of the national loan-claiming students (*Darlehnsnehmer*), not quite twenty thousand of them housed in the national archives of the Federal Republic, are consulted.[33] This has to be done with the utmost care, for the card registry not only does not constitute an exact mirror image of the student body as a whole but is not in itself complete. Porous as it is, by my reckoning it represents not even 2 percent of the entire student population in the Third Reich.[34]

In evaluating this loan-student file for the purpose of drawing inferences regarding the entire Third Reich student body, some limiting considerations are mandatory. The sample appears biased on several counts. First, it contains significantly fewer females than in the overall student population, especially for the late war phase, when a tremendous number of women entered disciplines like medicine. Thus in the sample of 2,019 medical students from 1933 to 1945 analyzed for this study, women prove to be consistently underrepresented in 1934–35, 1938, and 1941, for which years there are hard statistical data; only for 1943–44 is there a fairly close match of census and loan-student data.[35] The reason for the dearth of women in the loan-student sample might be that especially in medicine, more females than males tended to come from the elite class and therefore did not require loan assistance; yet the sample is still skewed toward male students.

Second, the loan-student sample is obviously representative of an economically weaker student cohort contained in the student body as a whole, with distinct implications regarding Nazi political choice. One may reason that because students had to be seen to be politically active as a precondition for receiving loans,[36] these students must have been more involved in politics than the general student rank and file. This would preclude any generalization, with respect to political behavior, from the loan-student sample to Third Reich students as a group.

Third, the loan-student sample is biased in favor of the early regime years because during World War II, fewer grants were handed out. This paucity of grants is documented in the contemporary literature, with economic improvement cited as an official rationale.[37] In the case of medicine, the improvement possibly was based on the support male students in medical platoons were receiving from the Wehrmacht. This condition, whatever its cause, is reflected in the combined figures of loan students for medicine, dentistry, and law, which fell off noticeably from 1940 on.[38]

A fourth argument against the viability of the sample would center on the nature of medicine as a discipline long known to be the most expensive to pursue and therefore accessible only to children of relatively wealthy parents, regardless of gender. Indeed, in the Third Reich as earlier in the republic on average one semester at medical school could be three times as expensive as a nonmedical semester.[39] Because medical students customarily had access to more money to begin with, a disproportionately smaller share of them would join the loan-student cohort, hence rendering the loan-student premedical and medical candidates untypical of the majority of those whose parents were able to finance this expensive program of instruction.

Each of the above considerations deserves a response, however haphazardly formulated. The first caveat might be defeated by restricting the analysis of data merely to the male students, who still made up the majority of university students in the Reich. Their participation in Nazi politics also was much greater than the women's, who were not, for instance, represented in such pace-setting organizations as the SA and SS. In addition, this would make the selected loan-student data presented here more easily comparable with the data presented, for all disciplines, in Gerhard Arminger's pilot study in which he focused on males.

The second argument might be weakened by the political involvement of loan students of medicine, dentistry, and law combined, sometimes at a hefty rate, before the onset of the Third Reich, in other words, before the loan scheme administrators turned political commitment into a requirement for financial assistance. Table 5.2 illustrates that of the total of loan students of both sexes in law who joined a Nazi formation during their period of studies, for instance, almost 23 percent did so before the advent of the Third Reich. Of those who became party members till 1945 42 percent of all law students and 43 percent of all dental students actually took that step during the last years of the republic. Of course, one may counterargue that because those students had joined the party as early as 1930 or 1932, they knew they would be eligible for a grant from the Nazi government, hence they applied for and received one, whereas the politically ingenuous would hardly dare to ask for money. Yet a rebuttal could be that it was not impossible for politically neutral students to be awarded money, right through the Reich, when political allegiance was said to matter; Table 5.3 shows that almost one-fifth of the loan-student cohort in all three disciplines had no political affiliation.

Third, the relatively low frequency of loan students after the beginning of the war arguably resulted in the weak political distribution for this period as exhibited in Table 5.2 (medicine, law, and dentistry). But one can also hold that these thinned-out political frequencies were a function of general fluctuations in Nazi membership observed for the entire span of the regime. NSDAP and related auxiliary memberships tended to subside after 1939, for people above a certain age at least, as the regime leaders were favoring recruits mostly from the younger Hitler Youth.[40] As Figure 2 demonstrates, the rate of initial political participation vis-à-vis inactivity per year decreased after 1940, falling precipitously in 1943 and 1944. After the outbreak of the war the NSDAP alone acquired an increment of only about 50 percent of what it had managed to pick up from 1925, until that time, per year.[41] Hence those low political percentages after 1939, judged within the parameters of the entire period, in Table 5.2 and the falling off of initial Nazi involvement as portrayed in Figure 2 might not be peculiar to the loan-student sample, but rather could be characteristic of the entire student body.

Fourth, although it is beyond dispute that because of the expense involved, children of relatively well-off parents would be more likely to study medicine than those of poorer parents, penurious adolescents of both sexes enrolled in that field and therefore availed themselves of the loans; their sociocultural backgrounds were no different from those of their more affluent peers. One could deduce that it was precisely *because* medical studies were so expensive that medical students needed loans (amounts, in fact, which visibly topped those for the law and dental students), a point that was frankly alluded to by the loan officers themselves.[42] In Würzburg in 1934 more than one-third of all the medical students benefited from university fee reductions; at the same time, students of subjects other than medicine were complaining that medical clinicians in training were enjoying public transportation discounts, at the expense of nonmedical students.[43] On the other hand, it was generally acknowledged that medicine was underrepresented in the loan-student scheme, with law being found roughly proportional and dentistry not mentioned.[44]

To recapitulate, it must be taken into account that loan recipients were not immediately identical with the rest of the student body, mostly because economic pressures forced them to enter more readily into opportune political arrangements, whether they were personally agreeable or not. Therefore, one may argue that the pattern of distribution, meaning the differentials as they applied to social class and perhaps also to political association per discipline, was dissimilar for both the students in the loan category and those not receiving loans.

Even after examining only the data for the male cohort (because for comparative purposes figures for it are more easily processed than for both student genders combined), inferences to be derived from the loan-student sample can surely be made only through careful adjustments. In Table 5.4, the upper-class percentage in the male student-loan sample is lower than in the entire group of male students for 1934–35 because the sons of the wealthier elite were not in need of financial grants. Conversely, the lower-class percentage is higher (columns G and H). It can now readily be seen that though in the student body as a whole for the disciplines of medicine and law, upper-class students are overrepresented and lower-class students are underrepresented, these relationships are directly reversed in the case of the loan-student sample.[45] Dentistry presents a mixed picture because the differentials for the upper and upper middle class are the same for both groups of students, but those for the lower class are inconsistent.[46]

Nonetheless, if politics for the lot of Third Reich university students was a vehicle of career advancement, including the goal of study and subsistence money, then there is no reason why the differentials between the major political formations, pertaining to medicine, dentistry, and law as shown for the male loan-student cohort in Table 5.5, ought not to have been valid for the student body as a whole. That is, a loan student, once determined to join a formation, could have chosen the party for the same reason as a non-loan student, or the SA, or the SS. To express this in arbitrary numbers, one may assume that if fifteen loan students favored the party, ten the SA, and five the SS, then nine regular students probably were in the party, six in the SA, and three in the SS. On this premise, perceived differences in the political behavior between the three academic disciplines will attain validity.

Hence it is clear from Table 5.5 that the SA was the favorite political platform for members of all three disciplines in the loan group (certainly till mid-1934—see Table 5.2), as it was for the entire loan-student body; but dental students were attracted to it in even greater measure than were students of medicine or of law (or, for that matter, of most other disciplines). The same obtained for the SS, although here the general student average was higher than that for dental students. In the NSDAP and other auxiliaries, however, law and medicine students topped dental as well as most other students. This could be interpreted to mean that students of dentistry, a discipline still held in contempt by the lawyers and physicians, found the SA as well as the SS, both martial in their paramilitary apparel, best suited to propel their social ambitions and transport these to quick realization in a regime with a pronouncedly military mien. Keeping the above consideration in mind, this verdict may cautiously be extended from the loan-student sample to the general student universe.

In comparison, representatives of the respected professions of medicine and law were customarily relaxed. Relative to dental students, who hailed from the privileged classes to a much lesser degree (Table 5.4), they were confident of their social superiority and had no need to flaunt it through uniforms, brown or black. What is significant, however, is the mutual proximity of medicine and law in this regard, for their political allegiance percentages as shown in Table 5.5 correlate extremely positively.[47] The fact that politically, medical students behaved much more like law students is proof that both groups were tightly joined by sociocultural bonds, to the extent that their individual self-images still were virtually interchangeable.

Puzzling at first sight is the discrepancy, in the case of medicine (about law no judgments may be made for lack of supplemental data), between students and mature doctors: 28.6 percent of men students joined the party, as against 49.9 percent of men physicians; 32 percent of students served in the SA, as opposed to 26 percent among physicians; 5.8 percent of students favored the SS, compared with 7.2 percent of the licensed doctors (males only). The explanations would seem to lie in the progressive odiousness of the SA, after the Röhm crisis of June

30, 1934, as exemplified in Table 5.2. Upon graduation, students who had been pressured into the SA by the notorious SA-Hochschulamt[48] eventually left the Brown Shirts only to swell the ranks of the Nazi party and SS. Thereupon this circumstance manifested itself in the figures of the Reich Physicians' Chamber files that were evaluated for Chapter 2.

Finally, Table 5.6 attempts a comparison of medicine with dentistry and law by class and Nazi affiliation. But because the class divisions as crystallized in the loan sample probably were at variance with the general student situation, inasmuch as loans were a function of socioeconomic background, generalizations are once more risky. According to the tabulated figures, it now turns out that in the loan-student group at least the popularity of the SS with dental students may be credited to the predilection of whatever elite-class members there were among them, and of the SA to the ambitions of the lower-middle-class future dentists (columns G, H, J). And though the SS still shows up remarkably strongly in the subgroup of upper-class medical and particularly law students (columns C, E, M, O), the notable firmness of the NSDAP within medicine appears to be traceable to the lower middle class, and within law to both that class and the elite (columns A, E, K, O). The SA, as long as it endured, was most firmly rooted within lower-middle-class dental students, less so in lower-middle-class medicine and law student groups, and was neglected by future physicians and lawyers of the elite segment (columns B, E, G, J, L, O).

Interestingly, the only lower-class stratum in which the Storm Troopers seem dominant is that of the law students, while in the case of lower-class medical and dental students, as well as students of all subjects, their representation is proportional (columns B, E, G, J, L, O, Q, T). All told, if politics was an instrument of social mobility in the universities after 1933, then this analysis centering on just three select disciplines allows us tentatively to identify as the most upwardly mobile the following professional subgroups: medical students of the lower middle class who joined the NSDAP and of the working class who drifted into miscellaneous ancillary organizations; dentistry students of upper-class background who patronized the Nazi party and especially the SS, also those of the lower middle class entering the miscellaneous category and the SA, and lower-class NSDAP dentists; finally, lower-middle-class as well as working-class law students who were drawn to the SA. Obversely, both medical and law students with upper-class parents used the SS as a means of maintaining their treasured elite position, undoubtedly out of fear of being toppled from this august plane either by intrusive professional hopefuls from the two lower strata in their own disciplines or, more threateningly perhaps, by the collectively upwardly mobile profession of dentists. Again, this preliminary judgment may be applicable to the loan students and the vast majority of ordinary, economically secure students alike.

Overall, the Nazi formations sought out by male medical students in absolute numerical sequence were the SA, followed by the NSDAP (that order was starkly reversed after 1934), then the Hitler Youth, the Nazi Students' League, the SS, and the National Socialist Motor Corps as well as diverse lesser groups.[49] In these ranks, male students realized similar political-career ambitions as those already described for the women students. But since mandatory political chores were constantly interfering with studies, comparatively few male medical students were as active as a certain Friedrich Fleischmann, who had taken on a secondary career in the movement. Born in 1911 in Nuremberg, Fleischmann joined the SA and NSDAP in 1931. Probably studying medicine in nearby Erlangen by 1933, Fleischmann, who was described as a "climber and a fanatic" by his fellows, assumed a leading role in the local SA of Nuremberg. Stationed at the city's castle, the fifty men under his command in their capacity as auxiliary police arrested and interrogated political prisoners under torture. After being relieved of his SA duties, this man became a licensed physician in 1935.[50]

It is difficult to probe the political commitment of medical students from 1933 to 1945. All university students, medical ones included, started out in the Third Reich as a proved intellectual vanguard of the Nazi movement since the late 1920s, but to the degree that political obligations became more forceful, preventing serious study, their enthusiasm seems to have waned over time. This tendency to back away from Nazi politics as much as possible appears to have increased remarkably after the (displeasurable) outbreak of the war, with conscription interrupting potentially prominent careers in the professions, academia, the civil service, and industry.[51]

But even nominal political involvement could be a stepping-stone to success in a society that was governed by Nazi criteria of mobility. Thus once again one must admit to the possibility of opportunity and opportunism as twin factors in career planning—factors that called for a modicum of political involvement. Yet in the general student body as well as for the medical students specifically, the exact ratio between those who were merely formally active and those who wholeheartedly embraced service in the Nazi movement is still impossible to determine. That we should perhaps not underestimate the group of dedicated Nazi activists among the medical students is suggested by the inordinately high involvement of licensed physicians in the ranks of Hitler's organizations, some of whom, inasmuch as they were young enough, would have been persons who had emerged from biologistic medical-education brainwashing (New German Healing, *Rassenkunde*) in the medical faculties after 1932.

Whatever the career considerations may have amounted to then or later, there is ample evidence that medical students grumbled about the attempts to co-opt them into various activities of the *Fachschaften* for as early as 1934, even though formal membership could never be avoided. But if real opposition, for instance as an act of sabotage, was not encountered by the regime leaders, apathy and indifference were noticeable in various shapes and degrees. For instance, not to sign up for the study units' lecture training courses, labeled as voluntary ventures, was fairly common.[52] The *Fachschaft* leaders incurred much difficulty in dispersing the medical study units' tabloid, *Der Jungarzt*, for hardly anybody wanted to read it, even though it was free.[53] Judging from the situation in Würzburg, for which the most data are available, medical students tried to skirt not only the *Fachschaft*'s field-harvest work but also the hospital training practice, or they simply refrained from participation in door-to-door canvassing of donations for party purposes.[54] Characteristically, this neglect or even recalcitrance on the part of students was seldom interpreted by the *Fachschaft* chiefs as a sign of outright political opposition, for they realized that the multitude of *Fachschaft* offerings, which were optional, precluded simultaneous participation in all of them. As early as June 1934 in Freiburg, a student leader, paradoxically, was inclined to put the mounting indifference of his peers down to "the well-known tendency among medical students to exhibit a snobbish aloofness toward all matters somewhat out of the ordinary."[55] Very rarely was political motivation suspected, as occurred in 1935–36 in Rostock, where not enough students were said to be interested in voluntary enrollment for additional classes in *Rassenkunde*. Complained the convener wryly: "Either there is a deficit of National Socialism at this place or the university has degenerated to the level of a polytechnic."[56]

The medical students' collective attitude of inner detachment, sometimes compounded by personal annoyance, after the beginning of the war could not be monitored by the *Fachschaften* as they had done before because they lost their influence, and war planning and deployment directed by the army and the ministries took precedence over extracurricular party activities as those typical of the peacetime Alt-Rehse camp. It is certain that medical students were not seeking leave from service at the fronts because, as one Bonn geologist told British author Stephen Spender in the summer of 1945, they opposed the war on grounds of conscience, but rather because they were either fainthearted or refused to interrupt their careers for no good professional reason.[57] Sure enough, the ones who did stay home in the seminars and university laboratories often lacked the serious composure required of them in a time of national crisis.[58] Military companies of medical students (*Studentenkompanien*) stationed at some universities, whom party leaders such as Saxon Gauleiter Martin Mutschmann ideally viewed as paragons fit for the hard-pressed civilian population to admire, sometimes became restless, perhaps out of boredom or indignation about the regime's mounting bad fortunes in war, which tended to spoil their own chances for a happy professional future.[59] A Jena-based medical platoon, for example, whose members after excessive partying and much alcohol smashed a clay bust of the Führer to smithereens on July 2, 1943, was very likely driven not by hatred of Hitler but by a general sense of futility, exactly five months after the debacle at Stalingrad.[60] In 1944 lawyer Dietrich Güstrow consented to defend an advanced medical student, who as an officer at home on furlough after the horrors at the front, had gotten senselessly drunk and gone on a rampage in a residential district of Berlin.[61]

Staunch idealistic resisters to the Nazi regime among the medical students existed; once again they were chiefly to be found among the Marxists. They were willing to go to prison and concentration camp and to pay with their lives for their conviction. As early as March 1933 a woman medical student, daughter of a Bonn professor of dentistry, was jailed, after the Reichstag fire, for communist subversion.[62] Her costudent Donald Degenhardt met with a similar fate in Marburg.[63] Two years later in Berlin candidate of medicine Kurt Steude was maintaining a clandestine relationship with the communist circle surrounding the physician Karl Gelbke; Steude survived the regime in a Wehrmacht uniform.[64]

But there were also individuals with loose group connections who risked their lives for honor and decency and, perhaps, true medical ethos. Alexander Mitscherlich, attracted to Ernst Niekisch's circle in Berlin, moved to Zurich in 1935 to continue medical studies free from fear of the Gestapo. In 1937, to help the captured Niekisch, he crossed the Swiss-German frontier on a one-day pass. The police immediately apprehended him, and he spent eight months in a Nuremberg jail, to be released as capriciously as he had been seized without any formal indictment.[65]

Adherents to the White Rose resistance group that in late 1942 began its activities in Munich but had sympathizers in Hamburg, Berlin, and Freiburg justly have become the most celebrated German heroes: medical students Hans Scholl, Alexander Schmorell, Christoph Probst, and Willi Graf. These students and their friends were decapitated because they had condemned the Hitler regime on altruistic grounds using such audacious ploys as flyers and "open letters" distributed as handbills.[66]

The list goes on. Pathologist Professor Büchner writes about the students he met in his Freiburg seminars, many of them deeply religious, who during the war resented the regime increasingly, expressing these feelings in private letters to him from the front.[67] Karl Groeger, born in Vienna in 1918, was studying medicine in Holland when the war broke out. In 1943 he was part of an Amsterdam resistance group trying to shield Dutch Jews from deportation. Groeger died on the scaffold.[68] And Heinz Bello acted entirely on his own initiative, following the promptings of humanity the way he understood them as a disciple of Esculapius in Münster. He had already fought on the eastern front and courageously helped Münster civilians after bombing raids when in July 1943, surrounded by his comrades, he aired his disapproval of militarism, National Socialism, and the notorious corruption of the party brass. As a member of a student medical company he was tried before a Berlin military tribunal. He spurned several chances to escape. Bello was executed by a firing squad on June 29, 1944. That initially he had been denounced by two fellow students of medicine is indicative of the complex problem posed by the medical students' involvement in politics under Hitler.[69]

3. The So-called Jewish Question and the Quality of Medical Instruction

One of the avowed aims of National Socialist student leaders was to remove not only Jewish professors from the universities' faculties but also those Jewish students in their midst who were competitors for jobs. These students' goals were incorporated in a program for Nazi university reform.[1] In total accord with such sentiments, the highest regime leaders complied by imposing, in the first few months after Hitler's political takeover, closure on Jewish university students allowing them to attend institutions of higher learning only in direct proportion to their numbers in the civilian population. Hence by winter 1933–34, the proportion of Jewish students shrank to just over 1 percent of the student total, still slightly above the national share of (Mosaic-faith) Jews of less than 0.8 percent.[2] To give but one specific illustration in absolute numeric terms, in the department of dentistry at Würzburg by the fall of 1933 the number of Jewish students was reduced from about sixty to seven.[3]

In the winter semester of 1932–33 the Jewish share in the combined university and technical college student body had been 4.8 percent; in many disciplines, this proportion was higher; in statistics and the humanities, it was the highest. Medicine was the third highest at 7.8 percent; almost one-third of those students, however, were foreigners, mostly from the European East.[4] At the end of the Weimar Republic many Nazi doctors and students were calling for the removal of Jewish medical students as well as Jewish graduated physicians for reasons of competition; in some medical schools, such as Freiburg's and Erlangen's, the Nazi students' long-standing resentment of the Jews was intensified by the especially large contingent of them enrolled in medicine.[5]

But even though the Berlin government was prepared to take steps against Jewish university students, it did not act fast enough for a largely fanaticized student body that in driving out Jewish students would prove, in the coming years, to be always several steps ahead of appropriate Nazi laws. Because of the acute overcrowding in the profession and the visibility as well as qualitative excellence of Jewish doctors and students, this applied in particular to the field of medicine. For example, students in general would, as early as March 1933 (before any closure laws against Jewish students had been promulgated by the state), try to move against Jewish fellows who were receiving financial assistance, hoping to inherit their grants.[6] "Aryan" medical students, in sanctioning such action, would dissociate themselves from their Jewish peers in the lecture halls, insisting that Israelite students pursue their work in separate groups, as in a ghetto, before any government or even university regulation had been handed down.[7] At the University of Frankfurt in May 1933, medical students in SA uniform accosted their Jewish comrades, confiscated their student identity cards, and then chased them off the campus.[8]

These Nazi students were guided by their politicized *Fachschaften*, acting in the relentless spirit of Dr. Wagner, who was about to exert a formal influence on the medical schools on behalf of "revolutionary" Nazi party policy. But by late 1933 the government was beginning to issue pronouncements. Forthwith the existing non-"Aryan" medical students' professional future in the Reich was curtailed by prohibiting them from fulfilling any or all three of the mandatory requirements: final state examination, doctoral diploma, and licensure for practice. In early 1934 this rule was relaxed somewhat when it was stated that Jewish medical candidates who made clear their intention to migrate abroad would be eligible for doctoral convocation if they renounced their civil right to approbation in Germany. Later in the year yet another precondition for seemingly preferential treatment was, for German Jews, the voluntary renunciation of their original citizenship, once outside Germany.[9] German-Jewish students, however, were in a quandary. As long as they remained in the Reich, it was legally impossible for them to lose their citizenship, hence they could not receive their degrees; if they wished to emigrate to fill a job abroad, they had to have their doctorates in hand as a prerequisite for the post, yet this was denied them inside German borders.[10] Special consideration, which was theoretically provided for, was accorded only to partial "Aryans" (*Mischlinge*) and only after special dispensation from faculty and the Reich interior ministry.[11]

A new twist was added in February 1935, when licensure was generally disallowed for full or half Jews of German citizenship unless they had commenced their medical studies before the summer semester of 1933. Exceptions were possible only when the candidate had a valorous World War I record and a Nordic physique and composure. Students with only one Jewish grandparent were as yet not touched.[12] A further anti-Semitic measure at this time, affecting medical as well as other students, was the exclusion of Jews from nationally sponsored financial assistance.[13] A year later any German student applying for such funds had to produce a non-Jewish pedigree back to the year 1800.[14]

By then the question of how the remaining Jewish medical students should interact with their "Aryan" peers had become a point of strong contention among the staunchly Nazi *Fachschaft* leaders. They were seeking further ways to cut the hated Jews off, to isolate them, and then to expel them. Thus they seized upon the double issues of student practical training, the *Famulatur*, and of the race and gender of patients as training subjects. Implicitly, they were encouraged in their temerity by the indecisive rulings of various state administrations up to that time. Whereas the state of Baden had proscribed Jewish trainees for its government-sponsored institutions as early as April 1934, Prussian officials had still refrained from publishing such a ruling. As late as 1936 the Reich interior ministry was still of the opinion that *Famulatur* was an integral part of medical studies for everyone, including Jewish students. In gynecology and obstetrics, however, individual decisions should be rendered by the clinical directors as they saw fit.[15]

Thus in Würzburg in summer 1935, the local study unit ruled that non-"Aryans" could not be *Famuli* or interns at "German" hospitals but were free to gather experience in Jewish health care institutions.[16] Cologne's *Fachschaft* announced that Jewish students were not permitted to give "Aryan" women vaginal examinations and were to serve only Jewish female patients.[17] Leipzig, Hamburg, Frankfurt, and Jena followed suit, and Heidelberg still exercised restraint because its Jewish medical students were mostly foreigners.[18] Rostock did not have a single Jew enrolled.[19] Indeed, how much reduced to the level of principle the question was by that time is demonstrated by the extremely small number of Jewish students still left in all the medical schools: Würzburg had only three in a sea of about four hundred "Aryans."[20]

In the summer of 1937, when the alliance between the radical *Fachschaften* and Dr. Wagner's administration was being galvanized, not even a hundred non-"Aryans," including persons of mixed parentage, were enrolled in the Reich's medical schools.[21] By that time, the Nuremberg Race Laws of September 1935 were in force, in the preparation of which two powerful Nazi medical functionaries, Dr. Wagner and Dr. Gross, had wielded great influence.[22] By providing a "legal" definition of Jews for purposes of a protracted prosecution process that would ultimately transform itself into persecution, they implicitly presented a blueprint for radicalization of solutions to the "Jewish Question" that would include medical instruction in the universities. Hence Rudolf Hess's party office, particularly the tenacious Martin Bormann, in league with Wagner attempted to push the more conservative, still wavering Reich education ministry into more assertive action by laying down strict rules with respect to Jewish students in their contacts with "Aryan" patients and their role as *Famuli* in not exclusively Jewish clinics.[23] But as late as February 1938 Rust's officials insisted that because of the very few non-"Aryans" involved, the accelerated measures urged by Hess and Bormann were not called for. They also suggested to Frick's ministry that *Mischling* medical students, who had meanwhile all been placed in the category of full Jews, be treated as "Aryans."[24] In October Wagner intermittently conceded that quarter Jews, meaning Germans with one Jewish grandparent, again be admitted to the medical examinations, but that half Jews could avail themselves of that privilege only after special consideration by the interior ministry, in consultation with his own Reich Physicians' Chamber.[25]

In the end, this turned out to be a victory for the Nazi purists, Hess, Bormann, and Wagner himself, who had not long to live. After the November 1938 pogroms, which escalated Jewish harassment, the anti-Semitic restrictions effectively barring any full Jews of whatever original citizenship from medical school enrollment and examinations were embodied in the hitherto binding study regulation of spring–summer 1939.[26] Throughout the war, when German Jews were physically ghettoized and then evacuated for liquidation in the East, only quarter *Mischlinge*, with extremely few exceptions for half Jews, had any chance of studying medicine, for Wagner's October 1938 selection prerogative in regard to half-breeds was, after the Reich physicians' leader's death, faithfully exercised by the increasingly important NSDAP chancellery under Bormann, with Conti's acquiescence, and possibly assistance, in the interior ministry.[27] To all intents and purposes, the book on Jewish medical instructors and students had been closed.

This expulsion of Jewish medical students from German universities had similar consequences for the quality of medicine as a professional discipline as did the eviction of Jewish scholars from the field: a severe loss of substance. Jewish students were long known to be especially successful in examinations, hence they posed a grave competitive threat as future doctors. This explains the zeal with which "Aryan" medical students, before the war when they were still sufficiently fanaticized and had the opportunity to do so, hounded down their Jewish fellows and professors[28] alike, and why they enthusiastically underwrote the proscription of licensed Jewish physicians, zestfully pursued by Wagner's Physicians' League, as will be described in the next chapter.

This qualitative decline, which was to have grave import for the future of medicine in Germany after 1945, was predicated on additional factors not traceable to anti-Semitism. To begin with, the problem had a quantitative dimension in that whatever solid medical teaching had been left, as by unshakable coryphaei like Aschoff or merely competent instructors such as Hoff or Bürger-Prinz, was pressed into fewer hours than had been the case before 1933. This progressive curtailment of legitimate medical content commenced with the emergence of peacetime Nazi preoccupations for students and after 1939 led to martial supertasks. At the start of the regime, the students appeared to realize this as an impending problem when they admitted that the secret to professional success lay in the improbable but necessary combination of "meeting the tremendous challenges of our day and, at the same time, developing into first-class medical doctors."[29]

Thus, early in the regime precious time was deducted from needed study periods, especially before the premedical and final medical examinations, by the labor service imposed through the Nazi-coordinated student self-government, dispensation from which was possible only under exceptional circumstances.[30] Well into 1934, mandatory SA service, including physically demanding sports training and days-long stays in exercise camps, cut deeply into the study time of every male student, but especially medical ones because of their daily commuting between university and clinics. Psychiatry professor Oswald Bumke has estimated that as many as twenty-four hours per week were consumed by such activities in Munich.[31] After the grueling regimen of the SA subsided by late 1934, party organizations such as the SS, Nazi Student League, Hitler Youth, and NSDAP made demands on the students, which, in combination, could rival the original impositions of the Brown Shirts. The *Fachschaften* naturally supplied a work load of their own, even though medical students often tried to avoid it, which was often difficult. *Fachschaft* leaders conceded, however, that the imposition of their burdens, in excess of those by other cadres, weighed down on the students inordinately.[32] The inevitable result was shorter hours left for the study of medicine. Not surprisingly, *Fachschaft* functionaries themselves suffered. He was "feigning industriousness," wrote Würzburg's Hermann Lindgens from a Mülheim hospital, he was "playing doctor." "That's coming in very handy, for this way I can compensate for time lost earlier and bone up for the exam a bit."[33] Scrupulous teachers of medicine like Sauerbruch already saw the writing on the wall. At a party in the French Embassy early in February 1935 he grumbled about the low standard of the current crop of neophyte medical students. Their "intellectual state" was "appalling. They are picked because of their low membership card numbers, and preference is given to those with fathers in the party, and mothers in the National Socialist Womanhood. Five times weekly they have to attend marching and combat exercises, and lectures on the theory of race. Next morning they sleep through class, if they show up at all."[34]

The famous surgeon may have exaggerated the National Socialist family background of his charges, but his statement accurately prefigured the conditions of medical study under increased mobilization and then under war. The pattern of time constraints continued with the introduction of new study regulation in spring 1939, which stipulated that even though from then on there were two years less to complete one's studies, the same level of knowledge was expected of candidates upon graduation.[35] A similar rationale was employed a few months later to justify the trimester system, but as early as the end of 1939 it was realized that the trimester experiment was turning into a disaster because students were learning substantially less than ever before. The trimester system was ended, and at the height of the war, considerably sobered by the minimum qualifications of medical recruits at the fronts, de Crinis admitted it had been a mistake.[36] Especially after Hitler's attack on the Soviet Union in spring 1941, candidates in medicine who despite all procrastination did complete their curricula were rushed to the front straight from the examination hall, without the practical experience customarily provided by internship and without any chance to intensify their training on site, although they might return to a university for a few weeks of refresher courses.[37]

This system produced ramshackle physicians, whom even the wounded soldiers did not trust.[38] It can be persuasively demonstrated using the example of the surgeons. On one hand, specialism was discouraged or neglected so as to manufacture physicians with minimal general training in assembly-line fashion; on the other hand, the half-baked generalists were suddenly required to do mostly surgery in the field, a subject on which they had not had sufficient instruction. After a few months they would acquire a modicum of surgical technique without being expert specialists and would forget anything else they might have learned about medicine, including such areas of specialization as hygiene, physiology, or gynecology.[39]

Yet another aspect of negative curriculum change was that traditionally valid medical subjects were either shortened or abandoned to make room for useless fields like *Rassenkunde*, useless particularly in war. It will be recalled from the preceding chapter that race hygienics was progressively entrenching itself as a subject of research among scholars. That was tragic enough—for scholarship and for pure and applied science. But as a serious subject being taught in class, *Rassenkunde* had a potentially disastrous effect not only on the mental disposition but also on the professional ethics of the medical students. After *Rassenkunde* had become a proper topic for examination in 1936, more and more students engaged in it at the expense of legitimate subjects, and many young men and women wasted their time writing race-hygienic dissertations that formally qualified them as doctors.[40] This trend became even more threatening to tried and proven convention when the regime leaders decided, by 1938, that Reich Vocational Contest entries, which in the medical section were heavily saturated with *Rassenkunde*, ought to be counted as seminar papers and in lieu of doctoral dissertations.[41] Next, *Rassenkunde* became an integral part of the curriculum at every medical school, not just a few chosen ones. Pursuant to the new study regulation of April 1939, a medical examination candidate had to prove that he was "conversant with hereditary biology and racial hygiene" and that he knew about the "requirements of racial hygiene in practice."[42] This directive seems like a pep talk for the Auschwitz doctors! And in early 1944, when yet another curriculum revision was in the offing, Dr. Conti insisted that a proposed offering of *Rassenkunde* of two hours per week, to be taught in the tenth semester, be doubled to four hours, even though the somewhat more temperate de Crinis had not thought this necessary in light of the priorities of the battlefield. Conti still had enough influence to win the day on this point: course requirements in the final study regulation of October 1, 1944, did call for four hours of "race biology."[43] Therefore, with the mounting emphasis on ideology in medicine, it eventually had to come down to the pragmatic question of whether, behind the trenches, experts in *Rassenkunde* could save lives, as could experts in surgery, for instance.

The escalation of the war brought on further difficulties compounding the problem of decline in quality. Even before the conflict the hitherto healthy ratio between medicine students and medicine teachers had been changing to the detriment of the instruction process. After 1938, while the absolute number of students was increasing, the absolute number of professors was decreasing because many of the able-bodied were conscripted for war service. In Tübingen, for instance, whereas in 1935 28 percent of the faculty had been medical teachers instructing 34 percent of students who were in medicine, by 1939 44 percent of the students were in medicine being taught by 26 percent of the professoriate.[44] In Munich at that time, twenty-four students on average were forced to work on a corpse in the dissecting room at once, and surgical instruction was done partially over loudspeakers. Berlin resorted to the extension-speaker system in 1940, and Leipzig had it by 1942.[45] A related problem was that fewer and fewer books and teaching materials were available for an ever-growing throng of students.[46]

By February 1945 the discrepancy between faculty and students had become so great that in some universities dozens of candidates were examined by a single faculty member at one time. Because it was becoming evident that many students had entered examinations without formal preparation and certainly without official authorization, the process of screening as a function of medical qualification was placed in doubt.[47]

Indeed, the question may well be raised if throughout the years of the Third Reich examination standards had not been artificially lowered to accommodate the growing mass of factually ignorant would-be graduates. This is suggested by a juxtaposition of medical examination results and professorial assessments of the examinations as dependable instruments of selection. From 1932 to 1939, the more students scored highly in final medical examinations, the smaller the share of those who became preexamination dropouts. Faculty members in summer 1939 were making disparaging comments about the value of the tests.[48] That something was awry is suggested by Leonardo Conti's observation in November 1940 that even though the "performance" of medical students was noticeably receding, it would not be acceptable "to lower examination requirements and to evaluate positively any work that does not deserve it."[49]

Thereupon, medical examination standards appear to have been tightened somewhat, for eighteen months later the Security Service of the SS stated that outstanding results were very rare and that most medical graduates hovered at the level of "something like a midwives' training school."[50] By autumn of 1942 over half of all the candidates for a premedical examination did not pass at Freiburg; similar success rates were transmitted from Rostock.[51] At the end of the year Jena University surgeon Professor Nicolai Guleke complained that four times as many candidates had failed the finals than in 1938, and far fewer attained the highest rating, despite a lowering of standards. Germany, said Guleke, was well on its way to creating "second-rate physicians."[52]

As the regime's planners were gazing into the future, they realized that at war's end a sorry lot of largely inexperienced, one-sided young physicians—the cohorts that had been training over the last few years—would be returning from the fronts to start servicing the civilian population for the first time in their careers. That prospect was not good. Medicine might win the war in battles but would surely lose the victory at home, at least for the next thirty years, said one pundit.[53] There would be no specialists to help cure other than run-of-the-mill diseases, said another.[54] Perhaps one could comfort oneself with thoughts of medical school reform after the Final Victory.[55]

Reichsführer-SS Himmler was more cynical. He would rather not see any more new medical students in the universities, at least not of the present ilk. In July 1944 he informed the Führer's health plenipotentiary Professor Karl Brandt that it would be useless to proceed with a new plan for allowing military exemptions for secondary school graduates choosing to study medicine. The shortage of physicians would not be solved that way as long as the war was on, wrote Himmler. No one would want to rear a new generation of cowards, for it could not possibly be in the interest of the medical profession to keep attracting the "moral riffraff" of the nation.[56] Coming from the warlord of the concentration camps, which had done more than anything or anybody to pervert universal medical standards thus far, this was the saddest comment on the German medical profession in decades.

Chapter 6

The Persecution of Jewish Physicians

1. The Medicalization of the "Jewish Question"

The National Socialist proscription of German-Jewish doctors, a process of escalating intensity until its gruesome climax in the early 1940s, can be properly understood only against the background of the "biocracy" (Lifton's term)[1] that was part of the infrastructure of Hitler's state. In this biocracy, the German polity was treated, in typical organicist fashion, like a human body that was dependent for its continued existence on indigenous or extraneous factors capable of interfering with its functioning. The indigenous factors were said to be hereditary, the extraneous ones to derive from the environment or milieu. The equilibrium or well-being of the German organism was thus a function of negative, positive, or neutral roles those factors could assume in certain definable scenarios.

This physiological imagery was grafted onto the matrix of *Rassenkunde* as developed by the post-Darwinian German biomedical thinkers. I have already mentioned that physician Fritz Lenz's theory of racial inequality, however modestly formulated in its initial versions, made a strong impact on Adolf Hitler, who studied Lenz's text in the Landsberg prison cell in 1924–25. This theory, persuasive in its scientific guise, reinforced Hitler's much cruder notions about the superiority of blond-haired people over dark-haired ones, as he had derived them in his Vienna days from the primitive *Ostara* brochures of Lanz von Liebenfels.[2] Those syncretic thoughts congealed on the pages of *Mein Kampf*. Anything that Hitler wrote on race in this book appeared as instantly medicalized; conversely, any speculations that he ventured about medicine were informed by racist prejudice.[3]

More specifically, Hitler in his programmatic volume speaks of the German biological corpus (*Volkskörper*) as diseased and in need of radical cures. The ailments, as he sees it, are caused to "Aryans" by Jews, or, as Hitler simplifies it to great effect in the imagery of biopolitics, the Jew is disease personified. He is a "bacillus" or "parasite," ever ready to engage in "blood poisoning" inside the "national body." (Hitler referred to the Jew as a "bacillus" as late as July 1941.) The medical parabole is just as insinuating by association: the Jew is said to inhabit an "abscess," thus becoming a part of it. He advertises cultural "trash," which, as "pestilence," infests the German people thereafter. Perhaps Hitler's most revealing statement along those lines is his lamentation that the Jewish "poison was able to penetrate the bloodstream of our people unhindered and do its work, and the state did not possess the power to master the disease."[4]

Because of its biomedical content, one may assume that Hitler's book was ingested much more readily by *völkisch* physicians and racial theorists than by the population at large. The ideas the party leader had initially adopted from scientists like Lenz were, after enrichment with his own smatterings of thought and subsequent powerful vulgarization, adopted by Lenz's epigones. Since their outpourings once more influenced Hitler (as will be proved later using the example of Gerhard Wagner), there was thus a perpetual process of cross-fertilization, established firmly in the latter half of the 1920s and, as a genocidal dialectic, continuing to the point of Auschwitz.[5]

In the Nazi medical annals, from the inception of the regime, there is a continuous stream of metaphors equating Jews with disease. Respirologist Kurt Klare, cofounder of the Nazi Physicians' League, in March 1933 communicated to a colleague his opinion about the "decomposing influence of Jewry" within the German organism, as if Jewry were a sickness.[6] This theme of Jewish "racial decomposition" and the consequent "cleansing of our *völkisch* body" was graphically reiterated by Dr. Wagner and his medical aides on the occasion of the Nazi party rally in fall 1935—the fatal rally that introduced the anti-Jewish race laws.[7]

Dr. Dietrich Amende, another early physician follower of Hitler, drove home the lesson to be learned from Jewish "decomposition" once more in 1937.[8] Wagner, though relieved that the racial legislation had rendered "Aryan" German youth "immune" to the "Jewish poison," nevertheless went on to express his concern about "the biological danger the Jew is posing within our people" and uttered additional warnings against "Jewish parasites."[9]

After Wagner's death, Germany entered the martial phase, which was to mean a radicalization in the medicalized war against the Jews. Hence Hamburg physician H. H. Meier felt called upon to link the elimination of Jewish physicians, long under way in the profession, to the much larger problem of cauterizing the Jewish tumor in the German body when he wrote about the "elimination of Jewry from physiciandom and other facets of health leadership" as a medical precaution for the collective health of the nation.[10] Ernst Hiemer, an associate of Nuremberg Gauleiter Julius Streicher, who had his own strong views about medicine, published a repulsively suggestive primer dealing with bugs, tapeworms, and bacilli that were all identified with Jews. In the final chapter about "people's pestilence" Hiemer stated that from Poland, a country with millions of Jews, "these Jewish bacilli crossed over to us, bringing the Jewish sickness to our land. Our people almost died from this sickness, had Adolf Hitler not delivered us in the nick of time."[11]

This last phrase was an allusion to Hitler as healer, another well-honed paradigm used in the context of this biologistic allegory. This text, published in 1940, presents the vision of a final convergence of three complementary imagos:

the Jew as disease, the German people as patient,[12] and National Socialism (qua Hitler) as physician, at a time when the Jews of Europe were on the verge of extermination. Through the remaining war years, this triple theme would become firmly entrenched. Whereas Dr. F. Reichert spoke of the detrimental effect of the "parasitical intrusion of the Jews into the German host body" in 1940, his colleague Joseph Ruppert a year later dwelled on epidemics caused in vanquished Poland by disease-ridden Jews and stressed the Jews' immediate isolation.[13] Pointedly, Dr. Rudolf Ramm, an *Amtsarzt* on Conti's staff, wrote in 1942 that Jews had been putting the German people at risk through "the contagion of soul-poisoning ideas and the destruction of germinating life." Yet happily "today there are the blessings for our people resulting from the forcible removal of the Jew from the vital positions and offices of our state."[14] At a time when Leonardo Conti was publicly referring to Jews as "parasites" that could survive only "parasitically inside the peoples," Auschwitz killer physician Fritz Klein was lecturing a female inmate doctor that precisely because he was a doctor, he wanted "to preserve life." It was "out of respect for human life" that he would "remove a gangrenous appendix from a diseased body. The Jew is the gangrenous appendix in the body of mankind."[15]

Purely medical imagery had derivatives straddling the borders to morality or criminality. Sexuality possessed its medical as well as its (public and private) moral dimensions. The alleged bastardization of the "Aryan" race by Jews was a biological-medical problem by virtue of the entry of Jewish semen into the German female organism; it was also a moral one because of promiscuity. As early as the mid-1920s Hitler paired the two when he invoked the danger of the "parasites of the nation" debasing "our inexperienced young blonde girls." More viciously alluring was his characterization of the archetypal Jewish seducer, said to be as condemnable biomedically as he was morally evil: "With satanic joy in his face, the black-haired Jewish youth lurks in wait for the unsuspecting girl whom he defiles with his blood, thus stealing her from her people."[16]

Again in this instance, Hitler was further popularizing a partially medicalized image of the Jews that was not originally his own brainchild but had been around for some time.[17] It is possible that in this case he capitalized not only on the hearsay from Vienna or Munich but on the message in the popular novel by chemist Dr. Artur Dinter, who in the mid-1920s came to serve as the party's Gauleiter in Thuringia. Dinter had published, in many thousand copies as early as 1919, a novel, *Die Sünde wider das Blut* (The sin against the blood), replete with a pseudo-scientific appendix, in which he sought to document not only the sexual depravity of the Jews as they nested amid their German host people but also the calculated cunning with which they aimed systematically to impregnate as many innocent "Aryan" maidens as possible to bring down the Germanic race. Dinter wrote about a rich Hamburg-based Jew called Burghamer, originally from Galicia, who, while married to a beautiful blonde "Aryan," kept scores of stunning young Nordic mistresses in special apartments all over Germany, exchanging them for new blonde virgins as soon as they were pregnant with his bastard.[18]

Nazi physicians hastened to extemporize upon such pornography. The product of prolonged "Aryan" and Jewish sexual intercourse over time, volunteered Eugen Fischer in 1933, might produce a "very respectable culture," but never the same as that grown on purely German soil, never a German but a totally different one, a "half-Oriental" culture.[19] Dr. Walter Gross in the same year of Nazi political triumph expressed chagrin about the "alien blood laws" to which pure Germans had become beholden, to their undying detriment.[20] The year 1935, during which the Nuremberg Laws forbade all sexual relations between "Aryans" and Jews and also made marriage impossible, saw a plethora of polemics against "the influence of foreign blood" and "bastardization." Once more Wagner as author was in the lead, as he ruminated on the mutual union of Germans and Jews as "unnatural," as between two different species, in the image of perverse bestiality.[21] Three years later, when Jewish physicians were being decertified, it became opportune to speak of the elevated cousin of the common picture-book race defiler, namely the non-"Aryan" doctor who would disgrace his profession by performing illegal abortions on biologically worthy women.[22]

In 1939 the dynamics of the war lent added momentum to the development of this specific imagery, as any sexual immorality was said to be tantamount to "Jewish morality" per se.[23] Ramm, who in 1942 had composed a medical ethics text for the National Socialist doctor, remarked poignantly that Reich race legislation, long firmly in place, "would prevent for all times to come any further mingling of German-blooded people with the Jewish nether race."[24] This sexual imagery from the arsenal of Nazi ideology was cruelly inverted when in Auschwitz SS physicians such as Clauberg and Schumann took care painfully to sterilize Jewish women to prevent them from procreating ever again, and especially trained dogs snapped off the genitals of Jewish men in Treblinka, a death camp run, in its initial phase, by the physician Irmfried Eberl.[25]

As a variant of this theme, Nazi physicians identified Jews as both socially and physically in a sicker state than "Aryans." Again, Hitler himself had provided the cue. One of his favorite metaphors in *Mein Kampf* is of the Jew as a criminal, frequently, and race-specifically, as a "white-slave trader," aiding and abetting prostitution, which was of course a health-threatening infraction.[26] Later Gerhard Wagner went to great lengths in trying to delineate all the typically Jewish crimes, including pimping, but also drug-dealing and pickpocketing. In 1935 the Reich physicians' leader surmised that "due to their racial predisposition the Jewish people are particularly prone to commit serious crimes," and in 1938, when the Mosaic doctors had been professionally neutralized, he spoke of those former colleagues as "felons."[27]

Moreover, in the mold of Cologne medicine Professor Reiner Müller Jews were reported to be more disease-ridden than "Aryans," a condition that was attributable to the Jews' alleged lack of hygiene. "If the Jews were alone in this world, they would stifle in filth and offal," wrote Hitler in 1925, adding that dirty Vienna Jews, as he had known them, were at the fountain of all manner of disease.[28] Wagner and his acolytes then linked the Jews to an exceptionally high incidence of mental illness, which was classified as hereditary, and also observed a greater proclivity toward homosexuality among them than among "Aryans."[29] After the conquest of eastern territories, Jews living in the midst of ghetto filth in 1940–41 were judged, by SS physician Ruppert, to have fallen victim to exotic epidemics, to "diseases we are hardly familiar with any more in the Reich." Spotted fever at the end of 1941, explained Conti, was almost four times as prevalent among the Jews of occupied Poland as among ethnic Germans living there. Nevertheless, after the Jews' removal as a source of contagion "the danger has, for all practical purposes, been defeated."[30] Conti erred. In early summer of 1942 a fanatical Jew-hater at the University of Posen, anatomist Professor Hermann Voss, confided to his diary that his assistant, a Baltic nobleman, had died of spotted fever. This victim had caught the disease from one of several Jewish corpses, infested with typhus lice, in the anatomical institute.[31]

The removal of the Jews from the locus of disease in the widest sense, whether they be the cause, the carrier, or the essence of this disease, was the task of the "Aryan" as healer and, more precisely, the job of the Nazi physician. "Killing in the name of healing," as Lifton has explained the responsibility of SS doctors at Auschwitz,[32] was the ultimate function in a protracted and staggered program of excising cancers of race from a threatened Nazi body politic, the *Volksgemeinschaft*, but also from the corpus of the profession itself. Thus to the German doctor there was imputed a higher purpose than merely curing an ailing individual patient. According to Dr. Gross in 1936, the German physician also had the lofty mission of a racial warden. He would have to engage in "problem-solving in the area of natural selection, breeding and elimination, in short: in the preservation of our race."[33] Dr. Amende wrote a year later that "because I wish to be a physician, I have to be a National Socialist. The Nazi worldview and physicianship condition and complement each other. . . . From the very beginning I looked for connecting links in race science and applied racism, which form the basis for National Socialism and have been especially entrusted to the physician."[34] Wagner in 1938 was certain that an ever-growing number of German doctors were fighting in the front lines of the battle for the "preservation of our people's blood, the most precious thing we own and the only valuable which, once lost, can never be retrieved."[35] By dint of such reason Dr. Meier elevated the German physician to the level of a "people's leader," and during the war Conti and Ramm both emphasized the dual role of the doctor as population planner and race controller.[36]

From the beginning to the end, the Nazi solution to the Jewish Question was a medical one, in which German physicians played a key part. This larger international solution process involving entire populations was paralleled, that is, anticipated as well as emulated, at a lower, intranational plane by a social process of excommunicating and eliminating Jewish doctors from the German medical profession. This occurred not least because Jewish doctors were experts, the only experts capable of prolonging Jewish lives, the lives of the very men, women, and children who were to be annihilated by a far-reaching racial policy.

The key figures linking these two scenarios—the destruction of the European Jews and the proscription of German-Jewish physicians—were Dr. Wagner and Dr. Conti, for they became the executors of both schemes. When Hitler received Wagner and Alfons Stauder on that fateful April 5 in 1933, he commanded them to devote their future energies to the "race question."[37] Henceforth Wagner, and later Conti, and their medical staffers, Drs. Gross, Gütt, Blome, and Bartels, became instrumental not only in developing and introducing the Nuremberg race legislation but also in creating the severity with which its various enactments affected German Jews and the murderous ramifications thereafter. Indeed, if Wagner, who largely engineered the 1935 laws, had had his own way, half, quarter, and even one-eighth Jews would have suffered the entire impact of the provisions that struck full Jews after September of that year.[38] Wagner regarded the "Nuremberg Jew Laws" as the culmination of his systematic efforts over the years to cure the German public body of ills: sociopolitical diseases that resulted in the bureaucracy law of April 1933 and congenital disorders necessitating the law for the prevention of hereditarily sick offspring of July 1933.[39] Within Wagner's apparatus, first as the party's plenipotentiary for health and later Reich physicians' leader, two special offices were set up to control and monitor every German's racial pedigree and ferret out the Jews: the Office for Genealogical Research (Amt für Sippenforschung) and the Reich Genealogical Office (Reichssippenamt).[40] For Gerhard Wagner, the racial politics that produced the Nuremberg Laws was the "centerpiece of health policy" writ large, and at his funeral on March 27, 1939, it was aptly said that his entire life had revolved around the unceasing battle "to turn the Germans into the best people in the world, healthwise and race-wise."[41]

General health policy and racial planning remained interconnected from spring 1939 till the end of the Third Reich. It was under Reich Health Leader Conti that the "euthanasia" murders were commenced, and when the first selections took place, all the debilitated Jews were automatically chosen to die, but "Aryan" patients could still be exempt.[42] Auschwitz was the logical extension of sterilization and "euthanasia"; it became the racial clinic par excellence. For it was the exclusive prerogative of physicians to make selections for the gas chambers and to decide who among the Jewish prisoners was physically fit enough to continue living or ill enough to die.[43] This was knowingly alluded to by Dr. Ramm when he wrote that "the more quickly and thoroughly" the radical solution of the Jewish Question occurred, "the sooner and the better the shaping of the

European continent on a racial basis will take place."[44] One of the last racial health measures under consideration in Conti's office was, in August 1944, the abortion of quarter-Jewish fetuses.[45] It is unlikely that the Nazis ever possessed the wherewithal to implement this plan because they had not yet managed to prevent the birth of half Jews. But if nothing else, this bizarre proposal demonstrates the degree of radicalization toward the twin goals of racial and health planning of which Hitler's doctors were capable.

2. Precarious Legality: Till September 1935

In the Third Reich, the persecution of German Jews was a function both of regime planning and of populist actions that were always monitored and sanctioned by the authorities.[1] What happened to Jewish physicians from 1933 onward was therefore consonant with those separate but often interconnected approaches to the perceived problem, against the much larger backdrop of Nazi Judeophobic measures. This was shown early in the regime when high-placed functionaries of the Nazi Physicians' League, that anti-Semitic vanguard of the late republican years, made pronouncements that were expressions both of anticipated official policy and private sentiments shared by most of the *völkisch* doctors.

Thus league cofounder Dr. Kurt Klare, a week after Hitler's takeover, wrote ominously to a colleague that "Jews and philosemites ought to take note of the fact that Germans are masters of their own house once more and will control their own destiny."[2] Some three weeks later Dr. Conti, another founder, published the explicit warning that because no professional group in Germany had been harmed more by Jewry than the medical one, nobody ought to be surprised if the physicians now were shaking off the alien influence.[3] This view was freshly articulated in a programmatic article in the Nazi daily *Völkischer Beobachter*, penned by Gerhard Wagner himself, on March 23.[4] Dr. Hans Deuschl, a former deputy leader of the NSÄB, next called for the removal of all Jewish consulting physicians on contract with a private firm or panel insurance system (*Vertrauensärzte*).[5] Similar threats were issued by other members of the NSÄB leadership, Drs. Gütt, Kötschau, Reiter, and Gross, in the Nazi physicians' tabloid, *Ziel und Weg*. Of course, Gross was lying when he denied that "anti-Semitic hatred or economic jealousy" inspired the current Nazi polemics.[6]

The purge of Jews from the medical profession began in earnest in March, when Wagner, aided by Carl Haedenkamp and Alfons Stauder, initiated a process of dismissing Jewish functionaries from the national medical associations, as well as regional and local groups. Even before Wagner became the Nazi caretaker head of the two large unions, Hartmannbund and Deutscher Ärztevereinsbund, on March 24, *Sanitätsrat* Dr. Ludwig Steinheimer, secretary of the Nuremberg panel physicians' association, in mid-February was called to the office of Dr. Stauder, who still presided over both national bodies. Stauder told Steinheimer to go on an indefinite leave, thereby forcing him out of office.[7] Eventually, in Nuremberg, neurologist Dr. Wilhelm Stöcker took over, a man with the Golden Party Badge of the Old Fighters, who became the Nazi-style regional health commissar.[8] In Mannheim on March 18, the Jewish local physicians' association functionary Dr. Eduard Oppenheimer was summarily dismissed.[9] And in the capital every Jew had given up his seat in the Berlin Physicians' Chamber by March 29.[10] At the first joint meeting of the old Hartmannbund, the Deutscher Ärztevereinsbund, and the Nazi Physicians' League on April 2, Stauder, seconded by Wagner, proclaimed that the first measure all the functionaries had agreed upon was to cause all Jewish officials in the Reich to clear their desks. Wagner's National Socialist leadership principle was taking root.[11]

This was well-calculated state policy. But at the lower plane of popular opinion and spontaneously flagrant activity, Jewish physicians began to be hounded down in a much less organized fashion. Those events revolved around the infamous boycott orchestrated by Joseph Goebbels and Nuremberg Gauleiter Streicher for April 1. If the repulsive actions did not immediately follow those men's incitements, they preceded them and hence contributed to the hate-filled atmosphere that prompted the two Nazi leaders to implement their scheme.[12]

The perpetrators of the boycott demanded that all Germans unite in an ostentatious repudiation of Jewish businesses, including shops of all manner and lawyers' as well as doctors' services, following March 31, throughout Germany. Lists of Jewish proprietors and professionals were posted locally by the SA and fanatical party members. In Halle, for example, ninety-two stores, twelve lawyers' offices, and eleven practicing physicians were branded.[13] In Munich, Mayor Karl Fiehler instructed various party affiliates to apprise their members of the boycott; organized Nazi women were ordered to avoid Jewish doctors.[14] In northern Bavaria, the SA stuck black cardboard shields marked with yellow circles to the professional shingles of the Jews.[15] In Nuremberg, the heartland of anti-Semitism, a high-ranking Nazi said publicly and against all existing laws that municipal welfare offices would henceforth ignore, for reimbursement purposes, social insurance vouchers issued by Jewish doctors, and in Berlin, graffiti outside physicians' offices such as "Jewish Swine" proliferated.[16] Here, also, several Jewish doctors were temporarily rounded up, taken to the exhibition grounds near Lehrter Bahnhof, and shot in the legs during a roll call improvised by Nazi colleagues.[17]

How much of this activity was spontaneous is difficult to assess, yet it is certain that those individuals who stood much to gain by such harassments participated enthusiastically or else incited others. In the scenario of the doctors, they usually were *Jungärzte*, young physicians in search of employment or a panel practice, but also old, hardened anti-Semites like Klare. There is evidence to that effect from Breslau, where one complainant held that he had been turned down for a position at a local clinic, and from Munich, where personal denunciations occurred in great strength.[18] Significantly, the editorial office of *Ziel und Weg*, the NSÄB weekly, was receiving anonymous letters from disgruntled German physicians who wished to see their Jewish colleagues hurt because they were suffering from "being Jewed."[19]

There was much resentment against Jewish colleagues among the "Aryan" doctors, and much physical and psychological harm was done in the wake of the boycott. In Berlin, a twelve-year-old boy was having his appendix removed by a Jewish surgeon surrounded by non-Jewish colleagues. Anesthetized, the lad suddenly began to shout insults against the Jews from his subconscious, while the "Aryans" looked on dumbfounded.[20] As in Berlin at Lehrter Bahnhof, certain Jews were picked up by the SA or Gestapo and detained for a length of time all over Germany. This happened to Munich physician Ludwig Gluskinos, an orthodox Jew who had fought in a Bavarian regiment during World War I. Having been denounced by a Christian colleague, he was held in prison on the trumped-up charge of violating Germany's abortion law but let go after one week.[21] Others were much less fortunate. Berlin welfare physician Georg Benjamin, a well-known communist, was arrested on April 12 and held in the penitentiary till Christmas. On his release, his medical practice was abolished. Dr. Theodor Katz of Nuremberg, another decorated front officer, was taken to Dachau concentration camp in those weeks, where he served as inmate camp physician. By several accounts, he was killed by the SS because he had witnessed too many abuses. Just as his wife came to fetch him, clutching a visa for Palestine, she was told that her husband had committed suicide.[22]

Anticipating a body of anti-Jewish legislation, which by the spirit of the constitution that still formally governed the country was illegal, several municipalities and regional administrations were beginning to bar Jewish physicians from gainful employment, using questionable means. Top communal officials of Berlin and Munich, Julius Lippert and Karl Fiehler respectively, on their own accord broke legitimate contracts when they threw out all Jewish public health and welfare physicians.[23] Streicher's Nuremberg, not surprisingly, embarked on a similar measure.[24] The state of Bavaria discontinued all the Jewish doctors working for the public school system. Fürth prohibited Jewish and "Aryan" German doctors from deputizing for one another, Munich relegated Jewish physicians in hospitals to the treatment of Jewish patients, and Cologne suspended the reimbursement of municipal employees who had paid a Jewish doctor's bill.[25] Under the rabidly anti-Semitic health commissioner Eugen Stähle, Württemberg proscribed its Jewish public health officials, and Baden aimed to restrict all Mosaic panel physicians to their percentage in the population at large.[26] It was at this time that experts of the Reich labor ministry, at the instigation of Dr. Wagner, were toiling away to produce a set of laws designed to deal the first official blow to German-Jewish physiciandom.[27]

This ordinance was pursuant to a public declaration Wagner had issued in the presence of all ranking physician functionaries of the new order in Leipzig on April 2, to the effect that "in future no new Jewish doctors should be certified for panel practice."[28] The regulation was promulgated on April 22; technically it was a sequel to the Law for the Reconstitution of the Civil Service of April 7, 1933, which was used to remove all Jewish civil service physicians (*Amtsärzte*).[29] The April 22 ordinance stipulated that any existing agreements between the panel insurance funds and Jewish or partly Jewish physicians were to be canceled by July 1. (There was also a clause directed against "communist" doctors that has already been dealt with in Chapter 2.) As in the case of civil servants, the so-called Hindenburg exemptions were announced in the following weeks, applying to physicians who had established their practices before August 1, 1914, had seen front-line duty in World War I, had lost a father or son in that war, or had exposed themselves to lethal epidemics in quarantine camps.[30]

Next, every panel physician in Germany received a letter asking him about his pedigree, religion, and war record. If he was non-"Aryan," he was informed by Dr. Wagner's staff that his services were no longer required. Women were equally affected, with fewer chances for exception.[31] Later in the year, succession clauses were announced prohibiting collaboration between "Aryan" and non-"Aryan" physicians and abrogating contracts between Jews and private insurance funds beyond the panel system (*Privatkrankenkassen*).[32] Often, a male doctor's war record was not taken into consideration at first; he was told he could complain to the Reich labor minister in due course. But as the "black book" of the émigré Jews in Paris pointed out in 1934, even if he did so and was reinstated, this redress might come too late to do the practitioner any good, for in the meantime his patients had found a new doctor.[33] Sometimes the front-line-status clause did not work. Dr. Max Markus of Gottesberg in Lower Silesia was released from his contractual obligations as a *Knappschaftsarzt* (consulting physician for a mining company) despite his war record and an injury. After complaining to the minister, he was reconfirmed by Berlin but ended up outside the reconstituted panel practice system because ruses were construed to keep him out. The last incontrovertible trumped-up charge by the KVD against him, in September 1935, was of "continual unprofessional conduct."[34]

It is significant that in its plot against Markus, the KVD was eager to subdue this Jewish doctor with a vengeance, for should he have won his case in court, it would have served as legal precedent for a host of similar cases, in every one of which the KVD would have been caught in the wrong. Not least, the KVD hierarchy would have been liable to pay huge sums of restitution money to the Jewish victims, money that ultimately came out of the "Aryan" physicians' pockets.[35]

This issue was at the core of a fundamental difference of opinion between Wagner's functionaries and the officials in Franz Seldte's Reich labor ministry over how the matter of the Jewish physicians ought to be resolved. Typical of the government bureaucracy in those early years,[36] the conservative ministry officials were much more restrained than party stalwart Wagner and his cronies. The man who was to lock horns with Wagner and Conti in this matter was Dr. Oskar Karstedt, mandated by Seldte to process the Jewish complaint letters and finally to render a judgment on the contested cases. He was at a disadvantage at first, for KVD central (since August 1933) was empowered to cancel out the Jewish panel physicians immediately upon receiving their questionnaires if it saw fit, and hence it canceled out many more than Karstedt himself would have permitted. But when the action was over in the spring of 1934, Karstedt still had kept on a far larger number of Jewish physicians than Wagner and his entourage would have been willing to accept.[37]

Altogether by early 1934, twenty-six hundred physicians had been let go in the Reich, a very small minority of whom were communists. This translated into a noticeable percentage decline in that the level of non-"Aryan" panel physicians had sunk from 16.5 to 11.4 percent. The vacant spots were immediately assigned to "Aryan" *Jungärzte*.[38]

In any event, Wagner, on whose behalf this action was carried through by the Berlin Nazi physicians Erwin Villain and Martin Claus, and then nationally by KVD director Dr. Heinrich Grote, was furious at Karstedt and Minister Seldte for their timid interpretation of the law. As early as July 1933 he maintained that this was not the way to accomplish the National Socialist revolution and that, after all, the final law was "the well-being of the German people."[39] Leonardo Conti, then Berlin representative of the NSÄB, was equally dismayed about the irresoluteness of the government servants; he complained about the "large number" of re-admitted Jewish physicians and is said to have wanted to send Karstedt to a concentration camp by the fall.[40]

Undoubtedly to prevail over Karstedt by using intimidation tactics, the Berlin Nazi doctors decided in early July to arrest a random group of about four dozen male physicians, most of them Jewish and some also members of the SPD or KPD. Drs. Villain and Claus carried out the raid starting in the early morning of July 7. They kept the men in various Berlin prisons for a few days on vague charges of subversion, beating some of them for no apparent reason, such as the neurologist Dr. Kauffmann, the internist Dr. Cohn-Hülse, and the generalist Dr. Birnbaum. On July 11, Gestapo chief Rudolf Diels appeared, a man who has managed since then to whitewash himself in his memoirs as the innocent precursor of Reinhard Heydrich. Cynically, he told the physicians that they had been in "protective custody." Should they ever feel threatened again, they should voluntarily return to such custody. Meanwhile, Karstedt had been approached by Dr. Ruth Aron, the wife of one of the physicians and herself a dentist. Yet according to at least one of the doctors affected, it was not Karstedt who caused them to be freed but the still powerful Jewish congregation of Berlin.[41]

Because of its unusually high Jewish profile, Berlin was, of course, the fulcrum of anti-Jewish repression. Here, the newly appointed health commissioner Dr. Wilhelm Klein, in close association with Conti, was responsible for the brutal purge of Jewish doctors from hospitals and clinics.[42] Here also, the SA, SS, and Gestapo, backed by Nazi doctors, meted out individual harassment both to Jewish physicians who were forced to retire and to those who still had a period of grace. Capricious arrests and torture led to the violent death of Dr. Phillipsthal, who had poked fun at the Nazis before 1933, and Dr. Leopold, on the token charge that he had written an incorrect prescription.[43] Dr. Landsberg was said to have killed himself in prison—a sure indication that he was murdered, the consequence of personal revenge by Dr. Walter Ruppin, a violent Jew-baiter who had succeeded Landsberg as an official of the organized Brandenburg panel physicians. Ruppin, a Nazi party member since 1928, SA doctor, and Reichstag deputy, had accused Landsberg of an act of embezzlement that he had himself committed.[44] Dr. Ludwig Tietz did kill himself at the age of forty, and more than one Jewish physician died of shock or grief over the humiliations they suffered.[45]

Terror reigned against the Jewish doctors all over Germany, especially in the provinces, where there were fewer of them, which, ironically, made them even more visible. In Coburg, sixty-five-year-old Dr. Masur was apprehended and beaten by the hour for two nights, under the supervision of a public school teacher whom Bavarian Minister of Culture Hans Schemm was about to appoint as state secretary. The man thought he had been wronged by a medical commission once headed by Dr. Masur.[46] In Reichenhall a Dr. Stern, recuperating from a stroke in Meran, was replaced in his practice by a local Nazi doctor—a totally illegal action that caused great embarrassment to the party afterward.[47] This precipitous act was just another manifestation of the greed with which "Aryan" physicians pursued their Jewish colleagues in hope of inheriting their fortunes.[48] A tragic event occurred in Württemberg, where health commissar Stähle exercised his oppressive regimen with an iron hand. One of the local SS physicians turned out to have been raised by "Aryan" foster parents, whereas his natural father was revealed as a Jew. This Dr. M. became the victim of his own misguided ideology when he decided that a life without the SS, from which he was now evicted, was not worth living any longer and shot himself. Stähle ventured the terrible verdict that M.'s "Nordic hereditary mass had dominated to the point of victory."[49]

But in the German-Jewish community as a whole, the feeling was not yet altogether one of doom and despair. The successive measures after April 22, 1933, still had not destroyed Jewish physicians, mainly because of the formal exemptive (Hindenburg) clauses. Indeed, the majority of Mosaic doctors in Germany had either fought actively in World War I or had been practicing before August 1914. In November 1933 Karstedt pushed through still another decree favoring the physician widows of Great War front victims.[50] In Munich and Stuttgart relatively few Jewish doctors were concerned, and by 1935 over half of the capital's panel doctors still were Jewish—which was admitted by Jews and non-Jews alike.[51] Those Jews still allowed in the panel practice system were not losing their non-Jewish patients overnight because, contrary to the propaganda of Nazi physicians, they were generally held in high esteem and, as yet, no Nazi pressure was being applied to force German patients to stay away.[52] Moreover, those doctors who now endured the consequences of professional expropriation were aided, as best as was possible, by Jewish self-help organizations that mobilized the wealthier Jews' sense of collective solidarity.[53]

Until the Nuremberg race laws of September 1935, there were few additional enactments to complicate life for those Jewish physicians remaining within the panel insurance system and none to affect the forcefully opted-out ones who continued with private practice. A decree of May 17, 1934, reiterated the injunction of the previous year that no non-"Aryan" be admitted to panel practice and this time expressly mentioned "Aryan" physicians with Jewish spouses. German doctors were also at risk if they had married a Jew after July 1, 1933.[54] After February 13, 1935, German physicians were excluded from the insurance funds whose marriage to a Jew predated the July 1933 cutoff point.[55] This provision created hardship for some, but not necessarily right away. The Böblingen gynecologist Bernhard Heyde, for instance, who employed his Jewish wife as his assistant, was not forced to give up his practice until about 1937.[56] Others succumbed to Nazi propaganda and divorced their Jewish spouses, but some had done so even before 1935.[57] As a rule, mixed marriages were becoming a strain on both conjugal partners, whether they were Jewish or "Aryan." Private tragedies occurred. In Berlin the specialist Dr. Arthur Beer, a Jew, ended his life in spring 1935 to ease the situation for his Christian wife.[58]

If on a semiprivate level oppression of the Jewish physicians continued, this was a result of the half-measures taken by the government in banning them from panel practice in 1933. These measures had still made it possible for too many "Aryan" patients to go on seeing their trusted Jewish doctors and get reimbursed by the funds. Before harassing the Jews themselves, therefore, party agencies, including the KVD, but also German doctors, applied pressure to the patients to compel them to switch over to "Aryan" physicians.

Hence, while in the hospitals of large cities like Hamburg or Berlin so many Jewish staff members had been let go that "Aryan" doctors were called up to fill their places, doctors who, like the noted poet and sometime physician Gottfried Benn, would never have considered such service in normal circumstances,[59] many non-Jewish physicians blamed an apparent lack of patients on thriving Jewish practices. Thus some of them advertised their status by marking "German Physician" on their shingles.[60] Others complained to the authorities, who issued exhortations to Germans of all walks of life to leave the Jewish doctors to their Jewish patients.[61] This did not help much, for not only did many Germans prefer the Jewish experts for professional reasons but some also tended to visit them as an act of political disapproval.[62] In September 1934 the NSÄB chapter in Wiesbaden registered ruefully that in the past three months the twenty-four Jewish physicians still licensed for panel practice had been consulted by 8.5 percent of all the fund-insured patients who needed medical advice.[63] Small wonder if in July of the following year the radical party press was demanding the death penalty for all those Jewish doctors, not excluding the ones beyond the fund system, who still dared to treat gentile patients.[64]

But the regime had a much larger problem on its hands in that civil servants and even members of party organizations were reluctant to surrender their trusted Jewish doctors. To check the state officials, the NSDAP in Baden passed an edict in June 1935 announcing their exclusion from the German civil servants' union should they not drop their Jewish doctors (as well as lawyers). And in Ulm near Stuttgart, where the party had managed to obtain the patient lists of two Jewish panel physicians, the authorities were shocked by the large number of civil servants still frequenting those doctors.[65]

But the wrath of the Nazis knew no bounds when they found out how many of their own number still engaged Jewish doctors—those people were traitors, countermanding the ideology of race. The examples were ample. In Berlin, an Old Fighter with a bad leg was delivered to a Jewish private clinic, where the surgeons wished to call on Dr. Sauerbruch for the unavoidable operation. The Nazi himself, however, insisted on a Jewish surgeon. His wish was granted, but a postoperation infection later claimed his life.[66] The Jewish émigré physician Martin Gumpert relates in his memoirs that many Nazis came to see Jewish doctors more for psychological reasons, for here they could bicker away at their own regime without fear of discovery.[67] John Toland reports that after her suicide attempt in late May 1935 Eva Braun, the Führer's mistress, was treated by Munich's Jewish Dr. Martin Marx, for whom Eva's sister Ilse worked as receptionist. Reputedly, Hitler accepted Marx's diagnosis of "fatigue" as the official reason for a narcotics overdose, even though he probably guessed that Eva's real reason had been loneliness.[68]

The party agencies acted again. In Greater Wiesbaden, where 274 physicians, Jews and non-Jews, were officially registered by 1934–35, the Nazi Physicians' League issued a directive in late August 1934 admonishing all non-Jewish patients to see only "Aryan" doctors, of whom there were 161, conveniently listed in a separate, party-edited directory. Of those, almost 60 percent were carefully identified as members of the NSÄB, and it was strongly suggested that they be given preference. For all NSDAP as well as ancillary party members the observance of this list was made obligatory.[69] Moreover, in Thuringian Erfurt a few weeks later the local NSÄB and KVD functionary Dr. Curt Staeckert issued a circular complaining about the increasing popularity of Erfurt's sixteen Jewish panel physicians. Charging that those doctors had at least doubled their incomes (which he was in a position to know as local head of the KVD) and that the incomes of some "Aryan" physicians had receded accordingly, he vented his rage against the real culprit, the National Socialist patient: "If a communist or a reactionary goes running to the Jew, I can understand it, but if a party member or SA man in uniform visits a Jewish doctor, this is a breach of fealty to the Führer." Staeckert served notice that henceforth he would control the patients and would cause the immediate dismissal of recalcitrant party and SA members. Civil servants and even private employees would not escape his punishment either.[70]

All things considered, for the Jewish doctors of 1934–35 this phase was disconcerting, but relatively it still was one of calm before the storm. Periodically, there were signs of the tragedy ahead for those who did not close their eyes completely. Apart from social ostracism that many of them suffered at the hands of their "Aryan" colleagues,[71] individual Mosaic or baptized non-"Aryan" physicians still continued to fall prey to indiscriminate acts of private, semipublic, and official revenge, in the precarious legality that affected the lives of all Jews in the Reich at that time.[72] Any Jewish doctor could be singled out by real or self-appointed agents of the regime for vindictiveness or sport. Thus in the first half of 1934 fifty-seven-year-old Berlin gynecologist Max Hirsch from Berlin received a night call summoning him to a rich patient. He was ushered into a limousine, driven to Grunewald, viciously beaten, and told to take himself away "to Palestine."[73] The days surrounding the Röhm crisis raised the specter of lawlessness to an unusual degree even for Hitler's Germany. It stood to reason that Jews would suffer exceptionally, physicians among them, some of whom were groundlessly maligned and even shot.[74] In November 1934, Berlin chief physician Paul Lazarus, who was responsible for a wing at the private St. Anthony hospital, where patients with lung ailments were served desserts of pudding with sculptured swastikas—a brave if foolish attempt to mock the Nazis—was earmarked for a "rope-tightening" by the party before "repatriation to fresh air."[75] Time and again, Jewish doctors were picked up at their homes or from the street and taken to camps or jails, sometimes never to be seen again.[76]

Also, the fundamental disagreement between the Reich labor ministry and the Nazi-controlled KVD was still haunting the Jewish doctors, as the originally intended victims. The KVD was continually embarrassed because the final rulings of the labor ministry served as the legal basis for financial redress claims in cases of Jewish physicians who had been rashly discriminated against by KVD officials.[77] With this as a motive, and certain of the backing of most "Aryan" doctors in the land, the revengeful KVD officials were doing everything in their power to continue skirting or breaking the existing laws. In one instance a doctor was to be pushed out of the regional hospital of Pomeranian Belgard, although he was Hindenburg-exempt and had done no wrong. The local KVD pressured the region's administration and then the Reich ministry of the interior to force the man's expulsion, without ultimately succeeding.[78] In the second instance, Dr. Staeckert of Erfurt not only chastised his party comrades but sought to defame the sixteen Jewish panel colleagues to such a degree as to rob them of their livelihood. He even wished to harm the privately practicing Jews. Along with Dr. Carl-Oscar Klipp, the regional KVD superior, Staeckert concocted a charge of conspiracy to ship the doctors and their Jewish lawyers off to jail. Finally, even KVD central in Berlin realized that this matter had gone too far and ordered a close to the affair.[79] Ominously, KVD director Dr. Grote said in a public forum, addressing the loyal NSÄB members in Hanover on June 29, 1935, that the German medical profession still had not been cleansed of Jewish elements and that this goal had yet to be attained.[80]

Grote knew well of what he spoke. He was privy to the planning by Wagner, Gross, and others in regard to the anti-Jewish race legislation to be announced two and a half months later. This legislation would precipitate charges of sexual misdemeanor of unprecedented proportions against Jews, many aimed specifically against doctors. This, too, was already in the wind. From the beginning of the persecution, Jewish physicians had been unjustly accused of taking advantage of their female patients (or receptionists), and that of course was fully in accord not only with the general stereotype of the Jewish persona as sexual predator, but, in the medicalized image of progressive ethnic spoliation, with the more narrowly specified picture of the Jewish doctor as master and manipulator of, in Nazi terms, ill-begotten life. In this largely pornographic scenario of harassment of Jewish physicians on sexual grounds, the gynecologists and obstetricians naturally had the most to suffer.[81]

This theme continued through 1934 and in 1935 led to the race pronouncements of the September party rally. In spring and summer 1935, particularly, those sexual accusations were stepped up, against the wider background of molestation of all the Reich's Jews on sexual counts.[82] Jewish physicians were increasingly arrested and dragged off for having performed abortions on "Aryan" women, for having sexually abused female patients, or for having turned them into permanent mistresses.[83] At this time, Streicher's rag *Der Stürmer* further publicized the image of the Jewish doctor as race defiler by printing the story of blonde, beautiful Inge, who trustingly went to see the fat Jewish doctor with the thick lips and the hooked, fleshy nose, and how he approached her indecently as she was lying anxiously on the examination couch. A coarse illustration left no doubt in the reader's mind as to the insidiously destructive power of the Israelites.[84]

3. Progressive Disfranchisement: From the 1935 Nuremberg Race Laws to Delicensure in September 1938

After Gerhard Wagner's connivance, Hitler announced the Nuremberg Race Laws in a public speech on September 15, 1935, at the climax of the annual Reich party rally in Nuremberg.[1] This comprehensive, complex legislation defined who was a Jew right down to one of the four grandparents, but despite Wagner's earlier insistence, only full Jews, those persons identified as having four Jewish grandparents, now were to suffer immediate and automatic encroachments. Although they soon lost their citizenship (and were henceforth derogatorily classified merely as "residents" of Germany), Germans of mixed parentage (*Mischlinge*) were still able to petition the interior ministry for Reich citizenship (unless the proportion of "Aryan" blood predominated, in which case they had citizenship automatically). Since noncitizens could not hold public office, all Jewish civil servants still officiating in the German Reich were to be dismissed by December 31. Germans and Jews were prohibited from marrying, and all extramarital sexual contact between them was made a punishable offense. No Jew was allowed to have in his or her employ female Germans under the age of forty-five.[2]

These regulations dealt the most devastating blow to German Jewry to date.[3] More precisely, they entailed several serious consequences for Jews in the profession of medicine. The most obvious one was that since all Jewish civil servants who had been Hindenburg-exempt had to be forcefully retired, albeit with a—later reducible—pension, the remaining professors of medicine, *Amtsärzte*, and other state-employed Jewish physicians were finally to be dismissed. But under this rubric, the Nazis now also took the liberty of referring to privately contracted chief physicians at public hospitals.[4] Since the category of *Mischling* was now more closely delineated in that some partially Jewish persons were counted as part of the Jewish minority (for instance half Jews of Mosaic persuasion or married to fully ethnic Jewish spouses), the group of nonexempt "Jewish" physicians was enlarged.[5] The Reich Physicians' Ordinance of December 13, 1935, stated unequivocally that no new Jewish (including *Mischling* down to a quarter Jewish) candidates could henceforth be licensed for medical practice in the Reich, as long as there was a danger that the proportion of Jews in the total of the Reich's physicians would exceed that of Jews in the general population. Even those *Mischlinge* who were allowed to be citizens, and non-Jewish physicians married to Jews, would continue to be excluded from the profession, by withholding of licensure generally, and also by disapproval for the panel funds specifically, as had been stated under the ordinance of May 17, 1934, unless they received individual dispensations from the interior ministry.[6] Jews exempted by the regulations of 1933 were permitted to remain as members of the fund insurance system, at least in theory,[7] and neither were they touched if practicing beyond the panel scheme, which was becoming ever more difficult from an economic point of view.

This comprehensive legislation was designed to cause further deterioration of Jewish physicianship in the Reich, and it achieved its purpose. For those Jewish doctors still permitted and sufficiently strong-hearted to practice after fall 1935, there were one or two not so obvious clauses of the Nuremberg Laws that proved, over time, to be particularly irritating. Depriving Jews of their Reich citizenship was to make it more complicated for privately practicing specialists, for instance, to travel to attend international professional meetings or give lectures at a university, not just because of passport difficulties but also encumbrances in getting the necessary hard-currency exchange.[8] Moreover, the provision calling for dismissal of female help under the age of forty-five often meant that Jewish doctors lost not only their trusted "Aryan" assistants, including highly trained nurses in private hospitals, but also maids needed for a busy household, and could not easily replace them with qualified Jewish ones.[9]

Until Jewish physicians' licenses were totally abrogated in fall 1938, the Nazis took care to chip away slowly but relentlessly at the bedrock of professionalism remaining for the Jewish colleagues. In March 1936, Dr. Wagner's agencies decided that Jewish, panel-practicing radiologists should lose that status. This enactment remained legally doubtful until years later when the highest Reich appeals court finally substantiated the KVD's position.[10] By August 1936, word was spreading in Berlin leftist opposition circles that fund privileges were not honored by the KVD; Jewish panel physicians who performed surgery on "Aryan" patients were not paid.[11] In a Saxon spa a few months later, three Jewish panel physicians previously attending to many Jewish convalescents were taken off fund practice, without being given any reasons.[12] In Augsburg at the end of the year the contract between the four remaining Jewish panel physicians and the municipal welfare office was scheduled for cancellation.[13] In May 1937 the Reich Physicians' Chamber curtailed the constitutional right of any Jewish physician to participate in disciplinary proceedings, such as on medical ethics boards.[14] And finally, on January 1, 1938, all Jewish physicians were removed from membership in the often lucrative supplementary (private) insurance funds (*Ersatzkrankenkassen*), which largely serviced upper-income business employees. A few intrepid Jews who argued against the KVD in court that these funds were on a par with the general funds and thus were governed by the same criteria of membership adherence (Hindenburg exemptions) were lectured by the judges that the KVD was an instrument of the Nazi regime and therefore beyond the law. All at once, this callous measure deprived three thousand Jewish physicians of their livelihood, close to a thousand of them in the capital.[15]

Because "Aryan" patients, including civil servants and party cadres, were still reluctant to leave their Jewish doctors, especially those within the fund system, the Nazi medical authorities had to devise new ruses to direct them to the German physicians instead.[16] This was problematical because the law still provided no basis for doing so. In Munich, the overly eager mayor Fiehler at the end of 1935 could do no more than threaten municipal officials and employees by promising disciplinary action later on and evidently did so by 1937.[17] In the Hamburg area, a retired state official and SA man was evicted from the Brown Shirts and told that his pension would be reduced if he did not repent and discard his personal physician, a privileged panel-practicing Mosaic one. Yet another civil servant near Hamburg, a policeman, was about to face eviction from the force for sending his gravely ill child to the same doctor when he insisted on this course of action for the future. After superiors had informed the patient's father that the state officials' sickness fund would under no circumstances pay the fees of a Jew, that Samaritan doctor treated the child free of charge.[18] Then, in October 1936, the Reich interior minister passed a law forbidding state officials to visit any Jewish physicians, including the traditionally privileged ones. To drive the point home, the names of longtime civil service patients of Jewish physicians were exposed in the daily press.[19]

It was even more difficult to restrain the ordinary citizens, particularly since the Jewish doctors they consulted were legally able to practice. The only tactic the regime could use was persuasion and harassment typical of totalitarian systems. Party formations intensified their pressure on the collective membership so that the Labor Front in Hamburg denied reimbursements for medical certificates from Jewish panel practitioners by July 1936.[20] A month later the local panel fund of Dresden intimidated patients by prompting them to choose only non-Jewish physicians from the valid list of panel practitioners, which—as was the law—officially did not distinguish between "Aryan" and non-"Aryan" doctors.[21] Near Hamburg in the fall of 1937, party members were standing guard in front of Jewish doctors' offices, registering every German visitor who entered.[22] Beyond all pseudo-patriotic rhetoric,[23] the ultimate and extremely dubious weapon of the racist doctors was defamation; by 1938, the rabid hate groups such as those around Streicher had published the names and places of work of "Jew-consorts" who had consulted their old physicians.[24]

Hence several conditions and processes intersected over the years to further the progressive disfranchisement of Jewish doctors as bona fide members of a traditionally respected profession: the vicious jealousy of the "Aryan" physicians, the official legislation mostly emanating from Berlin, the extralegal machinations of Wagner's agencies, particularly the KVD, the acquiescence or collaboration of the law courts, the evil acts of wanton denunciation from among the common people, and the perfidiousness of all manner of party cadres. The unavoidable result was that Jewish doctors were losing income, despite the energy they invested in their calling. Privately practicing physicians, who would not be reimbursed by the panel funds, found it increasingly difficult to attract wealthy patients who could afford to disregard health insurance; these doctors' numbers were growing as more and more of them suffered from discrimination and their clientele remained constant or on the decline. Thus independent establishments—once well-to-do practices or private clinics—were forced to close.[25] One can only surmise that those Jewish *Privatärzte* were earning next to nothing before they finally gave up. In the case of Jewish panel practitioners, we have KVD testimony for 1936–38. The situation may have been just bearable until the end of 1935. But judging from the case of three Jewish generalists in Upper-Silesian Neisse, incomes dropped disastrously after that. As reported by the KVD officials themselves, the combined annual fund earnings of the three doctors in question had been no more than 800 marks, plus what they may have been able to bill private patients. That came to under 300 marks per person, at a time when "Aryan" physicians were grossing over 13,000 marks on average a year.[26] Whatever "Aryan" patients these doctors still had more likely than not paid them private fees in monthly installments, for the panel funds would try to refuse coverage for any but Jewish-insured patients.[27]

One may well ask how under such dark skies German-Jewish doctors mustered the stamina to hold out. Their circumstances were worsening virtually by the week. Because of the essentially sexual nature of the Nuremberg "blood laws" (the Nazi jargon), namely that Jewish males be forever prevented from plying their trade as race defilers by impregnating "Aryan" women, the professional relationships between Jewish male physicians and German female patients were now more in jeopardy than ever before. In growing numbers, Jewish physicians would be charged with *Rassenschande* or race defilement after young female patients reported to the authorities that they had tried to kiss them or exhibited other prurient behavior. Not only were these charges almost always false, but it is known that in several cases the "patients" had been sent by Nazi enemies to trick the physician into a compromising situation, and to catch him *in flagranti*, party stooges would suddenly enter on cue.[28] In one particularly shameful incident in September 1937, Dr. Otto Schwabe of Hanau near Frankfurt, who once had a flourishing practice, was accused of indecent assault by the husband of a patient, after the doctor had helped the couple with its roofing business for years. This physician had just received emigration papers for himself and his family when he was taken away to police headquarters. There he took his own life by jumping from the building.[29]

In the spirit of the blood laws, it was also becoming much more common to combine sexual misdemeanor charges with accusations of abortion.[30] For offenses against criminal code paragraph 218 protecting unborn life, heavy punishment was meted out to Jews. Thus in Hamburg Dr. Martin Jakobowitz was condemned to six years in the penitentiary in late 1935 and, of course, his medical license was taken away.[31] After trial in Nuremberg, Dr. Ernst Seckendorf was to be incarcerated for ten years; he was one of those accused of both crimes at once.[32] By themselves, *Rassenschande* verdicts seem to have resulted in shorter jail terms,[33] but this did not mean much, for it may be assumed that after their release those unfortunate physicians were picked up by the SS at the prison gate and taken to a concentration camp. There the Jewish "race defilers" were subjected to special tortures, and hardly any survived.[34] Probably in anticipation of this fate, the wrongly indicted Jewish doctors continued to commit suicide at an alarming rate.[35] The blood laws had one other humiliating effect for both Jewish patients and doctors in that those patients, where they still were being admitted to municipal hospitals (not, for instance, in Hamburg or Düsseldorf), from 1937 on had to be sequestered from the "Aryans," ostensibly to prevent *Rassenschande*.[36]

The problem of the *Mischling* physicians and mixed-marriage physicians was now further compounded. By September 1935 the situation had deteriorated for some partial Jews and had improved for others. But because on a few salient points of definition the September laws had been less than lucid (awaiting a finite regulation planned for the future), for yet a third group in between the uncertainty continued, and these people were wondering whether they would finally be counted among the Jewish minority or the German majority.

Physician members of this last group began to assert themselves immediately after the Nuremberg Laws. For it was becoming clear that Wagner, the KVD, and party agencies, just as in the case of Wagner's feud with the Reich labor ministry earlier, would insist on a harsh interpretation of the term *Mischling*, in possible opposition to the Reich interior minister, to whose office recourse was possible. Thus in December 1935 seven doctors of Mannheim, who were either half or a quarter Jewish but nonetheless were being boycotted openly by party organizations, applied to Minister Frick for recognition as non-Jews. Frick evidently notified Wagner, who then had no choice but to order the deletion of those doctors' names from the illegally circulating party blacklists.[37]

In 1936 and 1937 the situation for partly Jewish Germans was still ambiguous so that the eugenicist Professor Otmar Freiherr von Verschuer of Frankfurt University, along with his assistant Dr. Josef Mengele, attempted to clarify matters for his own purposes, which at the time involved paternity judgments, usually weighing the Jewish heritage against the examinees.[38] Not surprisingly, some *Mischlinge* were still allowed to practice, among the doctors who were ordered before the courts for sexually related infractions.[39] Wagner unflinchingly believed that not the least objective of the Nuremberg clauses was "to make the mixed race, which is politically and biologically unwanted, disappear as soon as possible, for a mixling can never be a patriot."[40] Probably to have firmer control over the uneasy situation of *Mischling* physicians and to obviate their appeals to the Reich interior ministry, as specified by the Nuremberg Laws, Wagner decided on September 8, 1937, to render a partly Jewish doctor's access to panel practice contingent on his own analysis of the case.[41] A recent sampling of the records of the Reich Physicians' Chamber to ascertain the qualities of those physicians who passed Wagner's test revealed that he applied strict criteria before granting panel-practice privileges. Invariably, the "mixlings" of the first degree, that is the half Jews, had to be baptized, male, and with official veteran status,[42] while the "mixlings" of the second degree (quarter Jews) encountered no hurdles.

Physicians in mixed marriages continued to be at risk, too. "Aryan" doctors with Jewish spouses first fell under the blood laws, and then under Wagner's September 1937 ordinance they were often expelled from the funds unless they agreed to divorce.[43] Front veteran Dr. Keller of Hindenburg (Upper Silesia), who refused to leave his wife, lost panel privileges as early as spring 1937, after which the Jewish woman took her own life.[44] Others fared similarly.[45] German doctors with half-Jewish wives seem to have had no problems,[46] but Jewish physicians with "Aryan" spouses were sometimes worse off than those with Jewish wives because in the cosmology of disease and race they were regarded as perennial "defilers."[47] By 1937, there still appear to have been 350 *Mischling* physicians practicing in the Reich, half and quarter Jews, most of them probably bereft of all panel fund ties. There were also 210 physicians of mixed marriage, approximately 40 of whom were residing in Berlin, where they had formed a support group.[48]

Inter-Jewish self-help became an ever more important condition of survival for these physicians in trying times. In Berlin, within the framework of self-restrictive autonomy and cultural self-realization that the SS was allowing the Jews of Germany short of evacuation and liquidation, physicians and auxiliary personnel could train recruits and seek continuing education under the curatorship of a renowned bacteriologist, Professor Erich Seligmann.[49] Financial support from wealthier Jews also continued, as did the proceeds from the annual Physicians' Ball in the capital, but they were dwindling.[50]

Training courses were held in the few remaining Jewish hospitals, by far the most viable organizations in the support network of German Jews at that time. In 1931, there had been thirty-five Israelite hospitals throughout Germany, with more than twenty-five hundred beds to serve patients of both faiths.[51] Indeed, the standard of those hospitals was so renowned that even as late as 1933, some of them, like the ones in Hanover and Breslau, had looked after more Christian patients than Jewish.[52] Now, superb Jewish doctors such as Siegfried Ostrowski, Siegmund Hadda, and Paul Rosenstein selflessly dedicated their talents to strictly Jewish patients in the clinics not yet closed by the Gestapo, even though they were enduring incredible hardship, mostly from lack of funds and the departure of qualified nurses and orderlies.[53] There were also smaller Jewish health care institutions such as a children's sanatorium and a medical spa in Bad Kissingen, but they, too, soon were taxed beyond their capacity.[54]

All told, the period of progressive disfranchisement for Jewish physicians brought on more tribulations in a variety of ways, up to the point of professional decertification in fall 1938. If a number of Jewish doctors returned from exile at that time, it was because of the rays of hope that they discerned, falsely based on the nontypical exceptions. Even though it was said by one knowledgeable observer that "anti-Semitism was strongest among the intellectuals, and most virulent among the doctors,"[55] there were of course still German physicians who not only disliked what they saw being done to their Jewish colleagues but who actually stepped in to help.[56] In addition, as physicians were getting scarce throughout Germany, the remaining Jews among them were treated somewhat less harshly in regions with an acute shortage of doctors.[57]

Further encouraging were court pronouncements, by hitherto uncorrupted justices, who ruled in favor of persecuted Jewish physicians and against Gerhard Wagner's KVD.[58] In the aftermath of the quarrels it had had with the Reich labor ministry, resulting frequently in lawsuits that the Jewish plaintiffs thought they had a chance of winning, the KVD's guiding principle was to make compensation payments "only if the association has actually been forced by court order at the highest appeal level."[59] As their preserved correspondence shows, these officials foamed at the mouth whenever they were compelled to give in and cede an annual pension to a "Jewish scoundrel."[60]

But the main development of capricious as well as systematic oppression continued unabated. In late October 1935 Dr. Hans Serelmann of Saxon Niederlunkwitz was delivered by his "Aryan" colleagues to the Gestapo for having performed a transfusion of "Jewish" blood on an "Aryan" patient. Serelmann spent seven months in a concentration camp before being released and able to flee the country.[61] Such "Aryan" doctors now had virtually all taken care to mark their office shingles with bright-red letters.[62] They would also cause the outside of their Jewish colleagues' dwellings to be smeared insultingly, and they saw to it that such colleagues were prohibited from using taxis to get to hospitals and that their mortgages were foreclosed illegally, further to ruin them economically.[63] It was clear that the ongoing arrests and condemnations of Jewish doctors were in no small degree the result of the German physicians' collusion and outright cooperation with regime authorities.[64]

With the Anschluss of Austria to the Old Reich (Altreich) in spring 1938 the suffering of Jewish physicians entered its final stage before the regime's crackdown in autumn of that year. It has been well documented and described how the Nazi forces, combining viciousness with alacrity, sought out and manhandled Jews, particularly in Vienna.[65] Henceforth the Jews of Austria were to share the fate of the Jews in the Altreich, but they tended to be even more mercilessly treated because the Nazis rightly suspected among them a greater proportion of hated eastern Jewry, such as from Polish Galicia, once part of the Austro-Hungarian Empire. In the course of the Waldheim affair it is only now coming to light how enthusiastically Austrian Nazis assisted the German anti-Semites, working off racist prejudices which, in the Austro-Hungarian realm, were more traditionally and much deeper rooted than in Germany proper.[66] Characteristically, Hitler's personal notions of anti-Semitism hailed almost exclusively from turn-of-the-century Vienna, then the hub of the disintegrating Habsburg domain.[67]

In the ensuing persecution of the Austrian Jews, the more elevated members of society such as academic professionals were singled out for special harassment.[68] Among those were the physicians, who, as the Nazis were charging, amounted to rather more than 50 percent of all the doctors in the country, making them much more heavily overrepresented than in Germany proper, with approximately 65 percent in Vienna alone.[69] In the roundups that followed, Jewish physicians probably surpassed all the other professions as victims, including lawyers, who also fared very badly.[70] In Vienna, Jewish doctors, upon immediate dismissal from employment or having been chased out of their offices and homes, were made to perform demeaning tasks while their "Aryan" servants sat down, watching comfortably.[71] There were tragic suicides.[72] Those among the Jewish doctors who had not yet capriciously been beaten out of office, arrested, or even murdered could attempt to carry on with private medical practice. Officially, this was stopped in September 1938, when the final act of vengeance was perpetrated upon Jewish doctors in the Altreich.[73] By spring 1939 approximately two thousand Jewish physicians had been removed from Austrian society.[74]

4. The End of the Jewish Doctors

The total elimination of Jewish physicians in the Third Reich began with an order issued by Heydrich's SD on April 6, 1937, to compile systematic lists of all Jews active in the medical profession throughout Germany.[1] On June 14 the nefarious Wagner in an audience with the Führer impressed upon him the necessity of eliminating the Jewish physicians still in practice, whether they were attached to the insurance panels or not.[2]

This was the prelude to Hitler's ordinance of July 25, 1938, cosigned by Interior Minister Frick and Deputy Führer Hess, which was based on the Nuremberg Race Laws. It stipulated that by September 30 all Jewish doctors were to be decertified. Frick was empowered to make exceptions in the case of a few Jews who could continue to treat their spouses and legitimate children. As stated in previous statutes, no more Jews could be licensed. Jewish doctors' office leases could be canceled for December 31 by either side.[3] As was elaborated in subsequent commentaries, those Jewish doctors who were to be retained were no longer regarded as full-fledged members of the German medical community; they lost the designation of "physician" and all memberships in professional organizations. They were to be tolerated only in places with a high concentration of Jews such as Berlin or Vienna (because "Aryan" doctors should not treat Jews), always subject to the recall of their transitory "privileges." Moreover, the revocation of Jewish doctors' office leases was to be one-sided, solely to the advantage of the "Aryan" leasors; if the physician wanted to give notice, the leasor was shielded by a protection clause, but not vice versa.[4]

At the end of September, then, Jewish doctors, as the world had admired them for decades, to all intents and purposes vanished from the German medical scene. The delicensure figures for Silesia are indicative of the changing pattern in other regions of the Reich. Here, 312 practicing Jewish physicians had remained by the fall of 1938, 191 of them in the panel insurance system. As of September 30, merely 15 Mosaic doctors stayed on, to treat the Jews of Breslau through the facilities afforded by the Israelite hospital.[5] In Württemberg 55 Jewish physicians were discontinued, 30 of them panel doctors. Twenty Jewish medical men remained in Stuttgart, and by early 1939 only 10 of them remained in the considerably larger city of Munich. By that time there were only 285 Jewish doctors to practice among the Jews of the Reich; their official designation now was *Krankenbehandler*, or, derogatorily, "sick-treaters," in which capacity they were severely regimented through supervision by the public health departments.[6] This expulsion of the Jewish physicians was accompanied by Nazi expressions of derision and contempt, and this time the economic advantages arising from this action for "Aryan" doctors were bluntly admitted.[7]

In the months following September 1938 and until the war, a spate of directives was issued, some of them in the context of general anti-Semitic legislation affecting all Jews, which made life for the sick-treaters progressively miserable. Not surprisingly, the Reich Physicians' Chamber instantly excluded as many former Jewish practitioners from retirees' pensions as possible, insofar as those colleagues had contributed to a retirement plan at all.[8] At the beginning of October it was stated that the allowable pariah physicians could avail themselves of panel-practice privileges, as long as their Jewish patients were insured, but only provisionally and subject to future rulings.[9] Later in the month, Jews generally had to surrender their passports, which jeopardized further their opportunity to travel abroad.[10] In December, Police Chief Himmler forbade German Jews the use of automobiles and canceled their drivers' licenses;[11] this action severely hampered doctors who were on call. Only two sick-treaters were to be permitted in the newly acquired city of Danzig early in 1939, and all Jewish doctors were proscribed in the "protectorate" of Bohemia and Moravia, carved out of Czechoslovakia, by the end of May in that year.[12] A demeaning imposition on Jewish doctors and patients alike was announced in June, when medicinal spas were said to be off limits for Jews unless they had an illness certificate signed by the regional health office, not the doctor, and could be segregated at the site from "Aryan" visitors.[13]

Meanwhile, the difficulties of Jewish physicians in Germany had been further compounded, in two important respects, by the November 9 and 10, 1938, *Kristallnacht*.[14] First, Jewish doctors became victims of the pogroms that took place throughout the German lands and, in accordance with the "Aryan" medical counterculture that wished to see Jews dead, were, if anything, treated more brutally than nondoctors because they alone could help preserve Jewish life. Second, inasmuch as they were able to treat their fellow Jewish victims as patients to restore them to a state of health (hence counterchecking that "Aryan" culture), they were beginning to imbue their specific vocation with a new important meaning. Their Hippocratic action now and in the future would develop into an antigenocidal subtheme right to the worst climax in the history of the Holocaust.

Hence the Nazi bullies, aware of the crucial role of doctors in Jewish society, arrested a veritable multitude of them in Berlin, "in order to deprive a large number of Jewish sick persons of medical aid," as Ostrowski has correctly observed.[15] Here in the capital Nazi hospital surgeon Kurt Strauss tolerated Jewish casualties of the anti-Semitic violence only with great reluctance, after they had been admitted to the wards by a more compassionate "Aryan" doctor.[16]

Because they were most suspect by Nazi criteria, it was extremely risky even for legitimate Jewish physicians to be found practicing their profession in the days after November 10. If they did not go into temporary hiding, they were subject to immediate arrest and dispatch to a concentration camp, as almost happened to Ostrowski.[17]

Thus the Jewish physicians of the Israelite hospital in Leipzig were picked up and carted off; Buchenwald, Dachau, and Oranienburg-Sachsenhausen near Berlin, the destination of most November pogrom victims, took in many doctors. Here they helped their fellow Jews, under the most primitive conditions. Often they were too weak to do so, as was Dr. Fackenheim of Wiesbaden, who suffered from diarrhea in Buchenwald.[18] Other Jewish doctors lost faith and committed suicide, and in Burgdamm near Bremen seventy-eight-year-old Dr. Adolf Goldberg and his wife, Martha, were shot to death, without provocation, by marauding SA men.[19]

The patients Jewish doctors were treating in the Israelite hospitals of the large cities were either victims of Nazi hooligan attacks or survivors of suicides, and many of the latter group could not be saved despite all efforts. The tasks of the doctors were complicated by Black or Brown Shirts and Gestapo agents who would search the hospitals and harass patients and personnel alike. In Fürth, for example, many Jewish inmates of the clinic, including those who needed emergency operations, and their warders were forced to stand at attention for the SA for an entire hour.[20] The Jewish physicians also were under the threat of vandalism, as occurred in Berlin, where Nazi troopers demolished the Israelite hospital's interior and specialized equipment.[21] "It is a people's duty," said Professor von Verschuer after the pogroms to representatives of heavy industry, in an address saturated with medicobiological metaphor, "to reject such alien race elements, if it wants to preserve its own kind. Once such elements have entered, they must be forced out and destroyed. There is no denying that the Jew is of a different kind and hence is to be resisted, if and when he seeks to enter. It is a matter of self-defense."[22]

The ordeals of *Kristallnacht* for most Jewish physicians lasted for a few weeks, for some until early 1939. When matters had quieted down, the daily work of caring for the Jewish population's health was resumed in the few remaining private practices and, predominantly, in the Israelite hospitals. Of those, the one in Berlin was the most significant; it and the institution in Hamburg lasted the longest—till the end of the regime. Because more and more Jews were leaving Germany, either through emigration or, after October 1941, through evacuation to the East, there were fewer and fewer patients to inhabit these hospitals. Therefore, the first of two inevitable signs of decay for the Jewish health care delivery system in those years was the periodic change of venue for these hospitals, from the original, usually generous grounds owned by the Jewish congregations to less auspicious environs and, finally, to the most modest dwellings imaginable, always under the spiteful tolerance of the SS. The second sign was closure. With the two notable exceptions, the hospitals were shut down one by one by the authorities after 1939: Leipzig's in spring 1940, Mannheim's in autumn 1942, and Breslau's in June 1943.[23]

The courageous doctors in those clinics no less than the ones in private practice defied adversity to be all things at once for their patients, who looked to them not just for the curing of ailments. Among the dwindling members of the Jewish communities, many of which had already lost their rabbis, these physicians had to assume the functions of emotional healers and spiritual caretakers as well. More often than not, the Jewish patients were victims of wanton Nazi assault or broken men and women just released from concentration camps. Thus the status of the Jewish doctors approached the heroic, as they tried to make ends meet without regular medical supplies, and permanently under curfew and all manner of constraints by the Gestapo and SS. In these curative situations frequently bordering on emergencies, the ethical value system of the doctors was in great danger of shifting away from its usual center of gravity, for life and death had taken on somewhat different meanings: was it right to keep alive a near-suicide victim who would be delivered to potential death once fully nursed back to health? The physicians themselves sometimes cracked under the tremendous strain, and then they would take their own lives.[24]

Nor were they immune from persecution by the regime's uniformed squadrons and twisted lawmakers outside the hospital walls. Tough sentences against Jewish doctors for "race defilement" continued to be pronounced. In one case, a doctor received a stiffer judgment than usual because his medical knowledge should have equipped him better to adhere to the blood laws.[25] Such physicians were to be found as inmates of concentration camps like Dachau, where they, nevertheless, unflaggingly practiced their vocation among their fellow prisoners.[26] An untypically sad case at the height of the war was that of Dr. Georg Benjamin, who, after release from Brandenburg penitentiary in summer 1942, was committed to a work camp, then transferred to the infamous Mauthausen camp, where a few weeks later he was brutally murdered.[27]

There is no denying that the National Socialist doctors saw their final goal, complete riddance of the Jewish competition, being realized. This was evident from various public remarks made by the Nazi physicians' leaders, in particular Conti, after the death of his erstwhile rival Wagner. At the climax of the war, the Reich health leader may have visited the Israelite hospital in Berlin with great pomp and circumstance and feigned respect for Jewish self-administration, but what truly gave him away were his open reminiscences about "the devastating influence of Jewry on the medical profession" or about the deplorable effect of Jewish doctors on midwifery—now all allegedly of the past.[28] The economic motif once more became transparent, as Conti calumniated the former Jewish colleagues as those who always mixed medicine with business and still boasted of themselves as great saviors of men.[29] Such slander reverberated throughout the Nazi medical establishment.[30]

Nonetheless, even then the lines between the Jewish and the "Aryan" realms of medical activity were not yet clearly drawn, mostly because of the exigencies of war. At the high-level Nazi staff meeting called for November 12, 1938, after the violence of *Kristallnacht*, SD chief Heydrich had argued on behalf of separation of Jewish from "Aryan" patients in public hospitals. Although this had been the subject of a special decree in 1937, it had never been consistently carried out, for the Jewish hospitals were unevenly distributed and often out of reach.[31] Indeed, since German physicians still were under compunction to treat Jewish patients when their doctors were unavailable, some of these German professionals continued their accustomed practice not only of seeing non-"Aryan" patients but also of committing them to those public hospitals whose directors did not expressly forbid it. This was happening—despite Heydrich's remonstrances—right through early 1939, when Jewish patients were quartered in several public hospitals alongside the "Aryans." The incidence and strength of "Aryan" complaints are unknown, but in Württembergish Laupheim a Jewish man came to be bedded in the women's section, and in Bremen an SA man protested against a Jewish presence in his sickroom.[32] Still, in April 1939 the Dortmund Gestapo divined that because of a dearth of proper Jewish institutions, Jewish patients were to be put up in normal hospitals, ideally in a separate wing. Early in 1940, too, it was said for Hamburg that German doctors could not refuse Israelite patients if sick-treaters were unavailable.[33] Whether they were actually missing or not, Vienna was one place in the Reich where some twenty months later Jews were still being treated by "Aryans."[34] By summer of 1942, at least, under the already known exceptional circumstances Jewish patients were still allowed into "Aryan" doctors' offices, particularly if this meant keeping them fit for the war effort.[35] German hospital accommodation, too, was said to be possible, but cordoned off from the "Aryans."[36]

These partial inconsistencies vividly demonstrate the need of the Nazi leaders, during a protracted war, to modify their policy of absolute extinction of the Jewish "race" in accordance with the realities of logistics and the demand for human labor, a course of action that was observed in the concentration camp of Auschwitz, for example, where forced work regimens as in the Buna camp ran alongside the program for mass killings. This compromised philosophy, which might have been a shock to fanatical purists like Gerhard Wagner, perhaps explains the Nazis' extended indulgence of *Mischling* physicians in the service of the nation's health, as the regular medical reserves were attenuated because of front-line commitments.

Informed by the spirit of the Nuremberg Race Laws of 1935, the 1938 legislation had subsumed Mosaic *Mischling* physicians of the first degree under the concept of "full Jew," meaning that those laws' provisions would strike them with relentless force. This entailed total work stoppage for them, save in a capacity as sick-treaters, pending further legislation. But new enactments on the entire *Mischling* question, prodded on in 1941 by Dr. Gross and by Wagner's onetime crony Dr. Blome, now Conti's deputy, did not materialize, undoubtedly in part because the mixlings' labor potential for the war effort was recognized. Similar deliberations at the Wannsee conference in January 1942 regarding the question of second-degree *Mischling* status led nowhere, nor was any headway made in March and October of that year or in spring 1943 because of much disagreement on definitions and procedures.[37] Therefore, *Mischling* physicians of the first degree, if they were baptized, at the height of the war were deemed inexpendable by the Reich health leadership, to counteract the medical labor shortage, and were deployed in the Reich, as were, naturally, all *Mischling* doctors of the second degree (some of whom could also be drafted into the Wehrmacht).[38]

There is a possibility that even half-Jewish doctors of Mosaic faith, whose category—if only by default—was not scheduled for annihilation in the foreseeable future, were asked by the Reich health administration to contribute to the war effort, especially after the more pragmatic Dr. Brandt had begun to overshadow Conti in summer 1942.[39] We may conclude this from a directive issued in December 1943, specifying the use of Jewish *Mischling* physicians, presumably in the civilian area. One such person, Dr. A. W. of Vienna, was told to report for emergency work assignment in the Austrian capital.[40] Some Christian doctors with Jewish spouses were also employed in this way.[41] As far as is known, however, only one Jewish physician married to an "Aryan" managed to survive professionally, in a manner of speaking, for this Dr. Walter Lustig was a former *Amtsarzt* who had become medical liaison officer between the Jewish ghetto community in Berlin and the Gestapo. He played an inglorious role by and large and was summarily shot by the invading Russians in 1945.[42]

It is a truism to say that for Germany's Jewish physicians the end was tragic. Those doctors who had not emigrated usually were evacuated to the ghettos and camps of the East along with the patients in their hospitals, or were individual victims of the periodic roundups in Germany since fall 1941.[43] Some did not see a concentration or extermination camp right away because they were needed in the war and occupation economy.[44] Hence there were German-Jewish doctors looking after the medical needs of ghetto populations in Warthegau, that portion of Poland annexed to the Reich, or of Jewish work camps, in the Austrian Burgenland bordering on Hungary.[45] Several of them were relatively fortunate in being deported to the "model" concentration camp of Theresienstadt, where the chances of survival were somewhat better, provided one did not succumb to illness or be carted off to Auschwitz.[46] At one time, there were a thousand physicians among sixty-five thousand inmates, many of them German and still practicing.[47]

Most sick-treaters who were arrested along with their fellow Jews and then evacuated continued caring for the ailing from the roundup point till their arrival in the camps.[48] In those desolate places, they continued this important work and thus became foils for the treacherous SS physicians. Only one German-Jewish doctor, the Cologne gynecologist Maximilian Samuel, betrayed the Hippocratic Oath in Auschwitz by collaborating with the enemy. In civilian life, this would never have happened; Samuel was hoping, through his desperate deeds, to save the life of his nineteen-year-old daughter, who had been deported with him. But in the end, he was killed, as had been his wife before him.[49] About the fate of his daughter the chronicle is silent.

5. A Chronicle of Exile and a Demographic Reckoning

One may well ask why no more Jewish doctors emigrated to foreign lands, and among those who did go, what were the circumstances of their exodus. Part of the first question is easily answered by pointing to the statistics of Jewish emigration to be detailed in the last part of this section, which make it clear that the great majority of physicians were able to leave Nazi Germany before the Holocaust, probably because they could clear the first and most important hurdle, the financial one, as they were generally well off. The reasons why the minority who died through violence had no other choice were tied to a complex set of factors, a combination of economic and psychological variables that today are difficult to appreciate. A few Jewish physicians may indeed have been too penurious to emigrate. But others of some means paradoxically may have found it difficult to part with wealth, and thus they lingered in the country of their birth or abode, experiencing what Berlin physician Hertha Nathorff has called "the eternal conflict," always hoping for a change for the better, until it was too late.[1] Dr. Martin Gumpert relates the significant episode that made him decide to leave in 1935 and how he disposed of all his earthly possessions quickly so as not to be trapped by material considerations before he sailed for the United States.[2]

There is no denying that even for Jewish doctors totally disillusioned with conditions in Germany a powerful set of deterrents caused emigration to be delayed and sometimes altogether stayed. In this, however, the doctors were not alone; they shared the fate of other professionals like lawyers and dentists, who were progressively struck down in a similar manner, or the fate of the relatively few rich persons. After the initial shock of Hitler's takeover and the first anti-Semitic measures such as, for physicians, the removal from panel practice, a large wave of émigrés left Germany in 1933. At this time, moderately generous conditions of immigration offered by foreign governments still gave them reasonable expectations of success.[3] But soon thereafter, reports were reaching the Reich, carefully monitored, analyzed, and disseminated by the German-Jewish organizations, of difficult requirements and psychological adjustment problems in the new host countries. Although physicians were needed in certain spots like the United States countryside, they generally did not come under the rubric of desirable occupations such as trained craftsmen or farmers, which were not popular with Jews. Accounts of immense culture shock resulting from unfamiliarity with a new language and sometimes leading to suicides were also discouraging; culture shock became one of the prominent symptoms of failed integration in foreign lands. It soon was fairly common knowledge, too, that the older the doctor, the smaller his chances of being admitted and licensed and actually succeeding anew economically; as it turned out, approximately two-thirds of the physicians who were to leave Germany were under forty-five years old, and colleagues over sixty generally remained behind, unless emigrating children could take them along.[4]

Physicians who procrastinated in Germany in the four years after 1933 always could find new reasons to rationalize their decision to stay. In 1934, many Jews of all walks of life labored under the illusion that Hitler's radicalism had spent itself, an impression that for some was corroborated by his decisive action during the Röhm crisis in the summer of 1934. They felt vindicated because, especially in 1935, when the emigration figures were the lowest of the prewar phase, many Jews returned (at great risk to themselves, for they were usually sent to concentration camps, a fate other Jews were slow to comprehend). Generally, although office hours for Jewish doctors still working may have become shorter and their earnings lower, a handful of them were extremely busy, conveying a false picture of opportunity. One physician had so much to do that he bought himself a new car weeks before the blood laws that were to cancel its use. Moreover, because the Jewish self-help organizations were centered here and for its well-known anonymity as Germany's largest city, but also because chances of work locally still were surprisingly promising, Berlin received a flood of Jewish doctors in those years, mostly from the provinces, but those who returned from abroad as well. This led to a mistaken notion among many that hard times had all but passed, a notion that was to be rudely shattered, if again not lastingly for some, by the Nuremberg race legislation of fall 1935. Some of the damage of that legislation was once more neutralized, or at least seen to be so, by the relative quiet enveloping the 1936 Olympic Games. Amid all this, the Jewish agencies were cautioning professionals, especially doctors, about further restrictive quotas and poor working conditions in their fields of specialization abroad, which tempted several to stay longer than was good for them.[5]

For those physicians still in the country, it was not until delicensure and the pogrom of November 1938 that the inevitability of emigration fully impressed itself on their minds. Hence in 1938 the (estimated) figure for Jewish refugees generally jumped from twenty-three thousand in the previous year to forty thousand, and in 1939 it reached seventy-eight thousand, the highest ever.[6] The physicians' own movement paralleled that demographic trend. As a West German authority on the subject has recently observed, however, the initial porousness of the foreign professional strictures over time became inversely related to the need for Jewish medical personnel to relocate.[7] This meant that by 1939, one year after the international repatriation conference of Evian-les-Bains had ended in disaster,[8] this need was evidently greater than ever before, but the chances for Jewish doctors to reestablish themselves in a new country were the worst they had ever been.

The trials and tribulations connected with the physical action of emigrating from the Reich were enormous; stories about them circulated throughout the Jewish communities and frightened many would-be leavers. Usually, a foreign visa could be obtained only if one or all of three specific prerequisites were satisfied: falling into the category of a preferred occupation; being vouched for by a relative or other eligible, financially secure guarantor; or possessing sufficient transferable wealth to support one's livelihood without supplementary job earnings or making demands on a public purse. Failing those criteria in the case of many countries meant being placed on a quota list with long waits. It is true that physicians were likely to have sufficient wealth, but if they did they were affected by punitive hard-currency restrictions that culminated in the Reich Flight Tax (*Reichsfluchtsteuer*) of May 1934. The main stipulation of this treacherous law, which punished the Jews for "fleeing" the country, was that people with post-1931 incomes of 20,000 marks annually or taxable assets of more than 50,000 marks had to cede one-quarter of their property to the national revenue department. The Nazis invented numerous other devious methods of depriving emigrating Jews of their possessions, such as—for doctors—withholding their libraries or valuable special equipment. By 1938–39, when there was a rush to foreign consulates, up to 96 percent of one's assets could be claimed by the state before departure. The Reichsmark was considered soft currency at the time, so the migrants would get comparatively little in return, especially in America. The National Socialist government profited by collecting the Reich Flight Tax, to the tune of 900 million marks, up to and including 1940.[9] As Dr. Paul Rosenstein, the noted Berlin surgeon, was to find out, even the border guards would apply pressure on him until he bribed them with a large check as he was leaving for Holland.[10]

Jewish physicians, like other prosperous Jews, were encumbered if they wanted to sell property or businesses such as a private clinic or assign them in trust to "Aryan" relatives or friends.[11] And as was to be expected, the KVD would try to skirt its legal responsibility of sending on pension payments to the Jewish émigrés' new foreign addresses; in the one case that is fully documented Gerhard

Wagner's bureaucrats presented a very dubious claim in court before winning over the judges.[12]

In the end, therefore, few Jewish physicians were able to receive visas on the strength of their wealth alone. But a fair number of them had relatives, particularly in the United States, as did Hertha Nathorff, or, like Gumpert, they were allowed to benefit from the magnanimity of a solvent sponsor.[13] There were other Nazi harassments, however, such as the withdrawal of passports and the withholding of needed transfer documents.[14] At the level of human concern, much insult was added to injury. One young doctor's wife, upon learning that her husband had just been released from Dachau after *Kristallnacht* incarceration in late 1938, decided immediately that her family must emigrate. She arranged for a private dinner meeting with the French consul in Stuttgart, ready to compromise her virtue for a visa and finding the consul a man of ambiguous generosity.[15] Often the departing physicians left children or wives behind, who would be subject to human ransom.[16] Several doctors emigrated as former inmates of a concentration camp, humiliated yet incapable of articulating themselves, for fear of reprisals.[17] Lest her flight from Germany should fail and she herself would fall into the hands of the Gestapo, the former Berlin Marxist town physician Käte Frankenthal carried cyanide with her for weeks.[18]

Added to the mental anguish was the fear of safety in a foreign land. Even before the Anschluss of Austria, the specter of war loomed wide, for Hitler's imperialistic greed became more obvious with every year. When would Hitler overrun Czechoslovakia, Belgium, the Netherlands? As early as 1933, therefore, the well-known Berlin internist Johannes Plesch did not go to Holland, contiguous to Germany, although he favored that country above all others, but to England, where he felt safer. The Austrian Dr. Hans Brauchbar later fled Austria for the Serbian town of Sabac, but in the spring of 1941 Hitler's soldiers overran Yugoslavia. At the end of October, along with other former Austrian residents, Brauchbar was shot by Nazi troops in an antipartisan vendetta.[19]

At the end of World War II, of the Jewish physicians who were successful in escaping from Germany the majority would end up in the United States, even though, until restrictive legislation in 1935, they initially favored the British mandate of Palestine. By a conservative estimate, the United States took in less than five thousand refugee physicians from Europe, the majority presumed to be Jewish, from 1933 to 1945.[20] This meant, for example, that by 1945 thirty-three, or 44.6 percent, of Greater Stuttgart's Jewish doctors had relocated in the United States, whereas only 10.8 percent had gone to Palestine, which became home to the second highest number.[21] Apart from the United States, especially for ideological and emotional reasons, the Middle Eastern mandate was very popular, but the socioeconomic constellation there as well as the impact of British politics presented a barrier against a substantial influx of Jews.[22] It was disheartening that by 1935–36, when the mandate's entrance requirements were tightened, the

United States still held firm to its austere refugee admission policy. These intertwined developments had direct consequences for the physicians, some of which turned out to be fraught with tragedy.

The generally reticent tolerance sometimes bordering on hostility with which Americans welcomed German-Jewish physicians can be understood only against the wider background of America's immigrant tradition, which, in the pre-Hitler decade, had experienced significant change. America had been the classical land of freedom for European migrants of virtually all origins in the nineteenth and early twentieth centuries, but its post–World War I isolationism entailed a more self-centered concentration on its national identity, which in turn produced a tendency to reject further immigrants, particularly those from places bearing no historic relationship to the reputed, originally northwest European founders. In May 1921, legislation was enacted to the disadvantage of immigrants from eastern and southern Europe, but it proved so ineffective that in 1924 the U.S. Congress introduced a quota system for European countries, prejudicing the South and East, which President Calvin Coolidge signed into law. As Kansas Congressman J. M. Tincher said at the time, the law's purpose was to deter "Bolshevik Wops, Dagoes, Kikes and Hunkies" from entering the country.[23]

Henceforth "kikes" were among the less favored ethnic groups seeking entry into a nation that in the first seven years of the 1930s was suffering from the Great Depression and in the throes of a difficult recovery. Even though until 1937 more people were leaving the United States than were entering and the economy could have used resourceful newcomers, right-wing politicians continued to fume over undesirables, including Jews, whom, partially on the Nazi model, they were fond of equating with Bolsheviks. German Jews came under the quota for German nationals that was set at approximately twenty-five thousand immigrants per year, but this limit was never reached until 1939. The reasons were multifarious. Informal labor union and industry restrictions bolstered by capricious legislation in individual states curtailed opportunities for economic activity in many areas. It took time and effort for the Jews to find the needed relatives or sponsors. For many, language obstacles proved more insurmountable than had been believed at first. In addition, American consuls abroad were extremely strict but also unnecessarily cruel in interpreting a directive by President Herbert Hoover of 1930 advising rejection of candidates not deemed financially viable.[24]

In 1937, the Hoover directive was beginning to be relaxed, and an appreciably greater number of Jews were being allowed into the country. But the consuls' waiting lists were starting to fill up with names of German and Austrian Jews so quickly that for many, years of waiting were unavoidable.[25] Moved by Nazi terror after the Anschluss of Austria in March 1938, President Franklin D. Roosevelt proposed the plan for the summer conference at Evian, at which not just all the participating governments but his own as well failed to recommend selfless measures of pro-Jewish support.[26] It was only after a further horror, surrounding

Kristallnacht in November of that year, that Jews could finally take advantage of the full quota as German national immigrants, and they did so visibly both in 1939 and 1940.[27] But thereafter, America's joining the war, the Reich's repression (Himmler forbade Jewish emigration in October 1941), and continued xenophobic fulminations both at the U.S. political and the everyday human relations levels conspired to shut the door to further Jewish refugees and also to militate against a speedy integration of those already in the country.[28]

Against this backdrop, the chances and the progress of the Jewish physicians must now be briefly outlined. Quantitatively by 1945, those doctors constituted about 2.3 percent of the total of 132,000 Jewish immigrants from Germany and Austria into the United States since 1933.[29] Those among the 3,000 Jewish doctors who had made up their minds to enter the country before fall 1936 encountered the least difficulties, after having been granted entrance, in being admitted to medical practice in five eastern seaboard states that were known to be liberal: New York, Massachusetts, New Jersey, Connecticut, and Maryland, along with Illinois in the Midwest.[30] New York State was the most enlightened of all; it required merely a language examination for the establishment of private practice, whereas the rest of the states called for so many prerequisites as to frustrate most applicant physicians who wished to settle there: citizenship papers (attainable only after five years of permanent residence), residency papers leading to citizenship (so-called first papers), national or state licensing board certificates, and internship in a U.S. hospital.[31] After October 1936 the privileges were diminished for two main reasons. First, New York State, under pressure from reactionary, antialien doctors, introduced a stipulation that apart from the English-language test foreign physicians would have to pass a proper licensing board medical examination; and second, a conservative, constrictive trend among all the physicians in the United States led to an almost undefeatable barrier, the peak of which usually consisted in a demand for U.S. citizenship before a physician was allowed to take the state-sanctioned license test.[32]

It was sadly ironic that America needed more doctors at this time because its universities had, for decades, not been producing enough of them, relative to the population; this need became crucial during World War II. As in Germany and other European countries, there was a dearth of physicians in rural areas.[33] But in many of the southern or midwestern states endowed with such an infrastructure the bigotry of their inhabitants had resulted in some of the toughest entry specifications; Georgia, Alabama, Mississippi, and Idaho fall into this category.[34] Until 1945, they appeared to be leading the other states, not excluding New York, in an exercise of xenophobic execration.

Despite the pleading of enlightened medical bureaucrats, notably from the East Coast, to show generosity, and their insistence that it was not intended for the refugee doctors to seek employment in congested (urban) areas, the members of the individual state medical licensing boards would not soften but instead solidified further their stringent prerequisites.[35] "American doctors sympathize with the plight of colleague-victims of European discrimination," ran their philistine argument. "At the same time, they feel that the traditional generosity of American medicine should not be strained to the point where it would sacrifice our economic security for theirs."[36] By 1943 opportunities for the immigrants to take licensing examinations had been withdrawn by all the states except New York and Massachusetts.[37] This meant that most Jewish doctors, save those who had settled in New York State before October 1936 or in some of the other liberal eastern states, could not establish themselves properly in practice for years, often after distasteful unprofessional pursuits such as door-to-door selling or demeaning work in a hospital, before acquiring their citizenship papers and then passing the various medical examinations.[38] There were few exceptions, such as California, and its was not on moral grounds. For this Pacific state harbored Oriental residents and hence had to certify Oriental physicians to practice because white Americans would refuse to treat the Chinese. By this logic of inverted racism, Jews could not legally be kept from licensure; nonetheless, they, too, would find themselves in an unfriendly environment.[39]

All told, twenty-one of the forty-eight states categorically denied foreigners a medical practice within their confines.[40] And if it is maintained that by the end of the 1940s, at the latest, most Jewish physicians in the United States were doing well and some were extremely successful, to the point of being fully respected by the communities within which they worked,[41] this could not have been true without vast material sacrifices and unfathomable personal suffering beforehand.

Unfortunately, our history would be far richer if we knew what happened to certain physicians, beyond the fact that they left Nazi Germany for the United States and stayed there. Dr. Nathan of Nuremberg, Dr. Oskar Nussbaum of Bremen, and Dr. Simon Gideon of Stuttgart are examples. Nussbaum is on record as the last Jewish doctor to escape from that Hanse seaport, on August 26, 1939, and Gideon died in 1959 in Chicago, after establishing a gynecological practice there.[42] Pathologist Dr. Heinz Jacques Ahronheim, who had graduated from Berlin magna cum laude at age twenty-five in 1932, was one of those very few fortunate persons with a close relative in America, his mother in Chicago, where he was able to move in early 1936. He appears to have found immediate employment at the W. A. Foote Memorial Hospital in Jackson, Michigan.[43] Dr. Fritz Aron emigrated from Berlin in 1938 and died as a well-respected physician in America in 1962.[44]

Dr. Cäsar Hirsch of Stuttgart, however, killed himself while in the United States.[45] And although the reasons for his suicide have not been divulged, they may be surmised to have been the result of failed acculturation coupled with economic misery, which haunted so many of the medical newcomers. Of the first condition several physicians have complained in their memoirs, but no one has been able to evoke these feelings more effectively than the child of a German-

Jewish doctor: "New Yorkers in the early forties did not differentiate between immigrant Jews and Gentiles, and for many I was German, maybe even a Nazi; in any case an enemy."[46]

If Jewish physicians in the state of New York, especially in the melting-pot metropolis, fared better than anywhere else in the United States, then reports of their tribulations in that area today must be regarded as felicitously indicative of the realities of the struggle in the rest of the country. Hanns Schwarz writes of the cutthroat competition among New York doctors that gave no quarter to potential intruders.[47] Even the most able specialists from Germany, after having passed their language tests and before the stifling October 1936 regulation, were agonizing over difficulties in the path of establishing a new office, out of which to practice independently, so that secondary or tertiary medical jobs had to be accepted, in someone else's employ and for pitiful rewards.

Dr. Ludwig Teleky, once a senior public health officer in Düsseldorf, was over sixty years of age when he arrived in New York in 1939. He was offered a small position with the Rockefeller Foundation for a modest honorarium. Later Teleky would lose his wife, and by the early 1950s the doctor had withdrawn from the world, working away in some library, day in and day out.[48] Dr. Paul Rosenstein arrived too late to be spared the 1936 New York State Licensing Board examination so he could not practice independently. After barely passing the language test, he, too, was offered inferior employment, with a salary of next to nothing. After he had been told that the Memorial Hospital for Cancer Research that could well have used this famous surgeon's talents followed a strictly anti-Semitic policy, he became a lecturer in topographic anatomy at the First Institute of Podiatry, but once again without the privilege of private practice and no pay. Without means, unable to retake the required state examination, and sorely disenchanted with the lack of collegial cooperation in New York, Rosenstein eventually went to Brazil.[49]

Dr. Käte Frankenthal, also from Berlin, persisted and as a consequence endured unspeakable humiliations. She secured a license to practice medicine in New York before autumn 1936 but could not find employment, nor would anyone assist her in founding her own practice. After some curative work and lecturing in Connecticut, winter 1938–39 saw her back in New York City, where she took on a small research chore for ten dollars a week. In summer 1939 this fifty-year-old woman was selling ice cream in the streets. She then sold ladies' hose and Christmas cards door to door. In 1940 an émigré friend offered her the use of his office, for an hourly rent, so that she could hope to begin attracting some patients of her own. Only by the late 1940s would Frankenthal be fully established professionally.[50] Her recent biographers have judged that she never really became assimilated in the United States. Assuredly, her fate was not exceptional.[51]

Palestine presented different challenges to the German-Jewish physicians. Britain had been under obligation from the League of Nations to "facilitate Jewish immigration under suitable conditions" into its mandate since the early 1920s.[52] Hence as a matter of principle, Palestine welcomed immigrants, supported on historic grounds by the international Zionist movement. Influenced by Hitler's assumption of power and anticipating German pressure on Jewish citizens, immigration requirements were refined by the British mandate government, according to the criteria of economic status, occupation, and age established as far back as 1920. The administration of this policy was entrusted to the Jewish Agency for Palestine in Jerusalem. Altogether, about fifty-five thousand German Jews were able to come to Palestine.[53]

The German newcomers most favored for entrance into Palestine early on were those who, in accordance with the guidelines, had practical occupational experience and were willing to perform physical labor in building the country. This would include many young men and women who back in Germany could prepare themselves for a future in the land of Israel under the guidance of the pioneer organization Hechaluz, until they embarked on the settlement journey, the *Aliyah*, a ceremonial occasion of the highest order. For a few years Nazi authorities, eager to see as many Jews leave the Reich as possible, entered into semiofficial agreements with Jewish-Palestinian representatives to aid this scheme; German authorities were instructed by the SS to further it, and there even was a money transfer plan put in place by which German export-to-Palestine interests profited, as well as the migrating Jews. As a consequence, Palestine became the most important target country for German Jews, if only till 1936, when the political constellation changed.[54]

But since not just Jews but also Arabs were living in Palestine, there was ongoing unrest over competencies and the sharing of land and resources, to say nothing of cultural discrepancies. The turmoil culminated in early 1936, producing an Arab general strike, in the course of which the Arab leader, Jerusalem's Mufti Amin al-Hussein, demanded an end to all Jewish immigration. The British thereupon installed a royal commission under Lord Peel to study the matter, and it recommended, by July 1937, the creation of separate Arab and Jewish states in the area, rather than cohabitation between the two peoples. During a period of transition to forge these two new national entities, Jewish immigration should be halted. Still not satisfied, the Arabs rebelled further until the British put them down by force in 1939.[55]

Finally, in May 1939, London drew up a White Paper, the essence of which was tantamount to "a total reversal of the Balfour Declaration," which in 1917 had called for the creation of a separate home for the Jewish people.[56] The earlier idea of partition now was dismissed and the coexistence of Arabs and Jews was represcribed as a matter of high policy. After the failure of the Evian conference and the pogroms of *Kristallnacht* in 1938, and with war drawing nearer by the day, the British allowed for a further immigration of Jews for five years. A total of approximately seventy-five thousand were to be admitted.[57] Finding this quota wanting, clandestine Zionist organizations in Palestine, with their agents throughout Europe, engineered large-scale illegal immigration so that by 1939, out of 27,561 Jews coming into the country, 11,156 were clandestine entrants.[58]

The fate of would-be immigrant German-Jewish physicians fluctuated with the descending rules and regulations but also with demand for them in the marketplace. Initially, they were not favored by the C-type category of immigration, requiring manual labor skills for internal colonizations, and as academics they were not suitable for occupational adaptation and retooling. But they did have good chances under the A-type rubric stipulating independent economic status if they possessed 12,000 marks to infuse into the Palestinian economy.[59] And so in the first two years under Hitler about six hundred doctors appear to have entered the country legally, representing approximately one-third of all German-Jewish refugee physicians at that point. But significantly, because of the large numbers of physicians already in Palestine, only about two hundred of these were able to establish private practices without having to undergo laborious recertification;[60] another two hundred contracted some sort of medical employment, and the rest had to retrain for entirely different jobs. Until the 1935–36 watershed it was argued by German-Jewish auxiliary organizations like the Berlin-based Central-Verein that because the influx of immigrants into Palestine was still substantial and was judged to be continuing, a correspondingly large number of physicians would be needed to care for those migrants.[61]

That, however, was a miscalculation, for by 1935 there also were in the mandate some 600 nonimmigrant Jewish physicians as well as 200 Arab doctors; the ratio of 1 doctor per 174 Palestinian residents was among the densest in the world.[62] In the course of Arab anti-Jewish agitation leading to the Peel Report of 1937, the Arab doctors prevailed on the British high commissioner to reduce drastically the number of incoming German-Jewish immigrant doctors, and despite Jewish protests, the authorities agreed.[63] In a draft by Palestinian Attorney General H. H. Trusted of July 18, 1935, it was proposed that the hitherto valid Medical Practitioners Ordinance of 1928 be amended so that only citizens or permanent residents of Palestine before December 1, 1935, could be granted licenses to practice.[64] The Jewish Agency for Palestine issued a protest, reminding the British that "the immigration in recent years of distinguished Jewish physicians and surgeons, particularly from Germany, has already done much to raise the standards of the medical profession and is gradually making Palestine a medical centre for the neighbouring countries—a development of considerable utility to the country as a whole which will necessarily suffer a check in consequence of the proposed restrictions."[65] But this protest came to no avail, for the new ordinance was promulgated on October 30, marking December 1, 1935, as the cutoff date for the attainment of Palestinian citizenship as precondition for practicing medicine. As an element of small succor, an undetermined quota for new licensees was provided for, consonant with the arising need as assessed by the high commissioner.[66]

This ruling placed a serious damper on the hopes of all putative Jewish immigrant doctors, notably those who were considering illegal immigration to Palestine after the blood laws, and led to the stronger trend to go to America. Up to five hundred Jewish physicians, mostly from Germany, emigrated to Palestine in October and November before the ax fell. Unfortunately, it is not known exactly how many German-Jewish physicians henceforth entered the territory and how many of them were permitted to assume medical practice, but they could not have exceeded three hundred.[67] Some information for the liberal pre-December 1935 phase and for the difficult time thereafter may be gleaned from personal histories recorded in the pertinent literature and a few archives.

German physicians of Zionist persuasion who moved to Palestine before December 1935 possessed by far the best chances of success because they were usually prepared to retrain for a profession or occupation other than medicine if necessary.[68] It is virtually certain that Dr. Adolf Würzburger of Heilbronn and Dr. Max Cramer of Stuttgart, who were Zionists and acutely aware of the oversupply in the profession, and who left Germany in 1934, became both needed and esteemed medical practitioners in Palestine. In addition, ophthalmologist Cramer proved himself an enthusiastic settler and willingly treated the eye diseases of the indigenous Arab population.[69] The Stuttgart medical couple Drs. Edgar and Anna Heilbronner arrived in Palestine in 1933–34 and eventually became directors of the Alyn clinic.[70] Dr. Aron Sandler and Dr. Felix A. Theilhaber both were worthies of the Berlin Jewish congregation; they reached Palestine in 1935 and may be presumed to have been granted their new licenses without a problem.[71]

Possibly on the dark side of fortune was the surgeon Rosenstein, who visited Israel in 1936. Undoubtedly aware of the fall 1935 regulations, of which he tells the reader nothing in his memoirs, Rosenstein alleges to have considered accepting the directorship of the Bikur Cholim hospital. He says that he could not bring himself to do so because of the Arab-Jewish violence and the prohibitive cost of relocating himself and his family.[72] In historic hindsight, the first reason is plausible, but the last one does not make sense in the case of a man who for years had been accumulating a fortune in Berlin. Could it be that Rosenstein would have been barred on the basis of the 1935 proscription and was too embarrassed to admit this in his memoirs? Rosenstein eventually found refuge in Brazil.

Georg Peysack and Max Sadger left Germany for Tel Aviv in 1936 and 1937, respectively, and it is not known how they fared. Peysack was a thirty-three-year-old, barely graduated physician who may have found Palestine too inclement a professional climate, even if he came under a favorable quota. Sadger, however, was an eye specialist who, like Cramer, could have fulfilled an important service.[73] Siegfried Ostrowski arrived from Berlin in 1939, just a few days before the outbreak of the war, probably under the legitimate quota and possibly, because of his official work at the Israelite hospital, with the help or acquiescence of Nazi authorities. He is reputed to have continued his medical work in Israel.[74]

There are sad accounts concerning at least two doctors who wished to fashion a new future for themselves in Palestine but ran afoul of circumstances. Dr. Henriette Rotzinger migrated to Italy at the age of thirty-six in 1934. By 1942, after a stint in Siebenbürgen (Romania), she was on one of the notorious illegal immigration vessels attempting to dodge the British and land on the Palestinian shore.[75] Her ship was wrecked, and she was brought to Cyprus. Only in 1944 did she find her way to Palestine, probably legitimately, for she was employed there as a physician.[76] Her colleague Dr. Leo Gross almost surely became the victim of remigration to the Third Reich. In Palestine by November 1935 and qualifying for his new medical license under the October regulation, Gross was one of those unlucky émigrés deluded into returning to Germany in 1935–37. He seems to have traveled back to his native Kolberg, believing his residency status in Palestine to be sufficient protection in case of dire need. The last the Palestinian authorities heard of him was that he had been dragged off to a concentration camp. In 1940, when his case was reviewed, he was presumed to be dead and his license lapsed because he had been in the mandate for less than four weeks and had never claimed his papers.[77]

England was somewhat lower in the hierarchy of receiver nations for German-Jewish doctors, behind Palestine and France as early as 1934, even though it seems to have accepted about fifty thousand German and Austrian Jews of all social stations by the beginning of the war.[78] The growing sentiment for appeasement may have been a factor in British reluctance to accept Jews, certainly by 1938.[79] But, writes Bernard Wasserstein, the most knowledgeable expert on this subject, although Britain in the final analysis took in more Jews per capita than Palestine, it developed an indigenous opposition once those Jews had entered, in large part because of the crippling depression and high unemployment that plagued England for years. This internal anti-Semitism did not decrease; on the contrary, it increased at the beginning of World War II, escalating further during the later war years.[80]

Britain had much harsher regulations than either the United States or Palestine. No German-Jewish physician fleeing to England was allowed to practice without repeating years of study and a medical examination at one of the nation's universities. In the first two years of Hitler's rule close to two hundred physicians were admitted to the British professional reintegration process, with a view to allowing them to practice eventually, but a jealously restrictive national medical association in league with the Royal College of Surgeons clamped down on this policy of moderate tolerance by 1938,[81] and thereafter the war was on in any case. Britain, however, with its penchant for excellence in science and scholarship, seems to have extended preferential treatment to truly distinguished German-

Jewish physicians of the caliber of Johannes Plesch, who today is appreciative, if guardedly critical, of the English in his recollections.[82] This elitist British predilection notwithstanding, several ordinary Jewish physicians ultimately succeeded in England: Dr. Siegmund Weil of Stuttgart, Dr. Ilse Lehmann of the Jewish youth camp at Gross-Breesen, Dr. Paul Hes of Bremen, Dr. Ilse Friedheim of Hamburg (via India), and Dr. Rudolf Friedländer of Dideburg.[83]

Fate dealt the British a sadistic blow in 1941 when medical personnel were at a premium for reasons of war, but also, once again, showed off the folly of the Americans. The British government, requiring "about one thousand physicians for civilian and military purposes," could have taken advantage of émigré doctors then volunteering for these jobs from the United States. In the end, they were not acceptable to London, ironically because they lacked U.S. citizenship. Yet neither would Washington recruit these experts for service in the American Red Cross.[84] Chauvinism did triumph in these, the most enlightened of the Western democracies.

In spite of its conservative nationalism, it must be said that England still looked very good in comparison with the rest of the world, save the United States and Palestine. For besides England, very few European countries accepted Jewish doctors for the practice of medicine, and only with reservations. Fascist Italy had a virtually unrestricted immigration policy until September 1938; by 1935, approximately one thousand German Jews had moved there, including several physicians.[85] Among them were Dr. Werner Sandelowski and Dr. Dorothea Futter, both from Berlin, the former of whom migrated to the Riviera and the latter to Rome.[86] By mid-1935 some one hundred German-Jewish doctors had repeated their medical examinations in Italy and entertained hopes of being registered as medical practitioners.[87] Dr. Futter wished to set up a pediatric practice in Milan.[88] But the medical faculties had instigated a new law forbidding the relicensing of foreign doctors.[89] On September 7, 1938, new Italian race laws were in place, and a few months later the Italian government sternly warned foreign Jewish physicians that, because they were "doubly strangers in Italy and . . . enemies of Fascism," the authorities would not countenance their presence.[90] It is estimated that by September 1939 ten thousand German and Austrian Jews had left the country again for greener pastures, thus continuing their odyssey. Physicians, of course, were among them, such as Dr. Sandelowski, who shortly before the outbreak of the war was in Bolivia, and Dr. Rotzinger, who temporarily settled in Romania.[91]

In Europe, the last country of hope for Jewish doctors appears to have been the Soviet Union, at least theoretically, for two reasons. First, it suffered from a chronic shortage of physicians, and second, it would naturally welcome enemies of fascism, especially if they were Marxist-oriented.[92] But little is known about communist Russia as a haven for Jewish physicians, except that some German practitioners fled there, with an uncertain fate ahead of them, because, evidently, they were not to be exempt from Stalin's purges. But by 1939 Moscow had sent out word that German-Jewish doctors were not welcome in the realm, and one wonders what ultimately happened to a certain Dr. Alfred Stern, thirty-five years old when he arrived in the Soviet Union by August 1937.[93]

All the remaining European countries were less hospitable. Chief among them, because of its size and significance as a potential benefactor, was France. But this western neighbor of Germany became doubly precarious for Jewish doctors because of its own ingrained anti-Semitic tradition and the superimposition of fresh Judeophobic impulses, generated after 1939 by the German occupation in the north and the indigenous fascist regime in the Vichy-controlled south. Yet despite its known xenophobia, France, perhaps because of its reputed lifestyle, was a preferred country of refuge for German Jews as early as 1933, when in excess of eight thousand entered there. The physicians among them constituted more than one-tenth of all the Jewish émigré doctors in this early phase.[94] More Jews came to France in 1938–39, many of them from Austria and the Sudetenland, so that a total of approximately twenty-five thousand were present there just before the war, including several thousand illegals.[95]

Until the war the French government, under pressure from chauvinistic medical students and self-protective physicians such as the ones in colonial Tunis, was steadfast in not permitting any of the refugee doctors to practice and in withholding from them the opportunity to do so by the granting of relicensing privileges on the British model. Most Jewish professionals remained in France by dint of temporary residency papers only, meaning that doctors would chance deportation back to Germany if they were found to be practicing. Nonetheless, some doctors did just that, for instance as assistants to established French physicians, under disgraceful working conditions and with little or no pay. Realizing the futility of their situation, foreign Jewish physicians in France generally sought to move to another country, as did Käte Frankenthal (to Switzerland, Czechoslovakia, and finally the United States) and the Stuttgart homeopathic practitioner Dr. Friedrich Wolf (to Mexico).[96]

The situation for Jewish doctors in France deteriorated even more after the outbreak of war, when the Vichy government in the south inaugurated harsh anti-Semitic statutes, including one specifically directed against doctors, and later still when its authorities and the German occupation forces in the northern half of the country began rounding up all Jews for deportation. Two German-Jewish physicians who were known to be in the Paris area beyond the time of the formal surrender, albeit probably inactive, were said to be unaccounted for by the Nazi occupation authorities in 1942 and 1943. Kurt Schachtel, son of a Berlin tailor, was registered in Palestine by 1935 and in Paris thereafter. In summer 1942 the German embassy in Paris advised that it had no knowledge of Schachtel's whereabouts—meaning that he may have left surreptitiously, without renewing his German passport, and gone elsewhere. Or he may have been evacuated and murdered in a death camp. The same can be assumed about Dr. Bruno Meyerowitz, the son of a Königsberg lawyer, by January 1943.[97]

Few other countries, in Europe or elsewhere, were important for would-be émigré physicians. Switzerland's callously stringent immigration and residence policy allowed hardly any Jewish professionals to stay there, let alone resume practice legally. Defying these antialien regulations with a cunning that was as uncommon as it was admirable, Käte Frankenthal managed to be medically active under cover until her nerves gave out and she crossed over to Czechoslovakia.[98]

On the face of Europe or the entire Western Hemisphere, nary a country was left for the Jewish physicians to seek shelter in. Belgium, Holland, and the Scandinavian nations were all dangerously close to the German border, and though they might reluctantly offer asylum, no legal or gainful medical work was allowed there.[99] Czechoslovakia officially accepted refugees until the March 1938 Anschluss, which cast its shadow northeast, but no doctor could practice there either.[100] The British dominions of Canada and Australia not only had immigrant-restrictive legislation but expressly prevented Jewish physicians from setting up practice, Australia using the specious argument that German and Austrian medical standards were lower than her own.[101] The Latin American countries such as Argentina, Brazil, Mexico, and Chile were in need of agricultural laborers, and vituperative anti-Semitism allowed comparatively few Jews inside their borders, even though Brazil seems to have been more open-minded to physicians than any of the others.[102] Ironically, the last country remaining for the most desperate of Jewish doctors as for other Jews who still had some money for a ship's passage was Shanghai on mainland China, not really a country at all but an internationally administered Free Zone, for which no visas were required. Several Jewish doctors stayed there, even legally practicing medicine, some for a few years, until they could escape to other lands. Those who remained fell victim to the Japanese invasion that was part of the Far Eastern theater of war, but none are known to have perished.[103]

What are the statistics of this gruesome exodus? To justify their actions to an astonished world, Nazi leaders always exaggerated grossly the share of Jewish physicians (as of other Jewish professionals) in the population at large. For instance, on February 15, 1934, Reich Interior Minister Frick explained before the diplomatic corps that until the Nazi takeover in January 1933 48 percent of all the doctors in the Reich had been Jewish.[104] In reality, the figure was much lower, notwithstanding today's difficulty in arriving at exact percentages. These difficulties are partially contingent on the absence of census figures for non-Mosaic (baptized or religiously dissident) Jews in the Reich and partially on unreliable figures for emigration and deportation. Hence we can only estimate.

Although most historians credibly put the figure of Mosaic Jewish doctors in Germany at approximately sixty-five hundred for January–April 1933, some scholars have advanced the convincing argument that if non-"Aryans" of all descriptions (dissidents, baptized, and *Mischlinge*) are included, this figure would rise to nine thousand. According to their reckoning, these medical men and women would have amounted to between 15 and 17 percent of physicians in the country.[105] There is a loose consensus among experts that when the first ordinance struck Jewish doctors in 1933, between four and five hundred non-"Aryan" physicians decided to emigrate and that by January 1935 that number had risen to between fifteen hundred and seventeen hundred.[106] By this time fifty thousand Jews in all are reputed to have left Germany for other places.[107] For the following years, various estimates of the number of remaining Jewish doctors have been advanced. There were, more or less, five thousand practitioners left in 1936 and close to four thousand in June 1937. That last-mentioned figure still amounted to 10 percent of all physicians licensed to practice. In Berlin alone, up to 30 percent of all panel physicians still were non-"Aryans" by the terms of the 1935 blood laws.[108] After delicensure in the fall of 1938, merely 708 Jewish sick-treaters had been left in the Reich; that figure shrank to 285 by the end of the year.[109]

The final tally of dispersion and destruction of German-Jewish physicians serves as stark testimony of inhumanity for those "Aryan" doctors who devised the staggered race legislation, drove out their unwanted colleagues, and implemented the selections on the ramps. From 1933 to 1945, anywhere from forty-five hundred to six thousand Jewish physicians were expelled from the country, equaling as much as two-thirds of all non-"Aryan" doctors.[110] By one dependable count, from January 1933 on up to 5 percent, or several hundred, of the Jewish physicians may have committed suicide.[111] An indeterminable percentage may have died of natural causes, but undoubtedly, death was often induced or accelerated by the traumas of shock and grief. Be this as it may, even by the most conservative accounting, one is forced to conclude that no less than one-quarter of Germany's Jewish physicians, or over two thousand, perished in the Nazi Holocaust.

Conclusion: The Crisis of Physicians and Medicine under Hitler

At the end of a complex story, we cannot avoid the question, What was the historic place of the German physician in the Third Reich? In the final analysis this amounts to the problem of assessing his professional mores in a universal context. Among German doctors of the Nazi era, two easily identifiable extremes can be made out at either side of the spectrum of ideal types: the doctor who gave his life for his vocation and the one who killed in the name of it. In the middle, there stood the regular practitioner who tended his patients faithfully, as he had done before 1933 and would again after 1945.

Yet with reference to the Hippocratic ideal, this midpoint was not the same in 1942 as it had been in 1932, and it had shifted even further from the standard accepted at the turn of the century. As the Swiss historian of medicine Esther Fischer-Homberger has formulated it, the "norms" had changed, relative to which medical crimes against humanity—the ultimate that German physicians were to be capable of—faded in perniciousness as they became more ordinary than unusual.[1]

Naturally, this is not to imply that all doctors in the Third Reich took part in these crimes on a regular basis or even knew about them. But it does mean that their legitimate professional activities occurred in the shadow of those crimes and that there was a significant interaction between the misdeeds and daily medical practice, which, perhaps imperceptively but decisively in the long run, changed the professional ethos motivating all the doctors in Germany.

It is true that technically only a small number of physicians in Germany became tainted by crimes against humanity. At the time of the Nuremberg Doctors' Trials in the late 1940s, Chicago professor Andrew C. Ivy, the prosecution's expert, put this number at about 70, but it was soon revised upward to between 350 and 400.[2] For today's historian of medicine, the problem is not with those figures as such, for in principle it is irrelevant whether 50 or 500 doctors committed medical infractions in concentration camps and "euthanasia" stations. The problem, rather, is with the manipulation of these numbers by the great majority of post-1945 German physicians to exonerate themselves. Defenders of the West German medical establishment reason to this day that since the premier medical criminals have been caught and sentenced, all the uncomfortable questions that might have lingered have been answered and therefore things are back to business as usual. The implications of this view are that German medicine, at its crest in the 1920s, survived the Nazi period with a few unfortunate bruises but essentially intact enough to rebound to its prior international heights. The medical malefactors were extraneous intruders, not part of the hallowed German medical tradition and hence in no way typical.

The physicians who offer such an interpretation today are mostly older professionals, and they carry much weight. Ironically or perhaps significantly, in their youth they participated in the pre-1945 medical establishment in some capacity or grew up in Nazi society; presently they either feel or are *ex cathedra* called upon to comment on Germany's medical past. They include Dr. Karsten Vilmar, the current president of the West German Bundesärztekammer, Professor Hans Schadewaldt, historian of medicine at Düsseldorf University, and Dr. Günter Huwer, formerly chief gynecologist at the Wenckebach Hospital in West Berlin.

Karsten Vilmar was born in 1930, the son of a physician in Bremen; he was trained as a surgeon. In his official position as the ranking medical functionary in the Federal Republic since 1978 he announced that "only a minority of German doctors—one might justifiably call them a macabre 'order'—spoliated the reputation of our profession" and that the much-publicized crimes were "diabolic perversions."[3] Schadewaldt, a semiofficial court chronicler of organized German doctors and president of the International Society of the History of Medicine in 1988, was born in 1923 and studied medicine during the Third Reich. He found himself in the Wehrmacht at the end of the war and then for three years in a prisoner-of-war camp. In 1949 he completed his medical education, entered academe, and obtained a full chair in the history of medicine in 1965. His stand, too, is that the evil German doctors were a deplorable exception, but despite extant records, he places their number even below the one hundred mark.[4] Dr. Huwer was a thirty-three-year-old assistant physician in gynecology at the University of Jena when he joined the NSDAP in spring 1933—not in expectation of any rewards, as he averred in 1987, but because "everyone" in his unit did it and in recognition of Hitler's "previous success." (Yet also, one suspects, he had his eyes on possible spoils, for Hitler had been able to "encourage youth for the future, to instil it with self-confidence and idealism.") After his *Habilitation* in 1935 Huwer traveled to China, where he embarked on a university career, retaining his NSDAP status in the party section reserved for German citizens abroad. Eventually, he was made an adjunct professor in Jena on leave of absence, and he always maintained his contact with the Reich. After the war and the subsequent Chinese Revolution he moved on to South Korea, where in 1959 right-wing dictator Syngman Rhee bestowed on him a national medal. Having returned to West Berlin in 1960, Huwer accepted the Federal Republic's highest award (Bundesverdienstkreuz) and retired in 1966. This gynecologist has recently insisted that he learned about medical crimes in the Third Reich only after 1945. In 1938, when he visited Germany, "no one was in a situation to know that Hitler and a part of his retinue would turn into felons." Huwer's apologetic ruminations culminate in the assertion that "German physicians knew just as little about the [medical] crimes as the German people themselves. We are aware that a fraction of physiciandom became guilty. . . . In every occupation there were and there are those who abuse their calling."[5]

The salient point Huwer misses and one that complicates our present evaluation is that medical men and women like himself, who were nominal Nazi party members and possibly much more, were inadequately "de-Nazified" after 1945 because doctors were needed to prevent and cure all manner of disorders among a destitute civilian populace.[6] This also meant that former Nazis reoccupied or newly ascended to university chairs and that the medical bureaucracy was heavily infiltrated by experienced but politically compromised personnel.[7] From 1945 to the early 1960s, in the worst of cases, former killers or their assistants like Dr. Herta Oberheuser, Professor Werner Heyde, or Professor Anton Kiesselbach were allowed complete license to practice or teach, and, in comparatively harmless scenarios, scores of former party, SA, and SS members resumed regular office hours.[8] Both situations implied the continuation of political attitudes that even in a germinal state must have been dubious in a new democracy, even if judged on purely formal grounds. But more critically, such unqualified passage suggests the carryover of a medical mentality that had taken full shape against the background of the censored misdeeds, whether men like Vilmar, Schadewaldt, or Huwer today choose personally to detach themselves from them or not.[9]

It is important to understand that after 1933, German everyday medical practice to a large extent was an indirect reflection of academic medicine, its fluctuations and contortions that were a foreseeable consequence of a combination of two separate factors: overextended natural science on one side and the ideology of naturalism and race on the other. Insofar as the one was progressive, representing rationality pushed to questionable extremes without the temperate influence of ethics, the other was regressive, an offspring of irrational romanticism in the service of the *Volksgemeinschaft*.

Both developments may be traced back to the final third of the nineteenth century. After national unification in 1871 German medicine came under the powerful influence of the drive for *Grosswissenschaft*, which resulted in the buildup of mighty industrial complexes spurred on by the quick and overwhelming advances in natural science and inspired, simultaneously, by an unshakable belief in boundless materialistic progress. Primarily involved in this process were the state, which furthered the new advances for its own ends, and the universities, within which the new technologies could nestle.[10] Medicine used these developments; the *exakt-naturwissenschaftliche Einstellung*, the strictly natural-scientific approach, became one of the hallmarks of its professionalization. Both in the universities and semipublic research institutions such as the new Kaiser-Wilhelm-Gesellschaft men such as Robert Koch, Wilhelm His, Jr., and Paul

Ehrlich emerged as world-renowned pioneers of a scientifically oriented medical discipline.[11]

That trend continued through the Weimar Republic, even though funding for research and development was harder to come by.[12] The Great War was disruptive, but it also added momentum to the movement toward progress, for shortages, hardships, and strictures encouraged the creative processes in the direction of new inventions, for instance in the chemical area of synthetic substitutions, or prosthesis (the "Sauerbruch Arm") in medicine.[13]

Medicine now charged ahead in a positivistic and ultrarationalistic mood, using many of the attendant advances in related natural sciences such as chemistry and physics. Its objectives became bolder and bolder: not merely the prevention and extirpation of human diseases but, through the genetic science of biophysics, the improvement of the human species. German physicians had been leading the world for decades, and Germany in the 1920s also was prominent in this sector, although by no means isolated. There were geneticists in the United States, Scandinavia, England, and the Soviet Union. In Germany, one practical result of such research was a plan for the sterilization of hereditarily diseased people—it existed on the order book of the Prussian Landtag by 1932.[14]

One of the prerequisites that turned into a sort of fetish of this exact-scientific attitude was the experiment—it, too, a child of rationalization in the past century. At the universities, the theories had to be validated by experiments. It was unquestioned that advances in medicine (as in natural science) could be achieved only through the inductive method of formulating a hypothesis and testing it, by subjecting it to revision and verification in a controlled series of empirical observations.[15] Throughout the 1920s and well into the Third Reich, German medical scientists were ruled by a consensus that as desirable as human experiments were, for moral reasons animals had to suffice as objects of empirical experimentation.[16] In 1902, the Berlin neurologist Albert Moll had published a comprehensive catalog of taboos indicting medical experimentation on patients, whose ailments were not to be exploited by their doctors. At that time, it had never occurred to Moll that healthy persons could artificially be made ill for the sake of scientific knowledge, as happened later under Hitler (e.g., Heissmeyer).[17] After 1931, codification in Germany allowed for human experimentation only in complementation with that on animals, and on a totally voluntary basis.[18] By and large, right up to World War II the usual form of human experimentation by doctors was upon themselves, as practiced by the surgeon August Bier in 1899 for the improvement of anesthetics (lumbar injection) and thirty years later by Werner Forssmann, when he guided a catheter through a vein into his heart.[19]

Medicine as a science became complicated after 1933. On one hand, its positivistic aura continued, with researchers tending to conduct it for its own sake, beyond any ethically binding framework and moving it to the realm of scientism—a danger Sauerbruch knew about and decried in 1937, when he spoke of medicine's "one-sided rationally mechanistic mode."[20] On the other hand, precisely because *exakt-naturwissenschaftliche Medizin* was carried on like a positivistic discipline, ostensibly value-free, it was susceptible to usurpation by an unconscionable political regime that desired its services. The Nazi system commenced to conscript medicine not merely as an applied, but as a subservient science, a *Zweckwissenschaft*, prescribing for it a specially designed ethos dictated by the priorities of National Socialist governance and hence politicizing it.[21]

Under Nazi aegis, then, and especially with the onset and escalation of war, medicine felt free further to pursue its unlimited quest for knowledge and serve the state at the same time. Because animal experimentation was known to be a poor substitute for experiments on humans, for only analogous inferences could be drawn,[22] the crossover to human experimentation during the war became a logical consequence of prior practices that had been fettered. Unfettered, exact scientific medicine adopted a deterministic hue, stopping, for the sake of vivisection, only at the terminal experiment. For example, in the case of pressure-chamber research (pilots exposed to stress and vital insufficiencies) it had been speculated in 1935 that in heights over six thousand meters a person's lungs would "probably" be able to take in more air.[23] This theory anticipated pressure-chamber experiments by Luftwaffe physicians such as Walter Kreienberg on human volunteers in simulated altitudes of up to eight thousand meters, at the beginning of the war, and later Rascher's Dachau tests. When at the height of the conflict Rascher was performing vivisections on his helpless victims, altitudes of eighteen thousand meters were simulated, after it had been established that monkeys as experimental objects had outlived their value at twelve thousand meters. Through the use of human subjects, the state would benefit in the end, for the superior British high-altitude aircraft now might be vulnerable.[24]

Characteristically, all applications for human experimentation, for example in the SS, henceforth tended to be rationalized on the ground that animal tests had taken the researcher only so far, and better results would accrue only after transfer of the experiment to humans—as was argued in proposals by Brandt and Gebhardt (phosphor burns), Rose and Conti (typhoid fever), and Clauberg (sterilization).[25] In an atmosphere pervaded by contentment over seemingly incontrovertible evidence derived from human experimentation at war's end it was small wonder that medical scientists, not excluding Sauerbruch himself, who in ordinary circumstances never would have dared to substitute human for animal "material," could not help but be privy to some of the excesses, or even avail themselves of their fruits.[26]

To compound the difficulties, there was yet another trap. Because inviolable ethics were submerged, and because the state now took precedence, it was also possible for the exact-natural-scientific methodology of medicine to be faulted in the way it was carried out so that, ironically, what had once started out as objective, rational science in the end became its caricature. This could happen particularly when the inductive method, the constant careful testing of hypotheses, had been corrupted, for example, if a conclusion to be proved had been preconceived as a given and treated apodictically, in the manner of an axiom, even though the motions of the scientific process were observed. Nazi medical researchers became guilty of such pseudo-science in the course of their genetic (eugenic) research attempting to "prove" the dominance of hereditary over environmental factors. They did this because, once more, Nazi dogma imputed the desired results before experimentation had begun.[27] They used statistics based on pairs of twins to demonstrate that bearers of (allegedly) negative hereditary traits like a violently criminal disposition could not be rehabilitated and hence had to be neutralized, which could mean physical annihilation.[28] (Such "research" provided the justification not only for the radical solutions culminating in sterilization, castration, and "euthanasia," but also for increased penal treatment, such as the prosecution of "unreconstructable" homosexuals and rebellious juvenile offenders during wartime.)[29] The statistics, however, invariably were spurious, based on insufficient or wrongly selected samples, and the argumentation was specious, confusing cause and effect, mistaking a symptom for the condition whence it sprang, in short, generally putting the cart before the horse and specifically imparting falsehoods.[30]

In contradistinction to rationalized medicine, certain of the Third Reich's physicians paid tribute to the antiscientific, holistic variant espoused by the iconoclastic Danzig surgeon Erwin Liek, which was in essence irrational. The intellectual roots of its organicism lay in the cultural pessimism of Lagarde, Langbehn, and Nietzsche, with twentieth-century references to Moeller van den Bruck and Spengler.[31] Liek, who had been a racist, deeming the Negro to be at the bottom of the blood hierarchy, might have been Hitler's health plenipotentiary in the Time of Struggle and thus could have preempted Gerhard Wagner, had it not been for his failing health.[32] It will be remembered from earlier chapters that the goals of Liek's followers in the Third Reich were in keeping with an exaggerated naturalism and extreme antirationality, as were the sundry antispecialism, anticity, antiuniversity, antipharmaceuticals, and antihospital sentiments. Liek adepts tended toward homeopathy as developed by Samuel Hahnemann in the early nineteenth century and honed in the 1920s by Liek's compatriate Hans Much. In its regressionism, the Liekists' imagery of physiological equilibrium to be aided by the force of "Dr. Nature" was reminiscent of the ancient humoral pathology of the four body fluids that had been definitively laid to rest by Rudolf Virchow in the 1850s.[33]

Two elements of Liek's teaching had far-reaching effects on the development of the naturalist side of Nazi medicine and hence must be dwelled on at greater length: his specific interpretation of pain and his antagonism to scientific experimentation. Physicians of the Liek school contended that pain was a necessary by-product of the state of sickness as well as of the healing process and should not be artificially suppressed. Not only would pain, as a symptom of physiological imbalance, guide the diagnostician's hands (this was, of course, a long-held view and not especially outlandish),[34] but endurance of pain was a mark of character. Hence pain acquired a moral dimension. The ability of a patient to endure pain was said to be a measure of his personal prowess and, even more important, indicative of his race. The heroic type favored in Nazi ideology was expected to bear pain well—a notion that in part derived from the reckless abandon of World War I shock troops and the Freikorps and was glorified in literature as late as 1934 by the war-and-death enthusiast Ernst Jünger.[35] The Jew was believed to be less able to stand pain than the "Aryan" and hence not predisposed to heroism. "National Socialism's heroic man and the biologically perfect racial type—they are one and the same," wrote Karl Kötschau in 1935, the year of Liek's death.[36] Such conviction created the potential for lethal inversion, for pain could be applied deliberately to gauge the heroism and indeed the racial quality of any given person.

The second element in Liek's catechism was antipodal to the experimental attitude of the scientifically inclined physician. As Liek and his epigones were rejecting the "mechanistic" medicine of the faculties, they condemned their raison d'être, the empirically grounded experiment on animals and, by extension, humans. It is important to understand this feeling correctly. It originated not out of humanity, a love for humankind, nor one for animals in the manner of some overzealous animal-rights crusaders (the often-encountered theory that Nazis had spurned human life in preference for that of animals, in particular house pets, is without basis in fact—nonsuspect societies love pets also). Its mainspring was the Liekists' distrust of man's ability to mutate permanently what nature had originally shaped—a conviction that was well in line with their conservatism and retrograde romanticism.[37] It led them to a sort of fatalism, an unquestioned acceptance of what they thought to be natural or biological inequalities that could never be altered, such as the discrepancies between races. As a corollary, it meant that the truly sick, those who were denied a recovery of their balance by nature's power, were doomed to eventual perdition. To be ill, after all, was immoral.[38] As one of the surviving Third Reich physicians judged the Nazis scathingly: "They wanted to do away with the diseases by liquidating the sick."[39]

Under Liek's admirer Gerhard Wagner, the Liekists were noticeably strong in the beginnings of the Nazi health bureaucracy, until mid-1939. Liek's followers included Walter Schultze, Kurt Klare, Karl Kötschau, Ernst Günther Schenck, and Joachim Mrugowsky, and they were fond of repeating the master's epithet that conventional "mechanistic" training would produce medical technicians but never physicians.[40] With the exception of Mrugowsky, who was already moving in SS circles, all of them had some function in Wagner's establishment. Professor

Franz Wirz, the dermatologist, whose mission was to help Wagner infiltrate the high schools of medicine, was a fervent admirer of "our great Liek."[41] Sympathizers in high party echelons included Hess, Streicher, and, to a certain extent, Himmler, even though more prudent men would always pull him back from fantasy to empiricism.[42] Liek's greatest triumph was the posthumous institutionalization of his ideas within Wagner's creation, the system of New German Healing. And Liek bears an intellectual responsibility for his disciples' view of the Jews as elements endangering the healthy balance of the *Volksgemeinschaft*, a vision that helped to create Auschwitz.

Officially, Liek's era may be said to have ended with the death of Wagner, which, coincidentally, ushered in the second phase of public health administration under martial auspices that called for rationality, not mysticism. But rather than fading away quickly, the Liek tradition merged with the rationalist approach. Conti always exhibited a certain affinity for Liek's ideas, which, during the war, boldly manifested itself when he invoked Liek's memory in public addresses and insisted, in his own area of expertise and that of the maternal Reich midwife leader, that natural childbirth be encouraged and its inevitable pain be endured by the mother.[43] With Conti's sense of sufferance, naturalist-oriented publications beholden to Liek continued to appear, as did the journal *Hippokrates*; old stalwarts of New German Healing like Kötschau were allowed to publish their unchanged rhetoric as late as 1944; and in his own administration Conti retained original Liekists like Schenck and Dr. Hans-Dietrich Röhrs.[44]

And although exponents of the reigning exact-scientific school of medicine sometimes were fond of emphasizing their differences of opinion with Liek, as did the redoubtable Agnes Bluhm in 1936, and coryphaei like Heidelberg's Johann Achelis held forth about the physiology of pain without mentioning the Danzig surgeon,[45] his philosophy lived on tenaciously. In gynecological faculty circles, for example, where arch-conservatism triumphed, Liek's concept of natural childbirth was paramount even at the pinnacle of war.[46] The by then homeopathically inclined surgeon August Bier was held in high regard and in 1937 along with Sauerbruch won the *Nationalpreis*, the regime's greatest honor.[47] Rational Sauerbruch himself had his Liekist side.[48] Clinically educated Marburg hygienicist Wilhelm Pfannenstiel, yet another SS officer, waxed enthusiastic about the "equilibrium of extreme power sources" and sickness as an "attempt at auto-repair."[49]

Liek's long-term effects may have been insidious. Viktor Freiherr von Weizsäcker of Heidelberg, who after the war would denounce the Nazi medical crimes, in 1944 admitted to an empathy with "antimechanistic new healing."[50] In more recent times, a West German critic of the Nazi doctors has charged that in his therapeutic vision the seemingly unblemished Weizsäcker never was able to differentiate between therapy and destruction, only between justified and unjustified destruction.[51] Could this be read as an assault on Weizsäcker's belief in

Erwin Liek's fatalism, as epitomized by acquiescence in nature's practice of triage? As a psychiatrist, writes Peter Gay, Weizsäcker admired Sigmund Freud—a rare occurrence among Germans. But, continues Gay, he credited the great Viennese with "Asian wisdom" rather than with a universal intelligence.[52] Was that not another sign that Weizsäcker had internalized Liek's axiom of the irremovable natural differences, in this case between races?

Rassenkunde as described in Chapter 4 always was a specifically National Socialist phenomenon. In the main, it possessed a natural-scientific component, deriving from conventional anthropology and positivistic medicine, and an ideological component, culminating in the concept of an immutable hierarchy of blood. If this latter portion was not always owing to Liek, it certainly was begotten by the same neoromanticism as was the Danzig surgeon's *Weltanschauung*. The historic course of *Rassenkunde* from Ploetz to Koller has already been charted. Within this course, a narrower path can be mapped out that led directly from the experimental laboratories of the late nineteenth century to the gas chambers of Auschwitz. Four men were treading that path, all of them physicians, each one starting as a genuine disciple of science and veering increasingly toward the irrational as time progressed, eventually to cast shadows even beyond World War II. Their names were Theodor James Mollison, Eugen Fischer, Otmar Freiherr von Verschuer, and Josef Mengele.

In this corona, Theodor Mollison may be said to have been the senior, if only by age. Mollison was born in 1874 and socialized in the natural-scientific and imperialistic atmosphere of the Wilhelmine era. Licensed as a physician in Freiburg in 1898, he practiced medicine for three years in Frankfurt. He then took several semesters of natural science in Würzburg before setting out on a months-long study trip to the German colony of East Africa in 1904. Upon his return in 1905 he enrolled in anthropology at Zurich, which had been host to Agnes Bluhm and Ernst Rüdin only a few years earlier, obtaining his *Habilitation* there. He received an associate professorship in Heidelberg in 1916 and was appointed full professor of anthropology in Munich ten years later.[53]

In the present context, two aspects of Mollison's career are revealing: his regular *exakt-naturwissenschaftliche* training in medicine and anthropology and his conditioning in the abject racism observed by the German colonial masters, particularly the hypernationalistic physicians in the African territorial administration at that time.[54] It will be remembered that Philalethes Kuhn, another champion of Nazi *Rassenkunde*, had had a similar exposure to the seminal ideas of a Germanic master race in southwest Africa, where he took part in the genocidal war against the Hereroes in 1904.[55] Indeed, such racism is reflected in Mollison's prewar writings on the Maori, in German colonial Polynesia, despite the unquestioned scientific substratum. It was Mollison's objective to measure prehistoric and contemporary aboriginal (Polynesian) anatomical features to prove scientifically what he presumed to exist: "differences between separate races."[56] And indeed, in a publication of 1923, Mollison placed the Negro just above Neanderthal man and the Australian aborigine just below, in a rank order of "lower races."[57]

That article had been coauthored by Eugen Fischer, who was Mollison's junior by four months. Fischer, too, graduated as a physician in 1898, having studied in Freiburg, where he and Mollison could not have been strangers. He became an anatomist with a strong secondary interest in anthropology; by 1904, he was associate professor in Freiburg. In 1908, Fischer, like his friend Theodor Mollison, sailed for Africa to do "anthropological research." His resultant testimonial was the study about the "Rehoboth Bastards" (1913), a self-enclosed group of Dutch-Hottentot half-breeds in German southwest Africa, which for white supremacists around the world became a classic.[58] In many respects, the book read like a manual for white man's colonial rule over native tribes: their treatment must be "good, just, stern and not pampering," for even as mongrels, which placed the Rehobothers noticeably above the indigenous natives, they could not come close to the white race, judged by the indexes of intelligence, morality, or vitality.[59] In 1923 Fischer expanded on the Negro by judging condescendingly that he was "not especially intelligent in the actual sense of the word, and above all, bereft of any spiritual creativity or imagination . . . yet docile and clever. Prescience and spiritual independence are little developed. Of a cheerful disposition, the Negro indulges his carefree existence day in, day out."[60]

Not surprisingly, in the future the less aggressive Mollison remained in the backyard of world recognition, unlike his collaborator Fischer, who would rise to fame as Germany's preeminent interpreter of *Rassenkunde*. In 1927, Fischer accepted the directorship of the newly founded Berlin Kaiser-Wilhelm-Institut für Anthropologie und Eugenik coupled with a full professorship in anthropology at the university.[61] Nonetheless, Mollison, who during the Third Reich openly admitted to his expertise in *Rassenkunde* now that the term was fashionable, remained in close contact with Fischer, as was evinced in 1936, when he needed 2,000 marks for the processing of primordial skeletons from a foundation to be approved by his celebrated colleague.[62]

There can be no argument that in the passage of time Eugen Fischer's original exact-scientific fundament was overgrown by the irrational notions that had already inspired his early racist outpourings. Fischer may or may not have been noted for anti-Semitism before 1933.[63] In his stratified racist worldview, however, there certainly was room for Jews, as he would often show after Hitler's ascension. He admired the anti-Semitic Führer unreservedly if only because he followed a "qualitative population policy."[64] In 1933 the famous geneticist pronounced publicly against "international intellectualism" and in favor of "race and the conscious desiderate of the Nordic ideal-race of our Germanic forebears, a desire to annihilate ruthlessly anything of alien race." Concurrently, he turned against the "alien spirit" of the un-*völkisch* and condemned the immigration into

Germany of eastern Jewry.[65] And at the height of the war, the physician-cum-anthropologist assisted anti-Semitic theologians in identifying Jews as intruders into Egyptian civilization by classifying them arbitrarily: by something "in the Jewish facial features, which is not measurable," nonetheless of the "intellectual Jewish type," with the "insolent" (*frech*) expression typical of the intellectual Jew.[66] To be sure, race scientist Fischer never neglected to advance the empirical work of the biophysicists as based on studies of twins.[67] But he also partook in the assessment of the "Rhineland Bastards," those unfortunate post–World War I offspring of French colonial fathers and German mothers, just before their forced sterilization, and helped to plan the evacuation of all European Jews to Poland-based slave camps.[68]

Fischer's equal as a researcher and scholar was Otmar Freiherr von Verschuer, whose allusions to the master pervade his own work and who succeeded Fischer at Berlin in 1942, to become his lifelong friend thereafter.[69] Baron Verschuer, scion of an aristocratic Hessian family, was born in 1896 and hence belonged to that Freikorps generation which blamed the loss of the first war on Marxists, pacifists, and Jews. A demobilized first lieutenant in 1918, Verschuer was immersed in the racist, prefascist subculture of the period in a double capacity: as a fellow of the Verein Deutscher Studenten, long Germany's most extreme anti-Semitic fraternity, and as a member of the notorious Marburg student Freikorps that in cold blood shot dead fifteen alleged communists near Mechterstedt in 1920.[70] In his memoirs of 1936, the former commander of that Freikorps, Freiherr Bogislav von Selchow, a former imperial frigate commander, inveterate anti-Semite, and by then an ardent Nazi, speaks highly of the much younger Verschuer, who during the massacre was his aide-de-camp.[71]

Allowed time off for studying, Verschuer majored in medicine. He graduated as a generalist in 1923 and was certified as an internist in 1927. That year marked his rise to dubious stardom. He also managed his *Habilitation*, specializing in genetics, and, after a noted inaugural address at Tübingen, was installed as director of the anthropological section at Fischer's Berlin institute.[72] Here, goaded on by the scientific optimism of the day, he did much biophysical experimentation, publishing prolifically.[73]

Such work was carried into the Third Reich, and Verschuer became one of the chief protagonists of comparative twin research and a positive population policy based on whatever possibilities of genetic engineering then existed.[74] Since this was of interest not only to Germans, the baron traveled abroad and was quoted widely in international specialized publications.[75] His superiors and the new authorities smiled on him, and he rose to the challenge of full professor and chief of the new institute for hereditary science and race hygiene at Frankfurt University in 1935.[76] Logically, he was a party member by July 1940.[77]

But Verschuer, too, became more susceptible to irrational currents, and characteristically, it was his own prefigured racism that propelled him into the camp of the ideological fanatics. As Aryanization of German society proceeded, Verschuer could not help but have a hand in "scientifically" ascertaining the people's racial pedigrees.[78] In January 1939 the baron, in a Berlin public lecture, spoke in all seriousness about the "differences in the racial traits between Germans and Jews."[79] As he himself has reported, his institute cooperated in the training of future physicians under the auspices, and along the guidelines, of the SS.[80] His genetic insights became instrumental in—by universal standards—criminal medicine climaxing in sterilization and "mercy killing."[81] And his unsavory racism was even more radicalized when in 1944 he acknowledged that Germany was waging a "racial war" against "World Jewry" and demanded as a "political priority of the present, a new, total solution to the Jewish problem."[82]

Heinrich Wilhelm Kranz was in 1942 Verschuer's successor in Frankfurt. The baron knew him well as a comrade-in-arms of the Mechterstedt massacre.[83] Only a year younger than Verschuer, Kranz was as much in the baron's age cohort as Fischer had been in Mollison's.[84] I have already detailed the nefarious pseudoscientific activities of the onetime ophthalmologist.[85] Here it is important to point to the intragenerational as well as the intergenerational cross-connections between Kranz and Verschuer on one hand, and Kranz and Fischer on the other—this was a self-supportive network of a few insiders based on ongoing reciprocal fertilization.[86] In addition, it is well to emphasize Kranz's abject racism, specifically his anti-Semitism, which was discernibly in the Liekist mold.[87]

Doubtless inspired by Eugen Fischer, Kranz set for himself in his Giessen institute the task of examining "Aryan"-Jewish and "Aryan"-Gypsy "mixlings," to determine which component in them was stronger.[88] By the time Professor Kranz was making this objective public, a young scientist from Swabian Günzburg working with Baron von Verschuer some thirty miles south, in Frankfurt, was already deeply impressed by his own teacher's forays into *Rassenkunde*. He was probably aware that Verschuer had, in 1928, made a research excursion with Fischer to Romania to take anthropological stock of the German minority in Siebenbürgen to determine its true "racial constitution."[89]

Of the several assistants Professor Verschuer employed in 1939, Dr. Josef Mengele was his favorite.[90] Mengele started his academic career in Munich, where, at the age of twenty-four, he received a doctorate in anthropology under Professor Mollison in 1935, who at that time was gravely concerned about the impact of what he termed the Jewish mentality on the "racially uprooted."[91] Mengele's dissertation dealt with the jaws of four primeval groups, one among whom, the Melanesians, was recognized as racially the lowest and then used as the standard against which to measure the other three, so as to rank them all according to empirically perceived differences. By formal criteria, Mengele's work was in the *exakt-naturwissenschaftliche* vein his teacher Mollison had been schooled in, but it exhibited two disturbing elements of subjectivity that appear to have marred the budding scientist even then. One was the certainty that "races" would be different from one another (a view that concurred with the doctrines of Mollison and Fischer) and that, as a consequence, differing qualitative value judgments would govern each of them.[92] The other had to do with Mengele's privately motivated choice of his topic, for, as the Brazilian autopsy report has recently confirmed, he was born with a diastema between his upper central incisors, and, as may be gleaned from his SS dental chart, had upper bicuspids missing symmetrically on both sides.[93] Was it legitimate for an objective scientist to choose as the object of his scrutiny a problem that was tied to his personal pathology?

Mengele continued to mingle the rational with the irrational after he arrived in Frankfurt to accomplish his second doctorate under Verschuer, this time in medicine, by 1938. Again he decided to examine dental and palatal disorders of children who had been operated on in the university's surgical department of Professor Victor Schmieden between 1925 and 1935. Mengele amplified this "material" on the basis of data on persons in the Frankfurt area whom Verschuer had already registered in the demographic files of his institute. All told, Mengele examined 1,222 people, parents and their offspring, concluding that the irregularities were hereditary with the highest degree of certainty. Moreover, he found a positive correlation between those disorders and other hereditary malfunctions such as idiocy, propensity for dwarfism, and hydrocephaly.[94] To suppose that this correlation disturbed him personally would not be wide of the mark.

Before Mengele arrived in Auschwitz in spring 1943 to continue his research with a view to *Habilitation*,[95] he visited his teacher Verschuer in Berlin at the anthropological institute. There he processed data on Gypsy twins already assembled by one of Eugen Fischer's graduate students, Georg Wagner.[96] What is significant about Mengele's subsequent Auschwitz experiments in his capacity as Verschuer's Berlin assistant is the admixture of objective science, as manifested in exact anthropometry and the methodical dissections performed by classically trained Hungarian pathologist Miklos Nyiszli, on one hand, and subjective humbug, such as injecting dark eyeballs with blue dye, on the other.[97] In Mengele's Auschwitz work, the ultimate benefactor of which was Verschuer, the rational and the irrational congealed, only to render the end result useless, for exact science will not countenance even a trace of irrationality.[98] The new boundless opportunities for experiments on humans constituted one of the ideals of that novel breed of natural scientists that was ethically unrestricted; here Mengele made utopia reality. Mengele's use of twins as guinea pigs also manifested an extension of the overdrawn positivism in science as practiced by the originally serious and always deeply religious internist Verschuer, who touted twin methodology in his spectacular Tübingen lecture as early as 1927 and then put it to the test in Frankfurt, still without murder.[99] The fact that the Auschwitz-murdered twins were Jews and Gypsies pushed an already questionable methodology into the dual realm of the falsely scientific and the irrational, for in their case, that which was to be proven, their racial insufficiency (an irrational presumption), was already preordained (a methodic fallacy).[100]

There are additional aspects of Mengele's research in Auschwitz that seem to be more immediate repercussions of mystical Liekist thought. As reported by survivors, there was the double doctor's extraordinary indifference to, or sometimes fascination with, the physical pain he inflicted upon his victims.[101] In those instances, was Mengele exercising the naturalist dictum that pain was a mark of (racial) character? The ultimate irrationality probably derived from his apprehension regarding his own place in the racial pecking order. Did the gap between his upper front teeth and the absent bicuspids on both sides suggest to him the potential for his own eugenic worthlessness, the proneness for hereditary deformity, and hence the inevitability of self-destruction? One of the derivatives of Liek's school of nosology had been the immutability, the incurability of disorders Dr. Nature could not mend, notwithstanding all the success of the positivistic medicine men in the image of Fischer or Verschuer. Was Mengele such an avid feeder of Auschwitz ovens because he wished to quiet that inner voice of his which told him his right to life was forfeited? Was that the reason for tearfully crying out that "not one Jew should stay alive" after he had learned that the Americans had bombed his paternal home?[102]

In the person of Josef Mengele, the most terrible of all the doctors under Hitler, we are not just dealing with a monster, a sadistic killer, whose research was scientifically worthless.[103] Rather, as Lifton has written, with all his pathological predilection for cruelty Mengele was a physician trained in the medicinal *Zeitgeist* whose "dedication to the Nazi biomedical vision kept him always on the border between science and ideologically-corrupted pseudoscience," the product of a marriage between the rational and nonsense.[104]

Unmistakably, between 1933 and 1945 the Mengeles of Germany had their bearing on everyman's medicine. It was in a conventional medical culture infiltrated from one side by a science alienated from humanity and from another by charlatanry that young physicians in the Third Reich were raised to learn and prepare for practice, with many predestined to practice after 1945. In their own lifetime they had recourse to citations in the serious literature of the work by Mengele—though always out of context with the Auschwitz scenario—and they would continue to find such citations in the postwar era. This applied even more to the work of Mengele's mentor Verschuer, who once again became an esteemed university professor in 1951, lionized by the international academic set.[105]

At the risk of repetition, it cannot be emphasized enough in what strength potential physicians were exposed to Nazi racial doctrines in the classrooms of the universities, doctrines that then infused their working knowledge, even if the doctors privately derided them.[106] For instance, in early 1942 many if not most of the "younger doctors" were in accord with "euthanasia," on the terms propagated by the Nazis at that time and doubtless discussed in the nation's medical schools, whereas older doctors were more reticent.[107]

Verschuer's seminars in Frankfurt serve as further proof. The baron was broadly in charge of training medical students in "hereditary and race discipline" (*Rassenpflege*) and of acquainting them with applicable regime laws in that sector. Techniques in the examination of potential marriage partners for "conjugal fitness" (termed "congenital pathology") were as much a part of the Frankfurt curriculum as were "hereditary diagnosis," "hereditary prognosis," and sterilization assessment. In "race science," discrepancies between human "races" and miscegenation were studied, such as between "Aryans" and Jews. "Population policy"—always the ultimate aim of the Nazi state—remained the wider background for all of this.[108]

Nor was Verschuer alone in this respect. From his chair in Heidelberg Carl Schneider, the noted psychiatrist, clandestinely influenced medical students in the direction of an antihumanitarian treatment of the congenitally ill housed in the Bethel asylum as early as 1934. This was some five years before the "euthanasia" killings actually began to take their toll, possibly at the hand of some of Schneider's own students.[109] In an extramural training camp Dr. Walter Gross said to a throng of female medical students in 1936 that their entire labors in the future would have to consider only preserving the race: "selection, breeding, and elimination." In medical practice, "race" had to be "absolutely predominant." "To work toward the breakthrough of this concept is the duty of everyone who has grasped its meaning, man or woman, and in particular of those who are daily being brought into contact with the real people: the male and female physicians."[110] Many young medical men and women in those years were graduating on the basis of original research projects that were largely bogus, such as the dissertations on heredity and race, which in a formal sense qualified these physicians well beyond 1945.[111]

Medicine in Germany was well on the way to being brutalized early in the regime and not just in classroom instruction. At first this happened as a consequence of the naturalistic impingements of the Liek school to which the faculties never were entirely immune, as textbooks like Georg B. Gruber's and Reiner Müller's show.[112] The imperative to avoid "effeminization," so lastingly preached by Liek and his apostles, well agreed with the masculine self-image of medical teachers that had been traded down through decades.[113] After fall 1939, the war accentuated these tendencies; some of the professors were remartialized in the trenches, and also martialized were the *Jungärzte* returning from the front on study leaves. Neither can it be discounted that several professors took time off from teaching to engage in medical crimes, whose ghastly aura then could linger on in classrooms. Gebhardt, Clauberg, Kremer, and Hirt, to mention only the most heinous, as admired teachers all had occasion to impregnate their students with objectionable ethos.[114] Professor Hirt of Strassburg University, who among other vile acts conducted mustard gas experiments on inmates of Natzweiler concentration camp, employed as his assistant Dr. Anton Kiesselbach, who worked with him both in the camp and in the seminars.[115] And so what had been an abnormality in peacetime readily became the rule. To a far greater extent than was salutary, the future doctors became inured to atrocities. Thus a post-1945 British observer was shocked to find that even when the war was over, Berlin students were still using the severed heads of Hitler's political victims for dissection purposes in the Charité Hospital. In the Charité basement, there were so many heads they were bobbing about in large tubs of brine.[116]

Students who had become acculturated to brutalization in the classrooms upon graduation acted out this attitude in daily practice, at the fronts, and, not too few of them, in concentration camps. As early as 1935 patients were complaining in the Reich that medical insurance assessors were applying unduly harsh standards, and one year later physicians were observed treating their patients in an uncalled-for hurry and in the discourteous manner of military superiors.[117] During the war, not least for lack of time and nervous pressure, examples of medical inhumanity by practitioners toward civilians multiplied, notwithstanding all the documented little heroisms.[118]

I have already alluded to circumstances in which, behind the battle lines, military medics had to forgo doctor-patient relations obtaining in peacetime. But many doctors strained the tolerance of the wounded soldiers beyond ethical and even practical limits, especially when inflicting pain, the ability of which to bear was an assumed criterion of manliness in war, especially in a fascist German war.[119] After May 1943 separate battalions of soldiers suffering from stomach and ear ailments were organized to be reemployed in combat. All manner of sick warriors were to be reconscripted for active service, so as to replenish the reserves.[120] In the concentration camps, too, ruthlessness by doctors toward inmate patients was indicative of this progressive dehumanization of the medical profession.[121]

One of the most ordinary and simultaneously most reprehensible ways in which physicians under Hitler would have to compromise themselves was through the decreed observance of sterilization. It has been estimated that as many as four hundred thousand persons of both sexes were sterilized from 1933 to 1945, most of them involuntarily.[122] How many of them had been through regular doctors' offices and were denounced to the authorities by family practitioners, as opposed to those indicted by state-employed physicians, has not yet been ascertained.[123] What we do know is that the threat to the doctor implied by a failure to report was severe enough to spoil the normally confidential relationship between him and his patient. If, as was commonly recorded, patients were frightened away from a doctor's office because of fear of being determined a sterilization "case," they were in fact being deprived of comprehensive health care that normally was owing to them.[124] A health care system, however, that excluded patients from its benefits for whatever reason was inappropriately selective. In the Third Reich, this alone demonstrated the corruption of the entire medical profession by the fascist regime.

Ultimately this corruption was tied to the progress of professionalization affecting these doctors under Hitler. Such progress on the whole was negative. In 1974 the West German historian of medicine Paul Ulrich Unschuld listed nine formal criteria of professionalization in modern medicine that may cursorily be applied to the roster of accomplishments of the Esculapian vocation under Hitler. In nominal sequence he mentioned (1) remuneration; (2) job-specific vernacular; (3) occupational symbols and clothing (uniforms); (4) formal training; (5) ethos, which is interested not in the end result of the occupational activity but in the means used to achieve it; (6) monopoly on expertise and licensure; (7) corporate independence; (8) degree of internationalization; and (9) social status.[125]

In reviewing the entire history of doctors under Hitler as contained in the foregoing chapters, we can only conclude that in point 1 progress was positive, for points 2, 3, 6, and 9 it was mixed, and for points 4, 5, 7, and 8 there was a remarkable regression.

There is no denying that physicians were better paid in the Third Reich, especially after 1937, than they had ever been before and in comparison with similar groups like lawyers and dentists, even though they lost some of their gains once more during the war. After 1945, severe losses in earnings were incurred, but soon physicians rose to the second-highest income level, just below that of corporate executives.[126] In regard to job jargon little change took place; what change there was must have been negative through the intrusion of medically alien terminology into the profession such as blatantly racist concepts like *Rassenkunde*. The same caveat may be applied to symbols and functional clothing. Although the time-honored white smock was the usual sight, doctors in their offices dressed in SA or SS apparel were not at all uncommon, and on the smock, too, the party badge as a symbol of Nazi fealty often was prominently displayed.[127] In social status, the physicians rose if judged purely on materialistic grounds. The medical profession's popular prestige in 1932 had been at its nadir; its rise after January 1933 was tied to partial advances to be detailed under point 6.[128] As fascist society solidified, the doctor came to maintain a preeminent place as a technician of people's health, charged with preserving civilian and military manpower resources.[129] But because of the many inroads possible by the regime itself—for instance in abrogating doctors' licenses or even criminalizing them after violations of pronatalist policy—the careless physician always had one leg in prison.[130] This made all of them potential pariahs and detracted from their social standing as a peer group.

To judge progress in the area of monopoly on skill and licensure is more difficult because of the tight nexus between the corps of physicians and the regime on one side and formal advances in codification on the other. Although such codification took place in the shape of statutes governing the exclusive right to panel practice, qualification and honor rules as well as legal definitions embodied in the long-awaited Reich Physicians' Ordinance (December 1935) and Professional Statute (November 1937), the physicians failed in the end to keep the quacks in abeyance.[131]

Moreover, one might question whether advances, say toward monopolizing licenses, as dictated by representatives of the regime were simultaneously advances each one of the German doctors could sanction. Here it would depend on whether the historian counts a Wagner or a Conti among the politicians of state or among the colleagues of the professionals; this once more affects the question of guilt for Nazi medical coordination. Probably one can say that Wagner and Conti acted in a dual capacity, perhaps even schizophrenically, under split loyalties as did all their minions in the medical hierarchy, a status that rendered the majority of Nazi doctors responsible both as executors of a criminal regime and as healers concerned with professional corporate progress.

That leads us to the first blatant failure, in the area of status independence (point 7). Unschuld circumscribes such independence in the main as the ability by the professional corps to admit or exclude from its ranks whoever is chosen on the basis of, presumably, profession-specific qualifications, without outside interference. He also implies "independence" in definition of operational function—a condition touching on point 6 (professional monopoly).[132] Outside interference can easily be interpreted as any meddling by the state, unheard-of by Hippocrates, and this of course occurred in the form of orders to exclude Jews and Marxists from the medical profession, with the details of expulsion being left to the corps' own administrators. One might stretch this argument and aver that the inequitable treatment of female physicians throughout the regime, for example the ruthless neutralization of their union and disadvantaging of married panel doctors, also falls under this rubric. More obviously compromising were the regime's prescriptions as to what medicine was to consist of: its delineation of *Rassenkunde*, enlistment of doctors for sterilization, "euthanasia," and medical killing on the ramp. One of the worst offenses in this sector was the progressive deletion of medical confidentiality between a physician and his patient—in the service of the state.

With regard to "internationalization" (point 8), our verdict is clearly negative: insofar as the Nazi regime nationalized itself, German medicine became deinternationalized, and to its detriment. Similarly, in the formal training of its recruits (point 4) the medical profession in retrospect presents a picture of near failure in the Third Reich. At one time during the course of the war, medical educators even deliberated the abrogation of the doctorate for physicians, hence infringing on point 6.[133] This criterion, point 4, also heavily intersects with point 5, bearing on medical ethos. Of all qualifications, ethos is perhaps the one most closely geared to the original content of the Hippocratic Oath, and also the most blatantly prostituted by doctors under Hitler.[134]

It is my contention that these ethical violations by themselves were sufficient to discount any nominal progress that might have been accomplished by the profession as detailed above, for ethics supersedes all other considerations. It was in the interpersonal relationship between healer and patient that German medicine corrupted itself, to varying degrees, between 1933 and 1945, to the extent that a metamorphosis in the art itself occurred. As has been shown above, in Nazi medical abuse the most important principle of the Hippocratic Oath was contravened, that which is embodied in the statement: "I will use treatment to help the sick according to my ability and judgment, but never with a view to injury and wrongdoing."[135] The true crisis of German medicine under the Nazis is that this covenant was stripped of its universal applicability. For even in the presence of so many goodwilled physicians and with the impressive scientific record of the past, this principle was trampled under foot, not in an incidental and haphazard fashion, but systematically, with potentially the gravest consequence for future medicine.

Appendix

Table 1.1. Percentages of Gross Income Groups by Selected German Professions and Occupations in RM 1,000, 1934 and 1937

Profession/ Occupation	Income group (A) 0–1.5	(B) 1.5–3	(C) 3–5	(D) 5–8	(E) 8–12	(F) 12–16	(G) 16–25	(H) 25–50	(I) 50+	(J) (total)
Physicians[a]	2.0	6.6	12.6	23.0	26.3	14.2	11.3	3.7	0.3	100
Dentists[a]	5.8	15.2	23.9	28.7	17.3	5.8	2.9	0.4	0	100
Lawyers[a]	5.8	14.5	17.7	20.7	16.7	9.7	8.8	4.8	1.3	100
All German self-employed[b]	19.2	33.7	20.5	11.5	7.0	2.9	2.6	1.7	0.9	100

[a] Based on figures for fiscal 1934 in *Deutsches Ärzteblatt* 67 (1937): 992. Excludes professionals of employee status earning less than RM 8,400, subject to automatic payroll tax deduction.
[b] Based on figures for fiscal 1937 in Table 23, *Statistisches Handbuch*, p. 564.

Table 2.1. Percentages of Selected NSDAP Joiners by Social Class and Professional Subgroup, and Recruitment Period, 1933–1945

Profession/ social group/ class	Recruitment period (A) 1933	(B) 1934–36	(C) 1937	(D) 1938	(E) 1939	(F) 1940–41	(G) 1942–45	(H) 1933–45	(I) 1933–45 (*N*)
Physicians[a]	32.9	2.6	43.4	2.6	3.9	11.8	2.6	100	76
Academic professionals[b]	37.1	5.2	34.1	2.2	6.0	12.4	3.0	100	267
Social elite[b]	39.5	4.0	30.9	2.1	6.2	13.4	4.0	100	1,021
All joiners[c]	22.0	2.8	27.2	2.0	7.7	20.6	17.7	100	15,916

[a] Physicians, excluding dentists and veterinarians.
[a–c] Percentages calculated on the basis of information in Kater, "Quantifizierung"; idem, *Nazi Party*, passim.
[c] Includes 2,759 socially unclassifiable joiners.

Table 2.2. Percentages of Selected NSDAP Joiners by Social Class and Professional Subgroup (in Total of All Classes Who Joined), and Recruitment Period, 1930–1945

Profession/ social group/ class	Recruitment period															
	(A) 1930–32 % in total of classes	(*N*)	(B) 1933 % in total of classes	(*N*)	(C) 1934–36 % in total of classes	(*N*)	(D) 1937 % in total of classes	(*N*)	(E) 1938 % in total of classes	(*N*)	(F) 1939 % in total of classes	(*N*)	(G) 1940–41 % in total of classes	(*N*)	(H) 1942–45 % in total of classes	(*N*)
Social elite[a]	9.2	180	12.2	403	9.7	41	8.0	315	9.0	21	6.3	63	5.0	137	2.7	41
Contained therein: academic professionals[a]	2.5	49	3.0	99	3.3	14	2.3	91	2.6	6	1.6	16	1.2	33	0.5	8
Contained therein: physicians[b]	0.3	6	0.8	25	0.5	2	0.8	33	0.9	2	0.3	3	0.3	9	0.1	2

a, b Percentages calculated on the basis of information in Kater, "Quantifizierung"; idem, *Nazi Party*, passim.

b Physicians, excluding dentists and veterinarians.

Table 2.3. Percentages of Physicians by Religion, Nazi Affiliation, and Sex, 1936–1945

Religion	(A) NSDAP members (male and female)	(B) NSÄB members (male and female)	(C) NSDAP members (male only)	(D) NSÄB members (male only)
Protestant	49.1	33.1	54.7	37.8
Catholic	35.2	25.2	39.8	29.4

Percentages based on absolute values in Kater sample (BDC, RÄK), 4,177 *N* (see n. 11, Chapter 2, 1). The percentages in this table have been adopted from cross-tabulation tables after application of statistical significance (X^2) tests. All percentages are significant ($P = 0.05$ or smaller).

Table 2.4. Percentages of Physicians by Nazi Affiliation and Medical Licensure Period, 1878–1945

Nazi affiliation	Medical licensure period (A) 1878–1918 $N = 100\%$	(B) 1919–24 $N = 100\%$	(C) 1925–32 $N = 100\%$	(D) 1919–32 $N = 100\%$	(E) 1933–38 $N = 100\%$	(F) 1939–45 $N = 100\%$	(G) 1878–1945 $N = 100\%$
NSDAP	39.1[a]	48.7[c]	53.1[e]	50.8[g]	43.2[i]	44.1[k]	44.8[m]
NSÄB	33.4[a]	45.6[c]	47.0[e]	46.2[g]	32.0[i]	7.4[k]	31.0[m]
NSDAP and NSÄB	30.8[a]	40.9[c]	44.1[e]	42.4[g]	27.7[i]	6.8[k]	27.9[m]
SA	15.6[b]	26.5[d]	30.6[f]	28.4[h]	36.6[j]	21.8[l]	26.0[n]
NSDAP and SA	9.9[b]	18.2[d]	20.4[f]	19.2[h]	22.0[j]	15.7[l]	17.0[n]
SS	1.9[b]	5.8[d]	9.4[f]	7.4[h]	9.2[j]	11.0[l]	7.2[n]
NSDAP and SS	1.1[b]	4.6[d]	7.2[f]	5.8[h]	5.8[j]	8.7[l]	5.2[n]
HJ	3.3[a]	4.5[c]	7.0[e]	5.7[g]	12.3[i]	16.2[k]	9.3[m]
NSDAP and HJ	2.8[a]	2.8[c]	3.4[e]	3.1[g]	5.5[i]	5.0[k]	4.1[m]

Percentages are based on absolute values in Kater sample (BDC, RÄK), 4,177 *N* (see n. 11, Chapter 2, 1). The percentages in this table have been adopted from cross-tabulation tables after application of statistical significance (X^2) tests. All percentages are significant ($P = 0.05$ or smaller). Percentages pertaining to SA and SS are for males only.

[a] = 876; [b] = 842; [c] = 662; [d] = 598; [e] = 580; [f] = 500; [g] = 1,242; [h] = 1,098; [i] = 1,105; [j] = 862; [k] = 954; [l] = 678; [m] = 4,177; [n] = 3,480.

Table 2.5. Ages of Selected NSDAP Joiners by Social Class and Professional Subgroup, and Recruitment Period, 1933–1945

Profession/ social group/ class	Recruitment period													
	(A) 1933		(B) 1934–36		(C) 1937		(D) 1938		(E) 1939		(F) 1940–41		(G) 1942–45	
	Age	(*N*)	Age	(*N*)	Age	(*N*)	Age	(*N*)	Age	(*N*)	Age	(*N*)	Age	(*N*)
Physicians[a]	42	25	36	2	41	33	27	2	35	3	40	9	37	2
Higher civil servants[b]	40	93	43	6	40	74	—	—	46	5	49	39	42	4
Academic professionals[b]	39	99	40	14	38	91	30	6	39	16	36	33	38	8
Social elite[b]	39	403	38	41	39	315	30	21	40	63	44	137	34	41
All joiners[c]	36	3,502	37	450	38	4,330	26	314	35	1,231	36	3,271	22	2,818

[a] Physicians, excluding dentists and veterinarians.

[a–c] Ages and frequencies (*N*) on the basis of information in Kater, "Quantifizierung"; idem, *Nazi Party*, passim.

[c] Includes 2,759 socially unclassifiable joiners.

Table 2.6. Percentages of German Physicians, NSDAP Joiners and Established Members, and Nazi Kreisleiter, by Age Group, 1934–1937

Age group	(A) All German physicians 1937[a]	(B) Physician NSDAP joiners 1937[b]	(C) Registered RÄK NSDAP physicians 1937[c]	(D) All established NSDAP members Dec. 31, 1934[d]	(E) Kreisleiter Dec. 31, 1934[d]
30 and under	16.4	18.2	23.9	37.6	14.2
31–40	25.0	33.3	30.9	27.9	55.7
41–50	27.1	33.3	28.4	19.6	26.4
51–60	14.2	9.1	11.2	11.2	3.4
61 and over	17.3	6.1	5.5	3.7	0.3
Percent (total)	100	100	100	100	100
Frequency (*N*)	55,443	33	1,343	2,493,890	776

[a] Percentages calculated on the basis of information in Kann, "Altersaufbau, 1937," p. 208.

[b] Percentages calculated on the basis of information in Kater, "Quantifizierung"; idem, *Nazi Party*, passim (dentists and veterinarians excluded).

[c] Percentages calculated on the basis of absolute values in Kater sample (BDC, RÄK), 4,177 *N* (see n. 11, Chapter 2, 1).

[d] Adopted from Table 13 in Kater, *Nazi Party*, p. 261.

Table 3.1. Percentages of Physicians by Sex and Medical Licensure Period, 1878–1945

	Medical licensure period				
Sex	(A) 1878–1918	(B) 1919–24	(C) 1925–32	(D) 1933–38	(E) 1939–45
Male	95.2	90.0	84.2	73.6	72.7
Female	4.8	10.0	15.8	26.4	27.3
Percent (total)	100	100	100	100	100
Frequency (*N*)	378	249	273	440	447

Percentages calculated on the basis of absolute values in Jarausch sample (BDC, RÄK), 1,808 *N* (see n. 6, Chapter 3, 1). The percentages in this table have been adopted from cross-tabulation tables after application of statistical significance (X^2) tests. All percentages are significant ($P = 0.05$ or smaller).

Table 3.2. Percentages of Physicians According to Panel Practice Certification, by Sex and Medical Licensure Period, 1878–1945

	Medical licensure period					
Sex	(A) 1878–1918	(B) 1919–24	(C) 1925–32	(D) 1933–38	(E) 1939–45	(F) Frequency of physicians (*N*)
Male	70.6	79.8	68.7	22.5	0.6	1,462
Female	66.7	44.0	41.9	12.9	1.6	324
Differential index number	1.05	1.81	1.63	1.74	0.37	—

Percentages calculated on the basis of absolute values in Jarausch sample (BDC, RÄK), 1,808 *N* (see n. 6, Chapter 3, 1). The percentages in this table have been adopted from cross-tabulation tables after application of statistical significance (X^2) tests. All percentages are significant ($P = 0.05$ or smaller).

Table 3.3. Percentages of Specialized Physicians by Sex and Medical Licensure Period, 1878–1945

Sex	Medical licensure period				
	(A) 1878–1918	(B) 1919–24	(C) 1925–32	(D) 1933–38	(E) 1939–45
Male	95.0	91.1	86.6	80.6	50.0
Female	5.0	8.9	13.4	19.4	50.0
Percent (total)	100	100	100	100	100
Frequency (*N*)	141	90	127	62	4

Percentages calculated on the basis of absolute values in Jarausch sample (BDC, RÄK), 1,808 *N* (see n. 6, Chapter 3, 1). The percentages in this table have been adopted from cross-tabulation tables after application of statistical significance (X^2) tests. All percentages are significant ($P = 0.05$ or smaller).

Table 3.4. Percentages of General Practice Physicians by Sex and Medical Licensure Period, 1878–1945

Sex	Medical licensure period				
	(A) 1878–1918	(B) 1919–24	(C) 1925–32	(D) 1933–38	(E) 1939–45
Male	95.4	89.3	82.2	72.5	72.9
Female	4.6	10.7	17.8	27.5	27.1
Percent (total)	100	100	100	100	100
Frequency (*N*)	237	159	146	378	443

Percentages calculated on the basis of absolute values in Jarausch sample (BDC, RÄK), 1,808 *N* (see n. 6, Chapter 3, 1). The percentages in this table have been adopted from cross-tabulation tables after application of statistical significance (X^2) tests. All percentages are significant ($P = 0.05$ or smaller).

Table 3.5. Percentages of University Students by Social Class, Sex, and Academic Discipline, 1932–1935

Social class	Medicine		Dentistry		Law		All disciplines (universities and Technische Hochschulen)	
	(A) Summer semester 1932	(B) Winter semester 1934–35	(C) Summer semester 1932	(D) Winter semester 1934–35	(E) Summer semester 1932	(F) Winter semester 1934–45	(G) Summer semester 1932	(H) Winter semester 1934–35
Male								
Lower	3.0	3.5	4.4	4.5	4.1	4.4	6.0	6.2
Lower middle	54.2	56.2	72.2	73.2	53.0	56.1	60.1	61.2
Elite	42.8	40.3	23.4	22.3	42.9	39.5	33.9	32.5
Percent (total)	100	100	100	100	100	100	100	100
Frequency (*N*)	18,783	16,724	4,996	3,765	16,691	9,501	100,017	68,651
Female								
Lower	1.2	1.3	1.8	1.8	1.7	1.0	2.8	2.6
Lower middle	43.1	45.6	58.0	62.3	33.9	35.3	49.9	49.8
Elite	55.7	53.1	40.2	35.9	64.4	63.7	47.2	47.6
Percent (total)	100	100	100	100	100	100	100	100
Frequency (*N*)	4,714	3,945	1,244	839	1,101	306	18,984	11,217
Male and female								
Lower	2.6	3.1	3.9	4.0	3.9	4.3	5.5	5.7
Lower middle	52.0	54.2	69.4	71.2	51.8	55.5	58.5	59.6
Elite	45.4	42.7	26.8	24.7	44.3	40.2	36.1	34.6
Percent (total)	100	100	100	100	100	100	100	100
Frequency (*N*)	23,497	20,669	6,240	4,604	17,792	9,807	119,001	79,868

Percentages and frequencies are based on information in Lorenz, *Zehnjahres-Statistik*, 1:356–71. Her original categories of "miscellaneous occupations" and "without job indication" for student fathers were excluded from this table.

Table 3.6. Percentages of University Students by Sex and Frequency of Nazi Political Choice, 1933–1945

Sex	(A) Students of all disciplines not involved politically 1933–42[a]	(B) Students of medicine not involved politically 1933–45[b]	(C) Students of medicine holding one or more Nazi positions 1933–45[b]	(D) Students of medicine holding two or more Nazi positions 1933–45[b]	(E) Students of medicine holding three or more Nazi positions 1933–45[b]
Male	18.0	11.3	88.7	44.3	14.9
Female	24.4	33.7	66.3	31.1	7.0

[a] Percentages based on values in Table 7 in Arminger, "Involvement," p. 20: $N = 557$; $X^2 = 27.13$; $df = 5$; $P = 0.01$; $C = 0.323$.

[b] Percentages based on absolute values in loan-student sample (BA), 3,693 *N* (see nn. 33, 42 of Chapter 5, 2). These percentages have been adopted from cross-tabulation tables after application of statistical significance (X^2) tests. All percentages are significant ($P < 0.0001$).

Table 3.7. Percentages of Medical Students by Type of Nazi Political First Choice and Sex, 1933–1945

Sex	(A) Women's organizations %	(A) (*N*)	(B) Hitler Youth (HJ, BDM) %	(B) (*N*)	(C) NSDStB/ ANSt %	(C) (*N*)	(D) Others %	(D) (*N*)	(E) NSDAP %	(E) (*N*)	(F) SA %	(F) (*N*)	(G) SS %	(G) (*N*)	(H) NSKK %	(H) (*N*)	(I) Frequency (*N*)
Male	—	—	10.4	162	9.5	148	2.2	34	32.6	506	35.6	552	6.6	102	3.1	48	1,552 (1,749 including political abstentions)
Female	20.1	36	29.1	52	32.4	58	0.6	1	17.9	32	—	—	—	—	—	—	179 (270 including political abstentions)
Frequency (*N*)	—	36	—	214	—	206	—	35	—	538	—	552	—	102	—	48	1,731 (2,019 including political abstentions)

Percentages based on absolute values in loan-student sample (BA), 3,693 *N* (see nn. 33, 42, Chapter 5, 2). These percentages have been adopted from cross-tabulation tables after application of statistical significance (X^2) tests. All percentages are significant ($P < 0.0001$).

Table 3.8. Percentages of Physicians by Nazi Affiliation and Sex, 1933–1945

Sex	Selected Nazi Cadres						
	(A) NSDAP	(B) NSÄB	(C) HJ/BDM	(D) NSDStB	(E) NSV	(F) Women's organizations	(G) Nazi affiliation of any kind
Male	49.9	35.3	7.0	1.8	1.8	—	72.6
Female	19.7	9.9	21.1	3.9	1.0	18.7	52.4
Frequency (*N*)	1,873	1,296	392	88	70	130	2,891

Percentages based on absolute values in Kater sample (BDC, RÄK), 4,177 *N* (see n. 11, Chapter 2, 1). These percentages have been adopted from cross-tabulation tables after application of statistical significance (X^2) tests. All percentages are significant with $P < 0.001$, except for the values in column E, where $P = 0.177$.

Table 3.9. Percentages of Physicians According to Nazi Political Inauguration, by Sex and Medical Licensure Period, 1878–1945

Sex	Medical licensure period					
	(A) 1878–1918	(B) 1919–24	(C) 1925–32	(D) 1933–38	(E) 1939–45	(F) Frequency of physicians (*N*)
Male	46.9	72.3	72.6	83.6	80.0	1,029
Female	50.0	40.0	53.5	53.4	60.7	178
Differential index number	0.93	1.80	1.35	1.56	1.31	—

Percentages based on absolute values in Kater sample (BDC, RÄK), 4,177 *N* (see n. 11, Chapter 2, 1). These percentages have been adopted from cross-tabulation tables after application of statistical significance (X^2) tests. All percentages are significant ($P = 0.05$ or smaller).

Table 5.1. Growth of Academic Disciplines at Universities and Technische Hochschulen, Winter Semester 1932–1933 to Winter Semester 1943–1944

	(A) Winter semester 1932–33[a]	(B) Winter semester 1933–34[a]	(C) Winter semester 1934–35[a]	(D) Winter semester 1935–36[a]	(E) Winter semester 1936–37[a]	(F) Winter semester 1937–38[a]	(G) Winter semester 1938–39[a]	(H) Autumn trimester 1939[a]	(I) Second trimester 1940[a]	(J) Winter trimester 1941[a]	(K) Winter semester 1943–44[b]
Medicine (*N*)	24,298	23,899	21,649	20,556	18,034	16,604	15,905	16,565	14,304	18,742	39,028
Percent of all university disciplines	26.2	29.2	31.8	34.2	37.0	38.3	38.6	57.7	47.1	50.5	71.9
Dentistry (*N*)	6,522	5,864	4,847	4,100	2,861	2,058	1,612	742	681	755	1,363
Percent of all university disciplines	7.0	7.2	7.1	6.8	5.9	4.7	3.9	2.6	2.2	2.0	2.5
Law (*N*)	16,175	13,443	10,130	8,026	5,740	4,891	4,930	2,826	2,978	2,981	3,625
Percent of all university disciplines	17.5	16.4	14.9	13.3	11.8	11.3	12.0	9.8	9.8	8.0	6.7
All university disciplines (*N*)	92,601	81,968	68,148	60,148	48,688	43,388	41,227	28,696	30,351	37,093	54,252
All TH disciplines (*N*)	20,431	17,104	13,099	11,794	10,776	9,466	11,029	6,184	7,112	6,955	8,516

[a] Figures adopted from Lorenz, *Zehnjahres-Statistik*, 1:152–59. Students inclusive of foreigners.
[b] Figures adopted from *Statistisches Handbuch*, pp. 622–23.

Table 5.2. Percentages of Medical, Dental, and Law Students by Type of Nazi Formation of First Choice and Period of Nazi Inauguration, 1925–1945

Nazi formation of first choice	Inauguration period																	
	1925–32			1933				1934		1935–37				1938		1939–45		
	(A) Med.	(B) Dent.	(C) Law	(D) Med.	(E) Dent.	(F) Law	(G) Med.	(H) Dent.	(I) Law	(J) Med.	(K) Dent.	(L) Law	(M) Med.	(N) Dent.	(O) Law	(P) Med.	(Q) Dent.	(R) Law
NSDAP[a]	34.9	43.2	42.0	32.5	40.9	37.5	4.2	—	0.9	14.5	11.4	10.7	8.4	4.5	4.5	5.4	—	4.5
SA[b]	5.7	7.5	9.6	75.7	84.4	76.2	9.9	5.4	5.8	4.1	2.7	4.8	3.9	—	1.9	0.6	—	1.6
SS[b]	6.7	3.7	7.3	52.2	74.1	50.9	7.8	11.1	5.5	11.1	7.4	18.2	12.2	—	10.9	10.0	3.7	7.3
Others[a]	16.1	15.5	35.9	25.2	33.8	27.6	13.6	14.1	9.7	30.0	26.8	11.5	7.3	1.4	5.5	7.7	8.5	9.7
All formations[a]	13.6	14.5	22.9	49.5	64.4	52.8	10.3	7.3	6.2	15.5	10.4	8.9	6.4	1.0	4.2	4.6	2.4	5.0

[a] Both male and female students.

[b] Male students only.

[a,b] Percentages based on absolute values in loan-student sample (BA), 3,693 *N* (see nn. 33, 42, Chapter 5, 2). These percentages have been adopted from cross-tabulation tables after application of statistical significance (X^2) tests. All percentages are significant ($P = 0.05$ or less).

Table 5.3. Percentages of University and Technische Hochschule Students without Nazi Affiliation by Sex, 1933–1945

Sex	(A) Medicine 1933–45[a]	(B) Dentistry 1933–45[a]	(C) Law 1933–45[a]	(D) All disciplines (university and Technische Hochschule) 1933–42[b]
Male	11.3	13.4	11.3	18.0
Female	33.7	55.1	48.3	24.4
Male and female	14.3	19.6	12.2	18.5

[a] Percentages based on absolute values in loan-student sample (BA), 3,693 *N* (see nn. 33, 42, Chapter 5, 2).

[b] Percentages based on values in Table 7 in Arminger, "Involvement," p. 20 (N = 557).

[a, b] Percentages have been adopted from cross-tabulation tables after application of statistical significance (X^2) tests. All percentages are significant (P = 0.01 or less).

Table 5.4. Percentages of Male University and Technische Hochschule Students by Social Class, 1933–1945

Social class	Medicine		Dentistry		Law		All disciplines (universities and Technische Hochschulen)	
	(A) Winter semester 1934–35[a]	(B) All semesters 1933–45[b]	(C) Winter semester 1934–35[a]	(D) All semesters 1933–45[b]	(E) Winter semester 1934–35[a]	(F) All semesters 1933–45[b]	(G) Winter semester 1934–35[a]	(H) All semesters 1933–42[c]
Lower	3.5	10.3	4.5	10.2	4.4	11.5	6.2	8.8
Lower middle	56.2	71.2	73.2	78.9	56.1	72.4	61.2	63.9
Elite	40.3	18.5	22.3	10.9	39.5	16.1	32.5	27.3
Percent (total)	100	100	100	100	100	100	100	100
Frequency (*N*)	16,724	1,711	3,765	393	9,501	1,152	68,651	498

[a] Percentages based on information in Lorenz, *Zehnjahres-Statistik*, 1:356–71.

[b] Percentages based on absolute values in loan-student sample (BA), 3,693 *N* (see nn. 33, 42, Chapter 5, 2).

[c] Percentages based on values in Table 11 in Arminger, "Involvement," p. 23 ($N = 498$).

[b,c] These percentages have been adopted from cross-tabulation tables after application of statistical significance (X^2) tests. All percentages are significant ($P = 0.05$ or less).

Table 5.5. Percentages of Male University and Technische Hochschule Students by Type of Nazi Formation of First Choice, 1933–1945

Sex	(A) Medicine 1933–45[a]	(B) Dentistry 1933–45[a]	(C) Law 1933–45[a]	(D) All disciplines (university and and Technische Hochschule) 1933–42[b]
NSDAP	28.6	23.4	26.6	14.5
SA	32.0	42.2	33.9	38.4
SS	5.8	8.1	5.3	12.4
Others	22.6	12.7	22.9	16.8
None	10.9	13.5	11.3	17.9
Percents (total)	100	100	100	100
Frequency (*N*)	1,711	393	1,152	498

[a] Percentages based on absolute values in loan-student sample (BA), 3,693 *N* (see nn. 33, 42, Chapter 5, 2). The percentages are statistically significant at $N = 3{,}256$; $X^2 = 35.383$; $df = 8$; $P < 0.0001$; $C = 0.01$.

[b] Percentages based on values in Table 11 in Arminger, "Involvement," p. 23 ($N = 498$). They are statistically significant ($P = 0.05$).

Table 5.6. Percentages of Male University and Technische Hochschule Students by Social Class and Type of Nazi Formation of First Choice, 1933–1945

	Medicine, 1933–45					Dentistry, 1933–45				
	(A)	(B)	(C)	(D)	(E)	(F)	(G)	(H)	(I)	(J)
Social class	NSDAP[a]	SA[a]	SS[a]	Others[a]	All medical students[b]	NSDAP[c]	SA[c]	SS[c]	Others[c]	All dentistry students[b]
Lower	9.4	10.2	9.1	11.9	10.3	14.1	10.2	9.4	6.0	10.2
Lower middle	72.7	71.7	71.7	70.5	71.2	72.8	82.0	68.8	86.0	78.9
Elite	18.0	18.1	19.2	17.6	18.5	13.0	7.8	21.9	8.0	10.9
Percent (total)	100	100	100	100	100	100	100	100	100	100
Frequency (*N*)	490	548	99	387	1,711	92	166	32	50	393

[a–d] Percentages based on absolute values in loan-student sample (BA), 3,693 *N* (see nn. 33, 42, Chapter 5, 2).

	Law, 1933–45				All disciplines (universities and Technische Hochschulen), 1933–42				
(K)	(L)	(M)	(N)	(O)	(P)	(Q)	(R)	(S)	(T)
SDAP[d]	SA[d]	SS[d]	Others[d]	All law students[b]	NSDAP[e]	SA[e]	SS[e]	Others[e]	All university and TH students[f]
10.7	12.6	6.6	11.0	11.5	12.5	8.9	6.5	8.3	8.8
72.6	73.8	63.9	72.0	72.4	68.1	66.0	58.1	63.1	63.9
16.6	13.6	29.5	17.0	16.1	19.4	25.1	35.5	28.6	27.3
100	100	100	100	100	100	100	100	100	100
307	390	61	264	1,152	72	191	62	84	498

c, d, e The percentages are statistically significant only at $P > 0.05$.

f Percentages based on values in Table 11 in Arminger, "Involvement," p. 23 (498 *N*).

Figure 1. Physicians' Gross Income, 1929–1937

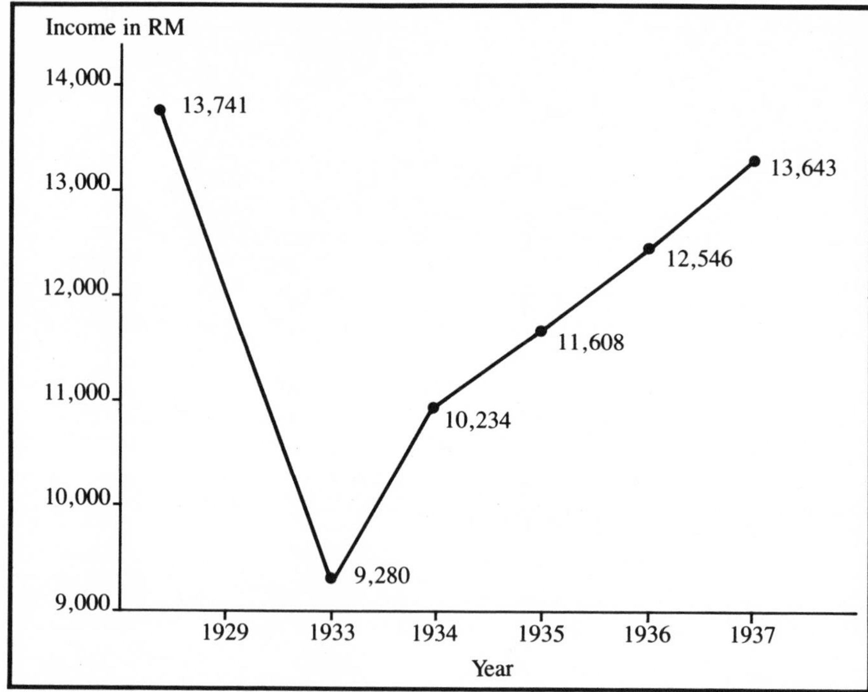

Source: Wuttke, *Herrschaft*, p. 200, n. 140.

Figure 2. Rate of Initial Participation in Nazi Formations by Medical, Dental, and Law Students, 1933–1944

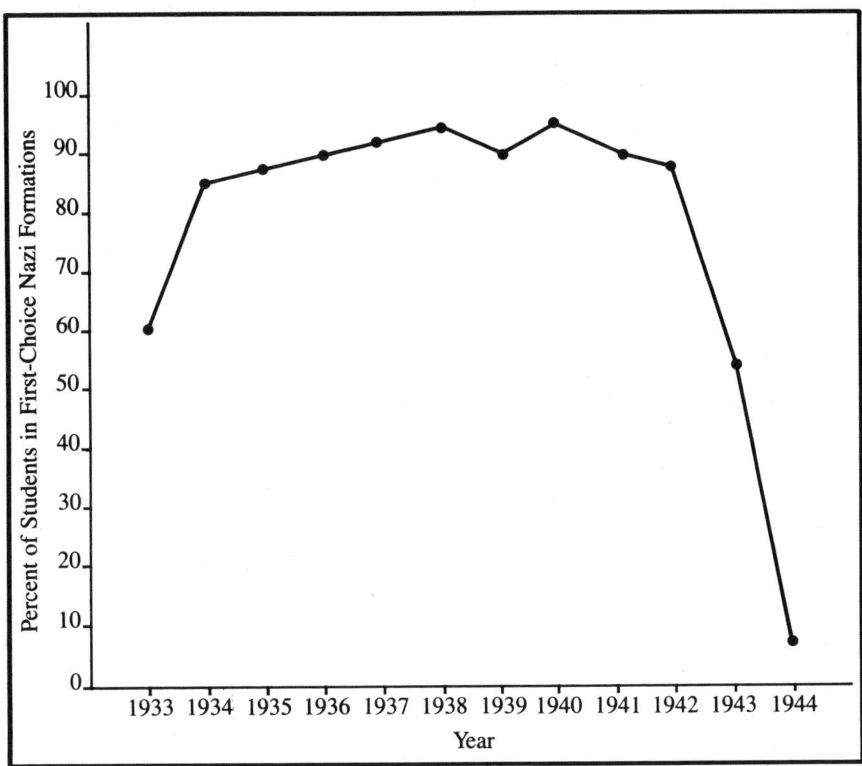

Source: Loan-Student Sample (BA), 3,693 *N* (see nn. 33, 42, Chapter 5, 2).
The percentages depicted are statistically significant at $N = 3{,}693$; $X^2 = 413.37$; $df = 11$; $P < 0.0001$; $C = 0.335$.

Notes

Abbreviations

In addition to the abbreviations used in the text, the following abbreviations are used in the notes.

AAWG	Archiv der Akademie der Wissenschaften Göttingen
ARW	Archiv der Reichsstudentenführung und des Nationalsozialistischen Deutschen Studentenbundes, Universität Würzburg
BA	Bundesarchiv Koblenz
BDC	Berlin Document Center
DAÖW	Dokumentationsarchiv des Österreichischen Widerstandes Wien
GLAK	Generallandesarchiv Karlsruhe
HHSAW	Hessisches Hauptstaatsarchiv Wiesbaden
HIS	Hoover Institution on War, Revolution, and Peace, Stanford
IfZ	Institut für Zeitgeschichte München
ISA	Israel State Archives
LBINY	Leo Baeck Institute, New York
NA	National Archives, Washington
NHSA	Niedersächsisches Hauptstaatsarchiv Hannover
SAM	Staatsarchiv München
SAMs	Staatsarchiv Münster
UK	Unterlagen der Kassenärztlichen Vereinigung Deutschlands und der Reichsärztekammer (photocopies at York University Archives)
UNANY	United Nations Archives, New York

Introduction

1. *B.Z.*, October 27, 1955, 12; Luther and Thaler, *Ethos*, p. 129; Lifton, *Nazi Doctors*, pp. 277–78; n. 114 in Conclusion to this book.

2. *Der Spiegel*, January 16, 1984, 86–88; *Wer ist Wer?* (1970), 79; *Frankfurter Allgemeine Zeitung*, May 27, 28, 1988. Bernbeck, born September 15, 1916, joined a Nazi Aviation Corps (NSFK) support group in August 1938 and the NSDAP in April 1942 (BDC, PK Bernbeck).

3. Kater, "Medizin und Mediziner," p. 325, n. 88. As far as could be ascertained, Szagunn was not a formal party member. But she was an anti-Semite: she endorsed Nazi race science (*Rassenkunde*) and in March 1941, upon the death of her predecessor, Edith von Lölhöffel, she commended that physician-editor for her "positive commitment to race and *Volk* through conscious rejection of Jewish elements and Jewish influence." See Szagunn, "Vierte Wiener Medizinische Woche," p. 404; Sza-

gunn, "Edith von Lölhöffel zum Gedächtnis," p. 96 (quotation). See also Szagunn, "Sportärztliche Erfahrungen"; Szagunn, "Dritte Wiener Medizinische Woche."

4. Szagunn, "Wandlungen im Krankheitsbegriff," esp. p. 331. Also see Kater, "Burden," pp. 45–46; Klee, *Was sie taten*, pp. 25, 139–43, 284, 312–13.

5. Kreienberg, "Auswirkungen," esp. pp. 3, 5.

6. BDC, MF and RÄK Kreienberg.

7. File Kreienberg (1944), BDC, Research Kreienberg. Also see text in Conclusion at n. 24.

8. *Wer ist Wer?* (1986), 743.

9. Hanauske-Abel, "Unfähigkeit zu trauern," p. 34.

10. *Who's Who in Germany*, p. 1408; vita, "Generalarzt Prof. Dr. Ernst Rodenwaldt," Bad Nauheim, July 26, 1944, BDC, Research Rodenwaldt. According to BDC, MF Rodenwaldt, this scholar joined the NSDAP on March 1, 1932, and left it on February 25, 1933. Also see Rodenwaldt's memoirs, *Tropenarzt*.

11. See Rodenwaldt, "Rückwirkung der Rassenmischung" (quotations pp. 385, 388, 389); Becker et al., "Einblicke in die Medizin," pp. 322–23.

12. Vita (as in n. 10). Cf. Rodenwaldt and Zeiss, *Einführung*, pp. 15–40.

13. Becker et al., "Einblicke in die Medizin," p. 323.

14. BDC, MF and RÄK Jungmann; Kater, *Politiker*, p. 169.

15. Kater, *Politiker*, pp. 169–70; *Wer ist Wer?* (1970), 582.

16. Jungmann, "Von der Fürsorge." The specifically Nazi character of *Vorsorge* as opposed to *Fürsorge* is explained in Kater, " 'Gesundheitsführung.' " On the Nazi career of Kötschau, see Chapter 2, 1, and passim.

17. BDC, MF, PK, RÄK, and SS files Sewering.

18. Sewering, "Ärztliches Zeugnis" Babette Fröwis, October 26, 1943, private archive Dr. Hans Halter, Berlin.

19. "Niederschrift über die Aufnahme der Babette Fröwis," Eglfing, November 1, 1943; death certificate Fröwis, Eglfing, November 18, 1943; telegram (death notification) Anstalt Eglfing to (mother) Barbara Fröwis, November 16, 1943, private archive Dr. Hans Halter, Berlin; Schmidt, *Selektion*.

20. *Deutsches Ärzteblatt* 82 C (1985): 857.

21. Kater, *Politiker*, p. 325.

22. *Der Spiegel*, November 8, 1976, March 21, 1977, June 19, 1978, May 14, 1979; *Deutsches Ärzteblatt* 82 C (1985): 857.

23. Berger, "Sozialversicherungsreform," pp. 73–74.

24. *Der Spiegel*, September 22, 1986, 120–27.

25. Klee, "Geldverschwendung"; *Der Tagesspiegel* (Berlin), May 27, 1986.

26. *Süddeutsche Zeitung* (Munich), June 25, 1986.

27. See Kater, "Hitler's Early Doctors," p. 42; entries for December 28–29, 1941, and January 15, 1942, in *Adolf Hitler*, pp. 157, 199–200. Among several, the best works on Hitler's illnesses and his relationship with personal physicians are Heston and Heston, *Medical Casebook*; and Bromberg and Volz Small, *Hitler's Psychopathology*.

28. Amende, "Arzt," p. 56. On Amende before 1933, see Kudlien, "Ärzte als Anhänger," p. 25; Kater, "Hitler's Early Doctors," p. 32.

29. Conti as quoted in *Deutsches Ärzteblatt* 73 (1943): 33.

30. Reiter, "Ärzte," p. 1016.

31. Falstein, *Martyrdom*, p. 267.

32. Lifton, *Nazi Doctors*, pp. 18, 43–44.

33. Alexander, "Science," pp. 44–45, quotation p. 45. Also see case of Dutch physician Hans Keilson as reported by Christian Pross in *taz* (Berlin), November 14, 1985.

34. See Kovács, "Luttes professionnelles"; "Politics," pp. 32–33, 41, 52.

35. *Globe and Mail* (Toronto), November 10, 1987; *Torture Report*, p. 10; Sheldon H. Harris, "Japanese Biological Warfare Experiments and Other Atrocities in Manchuria, 1932–1945: A Preliminary Statement," paper delivered at conference, "Medical Science without Compassion—Past and Present," Institut für Genetik, Universität zu Köln, West Germany, September 29, 1988.

36. Influential regime lawyer Dr. Falk Ruttke said: "I have been observing the undermining of law by Jews for some time now and shall . . . work especially toward the liberation of the German juridical system from the Jewish style of law" (letter to Hinkel, Berlin, July 26, 1935, BA, R 56I/89). Also see the superficial treatment in Müller, *Furchtbare Juristen*, pp. 67–75.

37. See Chapter 2, 1, n. 25.

38. This point is emphasized by Geuter, *Professionalisierung*, p. 34.

39. The Nuremberg Code and the "Principles for Those in Research and Experimentation" (1954) are reprinted in Etziony, *Physician's Creed*, pp. 82–86. Further see Moe, "Should the Nazi Research," p. 5; Baader, "Medizinische Menschenversuche," p. 41. The "lessons" of the Nuremberg Doctors' Trial are critically discussed, from today's perspective, in *Hastings Center Report*, special supplement (August 1976): 1–19.

40. *Torture Report*, p. 3.

41. Ibid., pp. 30–32.

42. Ibid., pp. 6–10, 13; Goldstein and Breslin, "Technicians of Torture"; *Der Spiegel*, January 7, 1984, 103; Geuter, "Psychiatrisch-psychologische Folter." See case of Asunción prisoner Napoleon Ortigoza Gomez in *Globe and Mail* (Toronto), December 21, 1987.

43. All this was accomplished at a two-day convention in Santiago (which I attended) that was monitored by Pinochet's agents, in December 1985. In mid-1986, ethical proceedings instigated by the Colegio were pending against fifteen Chilean doctors. See Christian, "In South America."

44. *Globe and Mail* (Toronto), April 23, October 14, 1985, December 14, 1987; *Torture Report*, pp. 6–10, 12–14; Wren, "Salvaging Lives." For Israel, see *Der Spiegel*, February 29, 1988, 134.

45. Novikov, *Politische Psychiatrie*; *Torture Report*, pp. 11–12.

46. *Torture Report*, pp. 14–17.

47. *Globe and Mail* (Toronto), March 1, 1988. Background in *Der Spiegel*, February 29, 1988, 161–66.

48. *Globe and Mail* (Toronto), October 24, December 13, 1986 (quotation). On the sterilization issue see *Sterilization*.

49. Gillmore, *I Swear by Apollo*; Lifton, *Nazi Doctors*, p. xii. The case of victim Linda Macdonald is reported in detail by *Globe and Mail*, December 23, 1987.

50. There are three versions of this book: *Diktat* (1947), *Wissenschaft* (1949), and *Medizin ohne Menschlichkeit* (1962).

51. Platen-Hallermund, *Tötung*.

52. Ternon and Helman, *Les médecins allemands*.

53. Wuttke-Groneberg, *Medizin*. See my review in *Archiv für Sozialgeschichte* 22 (1982): 672–74.

54. Klee, "*Euthanasie*."

55. Schmuhl, *Rassenhygiene*.

56. Kudlien, *Ärzte*. See the critiques of Rainer Appell in *Frankfurter Allgemeine Zeitung*, September 6, 1985; and William Coleman, "Physician in Nazi Germany."

57. Cocks, *Psychotherapy*. See my review in *Journal of the History of Medicine* 41 (1986): 371–72.

58. As examples of the former, see Thomann, "Otmar Freiherr von Verschuer"; and Weindling, "Preussische Medizinalverwaltung." As an example of the latter see Bartel, "Zur Entlarvung."

59. Müller-Hill, *Tödliche Wissenschaft*. This book is now available in an English translation (entitled *Murderous Science*) from Oxford University Press (Oxford, 1988).

60. Lifton, *Nazi Doctors*. See my review in *Bulletin of the History of Medicine* 61 (1987): 491–93; and the justly positive reviews by Harald Bräutigam in *Die Zeit*, September 11, 1987, p. 41; and by Neal Ascherson in *New York Review of Books*, May 28, 1987, pp. 29–33. Also see Arendt, *Eichmann in Jerusalem*.

61. Mielke died in 1959. Mitscherlich and Mielke, *Medizin ohne Menschlichkeit*, pp. 13–17; Mitscherlich, *Leben*, pp. 144–61, 188–92, 317; Kater, "Burden," pp. 37–38; Hanauske-Abel, "Unfähigkeit zu trauern," pp. 34–36.

62. Kater, "Burden," pp. 39–40.

63. Meyer, "Deathly Science," p. 6.

64. Hanauske-Abel, "From Nazi Holocaust."

65. Vita Hanauske-Abel, May 1987 (ms. with author); Stock, "Deutsche Ärzte."

66. *Deutsches Ärzteblatt* 84 B (1987): 847–59.

67. Hanauske-Abel, "Unfähigkeit zu trauern," esp. pp. 42–43; Becker to Staatsanwaltschaft bei dem Landgericht Köln, Marburg, August 17, 1987, private archive Hanauske-Abel (copy with author).

68. See Stock, "Deutsche Ärzte"; Johanna Bleker et al., "Sich der Wahrheit stellen: Medizinhistoriker kritisieren Vilmar," *Die Zeit*, November 6, 1987, p. 47. Also see the thoughtful letters by Drs. Faustmann, Fischer, Dörffer, Schmidt in *Deutsches Ärzteblatt* 84 B (1987): 1451–52, and Vilmar's predictably obstinate reply, pp. 1455–56; medical student G. Jette Limberg to Vilmar, as well as Vilmar's answer in *Rundbrief: Ärzte warnen vor dem Atomkrieg*, no. 23 (October 1987): 16; Renate Jäckle, "Ist die Vergangenheit wirklich bewältigt? Der Historikerstreit macht auch vor der Medizin nicht halt," *Süddeutsche Zeitung* (Munich), November 5, 1987, p. 48.

69. See Kater, "Burden," p. 40.

Chapter 1

1. Supply, Demand, and Deployment of Physicians

1. Kater, "Physicians in Crisis," pp. 49–59.
2. *Statistisches Jahrbuch 1932*, p. 404; ibid., *1934*, p. 510; ibid., *1935*, p. 496; ibid., *1937*, p. 542.
3. *Deutsches Ärzteblatt* 67 (1937): 903; *Ziel und Weg* 9 (1939): 88 (when possible, for numerical statements of this kind, the values compiled by the medicinal bureaucracy have been preferred over those compiled by the *Statistische Reichsamt* and officially published in *Statistische Jahrbücher*. The latter values were found to be at variance with the former and of only limited use, being too highly aggregated and inconsistent. In the case of medical students, for instance, dental students sometimes were included, sometimes not); Tennstedt, "Sozialgeschichte," p. 409.
4. Kann, "Zahl, 1942," p. 301.
5. Draft of letter Stadler to Conti, Munich, May 4, 1944, BA, R 18/3806.
6. *Ziel und Weg* 5 (1935): 232; ibid. 8 (1938): 573; Kollath, *Grundlagen*, p. 377; Bernhard to Oberpräsident Münster, Berlin, July 30, 1943, BA, R 18/3791; Holm, "Gedanken zur ärztlichen Planwirtschaft," Berlin, October 12, 1943, BA, R 18/3809; Grunberger, *Reich*, pp. 242, 252.
7. Kater, "Physicians in Crisis," pp. 52–53.
8. Diepgen, *Heilkunde*, pp. 269–71; Ramm, *Standeskunde*, pp. 82–83, 123–24; *Soziale Medizin: Zentralblatt für Reichsversicherung und Reichsversorgung*, no. 10 (1933): 155; "Erläuterungen zur Bestallungsordnung für Ärzte," [1939], BA, R 18/3764; "Fünfte Verordnung zur Durchführung und Ergänzung der Reichsärzteordnung," July 17, 1939, *Reichsgesetzblatt* (1939), I, 1287–88; Mersmann, "Ausbildung," p. 134; Klinger, *Wege*, pp. 74–75.
9. *Ziel und Weg* 7 (1937): 97, 225; Neumeister, "Lage," pp. 1265–66; Ramm, *Standeskunde*, pp. 86, 122; protocol, panel insurance hearing Dr. Ernst Bergmann (Thuringia), June 4, 1937; protocol, panel insurance hearing Dr. Hans Jordan (Breslau), January 18, 1938, UK, 130/118.02/4; Klinger, *Wege*, p. 72.
10. Ordinance Wagner, Berlin, February 22, 1937, in *Deutsches Ärzteblatt* 67 (1937): 221; ibid., p. 98.
11. "Notdienstverordnung," October 15, 1938, in *Reichsgesetzblatt* (1938), I, 1441–42.
12. Computation of average age at time of licensure on the basis of sample of 4,177 physician (compulsory) members of Reich Physicians' Chamber (*Reichsärztekammer*), 1936–45, comprising a total of approximately 79,000 file cards, in BDC, RÄK. Also see Neumeister, "Lage," pp. 1265–66; Ellersdorfer, "Auswirkungen," pp. 51–52; advertisement in *Ziel und Weg* 3 (1933): 274; sample of assistant physicians' contract, for Mannheim municipal hospitals, "Satzung über die Dienstverhältnisse der Assistenzärzte bei den städtischen Krankenanstalten," for January 1, 1933, [Mannheim], November 16, 1932, UK, 190; *Journal of the American Medical Association* 100 (1933): 830. See also the typical case histories in Forssmann, *Selbstversuch*, pp. 150, 162, 191; Bamm, *Menschen Zeit*, p. 159.

13. Stadler, "Arzt"; Bauer, "Arbeiter"; Schmidt, "Assistenzarzt"; Neumaier, "Krisis"; Oettingen, "Assistenzärzte"; Maassen, "Lebensverhältnisse"; and Julius Hadrich's remarks in *Deutsches Ärzteblatt* 67 (1937): 374–75.

14. Examples of advertisements are in *Ziel und Weg* 3 (1933): 138, 174, 206, 273, 544–45. Also see Mäding, "Ergebnis"; idem, "Nachwuchspflege."

15. Corr. Reichsverband Angestellter Ärzte e.V.-Conti, February–March 1933, UK, 190; *Ziel und Weg* 3 (1933): 26; Ellersdorfer, "Auswirkungen," pp. 56–58.

16. Ellersdorfer, "Auswirkungen," p. 55.

17. Ibid., pp. 51–53; *Ziel und Weg* 8 (1938): 571. Also see Groh to Reich interior minister, Berlin, June 9, 1938, BA, R 21/485.

18. See the examples in *Ziel und Weg* 3 (1933): 101, 205, 311.

19. Examples in Forssmann, *Selbstversuch*, pp. 172–76; Bamm, *Menschen Zeit*, pp. 146–47; *Ziel und Weg* 7 (1937): 97; Ellersdorfer, "Auswirkungen," pp. 58–59.

20. As indicated in "Entwurf eines Werbeschreibens," enclosed with Reichsstudentenwerk circular 50/39, Berlin-Charlottenburg, July 10, 1939, ARW, II, 280. Also see n. 24, below.

21. Klein, *Amtsarzt*, 3:20; *Ziel und Weg* 3 (1933): 543; ibid. 7 (1937): 273; Tennstedt, "Sozialgeschichte," p. 408.

22. *Ziel und Weg* 7 (1937): 476–77; ibid. 8 (1938): 77; Klein, *Amtsarzt*, 3:21; Klinger, *Wege*, p. 83; Seidler, *Prostitution*, pp. 12–17; Grunberger, *Reich*, p. 241.

23. "Prüfungsordnung für Kreisärzte" (effective April 1, 1934), Berlin, February 13, 1934, BA, R 18/3122; and the ads in *Ziel und Weg* 3 (1933): 102, 354.

24. See the revealing notice in *Ziel und Weg* 5 (1935): 337; and Gütt, *Gesundheitsdienst*, pp. 102–3; Ramm, *Standeskunde*, p. 67; as well as Wagner, "Stellung und Aufgaben," p. 779. In his officious 1942 publication, *Arzt*, p. 285, Nazi health official Dr. Kurt Blome intimated that as many as twenty thousand additional physicians were needed by May 1935. This figure appears far too high.

25. Gütt, *Gesundheitsdienst*, pp. 104–5; Regierungspräsident to Reich interior minister, Minden, May 12, 1939, BA, R 18/3122.

26. Until May 31, 1940, their induction rate was 20.1 percent compared with a rate of 33.9 percent for civilian doctors. Based on figures in Statistisches Reichsamt, VI, "Gesundheitswesen Männer und Frauen," n.d., BA, R 18/3715. Also see Conti to Göring, Berlin, August 1, 1940, BA, R 18/2956.

27. Cropp to OKH, Berlin, March 19 and April 23, 1942; Cropp to Reichsverteidigungskommissar Pommern, Berlin, April 8, 1943, BA, R 18/2958.

28. Conti to Länderregierungen et al., Berlin, September 25, 1939; Krahn to Cropp, Berlin, December 11, 1941; Krahn to Regierungspräsident Koblenz, Berlin, March 6, 1942; Ernst to Regierungspräsident Wiesbaden, Berlin, August 11, 1944, BA, R 18/3122; memorandum Josten, [Berlin], October 24, 1942; Cropp to Regierungspräsident Merseburg, Berlin, December 24, 1943, BA, R 18/2956.

29. Quotation Kauffmann to Conti, [Berlin], May 3, 1944, BA, R 18/3810. Also see Conti, "Jahre," p. 2.

30. Conti, "Jahre," p. 2; Conti to Göring, Berlin, August 1, 1940, BA, R 18/2956; unsigned memorandum, "Staatliche Gesundheitsämter," [Berlin, July 1941], BA, R 18/3715; Ernst to Reichsstatthalter Sachsen, Berlin, April 27, 1944, BA, R 18/2958.

31. See Petzina, *Autarkiepolitik*; Auerbach, "Volksmeinung," pp. 277–86; and text near n. 61 of section 4, below.

32. As in n. 11, above. Ramifications of this measure are outlined in follow-up orders (July 8 and September 15, 1939) listed in *Reichsgesetzblatt* (1939), I, 1204, 1775–76.

33. Individual case histories are detailed in Büchner, *Pläne*, p. 89; Neubert, *Arztleben*, p. 94; Hermann Radetzky's testimony in Albrecht and Hartwig, *Ärzte*, p. 220; Hoff, *Erlebnis*, p. 346; Schönberg, "Geschichte," pp. 122, 124; Bamm, *Menschen Zeit*, p. 163; Niedermeyer, *Wahn*, p. 454. The figures are from Statistisches Reichsamt, VI, "Gesundheitswesen Männer und Frauen," n.d., BA, R 18/3715. They may have been too low: see entry for December 15, 1939, in *Meldungen aus dem Reich*, 3:577. Naturally, there were local variations: in July 1940 in the Ruhr town of Hamm, about 60 percent of the doctors had been conscripted (doc. 133 [July 19, 1940] in Gersdorff, *Frauen*, p. 318), in Lusatian Zittau 50 percent by early 1941 (entry for March 25, 1941, in *Meldungen aus dem Reich*, 6:2144).

34. SD report 18, November 20, 1939, BA, R 58/145; *Bericht über das Bayerische Gesundheitswesen*, p. 9; Conti to RÄK, Berlin, September 14, 1939; Cropp to RÄK, Berlin, May 20, 1940, BA, R 18/3764; Lorenz, *Zehnjahres-Statistik*, 2:38; Berger, *Kulturspiegel*, p. 137; information service 41, Munich, September 21, 1944, SAM, NSDAP/31.

35. The general problem is alluded to in doc. 1 (October 1939) in Boberach, *Meldungen*, p. 6; information service 41, Munich, September 21, 1944, SAM, NSDAP/31.

36. Grote, "Tätigkeit," p. 56; KVD, circular 15/40, Berlin, June 25, 1940, BA, R 18/3785; Deneke and Sperber, *Jahre*, p. 95.

37. Case of ophthalmologist Dr. Ernst Jäger (Traunstein) (September–December 1940), BDC, PÄ Jäger.

38. Grote, "Tätigkeit," p. 56; *Deutsches Ärzteblatt* 70 (1940): 251. Example of *Hilfskassenarzt* Dr. Bernhard Heyde, married to the Jewish actress Ida Ehre, is in Klinger, *Wege*, p. 99; Witter, "Es hat doch auch."

39. Scholtz-Klink, report NSF, January–March 1941, BA, NS 22/860; KVD to Reichsverband der Betriebskrankenkassen, Berlin, April 15, 1942, BA, R 18/3785; information service 41, Munich, September 21, 1944, SAM, NSDAP/31.

40. Ordinance IV 6052/40 II of Reich interior minister, Berlin, January 2, 1941, BA, R 21/484.

41. Ibid. For a model example of application for *uk-Stellung*, see file Dr. Paul Eduard Kyrle (university clinic Vienna) (February 1941), DAÖW, 4100. Also see Cropp to Vorsitzenden der Ausschüsse für ärztliche Prüfung in Preussen, Berlin, February 11, 1942; Cropp to Regierungen der Hochschulländer et al., Berlin, October 29, 1941, BA, R 18/3764; [Conti], "Begründung," [Berlin, 1942], BA, R 18/5576.

42. [Conti], "Begründung," [Berlin, 1942], BA, R 18/5576; Cropp to Oberbürgermeister et al., Berlin, May 2, 1942, BA, R 18/3764.

43. Göring, Frick, Lammers, "Verordnung zur Sicherstellung der ärztlichen Versorgung der Zivilbevölkerung," May 27, 1942, in *Deutsches Ärzteblatt* 72 (1942): 241.

44. Memorandum Cropp, Berlin, December 10, 1942, BA, R 18/2958; memorandum Ehle regarding consultation with Korpsarzt XI on November 24, 1942; Sievers to Bruns, Hanover, December 4, 1942, NHSA, Hann. 122a, XII, 32m.

45. Conti to Reichsstatthalter et al., Berlin, January 11, 1943, BA, R 21/484; Holm, "Gedanken zur ärztlichen Planwirtschaft," Berlin, October 12, 1943, BA, R 18/3809.

46. See case of Dr. Karl Loeprecht (Monheim), in RÄK Bayern to Conti, Munich, April 16, 1943, BA, R 18/3810.

47. Information service 41, Munich, September 21, 1944, SAM, NSDAP/31; Reichsgesundheitsführer, newsletter 2/43, Berlin, December 20, 1943, BA, R 18/3766a.

48. Conti to Pfundtner, Berlin, June 16, 1943, BA, R 18/5576; Conti to Reichsverteidigungskommissare, Berlin, July 5, 1943, BA, R 18/3791.

49. "Erlass des Führers über das Sanitäts- und Gesundheitswesen," Führerhauptquartier, July 28, 1942, in *Reichsgesetzblatt* (1942), I, 515. Background is in Kater, "Doctor Leonardo Conti," p. 314.

50. Kater, "Doctor Leonardo Conti," pp. 318–19.

51. Ibid., pp. 319–21. Also see the telling example of the deployment of *Hilfskassenarzt* Dr. Müller (Einswarden), corr. June 1943, BA, R 18/3810.

52. Conti's speech of March 19, 1940, in *Deutsches Ärzteblatt* 70 (1940): 147; ibid. 72 (1942): 3.

53. Reichsgesundheitsführer, information 3/44, Berlin, January 20, 1944, BA, R 18/3766a; Himmler to Reichsverteidigungskommissare and Gesundheitsämter, Berlin, April 3, 1944, BA, R 18/3764.

54. Reichsgesundheitsführer, information 5/44, Berlin, March 20, 1944; Reichsgesundheitsführer, information 6/44, Berlin, April 25, 1944; Reichsgesundheitsführer, information 16/1944, Berlin, January 20, 1945, BA, R 18/3766a.

55. Memorandum, Berlin, June 20, 1944, BA, R 21/484.

56. Entry for March 23, 1945, in Goebbels, *Tagebücher*, p. 359.

57. Reichsgesundheitsführer, information 16/44, Berlin, April 25, 1944; Reichsgesundheitsführer, information 15/1944, Berlin, December 13, 1944, BA, R 18/3766a; information service 41, Munich, September 21, 1944, SAM, NSDAP/31. Also see nn. 11, 32, above.

58. [Conti], "Begründung," [Berlin, 1942], BA, R 18/5576; Krüger to Reichsstatthalter and Oberpräsidenten, Berlin, November 4, 1942, BA, R 18/3764; Brandt to Pleiger, Berlin, May 24, 1943, BA, R 18/3809.

59. Holm, "Gedanken zur ärztlichen Planwirtschaft," Berlin, October 12, 1943, BA, R 18/3809. Hitler's personal thoughts at this point are not known.

60. Reichsgesundheitsführer, information 2/43, Berlin, December 20, 1943; Reichsgesundheitsführer, information 5/44, Berlin, March 20, 1944, BA, R 18/3766a; list of co-opted physicians, Brunswick area, in KVD, "Saldenauszug aus dem Ärztekontokorrent," December 31, 1943, UK, 106. Also see Liebling, *Republic of Silence*, p. 216; BDC, RÄK Danilo Valentini (Italian), Panagiotis Nassuphis (Greek), Franz Piaseczynski (Polish), Dscheng Huang (Chinese), Assen Philippoff (Bulgarian), Manuel Picardo Castellon (Spanish).

61. Reichsgesundheitsführer, information 12/44, Berlin, September 20, 1944; Reichsgesundheitsführer, information 15/1944, Berlin, December 13, 1944, BA, R 18/3766a.

62. Wanjek to NSDAP-Amt für Volkswohlfahrt, Ibbenbüren, March 29, 1944; Sprakel to NSDAP-Amt für Volkswohlfahrt, Gau Westfalen-Nord, Münster, April 22, 1944, SAMs, Polit. Polizei, 3. Reich, 109.

63. Brandt's scheme was called *Jäger-Programm.* Conti to Speer, Berlin, May 6, 1944, BA, R 18/3122; Handloser to OKH et al., Berlin, October 20, 1944, BA, R 18/3764; Seidler, *Prostitution*, p. 54; n. 5 above.

2. The Nazi Reshaping of the Professional Organization

1. The process of *Gleichschaltung* has been outlined in Bracher et al., *Machtergreifung*, pp. 186–93 and passim.

2. On the founder of the NS-Ärztebund, *Sanitätsrat* Dr. Ludwig Liebl of Ingolstadt, see Pridham, *Rise*, pp. 110–13. Also see Kater, "Nazi Physicians' League"; idem, "Physicians in Crisis," pp. 67–68. Short vitae of Wagner are in *Völkischer Beobachter*, August 18, 1938; *Ziel und Weg* 8 (1938): 421.

3. Grote, "Entwicklung," p. 338; Diepgen, *Heilkunde*, p. 281; *Nationalsozialistisches Jahrbuch* 18 (1944): 208.

4. In summer 1933 Wagner expressed the benevolent aspect of his strategy: "If we want to get down to business . . . we have to adopt the political policy of compromise and, in matters of the medical profession, let bygones be bygones. In the interest of the community this includes, if necessary, offering our hand to our erstwhile political adversary and making him cooperate with us" (Wagner to Hartz, Munich, July 20, 1933, UK, 196/1).

5. See Lammers's return telegram of March 29, 1933, printed in *Deutsches Ärzteblatt* 62 (1933): 141. Vita Stauder in Fischer, *Lexikon*, 2:1496.

6. *Deutsches Ärzteblatt* 62 (1933): 141–43; Haedenkamp, "Die Gesamtvorstände," p. 309; Pfundtner to Wagner, [Berlin], April 29, 1933, in *Ärztliche Mitteilungen* 34 (1933): 415.

7. Ackermann, "Nachwuchs," pp. 126–27; Zapp, "Untersuchungen," pp. 90–93. The goals of Deutscher Ärztevereinsbund are sketched in Modersohn, "Führerprinzip," p. 49.

8. Quotations *Deutsches Ärzteblatt* 62 (1933): 142. Also see Haedenkamp, "Gesamtvorstände."

9. Ramm, *Standeskunde*, p. 45; *Ziel und Weg* 3 (1933): 78, 115; Parlow, "Zum Faschisierungsprozess," p. 169; Zapp, "Untersuchungen," pp. 95–96.

10. Par. 87, "Reichsärzteordnung," December 13, 1935, BA, R 18/5574; *Deutsches Ärzteblatt* 66 (1936): 517–18; Ramm, *Standeskunde*, pp. 45–46; Parlow, "Zum Faschisierungsprozess," pp. 169–71; Zapp, "Untersuchungen," pp. 97–99.

11. For three examples of the former, see Langbein, "Die Entstehung," pp. 89–90; Schadewaldt, *Hartmannbund*, pp. 133–42; and most recently, Dr. Karsten Vilmar, president of the German Federal Physicians' Chamber, in *Deutsches Ärzteblatt* 84 B (1987): 856. For an example of the latter, see Parlow, "Zur Integration," pp. 78–80;

idem, "Zum Faschisierungsprozess," pp. 168–71.

12. Schadewaldt has gone to great lengths to whitewash Stauder and, in particular, Haedenkamp. For his unconvincing arguments, see his undocumented book *Hartmannbund*, pp. 134–36. In his attempt to write the "official" history of Hartmannbund, Schadewaldt has obviously overlooked Wagner's letter to Hartz, Munich, July 20, 1933, UK, 196/1, in which Wagner lauds Haedenkamp's stance: "[Haedenkamp] . . . always stood in line with us, honestly and with integrity, and, in my opinion, from inner conviction, since the National Socialist revolution." Haedenkamp's subsequent actions and writings evidently justified Wagner's confidence. See p. 12 of Haedenkamp, *Neuordnung*; idem, "Gesamtvorstände"; *Deutsches Ärzteblatt* 63 (1933): 556–58; *Journal of the American Medical Association* 100 (1933): 1706. A short vita is in Knüpling, "Untersuchungen," p. 49. Also see the critical treatment in Wuttke-Groneberg, *Medizin*, p. 337, and docs. 220,2–220,5, pp. 377–84; Labisch and Tennstedt, *Weg*, 1:234–35; Kater, "Burden," pp. 35–36.

13. Vita Grote is in *Ziel und Weg* 8 (1938): 139; vita Bewer is in Knüpling, "Untersuchungen," p. 48. Quotation Zapp, "Untersuchungen," p. 103.

14. Characteristic rhetoric is in Grote, "Entwicklung," p. 339; idem in *Deutsches Ärzteblatt* 73 (1943): 178.

15. *Deutsches Ärzteblatt* 66 (1936): 517–18. According to par. 17 (2) of Hartmannbund's statute, in case of dissolution its assets were to accrue to the Ärztevereinsbund. "Geschäftsführung," September 19, 1929, enclosed with "Satzung des Verbandes der Ärzte Deutschlands (Hartmannbund)," June 16 and 17, 1931, UK, 190. The assets of Ärztevereinsbund went to the Reich Physicians' Chamber (*Deutsches Ärzteblatt* 66 [1936]: 517–18, and text after n. 21, below).

16. Tennstedt, "Sozialgeschichte," p. 401; Schadewaldt, *Hartmannbund*, pp. 123–27.

17. See text in section 1 near n. 7, and the following: [revised] "Satzung der Kassenärztlichen Vereinigung Deutschlands," Berlin, January 27, 1941, in Ramm, *Standeskunde*, pp. 267–70; ibid., pp. 47–49, 126; "Zulassungsordnung," Berlin, May 17, 1934, in *Deutsches Ärzteblatt* 64 (1934): 547–55; Grote, "Entwicklung," p. 338; *Ziel und Weg* 7 (1937): 370, 374; Wagner, "Stellung," p. 397; Haedenkamp, *Neuordnung*, p. 11; Parlow, "Zum Faschisierungsprozess," p. 171.

18. Par. 4 in [revised] "Satzung der Kassenärztlichen Vereinigung Deutschlands," Berlin, January 27, 1941, in Ramm, *Standeskunde*, pp. 267–70; par. 48 in [revised] "Zulassungsordnung," September 8, 1937, ibid., pp. 292–93; Klein, *Amtsarzt*, 3:13; Wagner, "Reichsärzteordnung," p. 3; Zapp, "Untersuchungen," p. 100.

19. Par. 2 (8) in [revised] "Satzung der Kassenärztlichen Vereinigung Deutschlands," Berlin, January 27, 1941, in Ramm, *Standeskunde*, pp. 267–70; ibid., pp. 48–49; Grote, "Entwicklung," p. 339.

20. The jurisdiction of the Reich labor ministry over matters affecting the KVD (in this case, its statute) may be gleaned from Syrup's statement of February 15, 1941, in Ramm, *Standeskunde*, p. 270. Also see Wagner, "Reichsärzteordnung," p. 3; idem, "Stellung," p. 397; *Deutsches Ärzteblatt* 73 (1943): 179. Evidence of friction between Wagner and officials of the labor ministry as early as spring 1933 is in Tennstedt and Leibfried, "Sozialpolitik," p. 219.

21. *Deutsches Ärzteblatt* 64 (1934): 254–55; ibid. 66 (1936): 334; Ramm, *Stan-*

deskunde, pp. 71–72; Kater, " 'Gesundheitsführung,' " p. 353; Labisch and Tennstedt, *Weg*, 1:231–32.

22. Grote, "Entwicklung," p. 338; Diepgen, *Heilkunde*, p. 280; Ramm, *Standeskunde*, pp. 42, 52. See also *Ärztliches Vereinsblatt* 58 (1929): 48. Critical in principle are the post-1945 evaluations in Fromm, "Berufsvertretung," p. 268; Atzbach, "Grundfragen," pp. 13–14; Knüpling, "Untersuchungen," pp. 43–45; Lüth, "Subkultur," pp. 368–69; Zapp, "Untersuchung," p. 101.

23. "Reichsärzteordnung," December 13, 1935, BA, R 18/5574; *Deutsches Ärzteblatt* 66 (1936): 517.

24. "Reichsärzteordnung," December 13, 1935, BA, R 18/5574; "Zugehörigkeit zur Reichsärztekammer," March 27, 1936, in Ramm, *Standeskunde*, pp. 228–29; ibid., pp. 56–58; "Zweite Verordnung zur Durchführung und Ergänzung der Reichsärzteordnung," May 8, 1937, in *Reichsgesetzblatt* (1937), 1:585–87; "Berufsordnung für die deutschen Ärzte," November 5, 1937, in *Deutsches Ärzteblatt* 67 (1937): 1031–37; ibid., pp. 1038–41; Wagner, "Reichsärzteordnung," p. 4; *Ziel und Weg* 7 (1937): 357; Klein, *Amtsarzt*, 3:23–24.

25. "Reichsärzteordnung," December 13, 1935, BA, R 18/5574; "Berufsordnung für die deutschen Ärzte," November 5, 1937, in *Deutsches Ärzteblatt* 67 (1937): 1031–37; ibid., pp. 1038–41; Wagner, "Reichsärzteordnung," pp. 2, 4; Ramm, *Standeskunde*, p. 52; Schadewaldt, *Hartmannbund*, p. 141. The concept and practice of Nazi *Gesundheitsführung* are explained in Kater, " 'Gesundheitsführung.' "

26. *Deutsches Ärzteblatt* 62 (1933): 142; Wagner, "Reichsärzteordnung," p. 3; Ramm, *Standeskunde*, p. 53; Klein, *Amtsarzt*, 3:23; Atzbach, "Grundfragen," p. 16. Lüth, "Subkultur," p. 369, underestimates Wagner's position within the confines of his office. The influence of the Reich interior minister is documented in Grote, "Entwicklung," p. 338; *Deutsches Ärzteblatt* 66 (1936): 501. For Wagner's actual role in the race legislation see Chapter 6 below.

27. Obituary in *Ziel und Weg* 9 (1939): 206. Also see Röhrs, *Hitlers Krankheit*, p. 126.

28. Background in Kater, "Doctor Leonardo Conti," pp. 304–8.

29. For Gütt's early vita and Third Reich activities, see Stockhorst, *Köpfe*, p. 168; and Stürzbecher, "Konzeption," p. 1075; Labisch and Tennstedt, *Weg*, 1:236–78; 2:281–344. The state health administration, inherited from the Weimar period, also experienced an ongoing Nazi revision from 1933 on. See *Ziel und Weg* 3 (1933): 79; Gütt, "Aufbau"; "Gesetz über die Vereinheitlichung des Gesundheitswesens," July 3, 1934, in Boschan, *Familiengesetzgebung*, pp. 261–73; Frick's remarks in *Der Öffentliche Gesundheitsdienst* 3 B (1937): 206–7; Labisch and Tennstedt, vols. 1 and 2, passim. Gütt's ambitions may be gleaned from Gütt to Minister [Frick], Berlin, April 5, 1939, BA, R 18/5583. An inveterate enemy of Wagner, Gütt had been looking forward to the creation of an autonomous Reich health ministry, presumably under his own leadership, since 1924. See Stürzbecher, p. 1076; Labisch and Tennstedt, 2:344–46; Röhrs, *Hitlers Krankheit*, pp. 126–27.

30. See Reiter, *Ziele*, esp. pp. 104–10.

31. Kater, "Doctor Leonardo Conti," pp. 309–12; Prinz, *Vom neuen Mittelstand*, pp. 298–302.

32. Kater, "Doctor Leonardo Conti," pp. 311–21; Conti, "Gesundheitsführung—

Volksschicksal: Rede des Reichsgesundheitsführers Dr. Conti auf der Kriegstagung des Hauptamtes für Volksgesundheit der NSDAP," Munich, March 28, 1942, BDC, OPG Emil Ketterer (pp. 10–11).

33. See text in section 1 near n. 49.

34. Kater, "Doctor Leonardo Conti," pp. 319–20.

3. Medical Specialization and Income

1. See Hadrich, "Zahl der Allgemeinpraktiker, 1929"; idem, "Zahl der Allgemeinpraktiker, 1930."

2. This ideal is well explained in Krannhals, *Weltbild*. That book in two volumes was one of the cornerstones of Nazi *Weltanschauung*, certainly for the educated, ever since the time of its first publication in 1928. See *Mitteilungen des Kampfbundes für deutsche Kultur* 1 (1929): 22–25.

3. On this see Kater, *Nazi Party*, pp. 184–89.

4. Par. 33 in "Berufsordnung für die deutschen Ärzte," November 5, 1937, in *Deutsches Ärzteblatt* 67 (1937): 1036; Kötschau, "Vorsorge," p. 245; Knoll, "Arzt," pp. 436–37; Grote, "KVD," p. 12; Hadrich, "Zahl und Verteilung, 1936," p. 1059; Bartels, "Gesundheit und Wirtschaft," p. 530; Wagner, "Gesundes Leben," p. 553; Berger, *Kulturspiegel*, pp. 108–9; *Nationalsozialistisches Jahrbuch* 18 (1944): 209; Tennstedt, *Selbstverwaltung*, p. 221. On the generalists' functions as Nazi informers, see *Deutsches Ärzteblatt* 64 (1934): 30. Functions of political block wardens (Blockleiter) are explained in Kater, *Nazi Party*, pp. 192–93, 208, 222, 227.

5. Wagner, "Ziele," p. 492.

6. Günther, *Bauerntum*; Scheda, *Deutsches Bauerntum*. Critically important is Bergmann, *Agrarromantik*.

7. See text in section 1 near n. 9; *Ziel und Weg* 7 (1937): 368–74, 416–20; Berger, *Kulturspiegel*, pp. 35–37.

8. *Ziel und Weg* 5 (1935): 100.

9. See text in section 1 near n. 9, and the following: Hadrich, "Zahl und Verteilung, 1936"; *Deutsches Ärzteblatt* 67 (1937): 98; *Ziel und Weg* 9 (1939): 50; Berger, *Kulturspiegel*, p. 110.

10. *Ziel und Weg* 7 (1937): 368.

11. Nanna Conti, "Die Mitarbeit"; idem, "Hebammenwesen"; *Die Ärztin* 17 (1941): 154; *Ziel und Weg* 5 (1935): 100. Also see Leonardo Conti to Oberpräsidenten et al., Berlin, December 16, 1939, BA, R 18/3766; *Deutsches Ärzteblatt* 70 (1940): 174. Stoeckel, *Erinnerungen*, pp. 242–43, probably overestimates the influence of Nanna Conti on her son.

12. Conti to Oberpräsidenten et al., Berlin, December 16, 1939, BA, R 18/3766; doc. 133 (July 19, 1940) in Gersdorff, *Frauen*, p. 318; Scholtz-Klink, report NSF, January–March 1941, BA, NS 22/860; Conti, "Hebammenwesen"; "Jahreslagebericht 1938," in *Meldungen aus dem Reich*, 2:113; Grunberger, *Reich*, pp. 252–53; Kater, *Nazi Party*, pp. 122–23.

13. Entry for April 10, 1940, in *Meldungen aus dem Reich*, 4:988; memorandum Florian, [Düsseldorf], January–February 1940, BA, R 18/3781; quotation Conti, "Gesundheitsführung—Volksschicksal: Rede des Reichsgesundheitsführers Dr. Conti

auf der Kreistagung des Hauptamtes für Volksgesundheit der NSDAP," Munich, March 28, 1942, BDC, OPG Emil Ketterer (p. 13).

14. Graf von Baudissin to Führerinnen der DRK-Bereitschaften, Züllichau, August 17, 1942, BA, R 18/3781; Cropp to Reichsstatthalter et al., Berlin, September 24, 1942, and January 6, 1943, BA, R 18/3766.

15. Anon. report, Cologne, [1942–43], BA, R 18/3781. Also see memorandum Florian, [Düsseldorf], January–February 1940, ibid.

16. Memorandum Florian, [Düsseldorf], January–February 1940, BA, R 18/3781; memorandum Hansen, Lübeck, February 23, 1943, BA, R 18/3781.

17. Kreisamtsleiter to Gauamt für Volksgesundheit Münster, Ahlen, March 9, 1943, BA, R 18/3781. Also see *alltägliche Faschismus*, pp. 188–89.

18. Grote, "KVD," pp. 12–13; Neumaier, "Krisis," pp. 17–18.

19. Hadrich, "Zahl und Verteilung, 1936," p. 1058; *Deutsches Ärzteblatt* 67 (1937): 904–5; ibid. 70 (1940): 449, 478; Kann, "Zahl, 1942," pp. 301–2. The assertion to the contrary in Grunberger, *Reich*, p. 241, is undocumented. For the proscription of the Jews, see Chapter 6 below.

20. Figures for 1937 are from *Deutsches Ärzteblatt* 67 (1937): 905. In 1942, for instance, the ratio between Berlin and Schleswig-Holstein had shifted slightly in favor of the province (doubtless because of the final removal of large numbers of Jewish Berlin specialists), whereas in the case of Hamburg and East Prussia the city had gained on the province. See the figures in Kann, "Zahl, 1942," p. 302; and *Deutsches Ärzteblatt* 70 (1940): 449–50. The Nazi functionaries' prejudice against city doctors' usefulness in the countryside at the height of the war is apparent from Reichsgesundheitsführer, communication 4/44, Berlin, February 20, 1944, BA, R 18/3766a.

21. Par. 29–34 in "Berufsordnung für die deutschen Ärzte," November 5, 1937, in *Deutsches Ärzteblatt* 67 (1937): 1035–36. Also see commentaries, ibid., p. 1040; and Ramm, *Standeskunde*, pp. 83–85.

22. For the eminent position of the (male) surgeon in German society before 1933 and after 1945, see Kater, "Professionalization," p. 685; Geyer-Kordesch, "Diskriminierung," p. 228.

23. Quotations from Dr. Wilhelm Josenhans in *Ziel und Weg* 3 (1933): 156; Seifert, "Ausbildung," p. 372. Also see Conti's speech of March 19, 1940, in *Deutsches Ärzteblatt* 70 (1940): 149; Hadrich, "Fachärzte," pp. 802–3; Professor K. H. Bauer's eulogy in honor of Martin Kirschner, January 16, 1943, in *Der Chirurg* 15 (1943): 129; Hoff, *Erlebnis*, p. 212; Forssmann, *Selbstversuch*, p. 179.

24. Par. 30 in "Berufsordnung für die deutschen Ärzte," November 5, 1937, in *Deutsches Ärzteblatt* 67 (1937): 1035; Klein, *Amtsarzt*, 3:15.

25. Computations based on figures in *Deutsches Ärzteblatt* 67 (1937): 905; ibid. 70 (1940): 450, 478. In this case, a comparison with corresponding pre-1933 values, though desirable, is impossible because of a partial combination of index figures for surgeons with those for gynecologists. See the example in Hadrich, "Zahl der Allgemeinpraktiker, 1930," p. 386.

26. Exposition and figures in *Deutsches Ärzteblatt* 67 (1937): 904–5; ibid. 70 (1940): 450, 478; Hadrich, "Zahl und Verteilung, 1936," p. 1059.

27. See His, *Front der Ärzte*; Fischer, *Lexikon*, 1:637.

28. Exposition and figures in *Deutsches Ärzteblatt* 67 (1937): 905; ibid. 70 (1940):

450, 478; Hadrich, "Zahl und Verteilung, 1936," p. 1059.

29. See Jess, "'Chirurgogynäkologen'"; *Ziel und Weg* 5 (1935): 227–28; von Mikulicz-Radecki to Stadler, Königsberg, February 22, 1941, BA, R 18/3781.

30. Exposition and figures in *Deutsches Ärzteblatt* 67 (1937): 905; ibid. 70 (1940): 450, 478. Also see Kater, "'Gesundheitsführung,'" pp. 355–62, 372–73. Regarding the proclaimed eugenic significance of pediatrics, see "Erläuterungen zur Bestallungsordnung für Ärzte," [summer 1939], BA, R 18/3764; Gruber, *Einführung*, pp. 209–10. In this connection, note the function of head pediatrician for the SS-Lebensborn, Josef Becker, in Lilienthal, "*Lebensborn e.V.*," p. 55 and passim. On the attitude to HJ, see text in Chapter 2, 2, at n. 82.

31. As in n. 24, above.

32. As in nn. 24, 28, above. Also see Kater, "Physicians in Crisis," pp. 66–67; Gumpert, *Hunger*, pp. 43–44; Mitscherlich, *Ein Leben*, pp. 104–7, 124–25; Cocks, *Psychotherapy*, esp. pp. 15–16, 87–93; Bastian, *Von der Eugenik*, pp. 69–71. For the typical German pre-1933 view of Freud see Liek, *Arzt*, pp. 144–47; Ringer, *Decline*, p. 383; Decker, *Freud in Germany*; Whalen, *Bitter Wounds*, p. 62; Quinn, *Life*, pp. 138–42.

33. *Stabsarzt* Dr. Hans Zielke quoted in *Deutsches Ärzteblatt* 72 (1942): 350.

34. Cf. *Ziel und Weg* 7 (1937): 476–77.

35. Seidler, *Prostitution*, pp. 48–52. *Beratende Ärzte* for pathology, psychiatry, surgery, hygienics, and internism are mentioned in Büchner, *Pläne*, p. 79; Hoff, *Erlebnis*, p. 356; Forssmann, *Selbstversuch*, pp. 255–56.

36. Memorandum Schmidt, Berlin, February 7, 1941, BA, R 21/484; Stähle to Conti, Stuttgart, May 14, 1943, BA, R 18/3810; Fischer, *Erfahrungsberichten*, esp. pp. 1–15, 23–55; Klinger, *Wege*, p. 95; text near n. 105 of section 4.

37. The first two documents in n. 36, above; and anon. memorandum, February 24, 1941, BA, R 21/484; Forssmann, *Selbstversuch*, p. 219.

38. Feuchter, *Luftkrieg*, pp. 146–284; Golücke, *Schweinfurt*, pp. 99–224.

39. Geschäftsführender Präsident, Deutsches Rotes Kreuz, to Landesführer, Potsdam-Babelsberg, July 2, 1943; Reichsgesundheitsführer to Reichsverteidigungskommissare, Berlin, July 5, 1943; "Der Arzt im Luftkrieg," [Berlin], September 2, 1943, BA, R 18/3791; Cropp to lord mayors et al., Berlin, May 2, 1942, BA, R 18/3764; *Die Ärztin* 20 (1944): 59.

40. Public Health Office, Cologne, to Krahn, Cologne, May 15, 1941, BA, R 18/2956; Conti to Reichsstatthalter et al., Berlin, January 11, 1943, BA, R 18/2958; Reichsgesundheitsführer, communication 9/44, Berlin, July 25, 1944, BA, R 18/3766a; Handloser to OKH et al., Berlin, October 20, 1944, BA, R 18/3764.

41. See text in section 1 near n. 12.

42. Quotation from Kluge, "Lage," p. 1206. In the same vein, see Neumeister, "Lage," pp. 1265–66; Diepgen, *Heilkunde*, pp. 10–11; also the unspecified letter by regime opponent Dr. Neumann (1935), printed in Schadewaldt, *Hartmannbund*, pp. 143–44; and, post-1945 uncritically, Deneke and Sperber, *Jahre*, p. 89.

43. Details in Kater, "Physicians in Crisis," pp. 52–53, 68.

44. This is not the place to present a history of the sickness fund insurance system (*Krankenkassenwesen*) in the Third Reich. But the following fundamental details may be noted. Although realizing that this system was badly in need of repair, Nazi

officials were wise enough not to implement drastic changes. They largely removed and even persecuted the erstwhile republican SPD functionaries of the panel funds (*Krankenkassen*), replacing them with their own, in the beginning often corrupt and inefficient men. As well, they dissolved the ambulatory medical services (*Ambulatorien*) of the funds. But even among the patients, to say nothing of the conservative doctors, these were not necessarily unpopular steps. Partially as a consequence of the Law for the Reconstruction of Social Insurance of July 5, 1934, between 1933 and 1939 the number of individual funds was scaled down from 6,427 to 4,436. Although serious cost-cutting efforts were made, until the end of the regime all types of funds were essentially maintained, and attempts by Ley, the pseudo-socialist DAF leader, to reorganize the entire fund system radically in the interest of his Labor Front wards were effectively blocked by the more conservative-minded leaders of the regime. See Haedenkamp, *Neuordnung*, pp. 16–25, 54–63, 70–71; Scherler, *Querschnitt*, pp. 14–52; Seifert, "Krankenversicherung"; Ramm, *Standeskunde*, pp. 120–22; Klein, *Amtsarzt*, 2:68–77; and the documents regarding the forced retirement of fund-employed ambulatory physicians (1934–35), UK, 207; and plans for a more lasting reform of the fund insurance system during the war (1943–45), BA, R 18/3783; R 18/3809; R 18/3813. Critically, see *Deutschland-Berichte* (1935), 2:101–2; ibid. (1936), 3:631–39; Peschke, *Geschichte*, pp. 405–8; Tennstedt, *Selbstverwaltung*, pp. 181–216; Tennstedt, "Sozialgeschichte," pp. 405–10; Tennstedt and Leibfried, "Sozialpolitik," pp. 135, 138, 151; Hansen et al., *Jahrhundert*, pp. 299–410, 460–99.

45. Also see Wuttke, "Herrschaft," pp. 195, 200, n. 140. A similar curve for earnings as that depicted in Figure 1 is indicated by income figures for Eutin gynecologist Dr. Wolfgang Saalfeldt in Stokes, *Kleinstadt*, p. 792, n. 16. The set of gross income figures for 1935 provided by Neumeister, "Lage," pp. 1265–66, minimizes earnings, even though only (generally lower-earning) fund physicians are addressed.

46. Wuttke, "Herrschaft," p. 195.

47. P. 210 of "1941—DAF-Amt Gesundheit u. Volksschutz," BA, R 18/3797.

48. Calculations based on figures in KVD Augsburg, Ausweichstelle Burgheim, "Saldenauszug aus dem Ärztekontokorrent," for December 31, 1943, UK, 106. According to Hagen, *Auftrag*, p. 141, some panel doctors could expect to earn one-third of their fees from private patients.

49. Calculations based on figures in KVD Braunschweig, "Saldenauszug aus dem Ärztekontokorrent," for December 31, 1943, UK, 106.

50. As in n. 49.

51. As in n. 49. Those are the figures that may be believed because the frequency of doctors was sufficiently high. There are some aberrant values in the list which may or may not be significant. Three lung specialists on average made in excess of 36,000 marks each (with one of them down for RM 19,156.10 for the final 1943 quarter), suggesting high operating (x-ray) or private clinic (sanatorium) expenses. The same holds true for a solitary radiologist who is listed with RM 21,051.23 for the year's end quarter. Single figures for two individual stomach and orthopedic experts were not deemed to be reliable.

52. For details about the complicated and often changing system in which the KVD remunerated all categories of war doctors (excepting those employed full time by the Wehrmacht and SS) after August 1939, as well as for documentation concerning the

income loss, see Petersilie, "Honorarverteilung"; Conti's speech of March 19, 1940, in *Deutsches Ärzteblatt* 70 (1940): 145–53; Grote's declaration, Berlin, April 1, 1940, ibid., p. 157; ibid., pp. 197–99; Grote, "Kriegsbesoldung"; Grote, "Tätigkeit," p. 58; Schütt, "Mitteilungen der Wissenschaftlichen Gesellschaft der deutschen Ärzte des öffentlichen Gesundheitsdienstes" [December 1939], BA, R 18/3122. For the case of an Upper Bavarian ophthalmologist who lost RM 3,000 in the first three months of the war, see Jäger to Landratsamt Traunstein and Ärztekammer München, Traunstein, September 15, 1940, BDC, PÄ Jäger.

53. Although Kluge, "Lage," purposely overstates the issues at hand, he is essentially correct. Also see Petersilie, "Honorarverteilung," p. 27.

54. Table 23 in *Statistisches Handbuch*, p. 564.

55. Grote, "Entwicklung," p. 339; *Ziel und Weg* 7 (1937): 201; ibid. 8 (1938): 502.

56. Grote, "Anordnung über des Fürsorgewesen der Reichsärztekammer," Berlin, February 20, 1937, in *Deutsches Ärzteblatt* 67 (1937): 221–22; *Ziel und Weg* 8 (1938): 20, 502.

57. Klinger, *Wege*, p. 77.

58. Example in Berger, *Kulturspiegel*, p. 117. The fee structure for privately practicing physicians, though based on pre-1933 guidelines (*Preugo* and *Adgo*), was protected by the Nazi health bureaucracy. See Bewer, "Befugnisse," pp. 222–23; Ramm, *Standeskunde*, p. 112.

59. KVD Augsburg, Ausweichstelle Burgheim, "Saldenauszug aus dem Ärztekontokorrent," for December 31, 1943, UK, 106.

60. Wuttke, "Herrschaft," p. 200, n. 140. The figures mentioned here are gross figures before income tax. They are corroborated in Berger, *Kulturspiegel*, p. 114. Cf. Ostler, *Rechtsanwälte*, p. 275.

61. Computation based on figures in Wuttke, "Herrschaft," p. 200, n. 140, according to growth formula in Floud, *Introduction*, pp. 91–92.

62. *Deutsches Ärzteblatt* 67 (1937): 993.

63. Statistics from ibid., p. 992.

64. Ibid., p. 993; Table 1.1.

65. Berger, *Kulturspiegel*, p. 114.

66. *Deutsches Ärzteblatt* 67 (1937): 993.

67. The dentists' mean taxable income in 1936 was RM 7,300. See Wuttke, "Herrschaft," p. 200, n. 140; Berger, *Kulturspiegel*, p. 114.

68. Tax calculation based on figures in Table 23, *Statistisches Handbuch*, p. 564.

69. Sauerbruch, *Leben*, pp. 291, 372, 385; Nissen, *Blätter*, p. 120.

70. See the example of Hamburg physician Dr. Heinz Klinger, in Klinger, *Wege*, pp. 78, 81; the (Greek) tour descriptions offered by *Deutsche Gesellschaft für ärztliche Studienreisen* in *Die Ärztin* 12 (1936): 229; and the travel advertisements in *Die Ärztin* 13 (1937): 54, 334.

71. See Forssmann, *Selbstversuch*, p. 201; Maassen, "Lebensverhältnisse," p. 295.

72. Sauerbruch, *Leben*, p. 331; Forssmann, *Selbstversuch*, p. 165. Psychiatrist Hans Bürger-Prinz preferred elegant, sporty BMWs (*Psychiater*, pp. 274–75).

73. "Glückliche Reisen!," in *Ziel und Weg* 6 (1936): vi. Also in this context, the

revealing anecdote about the unaffordability of a 1931 used imported Chrysler, for young Hamburg practitioner Dr. Klinger, in Klinger, *Wege*, pp. 80–81.

74. Hagen, *Auftrag*, p. 143.

75. Grote, "Tätigkeit," pp. 57–58; *Deutschland-Berichte* (1940), 6:236; RÄK. Ärztekammer Berlin and KVD. Landesstelle Berlin, circular 3/1943, Berlin, July 1, 1943, BA, R 18/3781.

4. Practicing Medicine in the Third Reich

1. Par. 8 (2) in [revised] "Satzung der Kassenärztlichen Vereinigung Deutschlands," Berlin, January 27, 1941, in Ramm, *Standeskunde*, p. 269; par. 51–79 in "Reichsärzteordnung," December 13, 1935, BA, R 18/5574; sanctions implicitly threatening the physicians in every one of the thirty-nine paragraphs contained in "Berufsordnung für die deutschen Ärzte," November 5, 1937, in *Deutsches Ärzteblatt* 67 (1937): 1031–37; ibid. 73 (1943): 194; Bewer, "Pflicht"; Ramm, *Standeskunde*, pp. 56–58. A victim's testimony is in Buchinger, *Marinearzt*, pp. 169–70.

2. Ramm, *Standeskunde*, p. 91.

3. "Meldeordnung der Reichsärztekammer," Berlin, March 27, 1936, in Ramm, *Standeskunde*, pp. 229–30; *Deutsches Ärzteblatt* 70 (1940): 232–34; Bunz, *Arzt*, p. 18; Klein, *Amtsarzt*, 3:14.

4. Doc. VIII/15A (October 6, 1934) in Stokes, *Kleinstadt*, pp. 853–55; *Ziel und Weg* 6 (1936): 133–34; Bunz, *Arzt*, pp. 9–10, 29; "Betr. Todesfall an Bauchfellentzündung," summer 1939, BA, R 18/3781; *Deutsches Ärzteblatt* 70 (1940): 232–34; Ramm, *Standeskunde*, pp. 104–5. See esp. Dörner, "Nationalsozialismus," p. 138; Weitbrecht, *Psychiatrie*, pp. 13–14. Such provisions complemented appropriate sections of the Law for the Prevention of Offspring by the Hereditarily Diseased (July 14, 1933), see Gütt et al., *Gesetz*, pp. 138–39.

5. The two cases are documented in *Ziel und Weg* 5 (1935): 518; Stokes, *Kleinstadt*, passim. Also see par. 3 in "Berufsordnung für die deutschen Ärzte," November 5, 1937, in *Deutsches Ärzteblatt* 67 (1937): 1032, also p. 1038; Bunz, *Arzt*, pp. 48–49; Bewer, "Pflicht," p. 171; Klein, *Amtsarzt*, 3:10–11.

6. Par. 46 (1), 4 in "Reichsärzteordnung," December 13, 1935, BA, R 18/5574; par. 3 in "Berufsordnung für die deutschen Ärzte," November 5, 1937, in *Deutsches Ärzteblatt* 67 (1937): 1032.

7. Grote, "KVD," pp. 12–13; *Ziel und Weg* 6 (1936): 290; Ramm, *Standeskunde*, p. 106.

8. Blome, *Arzt*, pp. 275–79; idem, "Fortbildungswesen"; *Ziel und Weg* 5 (1935): 445; ibid. 6 (1936): 289–90; Grote, "KVD," pp. 12–13.

9. Blome, "Fortbildungswesen"; idem, "Neuordnung," p. 7; *Ziel und Weg* 7 (1937): 74; ibid. 6 (1936): 290; Ramm, *Standeskunde*, pp. 106–8; Buchinger, *Marinearzt*, p. 164.

10. Quoting Professor Karl Eimer in *Deutsches Ärzteblatt* 67 (1937): 49. Also see ibid. 66 (1936): 13; and Blome, *Arzt*, p. 278.

11. "Reichsärzteordnung," December 13, 1935, BA, R 18/5574.

12. See "Begründung zu dem Gesetz über die berufsmässige Ausübung der Heil-

kunde ohne Bestallung," [1939], BA, R 18/5575; Wagner, "Volksgesundheit," pp. 138–39; Gersbach, *Bürgermeister*, p. 22; Klein, *Amtsarzt*, 3:81; *Journal of the American Medical Association* 100 (1933): 351, 1355.

13. A dedicated Nazi doctor's opposition to quacks is evident from letter from Dr. Kurt Klare to Frau H., Scheidegg, November 10, 1933, in Klare, *Briefe*, pp. 147–49.

14. See Berger, *Kulturspiegel*, p. 17; Gruber, *Einführung*, pp. 218–20; Wuttke-Groneberg, "Leistung," p. 49.

15. "Dritte Durchführungsverordnung zum Gesetz über die Vereinheitlichung des Gesundheitswesens," March 30, 1935, in Goetze and Meeske, *Reichsgesundheitswesen*, p. 15; *Ziel und Weg* 6 (1936): 341.

16. Wagner, "Reichsärzteordnung," p. 2.

17. *Ziel und Weg* 6 (1936): 341.

18. See *Deutsches Ärzteblatt* 67 (1937): 1038–39.

19. "Gesetz über die berufsmässige Ausübung der Heilkunde ohne Bestallung (Heilpraktikergesetz)," February 17, 1939, in *Reichsgesetzblatt* (1939), I, 251–52; Gersbach, *Bürgermeister*, pp. 22–30; Wagner, "Volksgesundheit," p. 139; Ramm, *Standeskunde*, pp. 60–61; "Begründung zu dem Gesetz über die berufsmässige Ausübung der Heilkunde ohne Bestallung," [1939], BA, R 18/5575; Gumpert, *Hunger*, p. 96; "1. Vierteljahreslagebericht 1939," in *Meldungen aus dem Reich*, 2:272.

20. Conti's remarks in *Ziel und Weg* 9 (1939): 336; Ramm, *Standeskunde*, p. 92.

21. Quotation from Pychlau to KVD.-Bezirksstellen-Leiter, Kolmar, April 15, 1942, BA, R 18/3785. Also see Falkenberg, "Misstände," pp. 38–39; Klein, *Amtsarzt*, 3:81–84.

22. Par. 13 (1) in "Reichsärzteordnung," December 13, 1935, BA, R 18/5574; par. 2 in "Berufsordnung für die deutschen Ärzte," in *Deutsches Ärzteblatt* 67 (1937): 1031. Commentary in Syroth, "Berufsgeheimnis"; Ramm, *Standeskunde*, pp. 100–101, 172.

23. Syroth, "Berufsgeheimnis," pp. 1470–71; Klein, *Amtsarzt* 3:9.

24. *Deutsches Ärzteblatt* 70 (1940): 124.

25. Quotation is my translation of *gesundes Volksempfinden*. See par. 13 (3) in "Reichsärzteordnung," December 13, 1935, BA, R 18/5574. Clause is repeated in par. 2 of "Berufsordnung für die deutschen Ärzte," in *Deutsches Ärzteblatt* 67 (1937): 1031. Also see Syroth, "Berufsgeheimnis," p. 1472.

26. Syroth, "Berufsgeheimnis," p. 1472; Ramm, *Standeskunde*, p. 101; text near n. 4, above.

27. Conti, "Gesundheitsführung—Volksschicksal: Rede des Reichsgesundheitsführers Dr. Conti auf der Kreistagung des Hauptamtes für Volksgesundheit der NSDAP," Munich, March 28, 1942, BDC, OPG Emil Ketterer (p. 11). Also see Kater, " 'Gesundheitsführung,' " pp. 357–58.

28. Cropp to Oberpräsidenten et al., Berlin, January 14, 1943, BA, R 18/3764; quotation from Vescovi, "Bedeutung," p. 228. For the modern ethical ramifications of medical confidentiality see Davidson, "Professional Secrecy."

29. An apologetic account of the Weimar friction from the physicians' point of view is presented in Schadewaldt, *Hartmannbund*, passim. Also see Kater, "Nazi Physicians' League," pp. 160–71.

30. As one example see Wagner, "Reichsärzteordnung," p. 3.

31. Kater, " 'Gesundheitsführung,' " pp. 372–73; Wagner, "Ziele," p. 492.

32. *Deutsches Ärzteblatt* 70 (1940): 49, 95; ibid. 72 (1942): 1; Berger, *Kulturspiegel*, pp. 138–39.

33. See Hartmann to Conti, Leipzig, November 28, 1940; Ley to Conti, Berlin, January 14, 1942, BA, R 18/3814; Conti to Gauamtsleiter, Munich, February 13 and March 31, 1942, BA, R 18/3785; memorandum [Kauffmann], [summer 1943], BA, R 18/3809; Kater, "Doctor Leonardo Conti," pp. 309–13; text in section 2 near n. 31.

34. *Deutsches Ärzteblatt* 72 (1942): 1–3; Möschler to KVD-Reichsführung, Weimar, September 21, 1943, UK, 130/118.02/3.

35. Doc. 373 (April 5, 1943) in Boberach, *Meldungen*, p. 381; doc. 345 (August 8, 1944) in Heiber, *Reichsführer*, p. 283; memorandum Kauffmann, Berlin, August 24, 1944, BA, R 18/3783.

36. My judgment concerning the international comparison is according to Grunberger, *Reich*, pp. 248–54. For the intra-German comparison, see the frequency of hospitalized patients: 388,492 in 1932, 425,058 in 1935, and 470,988 in 1938. Table 3, *Statistisches Handbuch*, p. 609; and Wuttke-Groneberg, "Leistung," pp. 22–24.

37. Seifert, "Krankenversicherung," p. 80; [draft], "Grundsätze für die Gestaltung der Leistungen der Krankenhilfe," May 14, 1942, BA, R 18/3785; *Bericht über das Bayerische Gesundheitswesen*, pp. 11, 17; Diepgen, *Heilkunde*, p. 11.

38. *Ziel und Weg* 8 (1938): 281, 633; *Deutsches Ärzteblatt* 70 (1940): 174; Conti, "Leistung," pp. 22–25; Conti, "Stand der Volksgesundheit im 5. Kriegsjahr," [January 1944], BA, R 18/3805 (pp. 8–9); Kelting, "Tuberkuloseproblem," p. 65; Kater, " 'Gesundheitsführung,' " pp. 363–64.

39. *Bericht über das Bayerische Gesundheitswesen*, p. 7; *Deutsches Ärzteblatt* 70 (1940): 174; Conti, "Leistung," pp. 17, 25; Conti, "Stand der Volksgesundheit im 5. Kriegsjahr," [January 1944], BA, R 18/3805 (pp. 11–12); Grunberger, *Reich*, p. 253; Kater, " 'Gesundheitsführung,' " pp. 355–56.

40. *Bericht über das Bayerische Gesundheitswesen*, pp. 16–17; "Luftterror und Seuchenverhütung," [1944], BA, R 18/3686; Grunberger, *Reich*, pp. 249–50. Computation for Herne according to figures in Meyerhoff, *Herne*, p. 57.

41. This ideologically premised policy is explained in Kater, " 'Gesundheitsführung,' " pp. 351–52.

42. Ibid., pp. 366–68. The casualty rate in the Mansfeld mines grew an annual compound average of 1.6 percent from 1933 to 1939, calculated on the basis of figures in Jonas, *Leben*, p. 410, according to the formula in Floud, *Introduction*, pp. 91–92. For the Reich level in 1935–37, see Grunberger, *Reich*, p. 248.

43. See, for instance, "Luftterror und Seuchenverhütung," [1944], BA, R 18/3686.

44. Meinberg, "Gesundheitsbetreuung," p. 527; *Bericht über das Bayerische Gesundheitswesen*, p. 19. Conti's pronouncements are in *Völkischer Beobachter*, April 25, 1940; *Deutsches Ärzteblatt* 70 (1940): 174.

45. *Bericht über das Bayerische Gesundheitswesen*, p. 16; Koller, "Der Gesundheitszustand des deutschen Volkes im 3. Vierteljahr 1942," Berlin, November 13, 1942, BA, R 18/3809; Meier, "Erkrankungen an übertragbaren Krankheiten im Deutschen Reich in den Jahren 1939–1942," BA, R 18/3789 (p. 13); Conti, "Stand der Volksgesundheit im 5. Kriegsjahr," [January 1944], BA, R 18/3805 (pp. 4–5); Grunberger, *Reich*, p. 249.

46. Koller, "Der Gesundheitszustand des deutschen Volkes im 3. Vierteljahr 1942," Berlin, November 13, 1942, BA, R 18/3809; "Luftterror und Seuchenverhütung," [1944], BA, R 18/3638; Meier, "Erkrankungen an übertragbaren Krankheiten im Deutschen Reich in den Jahren 1939–1942," BA, R 18/3789 (pp. 11–12); Conti, "Leistung," pp. 21–22; Conti, "Stand der Volksgesundheit im 5. Kriegsjahr," [January 1944], BA, R 18/3805 (pp. 3–5); Grunberger, *Reich*, pp. 249, 251; Gatz, *Hospitäler*, p. 67.

47. *Bericht über das Bayerische Gesundheitswesen*, p. 18; Conti in *Völkischer Beobachter*, April 25, 1940; Schütz to Ziegler, [Berlin], March 3, 1942, and to Gèronne, [Berlin], March 4, 1942, BDC, OPG Emil Ketterer; Gutterer to Zschintzsch, Berlin, November 2, 1942, BA, R 21/475; Meier, "Erkrankungen an übertragbaren Krankheiten im Deutschen Reich in den Jahren 1939–1942," BA, R 18/3789 (p. 14); Conti, "Stand der Volksgesundheit im 5. Kriegsjahr," [January 1944], BA, R 18/3805 (p. 17); Grunberger, *Reich*, p. 249.

48. Cases of mothers' deaths at birth and miscarriages did not get out of hand, in spite of the strain imposed increasingly on working mothers, especially in the countryside. See *Bericht über das Bayerische Gesundheitswesen*, p. 11; interior minister to ausserpreussische Landesregierungen et al., Berlin, October 30, 1939, R 18/5582; SD report 28, December 13, 1939, BA, R 58/146; Conti, "Gesundheitsführung—Volksschicksal: Rede des Reichsgesundheitsführers Dr. Conti auf der Kriegstagung des Hauptamtes für Volksgesundheit der NSDAP," Munich, March 28, 1942, BDC, OPG Emil Ketterer (pp. 11–12); Koller, "Der Gesundheitszustand des deutschen Volkes im 3. Vierteljahr 1942," Berlin, November 13, 1942, BA, R 18/3809; Kreisamtsleiter to Gauamt für Volksgesundheit Münster, Ahlen, March 9, 1943, BA, R 18/3781; Meier, "Erkrankungen an übertragbaren Krankheiten im Deutschen Reich in den Jahren 1939–1942," BA, R 18/3789 (pp. 1–2, 15–16); "Die Volksgesundheit im Jahre 1943," Berlin, December 15, 1935, BA, R 18/3810; "Luftterror und Seuchenverhütung," [1944], BA, R 18/3686; Conti, "Stand der Volksgesundheit im 5. Kriegsjahr," [January 1944], BA, R 18/3805 (pp. 10–12); entry for February 3, 1941, in *Meldungen aus dem Reich*, 6:1970–71.

49. Meier, "Erkrankungen an übertragbaren Krankheiten im Deutschen Reich in den Jahren 1939–1942," BA, R 18/3789 (pp. 4–6); computation for Herne based on figures in Meyerhoff, *Herne*, p. 57 (annual average compound growth rate according to formula in Floud, *Introduction*, pp. 91–92). Also see *Bericht über das Bayerische Gesundheitswesen*, p. 15; Seuchenreferat to Cropp, Berlin, June 1943, BA, R 18/3686.

50. Koller, "Der Gesundheitszustand des deutschen Volkes im 3. Vierteljahr 1942," Berlin, November 13, 1942, BA, R 18/3809. For 1943, see entry for September 27, 1943, in *Meldungen aus dem Reich*, XV, 5813–14.

51. See report Conti, Berlin, November 22, 1943, BA, R 18/1504; Conti, "Leistung," pp. 22–23; Conti, "Stand der Volksgesundheit im 5. Kriegsjahr," [January 1944], BA, R 18/3805 (pp. 7–8); Kelting, "Tuberkuloseproblem," esp. pp. 64–69; entry for December 1, 1941, in *Meldungen aus dem Reich*, 8:3049–51; Kater, " 'Gesundheitsführung,' " pp. 364–65.

52. See the figures in Jonas, *Leben*, p. 410; Tenfelde, "Provinz," p. 361.

53. On the twin phenomena of industrial ailments and sickness absenteeism in

general, see *Deutschland-Berichte* (1940), 7:122; Grote, KVD circular 16/40, Berlin, June 26, 1940; Focke to Conti, Rostock, January 3, 1942; Conti to Leiter der Gauämter für Volksgesundheit, Munich, March 31, 1942, BA, R 18/3785; [memorandum Conti], "Massnahmen zur Senkung des Krankenstandes," [Berlin, March 1943], BA, R 18/3809; Prinz, *Vom neuen Mittelstand*, pp. 268–69. Specifically on women, see "Aus dem Bericht . . . über die Zunahme des Krankenstandes," [spring 1942]; Engelhardt to Wirz, Karlsruhe, May 11, 1942; [draft], "Grundsätze für die Gestaltung der Leistungen der Krankenhilfe," May 14, 1942, BA, R 18/3785; docs. (June 9, 1942, and May 1944) in Eiber, "Frauen," pp. 618, 630; entry for September 27, 1943, in *Meldungen aus dem Reich*, 15:5811–12.

54. Conti, "Gesundheitsführung—Volksschicksal: Rede des Reichsgesundheitsführers Dr. Conti auf der Kriegstagung des Hauptamtes für Volksgesundheit der NSDAP," Munich, March 28, 1942, BDC, OPG Emil Ketterer; Conti, "Leistung"; Conti, "Stand der Volksgesundheit im 5. Kriegsjahr," [January 1944], BA, R 18/3805.

55. In this context, "hospitals" are defined as in Coermann and Wagner, *Ärzterecht*, p. 141.

56. See text in section 3, at nn. 3–9.

57. Calculations on the basis of figures in Table 3 in *Statistisches Handbuch*, p. 609. Annual average compound growth computations according to the formula in Floud, *Introduction*, pp. 91–92. On the growth of hospitals in the decade before 1933, see *Journal of the American Medical Association* 100 (1933): 754.

58. Figures for Lübeck's Städtisches Krankenhaus Süd as in memorandum Hansen, Lübeck, February 23, 1943, BA, R 18/3781. Otherwise as in n. 56, above. Also see the figure for the university clinic in Düsseldorf in Schönberg, "Geschichte," p. 167.

59. See memorandum Hansen, Lübeck, February 23, 1943, BA, R 18/3781; Mayer, *Jahre*, p. 36.

60. Calculated on the basis of figures in "Krankenhausstatistik," as of April 24, 1943, BA, R 18/3809.

61. "Übersicht über die wesentlichsten Runderlasse über das Krankenhauswesen," [1943], BA, R 18/3809.

62. Ibid.; [memorandum Conti], "Krankenhausversorgung," [March 1943]; "Krankenhausstatistik," as of April 24, 1943, BA, R 18/3809.

63. As in n. 27 of section 1; *Bericht über das Bayerische Gesundheitswesen*, pp. 5–6; Professor P. Esch's remarks in *25 Jahre*, p. 31; Gatz, *Hospitäler*, p. 26.

64. See Conti, "Gesundheitsführung—Volksschicksal: Rede des Reichsgesundheitsführers Dr. Conti auf der Kriegstagung des Hauptamtes für Volksgesundheit der NSDAP," Munich, March 28, 1942, BDC, OPG Emil Ketterer (p. 12); Buchinger, *Marinearzt*, pp. 175, 177, 182–83; Schönberg, "Geschichte," p. 41.

65. See Pfundtner to Landesregierungen et al., Berlin, September 27, 1938, BA, R 18/2958.

66. Entry for March 18, 1941, in *Tagebücher*, p. 542.

67. Stoeckel, *Erinnerungen*, p. 246. For the increasing frequency of bombing raids, see *Der Zivile Luftschutz*, pp. 118–20.

68. Below, *Adjutant*, pp. 311–12. On the raids, see *Zivile Luftschutz*, pp. 121–24.

69. Calculations on the basis of figures in memorandum, "Betrifft: Krankenanstalten," as of October 1, 1942, BA, R 18/3809.

70. Text in section 1 at n. 49; Speer and Brandt to Conti and Baubevollmächtigte, Berlin, October 8, 1942; "Übersicht der wesentlichsten Runderlasse über das Krankenhauswesen," [1943], BA, R 18/1309; [de Crinis] to [Conti], Berlin, October 13, 1942, BA, R 21/476. A Göring order of December 1938 to construct new hospitals away from city centers or strategic landmarks (*Zivile Luftschutz*, p. 277) seems to have had no practical results. In bitter retrospection, the Munich University psychiatrist Oswald Bumke writes (1946): "While shelters for hospitals were prohibited, those for the Gauleiter were constantly reinforced" (*Erinnerungen*, p. 126).

71. "Krankenhausstatistik," as of April 24, 1943, BA, R 18/3809; Golücke, *Schweinfurt*, pp. 59–71. For the stepped-up air attacks see *Zivile Luftschutz*, pp. 124–27.

72. Below, *Adjutant*, p. 331; Stoeckel (who slightly predates the Berlin raid), *Erinnerungen*, p. 259. Regarding the fortification, see Sauerbruch's criticism in memorandum for von Rottenburg, Berlin, July 9, 1943, BA, R 21/476. For the example of an attack on a Lower Rhenish hospital, see Gatz, *Hospitäler*, p. 67.

73. From October 1942 to May 1943 the number of hospitalized patients in the Reich had jumped from 407,514 to 512,992. See memorandum, "Betrifft Krankenanstalten," as of October 1, 1942, and memorandum Bernhard for Cropp, Berlin, May 4, 1943, BA, R 18/3809. Also see the other relative documents (March–April 1943) in that folder; as well as Ideler to Conti, Berlin-Grunewald, April 14, 1943, BA, R 18/3810.

74. Wolzogen, "Übersicht über die Krankenhaus-Sonderanlagen (Organisation Todt)," as of June 15, 1943; enclosure I., Brandt to Lammers, Berlin, June 22, 1943; Ofterdinger to Conti, Hamburg, August 30, 1943, BA, R 18/3809; Bürger-Prinz, *Psychiater*, p. 113. On the bombing damage to Hamburg, July–August 1943, including hospitals, see Middlebrook, *Battle*, pp. 142–61, 252–80, 322–37; and from a physician's perspective Ponsold, *Strom*, pp. 174–76. According to Giles, *Students*, pp. 297–98, none of the university clinics' 1,800 patients was harmed because of prudent sheltering there. For the effects of an air raid on hospitals in the western city of Mülheim-Ruhr in late June, see Amtsarzt to Regierungspräsident Düsseldorf, Mülheim, July 11, 1943, BA, R 18/3791.

75. Protocol, Berlin, June 29, 1943, BA, R 18/3791; report Conti, Berlin, November 22, 1943, BA, R 18/1504.

76. See Holm, "Gedanken zur ärztlichen Planwirtschaft," Berlin, October 12, 1943, BA, R 18/3809; memorandum [Cropp], Berlin, September 30, 1943; Gatz, *Hospitäler*, pp. 26, 86.

77. De Crinis's submissions to Conti, Berlin, August 27, December 22, 1943, and December 30, 1944, BA, R 21/476; *250 Jahre Charité*, p. 45; Jaeckel, *Charité*, pp. 401–2; Sauerbruch, *Leben*, p. 398; Stoeckel, *Erinnerungen*, pp. 259–60; Bergmann, *Rückschau*, pp. 286–90.

78. Catel, *Leben*, pp. 42–44; Schönberg, "Geschichte," p. 41; Professor P. Esch's remarks in *25 Jahre*, pp. 31–32; docs. h (July 1944) and i (October 1944) in Bardua, *Stuttgart*, pp. 208–9, 232–33.

79. See Gatz, *Hospitäler*, pp. 106, 111–12.
80. See Chapters 4 and 5, below.
81. See Pfundtner to Landesregierungen et al., Berlin, September 27, 1938, BA, R 18/2958; "Übersicht der wesentlichsten Runderlasse über das Krankenhauswesen," [1943], BA, R 18/3809; Birnbaum, *Zeuge meiner Zeit*, p. 231.
82. See *Deutschland-Berichte* (1935), 2:538; ibid. (1937), 4:657–58.
83. Scherler, *Querschnitt*, p. 37; *Ziel und Weg* 8 (1938): 108; doc. 156 (spring 1939) in Mason, *Arbeiterklasse*, p. 952; Kater, " 'Gesundheitsführung,' " pp. 368–69.
84. SD report 27, December 11, 1939, BA, R 58/146; *Deutsches Ärzteblatt* 70 (1940): 428–29.
85. Entries for December 18, 1941, in *Meldungen aus dem Reich*, 9:3110; and June 25, 1942, ibid., 10:3878; and for September 21, 1942, ibid., 11:4225–26; *Deutsches Ärzteblatt* 70 (1940): 39–40. Also see docs. 102–28 in Wuttke-Groneberg, *Medizin*, pp. 187–229.
86. "Massnahmen zur Behebung der Versorgungsschwierigkeiten auf dem Glasgebiet," [April 30, 1943], BA, R 18/3809; Reck-Malleczewen, *Diary*, p. 168.
87. See the want ads placed by doctors to attract medical secretaries in *Deutsches Ärzteblatt* 71 (1941): ix–x; Cropp to Kommissar der Freiwilligen Krankenpflege et al., Berlin, May 30, 1942, BA, R 18/5576.
88. Blome, "Keine Ausstellung privatärztlicher Zeugnisse über Arbeitsfähigkeit," Munich, December 15, 1939, in *Deutsches Ärzteblatt* 70 (1940): 3; Pohlkötter to Speer, Berlin, April 13, 1942; "Aus dem Bericht . . . über die Zunahme des Krankenstandes," [spring 1942], BA, R 18/3785; Hürmayr, circular 68/42, Münster, June 22, 1942, SAMs, Gauleitung Westfalen-Nord, Gauamt für Volkswohlfahrt, 7; Winkler, *Frauenarbeit*, p. 95; Klinger, *Wege*, p. 100; Kater, " 'Gesundheitsführung,' " p. 369.
89. Quotation Scholtz-Klink, report NSF, January–March 1942, BA, NS 22/860. Also see doc. 133 (July 19, 1940) in Gersdorff, *Frauen*, pp. 317–18; Russ to Reichsärzteführer, Krems, November 29, 1940, BA, R 18/3122; Conti, "Rückschau," p. 1; Blome to Conti, Munich, July 26, 1941, BA, R 18/3806; [Conti], "Begründung," [1942], BA, R 18/5576; [de Crinis] to [Conti], Berlin, October 13, 1942, BA, R 21/476; Holm, "Gedanken zur ärztlichen Planwirtschaft," Berlin, October 12, 1943, BA, R 18/3809; entry for May 24, 1943, in *Meldungen aus dem Reich*, 13:5279–80.
90. Conti to Speer, Berlin, May 6, 1944, BA, R 18/3122; entries for December 17, 1942, and February 15, 1943, in *Meldungen aus dem Reich*, 12:4579–80, 4809–11; "Mitteilungen an die Ärzte Südhannover-Braunschweigs," Hanover, September 1, 1944 (p. 1); and January 1, 1945 (p. 1), NHSA, Hann. 122a, XII, 126; Schenck, *Berlin*, pp. 46–47.
91. Hafemann to lord mayor, Berlin, April 21, 1943; Conti to Hermann, Berlin, April 7, 1943; RÄK. Ärztekammer Berlin and KVD. Landesstelle Berlin, circular 3/1943, Berlin, July 1, 1943, BA, R 18/3781; Cropp to Reichsverteidigungskommissare, Berlin, September 21 and November 9, 1943, BA, R 18/3764; case of nurse Maria Kiermayer in corr. Jäger (December 1943), BDC, PÄ Jäger.
92. Conti, "Gesundheitsführung—Volksschicksal: Rede des Reichsgesundheits-

führers Dr. Conti auf der Kriegstagung des Hauptamtes für Volksgesundheit der NSDAP," Munich, March 28, 1942, BDC, OPG Emil Ketterer (p. 14); RÄK. Ärztekammer Berlin and KVD. Landesstelle Berlin, circular 3/1943, Berlin, July 1, 1943, BA, R 18/3781; Cropp to Reichsstatthalter et al., Berlin, November 15, 1943, BA, R 18/3715; doc. 48–49 (March 1944) in Wuttke-Groneberg, *Medizin*, p. 88; Kögler to Speer, Schönlinde, April 5, 1944, BA, R 18/3122.

93. Conti to Speer, Berlin, June 29, 1943; Geschäftsführender Präsident, Deutsches Rotes Kreuz, to Landesführer, Potsdam-Babelsberg, July 2, 1943, BA, R 18/3791; BDC, RÄK Edmund Schöbel; *Die Ärztin* 19 (1943): 184; Brugsch's testimony in Albrecht and Hartwig, *Ärzte*, p. 189; Niedermeyer, *Wahn*, pp. 457–60; docs. h (August 1944) and i (October 1944) in Bardua, *Stuttgart*, pp. 209, 234.

94. Entry for April 30, 1942, in *Meldungen aus dem Reich*, 10:3694; Weinrich to Brandt, Kassel, May 3, 1943, BA, R 18/3810; protocol, Berlin, June 29, BA, R 18/3791; Holm, "Gedanken zur ärztlichen Planwirtschaft," Berlin, October 12, 1943, BA, R 18/3809; Kreishauptamtsleiter to NSDAP, Amt für Volkswohlfahrt, Bad Driburg, April 11, 1944, SAMs, Polit. Polizei, 3. Reich, 109; information service 41, Munich, September 21, 1944, SAM, NSDAP/31; Bressler to Korpsarzt, [Munich], September 27, 1944, BDC, PÄ Obermaier; BDC, RÄK Wilhelm Bollmeyer, Karl Miesemer, Emil Ryska.

95. Weight units are converted from metric figures in the original. The information is very reliable because it was compiled by SS intelligence. See enclosure with letter SS-Standartenführer Schmitz to Conti, Berlin, September 25, 1943, BA, R 18/3809.

96. Forssmann, *Selbstversuch*, pp. 261–62.

97. Catel, *Leben*, pp. 42–44.

98. Entry for March 26, 1945, in Hoemberg, *People*, pp. 196–99.

99. Hoffmann, *Ringen*, pp. 250–51.

100. Wolff-Mönckeberg, *Briefe*, pp. 118–23. A case of suicide, by a despondent woman physician from Thuringia, is recorded in *alltägliche Faschismus*, p. 187.

101. Stoeckel, *Erinnerungen*, pp. 236, 264.

102. Doc. 1 (November 1944) in Berghahn, "Meinungsforschung," p. 97.

103. Ohlendorf to Klopfer, Berlin, [fall 1942], Ohlendorf to Thierack, Berlin, February 22, 1944, BA, R 22/4203; case Dr. Heiler in Beer to RÄK, Munich, August 27, 1943, BDC, PÄ Heiler; case Dr. Guttmann (1944) in BDC, PÄ Guttmann; SD report, March 2, 1944, BA, R 58/193 (pp. 86–88); entry for March 25, 1941, in *Meldungen aus dem Reich*, 6:2144; and for October 2, 1941, 8:2832; BDC, RÄK Margarete Naske. For examples of prewar morals charges, see case of Gera internist Dr. Donath (spring 1935), UK, 213; and of Lübeck ophthalmologist Dr. Walter Kreuzfeld (summer 1937), UK, 130/118.02. For the pre-1933 period, see *Kriminalität der Ärzteschaft*.

104. Examples in RÄK. Ärztekammer Berlin and KVD. Landesstelle Berlin, circular 3/1943, Berlin, July 1, 1943, BA, R 18/3781; Bürger-Prinz, *Psychiater*, p. 114; Hoffmann, *Ringen*, p. 271.

105. Ring, *Geschichte*, pp. 293, 307.

106. Hoff, *Erlebnis*, pp. 350–52; Forssmann, *Selbstversuch*, p. 245.

107. Military physicians in occupied territory such as France lived a bearable,

sometimes even opulent life. See Klinger, *Wege*, pp. 92–96, 106–8; testimony of Dr. Wertheim in Hagen, *Leader*, pp. 51–53.

108. Hoff, *Erlebnis*, p. 350; Berger, *Kulturspiegel*, p. 140; Ring, *Geschichte*, p. 306; Klinger, *Wege*, p. 111; Fischer, *Erfahrungsberichten*, p. 14; Forssmann, *Selbstversuch*, pp. 215, 237, 265.

109. Bamm [pen name for Dr. Curt Emmrich], *Flagge*, p. 175. Also see ibid., pp. 29, 138; "Das Hohelied des Arztes," [1941–42], HIS, 13/258; Forssmann, *Selbstversuch*, pp. 237–38, 245, 265; Georg Pietruschka's testimony in Albrecht and Hartwig, *Ärzte*, p. 149.

110. Entries for January 22, February 5, March 6, 1942, in *Goebbels Diaries*, pp. 50, 86–87, 136; Seidler, *Prostitution*, pp. 46–47; Ring, *Geschichte*, p. 293; Fischer, *Erfahrungsberichten*, p. 31; Forssmann, *Selbstversuch*, p. 252; Dr. Wertheim's testimony in Hagen, *Leader*, p. 54.

111. Seidler, *Prostitution*, pp. 233, 236–37; Bamm, *Flagge*, pp. 248–50; Forssmann, *Selbstversuch*, pp. 218–19. Also see Ponsold, *Strom*, pp. 193–95; Klinger, *Wege*, p. 111.

112. Forsmann, *Selbstversuch*, pp. 237–38; Bamm, *Flagge*, pp. 113–15.

113. Ring, *Geschichte*, p. 298; Georg Pietruschka's testimony in Albrecht and Hartwig, *Ärzte*, p. 157; Sauerbruch, *Leben*, p. 376.

114. Bamm, *Flagge*, pp. 139–45.

115. Georg Pietruschka's testimony in Albrecht and Hartwig, *Ärzte*, p. 171.

116. Letter of October 6, 1943, in Bähr and Bähr, *Kriegsbriefe*, p. 281.

117. Sauerbruch, *Leben*, p. 376.

118. Ibid., p. 377; Ring, *Geschichte*, pp. 294, 318–19; Fischer, *Erfahrungsberichten*, pp. 2, 9, 23, 25, 28.

119. Ring, *Geschichte*, pp. 294–95; Forssmann, *Selbstversuch*, p. 264; Fischer, *Erfahrungsberichten*, pp. 1–5, 11; Buchbender and Sterz, *Gesicht*, p. 17.

120. Ring, *Geschichte*, p. 317; Fischer, *Erfahrungsberichten*, p. 3; text in Chapter 4, 3, at n. 89.

121. Bamm, *Flagge*, pp. 201, 334; Forssmann, *Selbstversuch*, p. 215. For exceptions, see Hans Schadewaldt in *Deutsches Ärzteblatt* 83 B (1986): 1187. Also see Chapter 4, 3, after n. 83; Chapter 5.

122. The clinic was founded by Professor Viktor von Weizsäcker. *Deutsche medizinische Wochenschrift* 82 (1957): 926. Also see Fischer, *Erfahrungsberichten*, pp. 38–41, 47.

123. The British journalist Grunberger, *Reich*, p. 253, speaks of "the army medical corps' predilection for amputations." The East German historian of medicine Ring, *Geschichte*, p. 308, charges the opposite.

124. Quotation from Grunberger, *Reich*, p. 253.

Chapter 2

1. Doctors in the Nazi Party

1. Bamm, *Menschen Zeit*, p. 159. Hamburg's reputation, which has persisted into the post–World War II era (see Giles, *Students*, p. 13), was not entirely justified. Among thirty-two Nazi Gaue in the Reich in December 1934, Hamburg stood fifteenth in frequency of Nazi members per capita. See *Partei-Statistik*, p. 35.

2. Buchinger, *Marinearzt*, p. 147.

3. According to Schallwig, "Paracelsus' Bedeutung," p. 10.

4. See the figures in Table 2.1, which must be used with caution. Confidence interval tests at the social-scientifically acceptable probability (*P*) level of 0.05 in some cases indicate significant percentage fluctuations because of low *N*. Also see Kater, "Quantifizierung," pp. 478–81; Kershaw, *Popular Opinion*, passim.

5. Cf. Kater, *Nazi Party*, pp. 1–16.

6. Table 2.1. Background is in Kater, *Nazi Party*, pp. 72–115.

7. Table 2.1. In column C, the values of 43.4 and 27.2 percent represent increases of 24.2 and 19.1 percent over the corresponding percentages in column A, respectively, and the values of 34.1 and 30.9 percent represent decreases of 8.1 and 21.8 percent.

8. Details are in Chapter 6.

9. The values in Table 2.2 are subject to the same considerations as apply to the values in Table 2.1, mentioned in the first part of n. 4.

10. In my NSDAP sample, I counted a total of 76 physicians, 1933–45 (excluding, of course, dentists and veterinarians, and possibly, for failure to detect them in the membership cards, professors of medicine) among a total of 13,157 new Nazi joiners with classifiable professions 1–14 (listed in Table 1 of my book, *Nazi Party*, p. 241. Also see pp. 252–53). Sampling procedures and the overall significance of the larger BDC master sample, 1925–45, are explained in my article, "Quantifizierung." Physicians in the Reich population were counted as in *Berufszählung, 16. Juni 1933*, pp. 48–51. For the procedure of identifying 27,047,899 socially classifiable persons in 1933, see Kater, *Nazi Party*, pp. 6–12.

11. For recent documentation of the last-mentioned, see Kershaw, *Popular Opinion*, pp. 156–223; Falter, "Wähler," pp. 52–53; Falter et al., *Wahlen und Abstimmungen*, p. 200; Childers, *Nazi Voter*, pp. 188–90, 258–66; and, with regard to SA leaders, Jamin, *Zwischen den Klassen*, pp. 89–92. The sample of 4,177 doctors, on which Table 2.3 is based, is out of a total (estimated) universe of approximately 79,000 cases, all members of RÄK, 1936–45, contained on file cards in the BDC (Kater sample. My estimate is higher than that of the BDC: 72,000. See *Der Spiegel*, February 22, 1988, p. 29). The values in Table 2.3 indicate that 49.1 percent of all Protestant and 35.2 percent of all Catholic physicians joined the NSDAP.

12. Given a universe of 4,177 *N*, a confidence interval test (see the first half of n. 4, above) shows that the percentage of 44.8 (column G of Table 2.4) may have been as high as 46.3 and as low as 43.3.

13. The professional plight of the 1919–32 group is described in Kater, "Physicians in Crisis." Confidence interval tests (see first half of n. 4, above) show the

percentages in columns C and D in Table 2.4 to have been larger, after allowing for fluctuations plus or minus, than those in columns A, E, F, and G.

14. This more recent verdict of mine, based on new research, somewhat modifies my earlier contention that "the doctors' enthusiasm for the regime declined when the war broke out and continued to lessen as it progressed" (*Nazi Party*, p. 135). The percentages of 43.2 and 44.1 in columns E and F of Table 2.4 do not, by the test described in n. 4 above, display statistically significant differences, suggesting uniformity in value. For the relative strength of physician Nazi newcomers in 1940–41, also see the value of 11.8 percent in column F of Table 2.1; for their mature age see the mean value of 40 in column F of Table 2.5.

15. Columns A and C in Table 2.6. The value of 28.4 percent in column C must be held to have been neither more nor less than the value of 27.1 percent in column A because of significant confidence interval fluctuations (see the remarks in the first half of n. 4).

16. The statistical uncertainty derives from the low *N* of the sample examined in column B of Table 2.6 (see the remarks in the first half of n. 4).

17. Kater, *Nazi Party*, pp. 201, 215.

18. Columns A, C, D, and E in Table 2.6

19. According to the testimony in Padover, *Experiment*, p. 97.

20. Domeinski, "Zur Entnazifizierung," p. 251.

21. List of physicians for the Kreise of Laufen and Berchtesgaden, [February 1935], SAM, NSDAP/371.

22. As quoted by Wuttke-Groneberg, "Leistung," p. 14.

23. Ibid. At the end of 1934, of thirty-two Nazi Gaue, Baden was in twenty-eighth place in frequency of Nazi membership as measured against total Gau population. See *Partei-Statistik*, p. 35. Also see Chroust, "Social Situation," p. 60, n. 78.

24. Computations according to the figures in *Ziel und Weg* 7 (1937): 225. At this time, 6,319 physicians were said to exist in Berlin, of whom between 23.3 and 29.5 percent still were Jewish. At the end of 1934, Berlin was in twenty-seventh place in the rank order of Nazi frequency (see n. 23, above).

25. Professor Konrad H. Jarausch, University of North Carolina at Chapel Hill, to author, Bielefeld, May 25, 1987. Jarausch's current research on the professions in the Weimar Republic and Third Reich is expected to cast more light on this issue. So far, see his excellent pilot articles, "The Crisis of German Professions" and "The Perils of Professionalism." It is obvious that Güstrow's impressionistic verdict for prewar Berlin, *Strafverteidiger*, p. 12, constitutes a gross misjudgment: "no more than six" Nazi lawyers. Also see Kater, *Nazi Party*, p. 112; and Stokes, "Professionals and National Socialism," pp. 454–55; and the as yet unsatisfactory book by Müller, *Furchtbare Juristen*.

26. Details are in Kater, "Hitlerjugend," pp. 606–12; idem, *Nazi Party*, pp. 91–94, 106–9, 123–26, 131–32.

27. International research is behind in this area. Thus far, see Ludwig, *Technik*, esp. pp. 106–8; idem, "VDI"; and Speer, *Inside the Third Reich*, passim; and Herf, *Reactionary Modernism* (my critique of this suggestive book is in *Archiv für Sozialgeschichte* 27 [1987]: 795–97). Rauschning wrote in 1942 (republished in 1971): "It is curious to note how many engineers Hitler drew into his select circle" (*Men of*

Chaos, p. 230). Further see Kater, *Nazi Party*, pp. 111–12. Jarausch has promised to extend his survey to the engineers, including architects. See his two articles mentioned in n. 25.

28. See the tentative, less than exhaustive article by Schröder, "Pharmazie," esp. p. 184, n. 17.

29. The exception is pre-1933. It was Dr. med. Gustav Schmischke, a generalist in Anhalt, born in 1883, who served as Anhalt's Gauleiter from July 1925 to September 1926 (Tyrell, *Führer*, p. 375).

30. In alphabetical order, they were Bartels, Friedrich; Benn, Gottfried; Conti, Leonardo; Deuschl, Hans; Frey, Gottfried; Gütt, Arthur; Hamann, Erhardt; Haselmayer, Heinrich; Klein, Wilhelm; Klipp, Carl-Oscar; Luther, Hans; Otto, Helmut; Pauly, Erasmus; Peschke, Karl; Schlegel, August; Schottenheim, Otto; Schuster, Johann; Spanuth, Robert; Stähle, Eugen; Strauss, Kurt; Thomalla, Curt; Vonnegut, Franz; Wagner, Gerhard. Doctors of dentistry and veterinary medicine were of course excluded from this count. See *Deutsche Führerlexikon*, passim. Some of the professors of medicine listed there are dealt with in Chapter 4 and the Conclusion.

31. "Jahreslagebericht 1938," in *Meldungen aus dem Reich*, 2:111. Reflecting on the situation in the Federal Republic of Germany is Naschold, *Kassenärzte*, pp. 111–14.

32. For a sociogram of Nazi Old Fighters before 1933, see Kater, *Nazi Party*, pp. 169–89.

33. Biographical details of these men are in Kater, "Doctor Leonardo Conti," pp. 301–4; Stockhorst, *Köpfe*, pp. 62–63; *Deutsche Führerlexikon*, pp. 41–42, 86–87, 512; vita Bartels in Bartels, "Antrag auf OPG-Verfahren," Munich-Harlaching, August 18, 1939, BDC, OPG Bartels; *Völkischer Beobachter*, April 23, 1939. Also see Kater, "Hitler's Early Doctors."

34. *Deutsche Führerlexikon*, p. 469; Stähle, *Geschichte*, pp. 4–17.

35. *Deutsche Führerlexikon*, pp. 350–51.

36. Obituary in *Deutsches Ärzteblatt* 70 (1940): 365.

37. Ibid. 68 (1938): 144; *Ziel und Weg* 8 (1938): 139; and text at n. 13, Chapter 1, 2.

38. In a questionnaire of April 17, 1941, BDC, RSK Klare, Klare used the term *nordisch-fälisch* to describe his "race." Also see Klare to Hinkel, Scheidegg, March 18, 1939, BDC, PK Klare; *Wer ist's?*, pp. 819–20.

39. A corporate portrait of Ortsgruppenleiter is in Kater, *Nazi Party*, pp. 169–70, 172, 190–93, 209, 211, 221–23.

40. On Mennecke, see "Lebenslauf" Mennecke, Eichberg, June 13, 1937, BDC, SS Mennecke; Platen-Hallermund, *Tötung*, p. 92; Chroust, "Friedrich Mennecke"; on Saalfeldt, see Stokes, *Kleinstadt*, pp. 395, 406–7; on Krauss, see Fröhlich, *Herausforderung*, p. 158.

41. Details on Kötschau have been gleaned from his personal papers in BDC, SS file, TF, RÄK, and PK Kötschau. Further see n. 55 of Chapter 4, 1.

42. Berger, *Kulturspiegel*, p. 97; Frei, *Provinzpresse*, pp. 224–25, 227–30.

43. *Deutsche Führerlexikon*, pp. 344–45.

44. Grill, *Nazi Party in Baden*, pp. 438–39.

45. *Deutsche Führerlexikon*, pp. 348–49.
46. Ibid., pp. 173–74.
47. They were Drs. Gerhard Wagner, Walter Gross, Paul Hocheisen, Karl Peschke, Josef Ständer, and Walter Ruppin. See *Deutsches Ärzteblatt* 66 (1936): 501. Reichstag deputyships could be rotated. Thus between March and December 1933, Eugen Stähle had been a delegate (Stähle, *Geschichte*, p. 11; *Deutsche Führerlexikon*, p. 469). On Reichstag emoluments then see Kater, *Nazi Party*, p. 210.
48. *Deutsche Führerlexikon*, p. 169.
49. Cases of Drs. Helmut Otto, Otto Schottenheim, Wilhelm Schenk, and Wolfgang Saalfeldt in *Deutsche Führerlexikon*, pp. 344–45, 435; *Ziel und Weg* 7 (1937): 58; Stokes, *Kleinstadt*, p. 395.
50. Case of Dr. Kurt Uhlenbroock in Kaul, *Ärzte*, p. 86; case of Dr. Hans-Jochen Boye, in his personal files (1940–43), BDC, PÄ Boye; also see *Deutsches Ärzteblatt* 70 (1940): 85–86; as well as text after n. 53 of section 2, below.

2. The Nazi Physicians' League and Other Party Affiliates

1. Local exceptions were, of course, possible. Thus in the Upper Bavarian Kreise Laufen-Berchtesgaden in early 1935, sixteen out of thirty-two resident physicians were in the NSDAP, but thirty were in the NS-Ärztebund. See n. 21 of section 1.
2. Percentages of 33.4 and 46.2 in columns A and D, Table 2.4
3. Table 2.4, columns E and F. In the comparison of the figures from Table 2.4 the confidence interval test (as described in the first half of n. 4 of section 1) establishes real numerical differences, with one exception: the juxtaposition of 33.4 percent (column A) and 32.0 percent (column E).
4. See *Ziel und Weg* 8 (1938): 420; Zapp, "Untersuchungen," p. 50; Tennstedt, "Sozialgeschichte," p. 406.
5. *Deutsches Ärzteblatt* 64 (1934): 27; *Ziel und Weg* 4 (1934): 37; Ramm, *Standeskunde*, p. 73. In Table 2.4, see column G.
6. Althen to NS-Ärztebund Hessen-Nassau, [Wiesbaden], August 20, 1934; Althen to Wiesbaden NS-Ärztebund members, Wiesbaden, August 30, 1934; Schffer [sic] to NS-Ärztebund Hessen-Nassau, Wiesbaden-Bierstadt, September 15, 1934; Althen to Kreisleitung Rheingau, Rüdesheim, October 5, 1934, HHSAW, 483/3159; Nazi affiliate organizations (including NS-Ärztebund) list of NSDAP candidates for Kreis Berchtesgaden-Laufen, October 10, 1935, SAM, NSDAP/122; Orlow, *History*, p. 56; Kater, "Sozialer Wandel," p. 43. Generally, Germans could not enter Nazi organizations, including the party itself, if they had belonged to a Masonic lodge on January 30, 1933. Wagner's "amnesty" evidently applied to physicians who left the lodges between that date and the time of their final dissolution, in July 1937. See Wagner, "Amnestie des Leiters des NSD.-Ärztebundes für die Ehrengerichtsbarkeit des NSD.-Ärztebundes," par. 3, Munich, May 17, 1938, in *Ziel und Weg* 8 (1938): 292; Kater, *Nazi Party*, pp. 161–62; doc. VIII/40 in Stokes, *Kleinstadt*, pp. 945–47.
7. See Kater, "NS-Studentenbund"; Bölling, *Volksschullehrer*, p. 125; Volz, *Daten*, pp. 25–27.
8. Kater, "Sozialer Wandel," pp. 28–29; idem, *Nazi Party*, pp. 44–49.

9. Statute, Nationalsozialistischer Deutscher Ärztebund e.V., [1929–30], BA, Schumacher/213.

10. Liebl, "Satzungen des Nationalsozialistischen Deutschen Ärztebundes," Ingolstadt, [1930], BA, Schumacher/213; Conti, "Der Nationalsozialistische Deutsche Ärztebund," in *Mitteilungsblatt der Arbeitsgemeinschaft Gross-Berlin des Nationalsozialistischen Deutschen Ärztebundes*, 1, no. 1 (Berlin, January 1931), BA, NSD, 53/2; Klein, *Amtsarzt*, 2:54–55.

11. See Kater, "Physicians in Crisis"; idem, "Nazi Physicians' League."

12. Conti, "Der Nationalsozialistische Deutsche Ärztebund," as in n. 10, above.

13. The established physicians Liebl, Klare, and Wagner were born in 1874, 1885, and 1888 respectively. Since for Dr. Theo Lang (Munich) and Dr. Kratz (Cologne) no RÄK cards in the BDC are extant, they may be presumed to have been mature enough to be retired at least by 1936.

14. Lejeune led the junior doctors' lobby, the Reichsnotgemeinschaft deutscher Ärzte, at first in fierce opposition to, but later in a joint effort with the Hartmannbund. His NSDAP number (1925) was 3964. Before and after 1933, he was a university teacher in the history of medicine (Cologne and Vienna), poorly regarded by more prolific colleagues in this field. Characteristically, a Nazi dissertation was devoted to him and his pre-1933 organization in 1940. See Lejeune to Stumpf, Cologne, March 15, 1938; assessment Diepgen, Berlin, May 24, 1944, BDC, PK Lejeune; *Ärztliches Vereinsblatt* 58 (1929): 486; *Münchener Medizinische Wochenschrift* 77 (1930): 1218; Ackermann, "Nachwuchs"; *Wer ist's?*, p. 953; and Fischer, *Lexikon*, 2:868.

15. Corr. honor proceedings Conti-Deuschl, September 1932, BDC, PK Conti; *Ziel und Weg* 2, no. 5 (1932): 2 (the near expulsion is mentioned in Reichsleitung, NSÄB, "Disziplinarhof-Entscheid," sign. Holzmann, Schultze, Ketterer, Brunswick, September 17, 1932); Blome, *Arzt*, p. 263. On the problem of intergenerational conflict in the Weimar Republic, see Kater, "Generationskonflikt," pp. 217–29.

16. Corr. Ärztlicher Kreisverband Oberpfalz [Hartmannbund]-Strasser (September 1930), BA, Schumacher/213.

17. Text at nn. 1–28 in Chapter 1, 2; Table 2.4.

18. See *Ziel und Weg* 3 (1933): 134, 671; ibid. 6 (1936): 20; ibid. 7 (1937): 5; ibid. 9 (1939): 22; Diepgen, *Heilkunde*, p. 281.

19. The official status of the NS-Ärztebund, like that of the Nazi Teachers' League and Nazi Lawyers' League, was that of an associated formation of the NSDAP (*angeschlossener Verband*), rather than, like SA, SS, and HJ, an integrated one (*eingegliederter Verband*). See Huber, *Rechtsgestalt*, pp. 336–37. As such, it became one of the departments of Hauptamt für Volksgesundheit of the NSDAP after its formation in spring 1934. See text in Chapter 1, 2 at n. 21; and Ramm, *Standeskunde*, p. 73. The additional disciplinary prerogative of the league is evident from *Ziel und Weg* 3 (1933): 29–30; ibid. 5 (1935): 52–54, 288–95. Also see Zapp, "Untersuchungen," p. 48.

20. Althen to members of Wiesbaden chapter, NS-Ärztebund, Wiesbaden, October 1, 1934, HHSAW, 483/3159.

21. Althen to Quästur der Universität Heidelberg, [Wiesbaden], September 29, 1934; Althen to professional comrades, [Wiesbaden], October 9, 1934; Althen, "Veranstaltungen," [October 1934], HHSAW, 483/3159.

22. *Deutsches Ärzteblatt* 65 (1935): 144. Also see *Die Ärztin* 12 (1936): 52.

23. Entry for May, 1935, in *Deutschland-Berichte* (1935), 2:538. On Lepsius, see Stockhorst, *Köpfe*, p. 268.

24. Althen to members of Wiesbaden chapter, NS-Ärztebund, Wiesbaden, August 11 and 30, 1934; Althen to HJ, Bann 80, [Wiesbaden], October 5, 1934, HHSAW, 483/3159.

25. Althen to members of Wiesbaden chapter, NS-Ärztebund, Wiesbaden, August 11 and 30, 1934, HHSAW, 483/3159; Michaelis et al., *Kultur*, p. 267.

26. *Ziel und Weg* 3 (1933): 489; ibid. 6 (1936): 450; Althen to HJ, Bann 80, [Wiesbaden], October 5, 1934; Althen to professional comrades, [Wiesbaden], October 9, 1934, HHSAW, 483/3159.

27. For the erection of the camp, the Hauff estate was bought in 1934 by the Nazi medical leaders. For this purchase funds expropriated from the Hartmannbund were used, the onetime emergency chest to which German physicians had contributed during the pre-1933 depression. On this, see Waldheim to Landgericht Leipzig, Leipzig, December 7, 1931, UK, 112; *Ziel und Weg* 5 (1935): 231; Grote, "Entwicklung," p. 339; Dr. Neumann's letter of 1935 printed in Schadewaldt, *Hartmannbund*, p. 144. Also see Blome, *Arzt*, p. 283; Diepgen, *Heilkunde*, p. 282.

28. Quotation from Ramm, *Standeskunde*, p. 75. Also see *Deutsches Ärzteblatt* 65 (1935): 567–68; *Ziel und Weg* 5 (1935): 256.

29. *Ziel und Weg* 5 (1935): 256; Blome, "Neuordnung," p. 8.

30. For the forced humor in the report by a participant, see *Deutsches Ärzteblatt* 65 (1935): 569–70; and the charge in Neumann's letter of 1935, in Schadewaldt, *Hartmannbund*, p. 144. The naturalist and holistic ideals are briefly stressed in Diepgen, *Heilkunde*, p. 282. Anti-intellectual polemic is in Blome, "Rückblick," pp. 10–12. By writing that *all* German physicians were conscripted for schooling at Alt-Rehse, Fischer, "Arzt," p. 10, n. 3, obviously confuses this elite training with the continuing education programs mentioned in Chapter 1, 4, at n. 6. Clearly, conscription for Alt-Rehse was imposed only on NS-Ärztebund members.

31. Blome, "Neuordnung," p. 8; idem, "Rückblick," pp. 1–12; idem, *Arzt*, pp. 288–90; Grote, "Entwicklung," p. 339.

32. *Deutsches Ärzteblatt* 71 (1941): 114–15. Cf. Modersohn, "Führerprinzip," p. 36.

33. Amtsleiter NS-Ärztebund Gau Hessen-Nassau to Althen, Frankfurt am Main, August 2, 1934; Althen to Behrens, [Wiesbaden], October 5, 1934; Althen to Deutsche Volks- und Berufsgenossen, [Wiesbaden], October 9, 1934, HHSAW, 483/3159.

34. Case of Dr. Scholten, in *Ziel und Weg* 8 (1938): 430; case of Dr. Bach, in "Aufzeichnung," enclosed with letter Wagner to Wacker, Munich, November 24, 1937, BDC, PK Bach.

35. Stähle, *Geschichte*, pp. 18–19; Schadewaldt, *Hartmannbund*, p. 138; Conti's speech of April 24, 1942, printed in *Deutsches Ärzteblatt* 72 (1942): 200; Zapp, "Untersuchungen," p. 55.

36. *Nationalsozialistisches Jahrbuch* 17 (1943): 206; ibid. 18 (1944): 189–90, 208–9. See the Nazi addresses paraphrased or partially reproduced in *Deutsches Ärzteblatt* 70 (1940): 96, 123–24; ibid. 72 (1942): 200–201. Also see the report of November 6, 1939, in *Meldungen aus dem Reich*, 2:424. See Conti's futile attempt

summer 1942 to redefine the NS-Ärztebund's functions as an agent of population planning, Lilienthal, "*Lebensborn e.V.*," pp. 141–42.

37. Zapp, "Untersuchungen," p. 55; Röhrs, "Betrifft: Hauptamtliche Ärzte für die NSDAP," enclosed with letter Röhrs to Schrepfer, Munich, November 25, 1943, BA, R 18/3810. On consequences of "total war," see Teppe, "Der Reichsverteidigungskommissar," pp. 297–98. On the fate of the Nazi Teachers' League, see Kater, "Hitlerjugend," pp. 615–18; Feiten, *Lehrerbund*, pp. 197–99.

38. According to Table 2 in Kater, "Hitlerjugend," p. 609.

39. In contravention of this ruling, some male NSDAP candidates used SA membership as a convenient stepping-stone to regular party membership during periods of party closure after 1933. See Kater, "Sozialer Wandel," p. 43; idem, "Quantifizierung," pp. 478–79; Orlow, *History*, p. 56; and the example of Dr. Uhlenbroock in Kaul, *Ärzte*, p. 86.

40. After application of the confidence interval test, as explained in the first half of n. 4 (section 1), to those values in Table 2.4, column D. The values for the SA in this table obviously refer to male physicians only.

41. Whereas Fischer, *Stormtroopers*, pp. 25–81, has insisted on a more proletarian membership for the rank-and-file SA, the scholarly consensus to date points to an overwhelmingly, if by no means exclusively, lower-middle-class makeup. See Kater, "Ansätze," pp. 800–807; Bessel, *Violence*, pp. 33–45.

42. Werner, "SA und NSDAP," pp. 407–8, 505, 509, 514; *Der SA-Mann*, Munich, October 29, 1932; Jamin, *Zwischen den Klassen*, p. 57. On the shortage, see Blome, *Arzt*, p. 237.

43. *Deutsche Führerlexikon*, pp. 86, 345; *Völkischer Beobachter*, April 23, 1939; Blome, *Arzt*, pp. 245, 265; doc. I/34A (March 20, 1932) in Stokes, *Kleinstadt*, p. 288.

44. Paraphrase of recollection by Dr. S., in Lifton, *Nazi Doctors*, p. 129.

45. Examples of physicians who joined the SA in 1933 are in Althen to NS-Ärztebund Hessen-Nassau, [Wiesbaden], August 20, 1934, HHSAW, 483/3159; Kötschau, "Fragebogen zur Erlangung der Verlobungsgenehmigung," n.d., BDC, SS Kötschau; Kaul, *Ärzte*, p. 86; Dicks, *Mass Murder*, p. 144.

46. See Blome, *Arzt*, pp. 265–66.

47. See Grote, "SA-Lager-Ärzte und Krankenkassen," Berlin, May 14, 1934, in *Deutsches Ärzteblatt* 64 (1934): 524; Althen to Wiesbaden NS-Ärztebund members, Wiesbaden, October 1, 1934, HHSAW, 483/3159.

48. Coermann and Wagner, *Ärzterecht*, pp. 67–68.

49. See Hocheisen to SA troop leaders, Munich, July 28, 1933, SAM, NSDAP, 27 (SA); Klinger, *Wege*, p. 45; Michaelis et al., *Kultur*, p. 267.

50. Kater, "Ansätze," pp. 807–8; memorandum Schwitzgebel, Neustadt/Haardt, April 19, 1934, GLAK, 465d/1419.

51. See the examples of Schlegel, Standartenarzt 1934 (*Deutsche Führerlexikon*, p. 416); Schenk, Gruppenarzt, and SA-Oberführer 1937 (*Ziel und Weg* 7 [1937]: 58); Bartels, SA-Brigadeführer 1938 (BDC, PK Bartels).

52. Some, like Kötschau, made the changeover in the midst of the prepurge turmoil, which, to insiders, was obvious for months. He left the SA in March to join the SS in April 1934 ("Fragebogen," as in n. 45, above). Others left for the SS shortly

after the purge. See the example of Ernst Fromm, BDC, RÄK and SS Fromm. Also see Dicks, *Mass Murder*, p. 144. For the example of Wiesbaden (NS-Ärztebund member) Dr. Carmsen who was contemptuous of the SA after the Röhm purge, see Ruckes to SA-Standarte 80, Wiesbaden, August 6, 1934, HHSAW, 483/3159.

53. See Klinger, *Wege*, p. 45.

54. One cannot say for certain whether the figure of 11 percent (Table 2.4, column F) represents an increase over that of 9.2 percent (column E) because of confidence interval fluctuations as explained in the first half of n. 4 (section 1).

55. Table 2 in Kater, "Hitlerjugend," p. 609.

56. SS formations did not include applicants, Sicherheitsdienst (SD), Verfügungstruppe, and Totenkopfverbände. Calculations on the basis of values in *Berufszählung, 16. Juni 1933*, pp. 48–51; *Statistisches Jahrbuch der Schutzstaffel der NSDAP 1938*, IfZ, Dc. 01.06 (pp. 103–5). Also see Kater, "Hitlerjugend," pp. 609–10. Veterinarians could not be separated from my calculations because they were included in the SS count.

57. Calculations as in the first part of n. 56. On the jurists in the SS, also see Boehnert, "Sociography," pp. 164, 168, 172–88; and idem, "Jurists."

58. Kater, "Verhältnis."

59. For an illumination of some of these aspects, see Müller, *Furchtbare Juristen*; Preuss, "Perversion"; Johe, *Justiz*; Gruchmann, *Justiz*; Staff, *Justiz*, esp. pp. 146–59; Ostler, *Rechtsanwälte*, pp. 239–80; Güstrow, *Strafverteidiger*. Cf. n. 25 of section 1; Jarausch, "Perils of Professionalism," p. 129.

60. Lifton, "Medicalized Killing in Auschwitz," p. 286; also idem, *Nazi Doctors*, pp. 447–51.

61. "Lebenslauf" Ebner, Kirchseeon, March 6, 1937, BDC, SS Ebner; Lilienthal, "*Lebensborn e.V.*," p. 45.

62. See Höhne, *Orden*; Stein, *Waffen-SS*; Wegner, *Soldaten*.

63. Personal papers Treite, BDC, SS and PK Treite; Stoeckel, *Erinnerungen*, p. 254. Vita Stoeckel is in Fischer, *Lexikon*, 2:1518.

64. See Stoeckel's rather naive account, *Erinnerungen*, p. 254. From the SS point of view, the induction was logical and predictable. See Wegner, *Soldaten*, esp. pp. 124–25, 275.

65. Vita Treite, Ravensbrück, March 29, 1944, BDC, PK Treite; Stoeckel, *Erinnerungen*, p. 254. Some of Treite's crimes are detailed in IfZ, NO-864; Buchmann, *Frauen im Konzentrationslager*, pp. 19, 27–29, 73, 78–79; 111, 114–16; Zörner et al., *Ravensbrück*, pp. 118–20, 135–36, 139, 160.

66. Letter J. P. Adams, Lord Chancellor's Department, London, England, to author, September 21, 1982.

67. Koehl, *Black Corps*, p. 109.

68. *Deutsches Ärzteblatt* 69 (1939): 422.

69. See the details in Gelwick, "Waffen-SS," pp. 110–13, 268, 386–91; Seidler, *Prostitution*, pp. 19–22.

70. Himmler, "Befehl für die Organisation des SS-Sanitätswesens der SS und Polizei," Feld-Kommandostelle, August 31, 1943, BDC, SS Karl Gebhardt. Also see Klein, *Amtsarzt*, 3:22; Gelwick, "Waffen-SS," pp. 110, 113, 129; Seidler, *Prostitution*, p. 22.

71. Stockhorst, *Köpfe*, p. 199.

72. Gelwick, "Waffen-SS," pp. 329, 387–88; *Der Freiwillige*, no. 5 (1967): 9–10.

73. On the general situation, see Gelwick, "Waffen-SS," pp. 387–91.

74. BDC, PÄ Boye.

75. BDC, PÄ Fischer. Quotation from Leitender Polizeiarzt, "Beurteilung des Herrn J. Fischer," Munich, January 10, 1938, ibid.

76. BDC, PÄ Wenzel.

77. BDC, SS Entress. Quotation from RuSHA assessment of Entress, Unna, April 16, 1940, ibid. Also see Kaul, *Ärzte*, pp. 88–89; Lifton, *Nazi Doctors*, pp. 261–63.

78. BDC, SS Mengele. Quotations are from Dr. Rudolf Schwarz, "Fragebogen!," Greiz, November 23, 1938; SS-Standortarzt Auschwitz, "Beurteilung des SS-Hauptsturmführers (R) Dr. Josef Mengele," Auschwitz, August 19, 1944, ibid. Also see Kaul, *Ärzte*, pp. 90–91; Zofka, "KZ-Arzt Josef Mengele."

79. See Brandenburg, *Geschichte*, pp. 127–85; Kater, "Jugendbewegung," pp. 155–72.

80. Cf. values in columns E and F of Table 2.4 with those in columns A–D. On Kondeyne, born in 1903, see *Deutsche Führerlexikon*, pp. 251–52; Stachura, *Nazi Youth*, p. 231.

81. Coermann and Wagner, *Ärzterecht*, p. 69.

82. Althen to HJ, Bann 80, [Wiesbaden], October 5, 1934, HHSAW, 483/3159.

83. See Kater, "'Gesundheitsführung,'" p. 373; and the following documents: *Deutsches Ärzteblatt* 65 (1935): 143–44; Marxer and Lutze, "Dienstleistung von SA-Ärzten in der Hitlerjugend," Munich, November 13, 1935, in ibid., p. 1200; *Bremer Nachrichten*, January 22, 1936. By 1939, writes Rüdiger plausibly, as formerly the highest-ranking female HJ leader, in her otherwise wholly tendentious and obfuscating tome, the number of HJ staffers again was down to five thousand (not least, perhaps, as a result of the unpopular directive of that year that HJ physicians refrain from smoking: *Hitler-Jugend*, pp. 191–213, esp. pp. 195, 201). On the parallel example of teachers serving in the HJ (7.5 percent of the profession by May 1, 1936), see Kater, "Hitlerjugend," pp. 602–6.

84. According to the RÄK records in the BDC described in n. 11 (section 1), 9.8 percent of all male physicians registering with RÄK during the Third Reich belonged to the NSKK before and after 1933. On the NSKK, see Krenzlin, "NSKK."; and Seidler, "Kraftfahrkorps."

85. Percentage according to RÄK records in BDC described in n. 11 of section 1. On the NSV, see Althaus, "Nationalsozialistische Volkswohlfahrt." The NSV's organizational linkage with the Reich health administration is touched upon in Kater, "'Gesundheitsführung,'" pp. 353, 355, 362–63, 369.

86. The exact rate is 2,891 out of 4,177, equaling 69.2 percent. According to the RÄK records in the BDC described in n. 11 of section 1. For a gender breakdown see Table 3.8.

3. Forms of Resistance

1. Bittner, "Widerstand," pp. 1531–32; Schadewaldt, *Hartmannbund*, pp. 131–44. Engelhardt and Schipperges, *Verbindungen*, p. 85, have minimized the gravity of Nazi medicinal crimes with their unsubstantiated claim that "the variegated spectrum of National Socialist commitment [by German physicians] was matched by a similarly marked spectrum of conservation and resistance." Also see Kater, "Burden," pp. 31–40.

2. My remarks are directed against recent historiographic attempts to qualify the phenomenon of "resistance" to the Third Reich by seeking to differentiate between degrees of potency of "planned" actions, coupled with an examination of the original intent of the "resisters." As far as I can see, neither part of the analysis has been done systematically, and the problem of a synchronous linkage between motivation and action has not been solved. Timothy W. Mason and Martin Broszat in particular have attributed various descriptive terms to Third Reich collective or individual activities marked by some form of unrest or another through the use of words such as *resistance*, *opposition*, *protest*, and their German equivalents, leading to semantic confusion rather than a matrix for logical differentiation. See Mason, "Arbeiteropposition"; Broszat, "Resistenz und Widerstand"; and my more detailed criticism of this in *Archiv für Sozialgeschichte* 23 (1983): 692, 696–97.

3. Quotation from *Ziel und Weg* 7 (1937): 357. Also see Grote, "Entwicklung," p. 340; Klein, *Amtsarzt*, 3:13; and text in Chapter 1, 2, near nn. 18–19, 24.

4. KVD-Amtsleiter Plauen to Rechtsabteilung, KVD Berlin, Plauen, May 16, 1935, UK, 200.

5. Baerwolf to Reich labor minister, Gotha, July 21, 1934, UK, 100. Full file of Baerwolf's case, ibid.

6. Case of Sch. (1943) in BA, R 18/1504. See esp. memorandum Krause, Lüneburg, May 10, 1943.

7. Herlitschka file (1943–44), DAÖW, 3996.

8. See Schumann and Werner, *Menschenrecht*, esp. pp. 56, 66–67, 141, 193–94, 428–30; Table 7, column J, in Kater, *Nazi Party*, pp. 252–53. Professor Lawrence D. Stokes, Dalhousie University, Halifax, Canada, kindly supplied me with the details regarding Dr. Wittern and co-inmates. Also see Stokes's article, "Schutzhaftlager." Computation of ratios is in line with the technique described in n. 10 (section 1), based on values in *Berufszählung, 16. Juni 1933*, pp. 48–51.

9. Exemplary for *Amtsarzt* situation: Hagen, *Auftrag*, pp. 130–34.

10. *Ziel und Weg* 3 (1933): 79; Karstedt, "Durchführung."

11. Grote to Reich labor ministry, Berlin, October 15, 1934, and other docs. (1934–35) in UK, 200.

12. Karstedt, "Durchführung," p. 179.

13. This lack of differentiation characterizes historiography in Nazi medicine undertaken in the left-leaning camp of mostly younger West German scholars, notwithstanding all the other merits of their work. See my remarks in "Burden," pp. 55–56. The case of an obviously non-Jewish socialist victim of the purges is appropriately mentioned in Leibfried, "Stationen der Abwehr," p. 169.

14. Quotation from *Ziel und Weg* 3 (1933): 133. Also see Mausbach and Mausbach-Bromberger, "Anmerkungen," pp. 220–21; Kudlien, "Widerstand," p. 213; Parlow, "Über einige Aspekte," p. 52; Kater, "Ärzte und Politik," pp. 36–37.

15. See cases of Drs. Laber and Fritz Benesch (1934–35) in UK, 207; also n. 44 in Chapter 1, 3.

16. Also included in this group was Georg Groscurth, who, as a lecturer in medicine at the University of Berlin, is dealt with in Chapter 4, 3, near n. 50.

17. Steude, "Gelbke," pp. 194–95. Details about the process of KPD neutralization in spring 1933 are in Repgen, "KPD-Verbot." Regarding the KPD's position on health matters in the Weimar Republic see Hahn, "Positionen."

18. Pechel, *Widerstand*, p. 87; Paul's testimony in Albrecht and Hartwig, *Ärzte*, pp. 138–39. The activities of Red Chapel have been notoriously neglected in Western, especially West German, historiography because it was not counted among the "legitimate" resistance groups. On Red Chapel's and other illegal communist activity in Germany see Mehringer, "KPD in Bayern," pp. 67–286; Mammach, "Kampf," pp. 338–54; Biernat and Kraushaar, *Schulze-Boysen/Harnack-Organisation*, pp. 116–18; Trepper, *Wahrheit*, pp. 87–276.

19. Paul's testimony in Albrecht and Hartwig, *Ärzte*, pp. 138, 140–43. On Paul and Küchenmeister, see Biernat and Kraushaar, *Schulze-Boysen/Harnack-Organisation*, pp. 116–18. Paul's subsequent history is interesting enough to warrant mention here. After playing a leading role in the post-1945 organization of the East German health system, she became a professor of medicine at the Medical Academy in Magdeburg (DDR) in 1958. While there, she aided in the prosecution of four medical students who had tried to help Hungarian revolutionary insurgents by upholding a trumped-up charge. In retrospect it appears that this professional had learned nothing from her own sad totalitarian experience. See testimony of then Düsseldorf medical student Hans-Berthold Neumann, one of the accused at Magdeburg, in *Ärztliche Mitteilungen* 46 (1961): 2025.

20. Kühn, "Mediziner," pp. 214–17. Werle's account, "Formen," pp. 53–58, is based on Kühn's unpublished East Berlin dissertation (1966).

21. Kühn, "Mediziner," pp. 227–32; Werle, "Formen," pp. 35–39.

22. Kühn, "Mediziner," pp. 239–48; Neubert, *Arztleben*, pp. 113–14; Werle, "Formen," pp. 58–62.

23. Kühn, "Mediziner," pp. 237–38.

24. Schumann and Werner, *Menschenrecht*, pp. 66–67; Mausbach and Mausbach-Bromberger, "Anmerkungen," p. 223.

25. Brugsch, *Arzt*, pp. 338–39.

26. Mausbach and Mausbach-Bromberger, "Anmerkungen," pp. 223. Also see Amann, "Antifaschistische Kampf."

27. Hochmuth and Meyer, *Streiflichter*, p. 202.

28. Grossmann, "Milieubedingungen," p. 468; Hetzer, "Augsburg," p. 182.

29. With a view to the German social elite, especially in World War II, I have expanded on this general theme in my book, *Nazi Party*, pp. 160–65. Also see Kershaw, "*Hitler Myth*," pp. 76, 85, 103, 161–66.

30. See Klee, "*Euthanasie*"; Platen-Hallermund, *Tötung*; Schmuhl, *Rassenhygiene*.

31. Platen-Hallermund, *Tötung*, pp. 64, 121–23; Herrmann, "Agitation," p. 239. Also note the example of Dr. Victor Mathes in Klee, "*Euthanasie*," p. 25; and of Dr. Gerstering in Schmidt, *Selektion*, pp. 51–53.

32. Examples are in Platen-Hallermund, *Tötung*, pp. 100, 122. Also see Klee, "*Euthanasie*," p. 274.

33. Herrmann, "Agitation," p. 239.

34. Hölzel to director [of Eglfing-Haar asylum], Schwarzsee, August 28, 1940, published in *Die Wandlung* 2 (1947): 267. A partial reprint is in Platen-Hallermund, *Tötung*, pp. 127–28; but see the reflective interpretation in ibid.

35. A telling example of this is in Zorn, *Stadt*, p. 68.

36. Stemming from the post–World War I French occupation of the Rhineland and Ruhr, during which the Paris government employed colonial troops, resulting in the phenomenon of "Rhineland bastards." See Marks, "Black Watch"; Pommerin, *Sterilisierung*. The example cited is from p. 59 of Pommerin.

37. Hagen to Hitler, Warsaw, December 7, 1942; Conti to Brandt, Berlin, March 31, 1943, BDC, PK Hagen. Also see Hagen, *Auftrag*, pp. 197–207.

38. Doc. (October 26, 1943) in Broszat et al., *Bayern*, p. 654.

39. Behrend-Rosenfeld, *Allein*, p. 56; Müller, *Geschichte*, p. 215; Stern, *Pillar of Fire*, pp. 145–46.

40. Entry for September 1935 in *Deutschland-Berichte* (1935), 2:1037; Brugsch, *Arzt*, pp. 294–95; Werle, "Formen," p. 97; Ophir and Wiesemann, *Gemeinden*, p. 483. Until autumn 1935, the nontreatment of German Jews by Nazi doctors was expressly forbidden. See Althen to members of Wiesbaden chapter, NS-Ärztebund, Wiesbaden, August 11, 1934, HHSAW, 483/3159.

41. See entry for April 10, 1936, in Stresau, *Jahr*, p. 125; Behrend-Rosenfeld, *Allein*, pp. 33–35, 43–44; Herrmann, "Agitation," p. 240; Hadda, "Als Arzt," pp. 232–33; Leuner, *Compassion*, p. 86; testimony of Brugsch in Albrecht and Hartwig, *Ärzte*, p. 185; Ophir and Wiesemann, *Gemeinden*, p. 298; Weisenborn, *Aufstand*, pp. 105–6.

42. Stern, *Pillar of Fire*, pp. 129–31; Lifton, *Nazi Doctors*, p. 231; *Globe and Mail* (Toronto), February 5, 1985.

43. Gebhard, *Strom*, p. 57; *Alltägliche Faschismus*, p. 79.

44. Entry for July–August 1934 in *Deutschland-Berichte* (1934), 1:292; Ruckes to SA-Standarte 80, Wiesbaden, August 6, 1934, HHSAW, 483/3159.

45. *Alltägliche Faschismus*, pp. 104, 107. For the relative frequency of jazz in the Third Reich, see Schäfer, *Bewusstsein*, pp. 129, 132–39. Jazz as a form of social protest against the Nazi regime (which Schäfer fails to see) is discussed in Peukert, *Volksgenossen*, pp. 197–201, 236–40.

46. Leber, *Gewissen*, p. 28.

47. Mann, *School*, pp. 12, 18.

48. The incident is related in entry for August 2, 1941, in Hassell, *Deutschland*, p. 193.

49. Doc. 10 (October 4, 1934) in Schadt, *Verfolgung*, pp. 109–10.

50. The story is sympathetically told in the chapter regarding Dr. Carlo Peltz, in Güstrow, *Strafverteidiger*, pp. 145–66. In a private conversation I had with them in Toronto in the fall of 1960, both Dr. and Mrs. Carlo Pietz upheld the "resistance"

version, claiming that Mrs. Pietz had stolen the court documents masquerading as a building maintenance person. Also see BDC, MF and RÄK Pietz.

51. Herrmann, "Agitation," p. 240.

52. Buchinger, *Marinearzt*, pp. 148, 164–68, 171–72, 174–75, 178–81, 184.

53. Niedermeyer, *Wahn*, pp. 276, 283–84, 407–37, 445–47.

54. On this score, Bittner's argument, "Widerstand," p. 1530, is basically valid. But he strains it by claiming that the German physicians' presence at the military front was the major reason why none of them participated in the July 20, 1944, anti-Hitler plot (ibid.). As was shown in Chapter 1, there were still enough doctors left in the Reich who could have done so.

55. See text in Chapter 1, 4, at n. 111.

56. See the examples in *Alltägliche Faschismus*, pp. 114–15, and, far less credible, in Senger, *Kaiserhofstrasse*, pp. 197, 200–204.

57. Büchner, *Pläne*, p. 73.

58. Testimony of Ahlson, Oslo, May 13, 1965, and other relevant documents in DAÖW, 3136.

59. Testimony of Graf Soltikow, May 16, 1975, in Blank, *Augenzeugenberichte*, p. 14.

4. The Problem of Motivation Reconsidered

1. This was said with a glance at the great surgeon Ferdinand Sauerbruch, whose own antiregime stance has been acknowledged in the earlier postwar literature, but, in view of more recent analyses, is now very doubtful. See entry for November 6, 1943, in Kardorff, *Aufzeichnungen*, p. 75; and Chapter 4, 2, at n. 93.

2. The situation of teachers is sketched in Kater, "Hitlerjugend"; and idem, "Elternschaft."

3. The protest is recorded as a fact by Kühn, "Mediziner," p. 232, but alluded to merely as a possibility in Werle, "Formen," p. 37.

4. Klare to Dr. B., Scheidegg, March 31, 1933, in Klare, *Briefe*, p. 71; "Der Leser hat das Wort," in *Ziel und Weg* 3 (1933): 546.

5. Quotation from Gütt, "Arzt," p. 81. Also in this vein see *Ziel und Weg* 5 (1935): 139; Blome, "Neuordnung," p. 3; Wagner, "Reichsärzteordnung," p. 3; Amende, "Arzt," pp. 56–57; Hellmann, "Landpraxis," pp. 369–70; and Otto Dittmann's remarks in *Ziel und Weg* 8 (1938): 108–9.

6. This last provision is mentioned by Ackermann, "Nachwuchs," p. 135.

7. Althen to Wortmann, [Wiesbaden], November 9, 1934, HHSAW, 483/3159.

8. Dr. Ideler and Dr. Sonnenberg, "In der Streitsache der praktischen Ärztin Dr. med. Hanna Donnerberg," [Berlin, September 30, 1938], UK, 130.118.02/4. On this general principle see Rebentisch, "Beurteilung," esp. p. 114.

9. See the typical advertisements in *Ziel und Weg* 3 (1933): 101, 173, 273.

10. Examples in ibid., pp. 205, 274, 311–12. Sometimes Nazi movement affiliation was circumscribed, through the use of the expression "the national attitude" (*die nationale Einstellung*), as in a Berlin ad of August 19, 1933, a facsimile of which is in Frankenthal, *Fluch*, p. 195.

11. *Ziel und Weg* 3 (1933): 28, 101, 173–74, 205, 273, 311, 353.

12. "Willi" to "Hans," Ruhrort, November 10, 1936, BA, R 56I/83.

13. Quotation from NSDAP-Gauleitung München-Oberbayern to Steinbrecher, Munich, June 26 and August 13, 1942, BDC, PK Sewering; text in Introduction at n. 17. Also see the positive party verdict on Dr. H.O. (Starnberg) in Ortsgruppenleiter Munich to NSDAP Kreisleitung, Munich, January 18, 1937, SAM, NSDAP/28 (SA). For the government, see case Dr. B. (1936–41) in Reich interior minister, memorandum, Berlin, December 1941, BA, R 18/2958.

14. See my remarks in *Nazi Party*, pp. 207–12, 223–28; and n. 29 in section 3.

15. Dr. A.E. to Wust, Murnau, July 7, 1933, SAM, NSDAP/84.

16. Cases of Drs. Hu., Hü., N., and R. (1935–43) in BA, R 18/5576. Under Himmler as new interior minister, Pfundtner was isolated at his post in November 1943 (Stockhorst, *Köpfe*, p. 323).

17. On the general difficulty of gauging multifaceted motivations for intraparty behavior, see Kater, *Nazi Party*, pp. 157–59.

18. Gross, "Revolution," p. 822. Also idem, "Flamme," p. 115. Less acerbic but no less serious is the chastising of fair-weather Nazi colleagues by Wilhelm Josenhans in *Ziel und Weg* 3 (1933): 157.

19. Quotation ascribed to Stolberg Dr. Theodor Kerten, as in Padover, *Experiment*, p. 97. Further see Althen to HJ, Bann 80, [Wiesbaden], October 5, 1934, HHSAW, 483/3159; *Ziel und Weg* 5 (1935): 337.

20. Quotation according to Platen-Hallermund, *Tötung*, p. 100; also see Brugsch, *Arzt*, pp. 292–93.

21. Hermann Radetzky's testimony in Albrecht and Hartwig, *Ärzte*, p. 219; case of Dr. Adolf Sotier in Friedrichs to Hauptamt Ordnungspolizei, Berlin, July 22, 1940, BDC, PÄ Sotier. Also see the case of Dr. Wilhelm Hagen, *Auftrag*, p. 146, who says he joined the party to protect himself as a formerly committed Social Democrat.

22. Bamm, *Menschen Zeit*, p. 149; Berger, "Einzelheiten," p. 82.

23. For the case of Sievers, see Kater, "*Ahnenerbe*," pp. 313–38; for that of Gerstein, see Friedländer, *Gerstein*.

24. Neubert's statement to that effect rings hollow, *Arztleben*, p. 87. His was the role of the picture-book opportunist: SPD-aligned in the Weimar Republic, a nominal Nazi in the Third Reich, and a communist fellow traveler in the post-1945 DDR.

25. As was claimed by several Nazi euthanasia doctors after World War II, according to Platen-Hallermund, *Tötung*, p. 122; and Klee, "*Euthanasie*," p. 273.

26. See Lifton, *Nazi Doctors*, pp. 384–414.

27. Senger, *Kaiserhofstrasse*, pp. 113–17. The gist of the episode has been repeated in Kudlien, "Widerstand," p. 215; Kudlien, "Ärzte als Helfer," pp. 221–22.

28. Senger, *Kaiserhofstrasse*, pp. 117–18.

29. RÄK membership card Hanf-Dressler and supporting docs., BDC, show only that he was an "applicant" (*Anwärter*) for NS-Ärztebund membership. Even if the doctor had been received into that organization, he would not have worn an SA or any other Nazi uniform. No doubt Senger was able to construe his sensationalist story for the 1980 publication of his book because Hanf-Dressler, who died in 1971 (Senger, *Kaiserhofstrasse*, p. 118), could not have protested against his version.

30. Focke to Conti, Rostock, July 8, 1943, BA, R 18/3810; and other docs. regarding Dr. L., ibid.

31. Hoff, *Erlebnis*, p. 342; doc. VIII/13C (October 6, 1945), in Stokes, *Kleinstadt*, pp. 848–49.

32. While Gauger was in the party, Thomalla worked out of the SS. See Klinger, *Wege*, p. 46; Gebhard, *Strom*, p. 55; *Deutsche Führerlexikon*, pp. 490–91; Stockhorst, *Köpfe*, p. 422. Gauger's party career is detailed in Cocks, *Psychotherapy*, passim.

33. Klee, "*Euthanasie*," pp. 216–18.

34. Aretin, *Krone*, pp. 295–96.

35. Klein, "SA-Terror," p. 52.

36. Klee, "*Euthanasie*," pp. 86–87.

37. Siegert, "Flossenbürg," pp. 470–71.

38. Lifton, *Nazi Doctors*, pp. 303–36. On Münch see Neumann, *Auschwitz*, pp. 120–21; *Nazi Medicine*, 1:243.

39. Thévoz et al., *Darstellung*, p. 188.

Chapter 3

1. Demographic Trends and Tendencies

1. On pre-1918 female medical students in the German Reich see Schönfeld, "Einstellung"; Jarausch, *Students*, pp. 110–12, 146; and Albisetti, "Fight."

2. In 1908–9 only 23 women graduated and were certified as doctors, but that number rose to 148 in 1913–14. See Huerkamp and Spree, "Arbeitsmarktstrategien," p. 109. Percentages for 1907 and 1925 are according to figures in Bridenthal and Koonz, "Beyond *Kinder, Küche, Kirche*," p. 64, n. 107. On the misogyny and closure see Kater, "Krisis des Frauenstudiums," pp. 217–18; idem, "Professionalization," pp. 686–88. Also see Eckelmann and Hoesch, "Ärztinnen," pp. 158–65.

3. See Kann, "Zahl, 1940," pp. 285; idem, "Zahl, 1942," p. 303.

4. This estimate falls between the value established for the Kater sample (16.7 percent) and that established for the Jarausch sample (18.5 percent) (see n. 6).

5. Kuhlo, "Zum Jahre 1944," p. 1.

6. This last percentage calculation according to an RÄK sample of 1,808 *N* selected randomly by Konrad H. Jarausch in the BDC and generously offered to me for statistical processing. In the case under discussion $N = 1{,}807, X^2 = 86.39, df = 1, P = 0.0001, C = 0.214$. With infinitesimal exceptions, the RÄK did not list full Jews who, as members of both sexes, could have been idle.

7. Column E of Table 3.1. Licensure figures for male and female medical students, 1922–32, are in Hadrich, "Voraussichtliche Angebot," p. 568.

8. *Die Ärztin* 15 (1939): 128.

9. That is the meaning of the differential index figure of 1.74 (approaching 2) in column D of Table 3.2. The values for 1939–45 are statistically not reliable because of low *N*: the combined frequency for males and females in column E is 4.

10. Dr. Grote and Dr. Sonnenberg, "In der Streitsache der praktischen Ärztin Dr. med. Margot Gressler . . . ," [Berlin, September 5, 1940], UK, 130/118.02/4.

11. Calculations are based on figures in Hadrich, "Zahl der Ärzte, 1935," p. 700; Kann, "Zahl, 1942," p. 303.

12. According to Kann, "Zahl, 1942," p. 303.

13. See text at n. 35 in section 4.

14. Cropp to Regierungspräsidenten et al., Berlin, September 5, 1941, BA, R 18/3764.

15. As in Table 3.2, the values for 1939–45 are statistically unreliable because of the low combined frequency of 4 (Table 3.3, column E).

16. The percentage values for male and female generalists in Table 3.4, column E (72.9 and 27.1 respectively), are statistically reliable because of a high combined frequency of 443 *N*.

17. *Ziel und Weg* 9 (1939): 88; Glöcker, "Bestand und Entwicklung," p. 45. The total percentage of newly established female specialists during 1938 was 8.4 (vis-à-vis male colleagues) (*Deutsches Ärzteblatt* 70 [1940]: 478).

18. *Deutsches Ärzteblatt* 67 (1937): 906; Hadrich, "Zahl, 1935," p. 700; *Die Ärztin* 15 (1939): 128; Kann, "Zahl, 1942," p. 303. See text near n. 19 in Chapter 1, 3.

19. See Wilhelm Josenhans in *Ziel und Weg* 3 (1933): 157; "Die Medizinerin," Reichsstudentenwerk, Mitteilungsblatt no. 2/39, Berlin-Charlottenburg, January 1939, ARW, II, 280. For the survival of the stereotype of pediatrics as a feminine medical specialty beyond 1945, see Rodnick, *Postwar Germans*, pp. 46–48; Paul and Stirn, "Versorgung," p. 196.

20. Figures according to Hadrich, "Zahl, 1935," p. 700; *Deutsches Ärzteblatt* 67 (1937): 906; ibid. 70 (1940): 478.

21. Hadrich, "Zahl, 1935," p. 700; *Deutsches Ärzteblatt* 67 (1937): 906.

22. Thimm, "Agnes Bluhm"; Just, "Agnes Bluhm und ihr Lebenswerk"; Bluhm, "Zur Frage"; Bluhm, *Aufgaben*, esp. pp. 72–98. Also see Romann, "Sondertagung," p. 306. Regarding eugenics and women, see Bock, *Zwangssterilisation*, esp. pp. 116–39.

23. Figures as indicated in n. 21. Urology was considered a male specialty by association: it was concerned mostly with the male urinary and reproductive organs. In 1971, the percentage of female urologists had increased to 1.0, from 0.3 in 1937. See *Deutsches Ärzteblatt* 67 (1937): 906; Paul and Stirn, "Versorgung," p. 196.

24. See the case histories of Edith Heischkel (history of medicine), BDC, Research Heischkel; Hildegard Schönberg (pathology), BDC, PK Schönberg; obituary for Schönberg in *Die Ärztin* 15 (1939): 201; Elisabeth Nau (forensic medicine), BDC, RÄK Nau; *Die Ärztin* 17 (1941): 271.

25. As in n. 21.

26. See text at n. 22, Chapter 1, 3.

27. Ungern-Sternberg, "Wert," p. 45; protocol Ruppin from Rittmarshausen camp, April 1, 1936, ARW, I, 80 g 581/2.

28. Kelchner, *Frau*, pp. 20–21; Geilen, "Ärztinnen-Fortbildungslehrgang." On Kelchner, see further below at n. 25 of section 2.

29. See the example of plastic surgeon Dr. Elfriede Scheel, born in 1903, who

received her specialty training in Paris ("Lebenslauf" and "R.u.S.-Fragebogen" Scheel, BDC, SS Paul Körner).

30. BDC, RÄK Essig and Geisler.

31. BDC, RÄK Bergk, Wermter, Daniel.

2. Marriage, Motherhood, and Militancy

1. Rissom, *Fritz Lenz*, pp. 58–60; Kater, "Frauen in der NS-Bewegung," pp. 202–3; Winkler, *Frauenarbeit*, pp. 28–37, 42–54; Klinksiek, *Frau im NS-Staat*; Pauwels, *Women*, pp. 11–48.

2. Advertisements in *Ziel und Weg* 3 (1933): 138, 312, 353, 545.

3. Hadrich, "Zahl, 1935," p. 700; *Deutsches Ärzteblatt* 67 (1937): 905–6; Kann, "Zahl, 1940," pp. 284–86; Kann, "Zahl, 1942," pp. 302–3.

4. Hadrich, "Zahl, 1935," p. 700; Kann, "Altersaufbau," p. 211; *Deutsches Ärzteblatt* 67 (1937): 905–6.

5. Kann, "Zahl, 1940," p. 286.

6. Dr. Ideler and Dr. Sonnenberg, "In der Streitsache der praktischen Ärztin Dr. med. Hanna Donnerberg [born 1895]," [September 30, 1938], UK, 130/118.02/4. In August 1937 the Nazi physicians' tabloid *Ziel und Weg* still spoke of "all the men" congregated on the occasion of the International Congress for Continuing Medical Education then held in Germany, although the accompanying photograph shows at least one woman in the crowd of delegates (*Ziel und Weg* 7 [1937]: 435).

7. Lölhöffel, "Ärztin in der Front," p. 267; Berger, *Kulturspiegel*, p. 137; Winkler, *Frauenarbeit*, p. 124.

8. Kann, "Zahl, 1942," p. 303.

9. Kelchner, *Frau*, p. 42; Ackermann, "Nachwuchs," p. 134; Klein, *Amtsarzt*, 3:13–14; Kirkpatrick, *Nazi Germany*, pp. 246–47; Pauwels, *Women*, p. 24.

10. Kirkpatrick, *Nazi Germany*, pp. 247–49; "Die Medizinerin," Reichsstudentenwerk, Mitteilungsblatt no. 2/39, Berlin-Charlottenburg, January 1939, ARW, II, 280. Also see Klein, *Amtsarzt*, 3:13–14. I could find no evidence for Claudia Koonz's undocumented claim that "married women physicians lost their right to practice [Koonz is suggesting permanently] and by 1935, women physicians . . . could no longer receive payments from the state-sponsored health-insurance system" (*Mothers*, p. 145. Also see p. 186).

11. Bartels, "Berufstätige Frau," quotation p. 16. On Bartels's background and typology, see sources in Chapter 2, 1, n. 33.

12. Haedenkamp, "Grundlagen," p. 561. On Haedenkamp's background, see Kater, "Burden," pp. 35–36.

13. *Ärzteblatt für Norddeutschland* 2 (1939): 588; Berger, *Kulturspiegel*, pp. 112–13; Bach to Huber, Berlin, November 18, 1939, BA, R 21/484. On Bach see further in Chapter 4, 2, near n. 6.

14. My calculation on the basis of the figures in Graetz-Menzel, "Über die rassenbiologische Wirkung," Table 10, p. 143.

15. Hadrich, "Lage," p. 160.

16. According to *Ziel und Weg* 7 (1937): 427.

17. According to McIntyre [Stephenson], "Women," p. 200. Also see her book,

Stephenson, *Women in Nazi Society*, p. 166. Albisetti's opposite conclusion (that women physicians were relatively infertile), in "Women Students," p. 35, was obviously arrived at out of context.

18. Examples in *Die Ärztin* 17 (1941): 32, 81, 271, 412, 466; ibid. 20 (1944): 22, 51.

19. For this official view, see Wolff, "Politische Erziehung."

20. Orlopp-Pleick, "Organisation," p. 32. Also see BDC, RÄK Orlopp-Pleick.

21. Röpke, "Ärztin im Reichsmütterdienst," p. 44.

22. Romann, "Ärztin," p. 8. Also see idem, "Sondertagung," p. 306. Romann was born in 1914. She joined the party in 1937 and received her licensure in 1939, by which date she was married (BDC, MF and RÄK Romann).

23. *Die Ärztin* 15 (1939): 124. Lölhöffel was born in 1896. She was licensed and married in 1923 and died of illness in 1941 (Szagunn, "Edith von Lölhöffel").

24. See Deicke-Busch, "BDM.-Ärztin und Elternhaus," p. 217; Kuhlo, "Zum Jahre 1944," p. 2.

25. Kelchner, *Frau*, esp. pp. 20–21, 30–31, 36, 40, 44, 46–47, quotation p. 42. See BDC, MF Kelchner.

26. See Eichhoff, "Nationalsozialistische Stimmen," cols. 1246–47; Dr. Lotte Kürzel's views as paraphrased in Berger, *Kulturspiegel*, p. 86.

27. Kelchner, "Ärztliche Berufstätigkeit."

28. Bluhm, *Aufgaben*, pp. 72–98; *Ziel und Weg* 6 (1936): 291.

29. See Kater, "Frauen in der NS-Bewegung," pp. 233–34.

30. For an example of how this argument was applied by male professionals of the Weimar Republic against women rivals, in particular women physicians and medical students, see Kater, "Krisis des Frauenstudiums," pp. 219–30; idem, "Professionalization," pp. 686–88.

31. Hoffa, "Frauenstudium," pp. 204–5.

32. Kirkpatrick, *Nazi Germany*, p. 247.

33. "Aufgaben der Ärztin," [Rittmarshausen, 1936], ARW, I, 80 g 581/1. Reverberations of this position are in Heidepriem, "Ärztinnenlehrgang," p. 1057.

34. See Chapter 1, 1, at n. 36.

35. Representative is the case of Dr. Herta Russ in Krems. See Russ to Reichsärzteführer, Krems, November 29, 1940, BA, R 18/3122.

36. Conti, "Rückschau und Ausblick," p. 1.

37. Entry for May 13, 1941, in *Tagebücher*, p. 637. For background see Winkler, *Frauenarbeit*, pp. 102–21.

38. [Conti], "Begründung," [Berlin, 1942], BA, R 18/5576.

39. BDC, RÄK Schwang and Wohlfeil.

40. Memorandum Unterabteilung IV B, Berlin, November 6, 1942, BA, R 18/2956 (also see Russ to Reichsärzteführer, Krems, November 29, 1940, BA, R 18/3122; *Die Ärztin* 15 [1939]: 129; "Merkblatt," [1938/39], BA, R 18/2956; Gütt, *Gesundheitsdienst*, p. 159); case of Dr. Annemarie Lachmann-Sossinka (1937–42), BDC, PÄ Sossinka.

41. Reichsgesundheitsführer, information 2/43, Berlin, December 20, 1943, BA, R 18/3766a. Quotation is from document dated March 25, 1943, partially cited in Rebentisch, "Beurteilung," p. 120.

42. Reichsgesundheitsführer, information 6/44, Berlin, April 25, 1944; information 8/44, Berlin, June 23, 1944, BA, R 18/3766a.

43. Chapter 1, 4, at n. 100; entries for July 25 and August 7, 1944, in Wolff-Mönckeberg, *Briefe*, pp. 121–23, 126; BDC, RÄK Jolles-Hahn.

44. Cases of cand. med. R.G. and cand. med. E.H. according to Reichsgesundheitsführer, information 12/44, Berlin, September 20, 1944, BA, R 18/3766a; quotation Bäuml, information 41, Munich, September 21, 1944, SAM, NSDAP/31.

45. Reichsgesundheitsführer, information 15/1944, Berlin, December 13, 1944, R 18/3766a.

3. University Students

1. Table 1 in Kater, "Krisis des Frauenstudiums," p. 208; Hadrich, "Das voraussichtliche Angebot," p. 568; Pauwels, *Women*, pp. 33, 41–42. Both Pauwels and Albisetti rightly stress the continuity, from the Weimar era, of the misogynist factor (see the latter's "Women Students"). As an example, Göttingen pathologist Georg Gruber put himself on record as addressing only the male students in his lectures (*Einführung*, pp. 33, 203, 219, 226, 244, 252–53).

2. Table 9 in Pauwels, *Women*, p. 150; "Tätigkeitsbericht der Fachschaft Kliniker für das Sommer-Semester 1937," Würzburg, June 17, 1937, ARW, IV, 1-31/10. In winter semester 1936–37 the Würzburg percentage had still been 18.2. Calculation based on name list, "Fachschaft: Kliniker [Würzburg] Winter-Semester 1936/37," ibid. On the interrelationship between type of university and Nazi controls see Kater, "Nationalsozialistische Machtergreifung," pp. 70–74. About Berlin, the political *Fachschaft* complained: "Students are difficult to coordinate because they are dispersed throughout the large metropolitan area" ("Berichte der einzelnen Fachschaftsleiter über die bisher geleistete Arbeit," [March 1936], ARW, I, 80 g 581/1). On similar problems in Düsseldorf, see Haag, "Krankenträgerausbildung," p. 415.

3. See text in section 2 at n. 9.

4. Table 9 in Pauwels, *Women*, p. 150.

5. *Reichsstudentenwerk: Kurzberichte, 1935*, p. [48]. Contrast this with the openly restrictive statement in Hoffmann (of Munich student services), "Richtlinien für die Stellungnahme," appended to letter Hoffmann to Stäbel, Munich, July 22, 1933, ARW, I, 6 p 154. Also see text in section 2 before n. 7.

6. Kater, "Krisis des Frauenstudiums," pp. 213–15; Pauwels, *Women*, pp. 41, 149 (Table 8); *Reichsstudentenwerk: Kurzberichte, 1938*, p. 26; "Die Medizinerin," Reichsstudentendenwerk, Mitteilungsblatt no. 2/39, Berlin-Charlottenburg, January 1939, ARW, II, 280.

7. Calculations are based on figures in *Statistisches Handbuch*, pp. 622–23. Also see the figures for women law students, 1932–39, in Table 9 of Pauwels, *Women*, p. 150.

8. *Reichsstudentenwerk: Bericht, 1941*, p. 29.

9. Ibid.; "Frauenstudium," appendix to *Ich Studiere*, p. 2.

10. Typically, see *Reichsstudentenwerk: Bericht, 1941*, pp. 30–33; *Reichsstudentenwerk: Kurzberichte, 1939*, pp. 15, 28; entry for July 1, 1943, in *Meldungen aus dem Reich*, 14:5416–17; also Kater, "Frauen in der NS-Bewegung," p. 236.

11. See Huber to Bach, Berlin, November 20, 1939, BA, R 21/484; Blome as quoted in *Deutsches Ärzteblatt* 70 (1940): 513; Conti, "Rückschau und Ausblick," p. 1; Dammer, "Frauenstudium und Ausleseprinzip im Kriege." Walter Stoeckel's claim that during the war Conti attempted to disallow female medical students defies the facts (*Erinnerungen*, p. 255).

12. Calculations based on figures in *Statistisches Handbuch*, pp. 622–23. Also see the representative values in *Reichsstudentenwerk: Bericht, 1941*, p. 67. In absolute figures, the onslaught of female secondary-school leavers on the medical faculties at the end of the regime still was overwhelming. In summer semester 1944 in Königsberg, a total of 180 girls applied, of whom only 56 were accepted after careful screening ("Dienstbesprechung der Dekane der Medizinischen Fakultäten in Halle am 28. Juli 1944," BA, R 21/476).

13. See below in Chapter 5.

14. See Klecker, "Frauenvorbildung und Frauenstudium"; Pauwels, *Women*, p. 96; and the trend signified by the figures in Lorenz, *Zehnjahres-Statistik*, 2:37. On Latin as immutable prerequisite see Diepgen, *Heilkunde*, p. 31.

15. These values were arrived at after analysis of RÄK data in the Kater sample (total *N*, 1918–45: 4,002).

16. As in n. 15.

17. Kater, "Medizinische Fakultäten," p. 97.

18. See the examples of "cand. med." mentioned in Reichsgesundheitsführer, information 12/44, Berlin, September 20, 1944, BA, R 18/3766a. Also see text after n. 43 in section 2.

19. For the latter observation, see Jarausch, *Students*, pp. 114–34. For Weimar, see Kater, *Studentenschaft*, esp. pp. 56–73, Table 2 on p. 208. In these and the following deliberations, the three social classes are defined, with slight variations, as for that table.

20. Columns G and H. Also see Pauwels, *Women*, p. 39; *Frankfurter Zeitung*, January 1, 1937.

21. Pauwels, *Women*, pp. 45–46; Table 2 in Kater, *Studentenschaft*, p. 208; *Deutsche Hochschulstatistik*, p. XII; Table 3.5, cols. G, H; Lorenz, *Zehnjahres-Statistik*, 1:372; Cron, "Studentin," pp. 249–50; Altstädter, "Sippe," pp. 242–43, 245. On women in the Great Depression, see Hausen, "Unemployment Also Hits Women."

22. Table 3.5, cols. A and B. Figures published in *Wirtschaftstaschenbuch für Ärzte*, p. 525, yield aggregate statistics to show that in summer semester of 1925, 33.1 percent of all female medical students in Germany hailed from the upper middle class, while only 31.0 percent of all male medical students did so. Figures published by Tornau, "Medizinstudium und Berufsüberfüllung," *Deutsches Ärzteblatt* 64 (1934): 1097, for winter semester 1933–34 may be interpreted to read that approximately 55 percent of all medical students (male and female) were lower middle class, and 42 percent were upper middle class. Using this statistic as a yardstick, one may carefully interpret the results of cross-tabulation of data in a university student (loan recipients only) sample, sex by class, 1933–45 ($N = 1979$; $X^2 = 12.654$; $df = 2$; $P = 0.002$; $C = 0.08$), which reveals that whereas 18.5 percent of the male medical students came from the upper middle class, 25.7 percent of the female ones did. The corresponding figures for the lower middle class are 71.2 percent males, 69.0 percent

females; for the lower class, 10.3 percent males, 5.2 percent females. Naturally, the proportion of the upper class was lower in both cases than indicated in Tornau's table because of the comparative indigence of the loan students. Cf. Altstädter, "Sippe," pp. 248, 250. Regarding the women students in this context, see *Reichsstudentenwerk: Kurzberichte, 1937*, pp. 16–17. Overall, see the qualifications regarding the loan-student sample in Chapter 5, 2, nn. 33, 42.

23. The actual values are: 14.9 percent of all female medical students' parents were white-collar workers, compared with 9.6 percent for the male students; nonacademic professionals, 7.5 percent female, 4.1 percent male; higher civil servants, 11.2 percent female, 8.1 percent male; farmers, 3.4 percent female, 7.4 percent male. Cross-tabulation of data in loan-student sample, sex by parental occupation, 1933–45 ($N = 1979$; $X^2 = 35.712$; $df = 12$; $P = 0.0001$; $C = 0.134$).

24. See text at n. 36 of Chapter 5, 2. For women students specifically, see "Frauenstudium," appended to *Ich studiere*, p. 2.

25. Table 3.6, cols. A, B.

26. Ibid., cols. C, D, E.

27. Result of breakdown analysis of total sample of 1,640 medical loan students, first-time political joiners (1,470 males; 170 females), 1933–45 (BA, loan-student sample).

28. Table 3.7 (col. C); and the figures in Table 7 of Arminger, "Involvement," p. 20. The percentage of 32.4 (58 *N*) in Table 3.7 (col. C) translates into 21.5 percent of total female medical students, politically nonorganized ones included. This figure rings true and is an additional criterion for the goodness of fit of the loan-student model, for at Würzburg in summer 1937, 25.6 percent of all female medical students had joined the ANSt. See "Tätigkeitsbericht der Fachschaft Kliniker für das Sommer-Semester 1937," Würzburg, June 17, 1937, ARW, IV, 1-31/10.

29. Table 3.7, col. E; Table 7 in Arminger, "Involvement," p. 20.

30. Table 3.7, cols. A, B.

31. Hauptamtsleiterin VI, Hauptamt für Studentinnen, Studentenschaft Marburg, to Wolff, Marburg, June 30, 1935, ARW, I, 11 g 218/3; Pauwels, *Women*, pp. 75, 89. See text below, after n. 34.

32. Romann, "Sondertagung," p. 309; Pauwels, *Women*, pp. 75–76, 109.

33. "Fünfte Verordnung zur Durchführung und Ergänzung der Reichsärzteordnung (Bestallungsordnung für Ärzte)," par. 5 (3), July 17, 1939, *Reichsgesetzblatt* (1939), I, 1274; memorandum Mentzel, Berlin, March 25, 1943; Rust, "Medizinische Studienordnung," Berlin, August 1, 1944, BA, R 21/484.

34. Wolff, "Bericht über das III. Reichslager"; Romann, "Sondertagung," p. 311; Braun, "Tätigkeitsbericht der Sachbearbeiterin Studentinnen der Fachgruppe Medizin WS 37/38," Würzburg, February 17, 1938, ARW, IV, 1-31/10.

35. Giles, *Students*, pp. 75–76, 189.

36. See the testimony of a participant in *Ziel und Weg* 5 (1935): 276; also "Semesterbericht der Fachschaft Vorkliniker [Würzburg], Sommer-Semester 1937," ARW, IV, 1-31/10; Pauwels, *Women*, p. 75.

37. "Berichte der einzelnen Fachschaftsleiter über die bisher geleistete Arbeit," [n.p., March 1936], ARW, I, 80 g 581/1; "Tätigkeitsbericht der Fachschaft Kliniker für das Sommer-Semester 1937," Würzburg, June 17, 1937, ARW, IV, 1-31/10. Also

see DFW, Abteilungsleiterin Berlin, circular F.W., April 1936, ARW, I, 80 g 581/1.

38. Romann, "Zweites Medizinerinnenlager in Kiel"; idem, "Die Sondertagung."

39. Rothe to Frick, [Berlin], November 26, 1935; "Medizinerinnenausbildung," [1936], ARW, I, g 581/1; memorandum Zschintzsch, Berlin, October 31, 1936, BA, R 21/485.

40. Reichsfachgruppe Medizin to Vowinkel, [Berlin], October 4, 1935, ARW, I, 80 g 581/2; Simon to Klein, Freiburg, June 18, 1934, ARW, I, 33 g 178/4; Hauptamt für Wissenschaft, Referentin für Medizinstudentinnen to Ruppert, Berlin, July 31, 1936, ARW, I, 11 g 218/2; "Tätigkeitsbericht der Fachschaft Kliniker für das Sommer-Semester 1937," Würzburg, June 17, 1937; "Tätigkeitsbericht der Sachbearbeiterin Studentinnen der Fachgruppe Medizin W.S. 37/38," Würzburg, February 17, 1938, ARW, IV, 1-31/10.

41. Evidently, cand. med. and Nazi party member (since May 1932) Elisabeth Vowinkel benefited professionally from her very active *Fachschaft* membership. See Reichsfachgruppe Medizin to Vowinkel, [Berlin], October 4, 1935, ARW, I, 80 g 581/2; "Personalfragebogen," Berlin, March 11, 1936, BDC, PK Vowinkel. For the voluntary character see Manthey, "Aus der Medizinischen Fachgruppenarbeit," p. 52.

42. As in n. 39; Wolff, "Bericht über das III. Reichslager," p. 163.

43. "Semesterbericht der Fachschaft Vorkliniker [Würzburg], Sommer-Semester 1937," ARW, IV, 1-31/10; Pauwels, *Women*, p. 75.

44. Manthey, "Aus der Medizinischen Fachgruppenarbeit," p. 52; Wolff, "Bericht über das III. Reichslager," p. 164; entry for November 24, 1939, in *Meldungen aus dem Reich*, III, 494.

45. Kortum to Isi, Bonn, October 1, 1936, ARW, I, 11 g 218/1; "Aufgaben der Ärztin," [1936], ARW, I, 80 g 581/1; "Tätigkeitsbericht der Sachbearbeiterin Studentinnen der Fachgruppe Medizin W.S. 37/38," Würzburg, February 17, 1938, ARW, IV, 1-31/10; Wolff, "Bericht über das III. Reichslager," p. 163; Romann, "Sondertagung," pp. 306–7.

46. Kortum to Isi, Bonn, October 1, 1936, ARW, I, 11 g 218/1; "Tätigkeitsbericht der Sachbearbeiterin Studentinnen der Fachgruppe Medizin W.S. 37/38," Würzburg, February 17, 1938, ARW, IV, 1-31/10; Kubach, *Studenten bauen auf*, pp. 55, 71; Romann, *Die Ärztin*," p. 9. Also see samples of competition entries in ARW, III, B; and, on the overall nature of the competition, Kater, "Reich Vocational Contest."

47. "Runderlass des Reichsministeriums des Innern," Berlin, January 1, 1940, BA, R 18/3764.

48. Klingelhöfer to Unterrichtsverwaltungen der Länder et al., Berlin, May 10, 1941, BA, R 21/484. This stipulation was somewhat modified later on in the war. See "Runderlass des Reichsministeriums des Innern," Berlin, March 25, 1943, BA, R 18/3764.

49. Luther, "Landdienst—Gesundheitsdienst"; Miedzinski, "Kriegseinsatz"; *Deutsches Ärzteblatt* 70 (1940): 43.

50. Corr. Stöckmann-Klingelhöfer, January–February 1942, BA, R 21/485.

51. Pauwels, *Women*, pp. 115–16 (quotation p. 116); Kalb, "Facheinsatz Ost 1940"; Siebert, "Studentinnen."

4. Medica Politica

1. *Die Ärztin* 12 (1936): 4; Baecker-Vowinkel, "8. Schulungslehrgang," p. 261.
2. Finkenrath, *Organisation*, p. 46.
3. *Die Ärztin* 12 (1936): 4. For background, see the articles in Hauer, *Paragraph 218*; Bridenthal and Koonz, "Beyond *Kinder, Küche, Kirche*," pp. 40–44; Frankenthal, *Dreifache Fluch*, pp. 117–19; Grossmann, "Abortion and Economic Crisis," pp. 67–72. Grossmann also points out, "Berliner Ärztinnen," pp. 186–87, 207–9, that in Berlin in 1930, a majority of BDÄ members was for abortion, under justified conditions.
4. "Liste der dem Deutschen Frauenwerk angeschlossenen Verbände, Stand vom 10.8.34," BA, Schumacher/230; Stephenson, *Nazi Organisation of Women*, p. 120; Kater, "Frauen in der NS-Bewegung," pp. 218–19.
5. Baecker-Vowinkel, "8. Schulungslehrgang," p. 261; BDC, MF Thimm. "Nazification" included the purging of Jewish members. For that process in Berlin, see entry for April 16, 1933, in *Tagebuch Nathorff*, p. 40; Grossmann, "Berliner Ärztinnen," pp. 211–12. Also see Koonz, *Mothers*, p. 144.
6. Orlopp-Pleick, "Organisation," pp. 30–31; BDC, RÄK Orlopp-Pleick.
7. *Die Ärztin* 12 (1936): 27–28.
8. See text in section 2, near nn. 9–10, 32.
9. Haedenkamp, "Grundlagen," p. 561; Stephenson, *Women in Nazi Society*, pp. 165–66.
10. *Die Ärztin* 12 (1936): 112; BDC, RÄK Sauer and Hoffmann.
11. BDC, RSK von Lölhöffel; Szagunn, "Edith von Lölhöffel."
12. *Die Ärztin* 12 (1936): 51; BDC, RÄK Schubert and Geilen.
13. Kater, "Frauen in der NS-Bewegung," pp. 233–34.
14. See esp. par. 46, and 87 (3) of "Reichsärzteordnung," December 13, 1935, BA, R 18/5574.
15. Thimm, "Alt-Rehse," p. 187; *Die Ärztin* 12 (1936): 228.
16. Baecker-Vowinkel, "8. Schulungslehrgang," p. 261.
17. Ibid.; *Ziel und Weg* 8 (1938): 630. See BDC, MF and RÄK Kuhlo.
18. *Deutsches Ärzteblatt* 69 (1939): 407.
19. *Die Ärztin* 19 (1943): 3.
20. See ibid. 17 (1941): 176, 407; *Ärzteblatt für Norddeutschland* 2 (1939): 463; Kuhlo, "Zum Jahre 1944."
21. In this category belong the defiant birth notices by women doctors (see text in section 2 at n. 18). In spring 1941 *Ärztin* editor Edith von Lölhöffel urged women colleagues to supply personal details for publication in the journal, "in order to strengthen unity among the professional comrades and to increase the knowledge about ourselves" (*Die Ärztin* 17 [1941]: 130).
22. 69.2 percent of physicians of both sexes were Nazi-organized (n. 86 of Chapter 2, 2).
23. Cols. D, E.
24. On this phenomenon see Kater, *Nazi Party*, pp. 152–53, 235; idem, "Quantifizierung," pp. 480–84; idem, "Frauen in der NS-Bewegung," pp. 234–36.
25. *Die Ärztin* 12 (1936): 27; Orlopp-Pleick, "Organisation," p. 32.

26. Table 3.8, col. F.

27. See text in Chapter 2, 4, at n. 6.

28. *Ziel und Weg* 3 (1933): 101, 173; *Deutsches Ärzteblatt* 70 (July 13, 1940): X–XII.

29. As in n. 8 of Chapter 2, 4; and BDC, NSF Donnerberg.

30. See text in section 1 near n. 10. The document mentioned in n. 10 speaks of no Nazi affiliation whatsoever, and in the BDC, personal records for Gressler could not be found (suggesting political abstinence at the 80 percent probability level. For this reckoning, see Kater, "Quantifizierung," p. 454, n. 4).

31. *Die Ärztin* 15 (1939): 201; BDC, MF and PK Schönberg. Also see text in section 1 at n. 24.

32. Russ to Reichsärzteführer, Krems, November 29, 1940, BA, R 18/3122. Russ joined the NSDAP in Korneuburg, Lower Danubia, on May 1, 1938 (BDC, MF Russ). It is not known whether Conti acceded to her request.

33. Kreisleiter Bad Soden to Amt für Volksgesundheit, Bad Soden, June 27, 1942, HHSAW, 483/191; BDC, RÄK Tries.

34. On the latter aspect, see "Die Medizinerin," Reichsstudentenwerk, Mitteilungsblatt no. 2/39, Berlin-Charlottenburg, January 1939, ARW, II, 280.

35. See Pauwels, *Women*, p. 139. Specifically, on the school physician (*Schulärztin*) see Drexel, "Über schulärztliche Arbeit"; on the work service physician (*Reichsarbeitsdienstärztin*) see Crome, "Gesundheitsdienst"; Mayr-Weber, "Aufgabe"; on the sports physician (*Sportärztin*) see Lölhöffel, "Frauensport und Frauentum"; Hoffmann, "Sportärztliche Arbeitsgebiet"; Szagunn, "Sportärztliche Erfahrungen"; *Die Ärztin* 12 (1936): 219–21; ibid. 15 (1939): 128; on the factory physician (*Betriebsärztin*; *Werksärztin*), see Stalherm, "Betriebsärztin"; Dohrmann, "Aus dem Arbeitsgebiet"; *Die Ärztin* 15 (1939): 130; Winkler, *Frauenarbeit*, p. 112; Golücke, *Schweinfurt*, p. 328.

36. Rüdiger, *Hitler-Jugend*, p. 191; Kohte, "Als Obergauärztin." Examples of both (a) *nebenamtlich* and (b) *hauptamtlich* active BDM women physicians are (a) Dr. Bertha Essig (born in 1894), Dr. Erika Geisler (born in 1914), Dr. Lore Heidepriem (born in 1896), Dr. Elisabeth Schindler (born in 1907); (b) Dr. Ursula Kuhlo (born in 1909), Dr. Hertha Ryll (born in 1913); see BDC, RÄK Essig, Geisler, Heidepriem, Schindler, Kuhlo, Ryll.

37. Rüdiger, *Hitler-Jugend*, p. 195; Kuhlo, "Gesundheitsdienst," p. 199.

38. Heidepriem, "Ärztinnenlehrgang"; *Die Ärztin* 12 (1936): 218; Bambach, "Wie wir Alt-Rehse erlebten"; Blome, *Arzt*, p. 304.

39. Deicke-Busch, "BDM.-Ärztin und Elternhaus"; idem, "Soforteinsatz von Feldscheren"; Geisler, "Ziel und Wege"; Kuhlo, "Gesundheitsdienst"; Bilz, "BDM.-Ärztin."

40. Panhuizen, "Wie mache ich." See the example of Dr. Elsbeth Nathow (born in 1905), a *Schulärztin* active in the HJ (BDC, RÄK Nathow).

41. Kater, "'Gesundheitsführung,'" esp. pp. 351, 353, 355–57.

42. See Orlopp-Pleick, "Organisation," p. 32; Röpke, "Mitarbeit."

43. Hellpap, "NSV."; idem, "Erholungspflege"; Röpke, "Ärztin im Reichsmütterdienst." See the examples of NSV collaborators Dr. Gertraud Bolle (born in 1908) and Dr. Grete Schöffl (born in 1911), BDC, RÄK Bolle and Schöffl.

44. Bluhm, *Aufgaben*, pp. 89–92; Soeken, "Rassenpolitische Erziehung."

45. Leiter, "Über bisherige Tätigkeit," p. 223. Also see Nau, "Tätigkeit."

46. Barbara König's testimony in Reich-Ranicki, *Schulzeit*, pp. 133–34. The Amt für "Rasse und Volksgesundheit," which the author mentions, most likely was the Rassenpolitisches Amt. See Johanny and Redelberger, *Volk, Partei, Reich*, p. 94.

47. Lilienthal, "*Lebensborn e.V.*," esp. p. 187.

48. BDC, MF Oberheuser; Buchmann, *Frauen von Ravensbrück*, pp. 75–79; *Über menschliches Mass*, p. 19; Zörner et al., *Ravensbrück*, p. 116; Gebhardt to Grawitz, Hohenlychen, August 29, 1942, BDC, Research Gebhardt; testimony of survivor Inga Madlung-Shelton in recorded interview with author, London, May 9, 1988. After the war, Oberheuser was tried by a West German court but required to serve merely seven years of a twenty-year sentence. See Kater, "Burden," p. 44.

Chapter 4

1. Infection of Medical Science with Nazi Ideology

1. McClelland, *State*, pp. 162-321; Jarausch, *Students*, pp. 144–46; Keller, "Dozenten der Medizin," p. 695. Percentage calculations according to figures in Modersohn, "Führerprinzip," p. 25. Also see Ferber, *Entwicklung*, pp. 59, 61–62, 67, 69; Bracher et al., *Machtergreifung*, p. 566. For the increase at one particular school, Giessen University, 1940–44, see Chroust, "Social Situation," p. 41. For the rector's elevated position in the Third Reich, see Seier, "Rektor als Führer"; doc. 95 of August 21, 1933, in Schneeberger, *Nachlese*, pp. 113–15. On the potential for influence by the party, see Kelly, "National Socialism."

2. This is obvious, not least, from the proposal of some Nazi scholars to establish new chairs in race science, first in the medical faculties, then in the natural-scientific and philosophical ones (Kranz, "Entwicklung," p. 287).

3. On this important connection, see the authoritative works of Mosse, in particular *Crisis of German Ideology* and *Toward the Final Solution*, pp. 150–237; and Pulzer, *Rise of Political Anti-Semitism*.

4. For Mosse, as in n. 3; Lifton, *Nazi Doctors*. Also see Lifton, "Medicalized Killing in Auschwitz"; and Kater, "Professionalization."

5. For instructive critical background reading on *Rassenkunde* or *Rassenhygiene* in the Third Reich see Saller, *Rassenlehre*; Lilienthal, "Zum Anteil." For the Wilhelmine period, Weiss, *Race Hygiene*, is useful.

6. See Mosse, *Germans and Jews*, esp. pp. 3–76; Rürup, *Emanzipation*, pp. 74–114; Mann, "Sozialbiologie," pp. 24–31; Gasman, *Scientific Origins*, esp. pp. 157–59; Bock, *Zwangssterilisation*, pp. 28–29; Lifton, *Nazi Doctors*, pp. 441–42; Fischer, *Lexikon*, 1:561–62.

7. *Wer ist's?* p. 1222; *Ziel und Weg* 6 (1936): 125; Mann, "Sozialbiologie," p. 31; Bock, *Zwangssterilisation*, pp. 29–31; Labisch and Tennstedt, *Weg*, 1:153–54. On Social Darwinism see Conrad-Martius, *Utopien*, pp. 124–93; and Zmarzlik, "Sozialdarwinismus."

8. Ploetz, *Tüchtigkeit*, esp. pp. 130–42 (quotation p. 133). See Weingart, "Eugenik," p. 322.

9. Mosse, *Crisis of German Ideology*, p. 99. Also see Conrad-Martius, *Utopien*, pp. 124–41.

10. As in n. 7 and Grober, "Lehrstühle für Rassenhygiene," p. 337; Mann, "Rassenhygiene," p. 82; Mann, "Sozialbiologie," p. 33; Weingart, "Eugenik," p. 326; text near n. 22 in Chapter 3, 1, and n. 22 itself. Also see Ploetz, *Tüchtigkeit*, passim.

11. Fischer, *Lexikon*, 2:836; *Wer ist's?* p. 913; Jakobi et al., *Aeskulap*, p. 121; Kater, "Hitler's Early Doctors," p. 40. On stereotypical German medical-colonial views of the African Negro see Sadji, *Bild*, pp. 154–73. On physicians' racism in Southwest Africa see Parlow, "Über einige kolonialistische," p. 540.

12. *Wer ist's?* p. 913; Labisch and Tennstedt, *Weg*, 1:166; Kater, "Hitler's Early Doctors," pp. 40–41.

13. Fischer, *Lexikon*, 2:1284; *Wer ist's?* p. 1285; Kater, "Hitler's Early Doctors," pp. 34–35, 41.

14. Fischer, *Lexikon*, 2:890; *Wer ist's?* p. 956; Krausnick, "Judenverfolgung," p. 301; Kater, "Hitler's Early Doctors," pp. 38–39; Lifton, *Nazi Doctors*, pp. 23–24.

15. Grober, "Lehrstühle für Rassenhygiene," p. 337; Müller, *Lehrbuch der Hygiene*, "Vorwort"; Rissom, *Fritz Lenz*, p. 72; Kater, "Hitler's Early Doctors," p. 40, n. 51; Schmuhl, *Rassenhygiene*, pp. 79–80.

16. Aly and Roth, *Restlose Erfassung*, p. 97.

17. Kater, "Hitler's Early Doctors," p. 43.

18. As an example, see Hitler's letter to Kuhn of June 6, 1935, in Jakobi et al., *Aeskulap*, pp. 127–28.

19. *Wer ist's?* p. 956.

20. Kuhn, "Universität," pp. 10–11; Grober, "Lehrstühle für Rassenhygiene." See also Rissom, *Fritz Lenz*, p. 72.

21. Examples are Aufklärungsamt für Bevölkerungspolitik und Rassenpflege, directed by Dr. Walter Gross (*Ziel und Weg* 3 [1933]: 352); Amt für Geneologische Rassenforschung, represented by Dr. Achim Gercke (ibid.); Arbeitsgemeinschaft 2 für Rassenhygiene und Rassenpolitik, directed by Professor Ernst Rüdin (Maerz, "Quelle," p. 90); Rassenpolitisches Amt der NSDAP, Zweigstelle Düsseldorf, directed by F. E. Haag (Jakobi et al., *Aeskulap*, p. 128).

22. According to Platen-Hallermund, *Tötung*, pp. 34–35. See Schultze, "Die Bedeutung der Rassenhygiene."

23. Müller, *Lehrbuch der Hygiene*, pp. 273–74. On Müller, see Fischer, *Lexikon*, 2:1086; *Wer ist's?* p. 1111. On a similar note, see Gruber, *Einführung*, p. 167; and Professor Kürten's remarks in *Deutsches Ärzteblatt* 64 (1934): 990. Historically, Müller was correct in pointing to the greater proclivity of Jews toward diabetes (because of consanguinity in ghetto environs). But it was the suggestion that Jews were more prone to be sick for chronic lack of hygiene, in juxtaposition with a blanket ruling on the superior health of Germans, which was offensive. Müller could have stated, for instance, that northern Europeans are known to suffer a propensity for cystic fibrosis. See Sigerist, *Man and Medicine*, p. 154; *Harrison's Principles*, pp. 314–15. Also see text in Chapter 6, 1, at n. 28.

24. Böttcher, "Wer ist Jude?" p. 98.

25. Lilienthal, "Rassenhygiene," p. 124; Adam, *Hochschule*, p. 172. Quotation is from Fischer's laudatio in *Bekenntnis*, p. 9. On Hoffmann see Fischer, *Lexikon*, 1:648.

26. *Wer ist's?* p. 1613; Jakobi et al., *Aeskulap*, p. 134; Maerz, "Quelle," p. 49; Bumke, *Erinnerungen*, p. 144; Ostrowski, "Schicksal," p. 330; Mersmann, "Ausbildung," p. 78. For an international reaction, see Bauer, "Gefährliche Schlagworte," col. 635.

27. Professor Dr. med. Fischer, born in 1874, was director of the Kaiser-Wilhelm-Institut for anthropology in Berlin but also had a chair at the university. More details on him in Conclusion at n. 58. Also see medical student Georg Wildführ's testimony in Albrecht and Hartwig, *Ärzte*, p. 337. Further see Benno Müller-Hill's revealing interview with Fischer's daughter, in *Tödliche Wissenschaft*, pp. 119–27.

28. Ebner, "Bestallungsordnung," p. 502; Lilienthal, "Rassenhygiene," p. 124; Jakobi et al., *Aeskulap*, p. 142. Also see Georg Wildführ's testimony in Albrecht and Hartwig, *Ärzte*, p. 338; and Chapter 5, 3, at n. 40.

29. A good survey is provided in Jakobi et al., *Aeskulap*, pp. 32–39.

30. Reiter, "Vorschläge zur Neugestaltung," p. 17; Linden to Rust, Berlin, February 14, 1938, BA, R 21/485.

31. Entry for first quarter 1939 in *Meldungen aus dem Reich*, 2:269, 271.

32. Memorandum de Crinis, [Berlin], n.d., BA, R 21/485; de Crinis's comment of July 28, 1944, in "Dienstbesprechung der Dekane der Medizinischen Fakultäten in Halle am 28. Juli 1944," BA, R 21/476.

33. An example of *Rassenkunde* in practice, though by a teacher not a physician, is in Richarz, *Leben*, p. 236. Teachers partook in special *Rassenkunde* training also provided for practicing physicians. See Jakobi et al., *Aeskulap*, p. 126; and *Ziel und Weg* 3 (1933): 352.

34. Klee, "*Euthanasie*," p. 44.

35. Verschuer to Conti, Frankfurt am Main, June 19, 1942; Fischer to Conti, Berlin-Dahlem, June 24, 1942; Lenz to Conti, Berlin-Zehlendorf, June 27, 1942, BA, R 18/3792. On Conti, see Mitscherlich and Mielke, *Medizin ohne Menschlichkeit*, pp. 191–92, 203–11; Klee, "*Euthanasie*," pp. 83, 87–88, 109–10, 163, 303–4, 352.

36. I have described this type in my article "Hitler's Early Doctors."

37. *Wer ist's?* pp. 877–78.

38. Bleuel and Klinnert, *Deutsche Studenten*, pp. 72–78; Selchow, *Hundert Tage*, pp. 323–38 (on Kranz see p. 330); Jakobi et al., *Aeskulap*, pp. 130–31; "Aktenmässige Darstellung des Ergebnisses der vom 15.–19. Juni 1920 vor dem Kriegsgericht der 22. Inf. Division stattgehabten Verhandlung gegen Angehörige des Marburger Studentenkorps," n.d., NA, T-253/23, 1474115-24.

39. *Wer ist's?* p. 878; Jakobi et al., *Aeskulap*, p. 131.

40. *Wer ist's?* p. 878; Jakobi et al., *Aeskulap*, p. 131.

41. *Wer ist's?* p. 878; Jakobi et al., *Aeskulap*, pp. 131–37.

42. Jakobi et al., *Aeskulap*, pp. 132–33. Regarding Jaschke's own exploits in race

hygienics, see ibid., pp. 20–21. Also see Fischer, *Lexikon*, 1:704; *Deutsche Führerlexikon*, p. 213.

43. Jakobi et al., *Aeskulap*, p. 140; *Ziel und Weg* 7 (1937): 161.

44. Jakobi et al., *Aeskulap*, pp. 142–44, 156; Kranz, "Entwicklung."

45. The suicide version is Müller-Hill's, in *Tödliche Wissenschaft*, p. 183. Jakobi et al., *Aeskulap*, p. 156, merely speak of his death while a fugitive. Kranz's war-criminal status is documented in UNANY, CROWCASS Central Registry File No. 40465.

46. Kranz, "Entwicklung," p. 287.

47. Ibid., pp. 288–89; Jakobi et al., *Aeskulap*, pp. 144–45. See esp. the medical dissertation in 1937 of Rolf Ludwig Martin, a butcher's son, on the relationship between race and crime. Martin concluded somewhat shakily that for Hesse, the Nordic type was least prone to commit crimes (*Rasse und Verbrechen*, esp. pp. 36–37).

48. *Deutsches Ärzteblatt* 69 (1939): 246–47; Jakobi et al., *Aeskulap*, pp. 146–49; Höss, *Kommandant in Auschwitz*, pp. 107–11; *Nazi Medicine*, 3:1–45; Müller-Hill, *Tödliche Wissenschaft*, pp. 59–65; Döring, *Zigeuner*; Zülch, *Auschwitz*; Hohmann, *Zigeuner*.

49. Aly and Roth, *Restlose Erfassung*, pp. 98–100.

50. Ibid., pp. 105–9; Jakobi et al., *Aeskulap*, pp. 150–56; Kranz, "*Gemeinschaftsunfähigen*"; Kranz and Koller, "*Gemeinschaftsunfähigen*."

51. Platen-Hallermund, *Tötung*, pp. 12, 31–32.

52. See Kater, "Hitler's Early Doctors," pp. 47–48, for the *völkisch* critique. For background to the crisis as far back as World War I, see idem, "Physicians in Crisis."

53. See text at n. 2 in Chapter 1, 3.

54. Liek was born in 1878. See Fischer, *Lexikon*, 2:915; Liek, *Arzt*; idem, *Gedanken eines Arztes*. Also see the Nazi obituary for Liek in *Ziel und Weg* 5 (1935): 61.

55. See text in Chapter 1, 3, after n. 1. Also see Reiter, "Revolution," p. 426; Kranz, "'Einkehr' und 'Umkehr,'" p. 38; Wagner, "Heilkunde," p. 420; Wagner, "Gesundes Leben," p. 549. The fiercest proponent of the Nazi holistic view, even beyond the war, was Karl Kötschau. See his "Nationalsozialistische Revolution," p. 293; his book *Umbruch*, esp. p. 40; and "Sinnforschung." Also Introduction at n. 16.

56. Reiter, "Ärzte," p. 1016; Wagner, "Heilkunde," p. 420; Kötschau, "Nationalsozialistische Revolution," pp. 293–94; Kötschau, *Umbruch*, e.g. p. 40; Klare, *Medizin*, pp. 15–16.

57. Feickert, *Studenten*, p. 34; Kötschau, *Umbruch*, p. 40; Blome, "Neue Deutsche Heilkunde," p. 250; Reiter, "Ärzte," p. 1016.

58. Reiter, "Revolution," p. 424; idem, "Ärzte," p. 1015; Klare to chief physician Dr. B., Scheidegg, March 31, 1933, and to chief physician Dr. K., Scheidegg, April 22, 1933, in Klare, *Briefe*, pp. 73–74, 117–18; *Ziel und Weg* 5 (1935): 15; Kranz, "'Einkehr' und 'Umkehr,'" pp. 38–39; Gross, "Revolution," pp. 820–21; Knoll, "Arzt," p. 439; Kötschau, *Umbruch*, p. 68.

59. See text near n. 2 in section 2.

60. *Neue Deutsche Heilkunde* (NDH), summarizing all the goals of the new organicist medicine in programmatic fashion and to be established "officially" in April 1936 under the partial headship of Karl Kötschau. See *Ziel und Weg* 6 (1936): 230; Marburg professor Schwenkenbecher's remarks, ibid. 6 (1936): 231–37; Kötschau, "Vorsorge." On the eventual fate of NDH and Kötschau see Haug's not wholly convincing article, "Lehrstuhl."

61. The mixture of aggression and readiness for compromise may be discerned from the rhetoric of Wagner and his aide Dr. Kurt Blome in Wagner, "Heilkunde," pp. 420–21; idem, "Gesundes Leben," pp. 549, 553; Wagner as quoted in *Ziel und Weg* 8 (1938): 425–26. Also see Gumpert, *Hunger*, p. 93; and the early supportive sentences of Wagner's patron Rudolf Hess (1933) in doc. 85, 2, in Wuttke-Groneberg, *Medizin*, p. 160, as well as Maerz, "Quelle," pp. 66–67; Blome, "Neue Deutsche Heilkunde," p. 250; Blome, "Neuordnung," pp. 3–4, 10; Blome, "Freiheit," p. 242.

62. Maerz, "Quelle," pp. 42–47, 55–56.

63. Blome, "Neuordnung," p. 10; Wagner, "Heilkunde," pp. 420–21; *Ziel und Weg* 6 (1936): 338. Also see Haug, "Rudolf-Hess-Krankenhaus."

64. Blome, "Neuordnung," pp. 8–9, *Ziel und Weg* 5 (1935): 256.

65. *Ziel und Weg* 8 (1938): 125.

66. *Deutsches Ärzteblatt* 64 (1934): 989.

67. *Ziel und Weg* 5 (1935): 256.

68. *Ziel und Weg* 7 (1937): 75; ibid. 8 (1938): 21.

69. Vezina, *Heidelberg*, p. 167.

70. Seifert, "Ausbildung." See Fischer, *Lexikon*, 2:1435; *Wer ist's?* p. 1486.

71. Borst, "Forschung und Fortbildung." See Fischer, *Lexikon*, 1:151.

72. Diepgen, *Heilkunde*, p. 22. For vita, Fischer, *Lexikon*, 1:315. For more on Diepgen's Nazi persona see Nabielek, "Anmerkungen"; Kater, "Burden," pp. 46–47.

73. As paraphrased in Haedenkamp, "Gesamtvorstände," p. 311.

74. Hoff, *Erlebnis*, p. 328; testimony of Georg Wildführ in Albrecht and Hartwig, *Ärzte*, p. 336. Also see Kater, "Medizinische Fakultäten," p. 92.

75. Büchner, *Pläne*, pp. 51–54, also p. 61. See Fischer, *Lexikon*, 1:193.

76. Aschoff, "93. Naturforscher-Versammlung," p. 1371. See Fischer, *Lexikon*, 1:44.

77. Karlson, "Versammlungen," p. 63; Ackerknecht, *Short History*, pp. 232, 242.

78. Brugsch, *Ganzheitsproblematik*. In particular, see "Vorwort," pp. V–VI. Vita in Fischer, *Lexikon*, 1:185.

79. Krehl, *Arzt*. Vita Krehl in Fischer, *Lexikon*, 2:818–19.

80. Hartmann, "Mut," p. 170. On Emil Karl Frey see Fischer, *Lexikon*, 1:448; on Erwin Payr, ibid., 2:1184–85.

81. Hoff, *Erlebnis*, pp. 386–87. On Bergmann, see Fischer, *Lexikon*, 1:101–2.

82. This list of would-be professors should not divert attention from such SS types as Waldemar Hoven in Buchenwald, who had their medical dissertations written for them by prisoner doctors. See anon. to Hoffmann, n.p., n.d., DAÖW, 957; and Kater, "*Ahnenerbe*," p. 238.

83. "SS-Stammkarte," BDC, SS Schenck.

84. "Ausführliches Gesamturteil," Munich, November 6, 1942, BDC, PK Schenck; BDC, MF Schenck.

85. Corr. Schenck, BDC, PK Schenck.

86. See Schenck, "Gesundheitshaus der Deutschen Ärzteschaft in Kempfenhausen," Munich, May 21, 1939; Schenck to Conti, Berlin, January 9, 1941 (including attached document), BA, R 18/3786. Also see Conti's introductory remarks in Schenck, *Grundlagen und Vorschriften*, p. 4.

87. As in n. 83, above.

88. Pohl to Himmler, Berlin, September 9, 1942, BDC, SS Pohl. See Schenck, *Grundlagen und Vorschriften*.

89. Himmler to Pohl, Feld-Kommandostelle, March 11, 1943; Pohl to Himmler, Berlin, December 22, 1943, BDC, Research HO 2070.

90. Quotation from Pohl to Himmler, Berlin, August 16, 1943, BDC, Research HO 2099. Maršalek, "Teuflische 'Initiative,'" pp. 50–51; Wuttke-Groneberg, "Leistung," p. 53. These authors maintain that numerous Mauthausen survivors were gassed.

91. In 1965 "Prof. Dr. med. habil., Dr. phil. nat." Schenck, without explaining his own role in the Nazi system of oppression, wrote a book, in which he—hypocritically, it would seem, for nowhere is the change from Saulus to Paulus documented—decried that "millions and millions of innocent and just people fell victim to the latest fire storm in human history" (Schenck, *Menschliche Elend*, "Einführung").

92. Potsdam RÄK file card Heissmeyer, BDC, RÄK Heissmeyer; Prokop and Stelzer, "Menschenexperimente," p. 76; Schwarberg, *SS-Arzt*, pp. 10–12, 122.

93. Schwarberg, *SS-Arzt*, p. 10.

94. "Auszug Urteil . . . In der Strafsache gegen . . . Kurt Heissmeyer," I. Strafsenat, Bezirksgericht Magdeburg, June 30, 1966, DAÖW, 4799.

95. Schwarberg, *SS-Arzt*, p. 30.

96. Ibid., pp. 30–55; Staatsanwalt Münzberg to Schwarz, Hamburg, August 24, 1967; "Gutachten des Sachverständigen Prof. Dr. Karl Kampfert," n.d., DAÖW, 4748. Heissmeyer, tried before a Magdeburg court in 1966, received a sentence of life in prison and died in August 1967 of heart failure (Schwarberg, *SS-Arzt*, pp. 123–24).

97. "SS-Stammkarte"; "Lebenslauf" Kremer, Münster, April 19, 1939, BDC, SS Kremer; "Dokument der Schande," p. 71.

98. Entries for October 3, 10, and 15, 1942, in Kremer's diary, reproduced in Langbein, *Wir haben es getan*, pp. 84, 86. Also ibid., p. 85.

99. Kremer's diary as partially printed in Langbein, *Wir haben es getan*, and Langbein's own commentary, pp. 94–100, quotations on pp. 95, 99. After May 1945 Kremer was delivered to Poland for trial and spent from 1947 to 1958 in the penitentiary. Back in Münster, the West Germans tried him again but succeeded merely in annulling his academic titles (ibid., p. 104). He died in June 1965 ("Dokument der Schande," p. 71).

100. The babies were boys, to impersonate for Himmler Rascher's natural sons. Rascher's wife could not have children, and the doctor knew that a successful SS career depended on male progeny. See Kater, "*Ahnenerbe*," pp. 101–2, 231–43; Mitscherlich and Mielke, *Medizin ohne Menschlichkeit*, pp. 20–71; Pueschel, *Seenotverbände*, pp. 104–10. Also see text in section 2 at n. 37.

101. "Sachbetreff" von Verschuer, September 1943, Kaiser-Wilhelm-Institut für Anthropologie, file no. Ver 1/05, BDC, Research Verschuer; Zofka, "Der KZ-Arzt

Josef Mengele," pp. 250–55; Gilbert, *Holocaust*, pp. 756, 687–88; Nyiszli, *Auschwitz*, esp. p. 54; Müller-Hill, *Tödliche Wissenschaft*, pp. 23, 71–75; Lifton, *Nazi Doctors*, pp. 337–83.

102. Lifton, *Nazi Doctors*, pp. 358, 378.

2. The Mechanics and Essence of Faculty Politicization

1. On Wirz see Fischer, *Lexikon*, 2:1697.

2. Memorandum Conti, Berlin, March 6, 1934, BDC, OPG Emil Ketterer; "Vollmacht" Hess, Munich, February 13, 1935, BDC, OPG Heinz Lohmann; *Deutsches Ärzteblatt* 64 (1934): 254–55, 1194–95; Kelly, "National Socialism," pp. 194–202; Giles, *Students*, pp. 157–58; Kater, "*Ahnenerbe*," pp. 135–36; Ellersdorfer, "Auswirkungen," p. 22. Wirz's influence is documented in Wirz to Gau-Gericht, Munich, January 21, 1936, BDC, OPG Heinz Lohmann; Luther, "Durchsetzung," pp. 120–21, 128–29.

3. *Wer ist's?* p. 1457; "Lebenslauf" Schultze, April 29, 1935, BDC, SS Schultze; Giles, *Students*, pp. 157–58; Maerz, "Quelle," pp. 61–62.

4. The chiefs of Amt Wissenschaft (Amt W) were, successively, mathematician Professor Theodor Vahlen (1934–37), Baden minister of state Dr. Otto Wacker (1937 to May 1939), and chemist Professor Rudolf Mentzel (after May 1939). See Kater, "*Ahnenerbe*," p. 136; *Wer ist's?* pp. 1057, 1639, 1665.

5. Kunisch to Wacker, [Berlin], December 21, 1937, BDC, Research Bach; *Wer ist's?* pp. 752–53; Heiber, *Walter Frank*, p. 808. Quotation from Jansen admirer Kötschau, *Umbruch*, p. 45. A sympathetic if subjective assessment of Janssen [sic] is in Büchner, *Pläne*, pp. 59–60.

6. Schultze to Rust, Munich, July 3, 1937; Wacker to Rust, Berlin, July 6, 1937; "Personalkarte" Bach; Mezger to Rust, Munich, February 19, 1938; "Vorschlag zur Ernennung" Bach, Berlin, March 15, 1938, BDC, Research Bach; BDC, RÄK Bach; "Lebenslauf" Bach, n.d., BDC, PK Bach; *Deutsches Ärzteblatt* 64 (1934): 989–90. Jansen evidently died of cancer in 1937 (Büchner, *Pläne*, p. 61).

7. Wagner to Wacker, Munich, November 24, 1937, BDC, PK Bach.

8. Bach to Reichinger, Berlin, May 2, 1938, BDC, PK Bach.

9. Quotation from anonymous memorandum, [fall 1937], BDC, Research Bach. Also see Schultze to Wacker, Munich, December 14, 1937, ibid.; and correspondence of Bach, 1937–38, ibid.

10. Zschintzsch to Bach, Berlin, September 7, 1939, BDC, Research Bach. Also see correspondence of Bach, ibid.

11. Partial protocol [Wacker] regarding the discussion of November 13, 1937, BDC, Research Bach.

12. See Stockhorst, *Köpfe*, p. 401; Kelly, "National Socialism," pp. 237–38.

13. Wagner, "Volksgesundheit," p. 139; par. 2 (2) of "Gesetz über die berufsmässige Ausübung der Heilkunde ohne Bestallung (Heilpraktikergesetz) vom 17. Februar 1939," in *Deutsches Ärzteblatt* 69 (1939): 151; ibid. 70 (1940): 15; "Erläuterungen zur Bestallungsordnung für Ärzte," [summer 1939], BA, R 18/3764. Also see the text in Chapter 1, 4, near n. 19.

14. The differences are explained in detail in Kater, "Doctor Leonardo Conti."

15. Schultze did not switch from the SA to SS until 1936. He was, above all, an enemy of Himmler's protégé Professor Walther Wüst, first a dean at and then rector of Schultze's stomping ground, the University of Munich. See "Stellungsnahme," Berlin, April 24, 1937; "Tätigkeitsliste" Schultze, Munich, March 4, 1940, BDC, SS Schultze; Kater, "*Ahnenerbe*," p. 280. Schultze was to leave the SD of the SS in early 1943 because Himmler was of the opinion that his membership there had been merely "nominal" for a long time (Himmler to Schultze, Feld-Kommandostelle, December 19, 1942, BDC, SS Schultze).

16. Generally, see Kater, "*Ahnenerbe*," pp. 130–39, 273–90.

17. De Crinis's appointment was effective on January 1, 1940, but because Rust's ministry this time around wanted a jurist, that is, a trained bureaucrat, to be formally in charge of the medical unit under Amtschef W, *Ministerialrat* Paul Klingelhöfer (deputizing for a conscripted superior) was the nominal head of the unit, even though de Crinis came to do all the work. See Mentzel to Amtschef Z, Berlin, December 13, 1939; and Rust to de Crinis, Berlin, December 27, 1939, BDC, Research de Crinis. In his scholarship, it goes without saying that de Crinis adhered to Nazi tenets. See Güse and Schmacke, *Psychiatrie*, pp. 316–19.

18. "Lebenslauf" de Crinis, n.d., BDC, SS de Crinis; BDC, RÄK de Crinis; Fischer, *Lexikon*, 1:276; Cocks, *Psychotherapy*, pp. 172–73.

19. See Hoff, *Erlebnis*, pp. 359–60; Forssmann, *Selbstversuch*, pp. 259–60.

20. Quotation from "Bestätigung" Rauter, Munich, October 9, 1934, BDC, SS de Crinis; and see de Crinis's vicious attack against Freud in his letter to Kummer, Berlin, April 17, 1942, BDC, PK de Crinis. Also Cocks, *Psychotherapy*, pp. 172–73.

21. "SS-Stammkarte" de Crinis, BDC, SS de Crinis. For the connection with Schellenberg, who took him to Holland in fall 1939 in preparation for the kidnapping of the Britons Major Stevens and Captain Best ("Venlo Incident") see Schellenberg, *Memoiren*, pp. 82–84.

22. Such a comment is made in two separate SS documents: "Personal-Bericht" de Crinis, [1940]; and memorandum Reichssicherheitshauptamt, Berlin, September 13, 1943, BDC, SS de Crinis. On de Crinis, Schellenberg and Himmler, also see Höhne, *Orden*, p. 528; Cocks, *Psychotherapy*, p. 214.

23. Memorandum Reichssicherheitshauptamt, Berlin, September 13, 1943, BDC, SS de Crinis. Also see Bethge, *Bonhoeffer*, p. 728.

24. See de Crinis's characteristic remark regarding Professor Schorre (Greifswald) in his memorandum dated Berlin, January 18, 1944, BDC, Research Rostock; and the determined manner in which he pursued the issues of a move by Professor Max Clara from Leipzig to Munich (1942) and by Professor Werner Catel from Leipzig to Vienna (1944–45): correspondence of Clara, BDC, PK de Crinis; correspondence of Catel, BDC, Research Catel.

25. See de Crinis's characteristic letter in matters regarding Professor Hoff, to Magnus, Berlin, February 17, 1942, BDC, PK Hoff.

26. De Crinis's extensive wartime correspondence with Bach is located in BDC, Research Bach.

27. De Crinis's pro-Nazi bias is obvious particularly in the case of the objection-

able surgeon Kurt Strauss, whose promotion he favored (de Crinis to Bach, Berlin, January 21, 1942, BDC, Research Bach; also see text below, near n. 56). Further see his letter, concerning Professor Wilhelm Trendelenburg, to Rostock, Berlin, July 10, 1942, BDC, Research Rostock. Significantly, de Crinis became criminally involved in the "euthanasia" killings (Klee, "*Euthanasie*," p. 227) and as a putative war criminal committed suicide in May 1945 (Müller-Hill, *Tödliche Wissenschaft*, p. 82).

28. Forssmann, *Selbstversuch*, p. 200. Forssmann's timing is faulty as well. He writes in 1938, but Conti was not appointed Reich health leader until 1939.

29. See Kater, "Doctor Leonardo Conti," pp. 308–25; Conti to Mentzel, Berlin, December 19, 1942; de Crinis to Conti, Berlin, January 12, 1943; memorandum de Crinis, Berlin, January 12 and February 6, 1943, BDC, OPG Emil Ketterer; "Tagesordnung für die Besprechung der Dekane der medizinischen Fakultäten Grossdeutschlands am 13. und 14. April 1943," BA, R 21/476; also see *Deutsches Ärzteblatt* 70 (1940): 96; Conti's public remarks of April 24, 1942, in *Deutsches Ärzteblatt* 72 (1942): 206. Conti, who taught a course in public health in the Berlin medical faculty as early as 1937 (*Ziel und Weg* 7 [1937]: 75), attempted in October 1943 to commission orthopedics professor Lothar Kreuz of the Charité to act as his delegate in matters concerning the medical faculties and thereby, presumably, countermand de Crinis's influence, but Kreuz shrewdly referred Conti back to de Crinis (Kreuz to Conti, Berlin, October 1, 1943, BA, R 18/3810). Henceforth Conti's influence remained relegated, as before, to junior and middling personnel in university institutes and clinics. See Conti, information 10/44, Berlin, August 3, 1944, BA, R 18/3766a.

30. As evidenced by the correspondence between the two men (1942–45), preserved in BDC, Research Rostock. Also see memorandum Conti, [Berlin], September 26, 1944, BA, R 18/3809. For personal details on Rostock, see BDC, RÄK Rostock.

31. Kater, "*Ahnenerbe*," pp. 99–100.

32. Memorandum Oberregierungsrat, Berlin, December 7, 1937; memorandum Kunisch, Berlin, December 9, 1937, BDC, Research Bach.

33. Fischer, *Lexikon*, 2:1389; "SS-Stammkarte" Schittenhelm (born in 1874); Brandt to Georgi, Berlin, December 12, 1934, BDC, SS Schittenhelm; Maerz, "Quelle," p. 96; Kater, "Medizinische Fakultäten," p. 87.

34. Fischer, *Lexikon*, 2:1203–4; "SS-Stammkarte" Pfannenstiel; Erbprinz zu Waldeck to Grawitz, Arolsen, December 16, 1936, BDC, SS Pfannenstiel.

35. Frank to Persönlicher Stab, RFSS, et al., Munich, June 2, 1939, BDC, SS Pfannenstiel.

36. "SS-Stammkarte" Pfannenstiel, BDC, SS Pfannenstiel; Rothfels, "Augenzeugenbericht"; Friedländer, *Gerstein*.

37. Sievers to Brandt, Berlin, March 27, 1941, NA, T-580, 154/248; Kater, "*Ahnenerbe*," p. 238.

38. Greiser to Greifelt, Posen, June 2, 1942, BDC, SS Holfelder; Kater, "'Gesundheitsführung,'" p. 363. Vita Holfelder in Fischer, *Lexikon*, 1:652.

39. "SS-Stammkarte" Freerksen; "SS-Personalveränderungsblatt," Berlin, June 21, 1944, BDC, SS Freerksen; "Teilnehmerliste der Dozentenführer an der Besprechung am 30. und 31.10.43 in München," BDC, PK Freerksen. See case of hygienist Professor Walter Blumenberg, born in 1895, Nazi Lecturers' League Gau representative in Breslau 1935 and *SS-Untersturmführer* 1937: "SS-Stammkarte" Blumenberg;

"Fragebogen" Blumenberg, Breslau, August 18, 1937, BDC, SS Blumenberg. Also see Kelly, "National Socialism," pp. 330–31, 338–39, 379. For a plastic example of a regional Lecturers' League leader's influence in medical appointments see Schwietzke to Berlin rector, Berlin, January 21, 1941, BDC, Research Hartmann.

40. Gebhardt to Himmler, Berlin, January 13, 1945; Himmler's letters to Karl [Wolff], Lammers, and Bormann, Feld-Kommandostelle, January 8, 1945, BDC, Research Rostock.

41. Fischer, *Lexikon*, 1:531; Voswinckel, *50 Jahre*, pp. 14–19, 22, 101.

42. Himmler to Grawitz, [Berlin], February 3, 1941, BDC, SS Fahrenkamp; Himmler to Grawitz, [Berlin], March 18, 1942, doc. 99b in Heiber, *Reichsführer*, pp. 106–7. In his letter to Grawitz, [Berlin], September 30, 1942, doc. 141b in Heiber, pp. 145–46, Himmler writes wryly: "I am sure that you, who has received the title of professor and, if I am not mistaken, likes to put it to use, would have a chance during these [human] experiments to make your scientific contribution and thus lay the fundament for this professorial title ex post facto." Also see Göring to NSDAP-Reichsleitung, Berlin, August 20, 1932; "Lebenslauf" Grawitz, Berlin, June 17, 1941; Rust's appointment letter, Berlin, December 22, 1941; "SS-Stammkarte" Grawitz, BDC, SS Grawitz.

43. Brugsch, *Arzt*, p. 296; Kater, "Hitler's Early Doctors," pp. 33–34, 46.

44. Mrugowsky was born in 1905; he joined the SS in 1931. See "SS-Stammkarte" Mrugowsky; "Lebenslauf" Mrugowsky; Genzken to Chef Personalamt Waffen-SS, Berlin, March 1, 1941; Grawitz, "Beförderungen in der Waffen-SS," Berlin, March 24, 1944; Mrugowsky to SS-Personalhauptamt, Berlin-Zehlendorf, October 14, 1944, BDC, SS Mrugowsky.

45. But Mrugowsky was eager to publish Auschwitz prisoner doctors' research under his own name (Lifton, *Nazi Doctors*, p. 305).

46. Memorandum Brandt, Führerhauptquartier, July 1942; Gebhardt to Grawitz, Hohenlychen, August 29, 1942, BDC, Research Gebhardt; Forssmann, *Selbstversuch*, p. 206; *Über menschliches Mass*, pp. 37–40; Zörner et al., *Ravensbrück*, pp. 127–28.

47. "SS-Stammkarte" Gebhardt; "Lebenslauf" Gebhardt, February 8, 1937; Gebhardt to Schmidt, Königswinter, July 22, 1937; "Fragebogen" Gebhardt, Hohenlychen, October 27, 1937; Schmidt to Gebhardt, Berlin, October 26, 1939; memorandum for Mentzel, June 29, 1943; von Herff to Gebhardt, Berlin, September 14, 1943, BDC, SS Gebhardt. The largely apologetic article on Gebhardt by Beckenbauer, "Der Arzt Dr. Karl Gebhardt," misinforms by dint of its unscholarly quality.

48. "Bestätigung" Rauter, Munich, May 7, 1934; "Lebenslauf" Hartmann, [1941], BDC, PK Hartmann (quotation).

49. See Sauerbruch's favorable evaluation of Hartmann's *Habilitation* thesis, undated, in BDC, Research Hartmann. Also see Sauerbruch's opinion as cited in letter of dean to rector, Berlin, August 7, 1936, ibid.; REM to Hartmann, Berlin, September 3, 1936, ibid.; and the documents mentioned in n. 99, below.

50. "Lebenslauf" Hartmann, [1941], BDC, PK Hartmann. Quotations assessment Binder 1934–35, BDC, SS Hartmann; Göttingen rector, "Leistungszeugnis," Göttingen, November 8, 1935, BDC, Research Hartmann.

51. Professor Rudolf Stich wrote cautiously: "My own assistant I would certainly

advise to go on proving his academic mettle with a few more studies. What factors may have caused Sauerbruch to propose the premature appointment . . . already at this time, in spite of the numerically very modest scholarly output, escapes me" (Stich to Scheer, Göttingen, March 1, 1941, BDC, Research Hartmann). Heidelberg Professor Martin Kirschner thought Hartmann's papers "fairly good" but joined Stich in his skepticism (Kirschner to Scheer, Heidelberg, March 10, 1941, ibid.). Also see dean to rector, Berlin, January 16, 1941; REM to Hartmann, Berlin, July 20, 1941, ibid.

52. See Holm to Rostock, Berlin, September 13, 1944, BDC, PK Hartmann.

53. "Lebenslauf" Madlener, [1941], BDC, PK Madlener; "SS-Stammkarte" Madlener, BDC, SS Madlener.

54. Among other services for the NSDAP, Strauss, born in 1901 and a Freikorps veteran, had assisted Conti in the pre-1933 establishment of the NSÄB in Berlin. See Kater, "Nazi Physicians' League," pp. 159, 161.

55. Forssmann, *Selbstversuch*, pp. 202–8, 211–12; Pross in Pross and Winau, *nicht misshandeln*, pp. 206–8. The friendships are further documented in Ley to Goebbels, Berlin, October 12, 1944, BDC, Research Strauss. While Forssmann credits Professor Wilhelm Baetzner with Strauss's *Habilitation* in 1933, Ley credits Sauerbruch in 1935. *Wer ist's?* p. 1571, appears to corroborate Ley's account.

56. Forssmann, *Selbstversuch*, p. 232; de Crinis to Bach, January 21, 1942; Bach to de Crinis, January 28, 1942, BDC, Research Bach; de Crinis to Krüger, [Berlin], October 30, 1942; Schellong to de Crinis, Münster, April 27, 1942; Ley to Goebbels, Berlin, October 12, 1944, BDC, Research Strauss.

57. Marrenbach to Norddeutsche Holz-Berufsgenossenschaft, November 8, 1944, BDC, Research Strauss; "SS-Stammkarte" Strauss, BDC, SS Strauss.

58. They included, among others, Dr. Otto Buchinger (dismissal as *Dozent* from Kolonialschule Witzenhausen), Dr. Georg Rost (dismissal as full professor of dermatology from Freiburg University), Dr. Georg Blessing (suspension and dismissal as full professor of oral medicine from Heidelberg University). See Buchinger, *Marinearzt*, p. 146; Hoffmann, *Ringen*, p. 21; *Wer ist's?* p. 1330; Vezina, *Heidelberg*, pp. 52–53.

59. Bumke, "Nichtordinarienproblem," p. 255.

60. Dr. Elfriede Paul's testimony in Albrecht and Hartwig, *Ärzte*, p. 137; Klinger, *Wege*, p. 71; Hoff, *Erlebnis*, p. 317; Nissen, *Blätter*, pp. 182–83; Zondek, *Fusse*, p. 162; Büchner, *Pläne*, p. 48. For Weimar, see Kater, "Nazi Physicians' League," p. 169.

61. See Pascher, "Universitäten," p. 54; Jakobi et al., *Aeskulap*, pp. 54–55, 63.

62. Adam, *Hochschule*, p. 38; Hoff, *Erlebnis*, p. 328; Büchner, *Pläne*, p. 55; Hoffmann, *Ringen*, pp. 27–30; Catel, *Leben*, p. 63. On Bickenbach, see Simon to Klein, Freiburg, June 18, 1934, ARW, 1:33 g 178/4; Mitscherlich and Mielke, *Medizin ohne Menschlichkeit*, pp. 169–73; and the apologetic article by former Nazi member (September 1939) Deneke, "Deutsche Wissenschaftler." On Hoffmann, see Fischer, *Lexikon*, 1:647.

63. Schadewaldt is speaking for Düsseldorf, which in the Third Reich was in no way different from other German medical schools (*Universität Düsseldorf*, p. 69).

64. Text in section 1 at n. 36.

65. *Wer ist's?* p. 911; *Ziel und Weg* 3 (1933): 352; Piechocki and Kaiser, "Gelehr-

tenschicksale," p. 383. According to the reliable *Wer ist's?* Kürten did not become a professor at Halle before moving to Munich in 1934, as reported by Piechocki and Kaiser, and repeated uncritically in my own article "Medizinische Fakultäten," p. 83.

66. BDC, RÄK Willy Usadel; *Wer ist's?* p. 1638; *Der Führer*, November 6, 1932; Adam, *Hochschule*, pp. 128–29 (quotation). On Georg Usadel, born in 1900, see *Wer ist's?* p. 1638; and Kater, *Nazi Party*, p. 187.

67. Jaspers, "Erinnerungen," p. 9; *Wer ist's?* p. 1542; Vezina, *Heidelberg*, p. 62; Drüll, *Gelehrtenlexikon*, pp. 150, 260; Dr. Hermann Weisert, Universitätsarchiv Heidelberg, to author, Heidelberg, February 9, 1987; "Gedächtnis-Feier für Ludolf Krehl am 18. Juni 1973"; and unidentified Heidelberg newspaper clipping, June 19, 1937, Universitätsarchiv Heidelberg. Stein joined the SS in May 1933 and the NSDAP in May 1937 (BDC, MF and SS Stein).

68. Adam, *Hochschule*, pp. 79–80.

69. *Die medizinische Welt*, October 7, 1933, p. 1448; *Wer ist's?* p. 715; Kater, "Nazi Physicians' League," p. 159.

70. BDC, PK Klare; Kater, "Nazi Physicians' League," pp. 157, 163; text in Chapter 2, 1, at n. 38.

71. *Ziel und Weg* 5 (1935): 27; ibid. 7 (1937): 181; BDC, RÄK Boehm; *Wer ist's?* p. 149; "Liste der Herren, die zur Abgabe von Voten besonders geeignet sind. (Medizin.)," n.d., BA, R 21/477; "Liste für Strassburg," Berlin, July 19, 1940, BA, R 21/476.

72. Quoted for March 8, 1944, in Steinert, *Krieg*, p. 441. Figures illustrating Nazi political affiliation for Reich medical faculty members, 1933–45, do not exist. For Giessen it is known that in this time span 42 percent of medical professors of all ranks, excluding the dismissed victims of the regime, were members of the NSDAP. But for Hamburg (and Tübingen) this figure appears to have been much higher. See Jakobi et al., *Aeskulap*, p. 62; Giles, *Students*, p. 161; Adam, *Hochschule*, p. 153.

73. See Chapter 2 above; Kater, *Nazi Party*, pp. 153–65.

74. Secret Councillor (*Geheimrat*) Professor Oswald Bumke was born in 1877. He became a full professor in 1914. See Fischer, *Lexikon*, 1:199; *Wer ist's?* p. 228; Bumke, *Erinnerungen*, p. 143; quotation from Bumke's introductory remarks as published in *Deutsche Zeitschrift für Nervenheilkunde* 135 (1935): 187–88.

75. *Wer ist's?* p. 1283; "Antrittsrede des Rektors am 4. November 1933," in Reinmöller, *Ins Dritte Reich*, pp. 3–5.

76. Bumke, "Staat und die Geisteskranken." For a qualification, see Lifton, *Nazi Doctors*, p. 26. Also see the very informative book by Cocks, *Psychotherapy*, passim; and Kater, "Burden," p. 46.

77. Güse and Schmacke, *Psychiatrie*, pp. 356–63.

78. Text above near n. 62; Hoffmann, *Ringen*.

79. See, for instance, Hoffmann, *Ringen*, pp. 13–14, 24.

80. Ibid., p. 14; *Völkischer Beobachter*, March 4, 1933. Regarding this pro-Hitler professorial declaration, see Faust, "Professoren für die NSDAP," pp. 41–42.

81. BDC, MF Forssmann; Forssmann, *Selbstversuch*, pp. 134–35, 156–57, 164, 212; cf. Forssmann, *Experiments on Myself*, pp. 125–27, 151, 157–61, 197.

82. BDC, RÄK Forssmann.

83. Bürger-Prinz, *Psychiater*; idem, "Die Frühdiagnose der Erbpsychosen" (1935),

reprinted as doc. 176 in Wuttke-Groneberg, *Medizin*, p. 301.

84. Bürger-Prinz, *Psychiater*, pp. 99–102; BDC, MF and RÄK Bürger-Prinz.

85. See the correspondence (1941–43) in BA, R 22/1193, esp. Sieverts to Kümmerlein, Hamburg, December 29, 1941. Also see "Jugendliche Cliquen und Banden," enclosed with Reich justice minister to Oberlandesgerichtspräsidenten, Berlin, June 10, 1944, BA, R 22/1177; Schmuhl, *Rassenhygiene*, pp. 229, 441 (n. 30); Roth and Aly, "Die Diskussion," p. 59, n. 1. More on Heinze in Klee, "*Euthanasie*," pp. 379–81.

86. Quotation from Bürger-Prinz to Rostock, Hamburg, November 16, 1943, BDC, PK Degkwitz; Bürger-Prinz to Rostock, Hamburg, January 11, 1944, BDC, Research Degkwitz. On Degkwitz's case, see section 3 near n. 59.

87. Assessment by Professor Ewald Stier of July 10, 1944, in "Personalnotizen," Hamburg, July 1944, BDC, PK Bürger-Prinz. Bürger-Prinz possessed his *Habilitation* since 1930. See his "Lebenslauf," ibid.

88. Hoff, *Erlebnis*, pp. 331–32, 355, 359–61, 378–82, 395–96.

89. Correspondence in BDC, PK Hoff.

90. Hoff, *Erlebnis*, pp. 328–29, 336.

91. "Lebenslauf" Hoff, n.d.; Kreisgeschäftsführer to NSDAP Amt für Volksgesundheit, n.p., January 15, 1937; Ortsgruppenleiter Würzburg-Ost to Kreisleitung Würzburg, Würzburg, June 14, 1940; Ortsgruppenleiter Würzburg-Ost, political evaluation of Hoff, Würzburg, January 12, 1937, BDC, PK Hoff; BDC, TF and RÄK Hoff. Also Zink, activities report of clinicians' *Fachschaft* for summer semester 1937, Würzburg, June 17, 1937, ARW, IV, 1-31/10 (on the significance of this, see text in Chapter 5, 2, near n. 6).

92. Ortsgruppenleiter Würzburg-Ost, political evaluation of Hoff, Würzburg, January 12, 1937, BDC, PK Hoff. Entrance into the NSDAP without a lengthy and personally signed application was impossible; as far as is known today, there were no exceptions. See Kater, *Nazi Party*, p. 365, n. 96.

93. All of this by Sauerbruch's own admission: see his (generally unreliable) memoirs, *Leben*, pp. 331, 366, 369, 374–93. On Sauerbruch's World War II exploits, also see Forssmann, *Selbstversuch*, p. 266. On Bier and Nazism, see Vogeler, *Bier*, p. 56. Essential vitae of Bier and Sauerbruch are in Fischer, *Lexikon*, 1:116, 2:1365–66.

94. See Sauerbruch's blank RÄK membership card, BDC, RÄK Sauerbruch; Nissen, *Blätter*, p. 182; Sauerbruch's address at the ninety-fourth convention of Gesellschaft Deutscher Naturforscher und Ärzte, Dresden, printed in *Mitteilungen der Gesellschaft Deutscher Naturforscher und Ärzte* 94 (1937): VI, XI; Gross, "Versammlung," pp. 540–42.

95. One example of many is Georg Wildführ's testimony in Albrecht and Hartwig, *Ärzte*, p. 359.

96. Sauerbruch's own account in *Leben*, pp. 380–85, in this case is plausibly corroborated by Stoeckel, *Erinnerungen*, p. 193. Sauerbruch's argument with the Nazi art historian Wilhelm Pinder has been reported by Hassell, entry for May 29, 1941, in *Deutschland*, p. 185.

97. See, among others, Sauerbruch's remarks in *Mitteilungen der Gesellschaft*

Deutscher Naturforscher und Ärzte 94 (1937): VI–XI; and in *Ziel und Weg* 9 (1939): 213–17; Zondek, *Fusse*, pp. 166–68.

98. See Sauerbruch's impassioned pleas, "Kameraden! Kollegen! Volksgenossen!" in *Bekenntnis*, p. 21 (also published in French and English); and "An die Ärzteschaft der Welt! Ein offener Brief Prof. Dr. E. F. Sauerbruchs," in *Die medizinische Welt*, October 7, 1933, p. 1447. An example of Nazi abuse is in Rühle, *Dritte Reich, 1933*, p. 157. Also see *Die Ärztin* 13 (1937): 165.

99. Sauerbruch to NS-Dozentenschaft, Berlin, June 21, 1935; Sauerbruch to Magnus, Berlin, December 23, 1935, BDC, Research Hartmann.

100. Hoffmann's otherwise authoritative account is too suggestive regarding Sauerbruch's factual complicity in the plot of July 20, 1944. Here it is based mostly on Sauerbruch's own reminiscences and on the book by Kramarz, which tends to be more cautious. Since Sauerbruch always exaggerated, one may take his post-1945 self-assessment concerning the July 1944 plot at face value: "complete innocence" (Sauerbruch, *Leben*, p. 391). See also ibid., pp. 372–74, 385–90; Hoffmann, *Widerstand*, pp. 377–78, 442, 445, 780, n. 75; and Kramarz, *Stauffenberg*, p. 132.

101. Kudlien and Andree, "Sauerbruch," p. 221.

3. Anti-Semitism, Resistance, and the Future of Medical Academia

1. See Hartshorne, *German Universities*, pp. 98–100; Table 22 in Ferber, *Entwicklung*, pp. 145–46; text in Chapter 6, 5, near n. 105. On physics, see Beyerchen, *Scientists under Hitler*.

2. *Völkischer Beobachter*, March 23, 1933; Wagner, "Rasse und Volksgesundheit," p. 152. Also see Böttcher, "Wer ist Jude?" p. 98.

3. See *Ziel und Weg* 3 (1933): 79–80; Rühle, *Dritte Reich, 1933*, pp. 112–13; Hartshorne, *German Universities*, pp. 175–76.

4. Hartshorne, *German Universities*, pp. 30–31; Ostrowski, "Schicksal," pp. 330–31. Kurt Klare came to enforce this law on behalf of Dr. Wagner, as far as medical journals were concerned. See *Wer ist's?* pp. 819–20; Klare to Hinkel, Scheidegg, March 10, 1939, BDC, PK Klare; Deneke and Sperber, *Jahre*, p. 82.

5. As an example see the edict for Baden of April 8, 1933, doc. 51 in Walk, *Sonderrecht*, p. 13. Also Carmon, "Impact," pp. 148–49.

6. Zondek, *Fusse*, pp. 163–65; *250 Jahre Charité*, p. 95; *List*, p. 71.

7. Krebs, "Wie ich," pp. 366, 368.

8. Jakobi et al., *Aeskulap*, pp. 48–49; *List*, p. 65.

9. On this see Kater, "Everyday Anti-Semitism."

10. Nückel to Conti, Berlin, March 9, 1933, BA, R 56I/100. Vita Liepmann in Fischer, *Lexikon*, 2:915–16.

11. Nissen, *Blätter*, p. 141. Pre-1933 vita in Fischer, *Lexikon*, 2:1121–22.

12. Example of anatomist Professor Johannes Sobotta in Bonn, as in Hoffmann, *Ringen*, p. 18; example of internist Theodor Brugsch in Berlin, as in Piechocki and Kaiser, "Gelehrtenschicksale," p. 385.

13. Lubarsch, *Gelehrtenleben*; Jaeckel, *Charité*, pp. 342, 348; Forssmann, *Selbstversuch*, p. 47; *Ziel und Weg* 5 (1935): 26. See the obituary in *Journal of the American*

Medical Association 100 (1933): 1554. Also Fischer, *Lexikon*, 2:945–46.

14. Hartshorne, *German Universities*, pp. 175–77.

15. *Meldungen aus dem Reich*, 2:110.

16. Klein, *Amtsarzt*, 3:16.

17. *List*, p. 74; Vezina, *Heidelberg*, pp. 117–18; Bürger-Prinz, *Psychiater*, pp. 67–68; Stern, *Pillar of Fire*, p. 158; Macrakis, "Wissenschaftsförderung," p. 373. On Rüdin, see *Deutsche Führerlexikon*, p. 397; Seidelman, "Mengele Medicus," pp. 222–24, 233. On Mayer-Gross, Fischer, *Lexikon*, 2:1011.

18. Fischer, *Lexikon*, 1:588; *Wer ist's?* p. 611; Piechocki and Kaiser, "Gelehrtenschicksale," p. 386.

19. Stoeckel, *Erinnerungen*, p. 225; Hoffmann, *Ringen*, pp. 19, 57; *Wer ist's?* p. 659; *250 Jahre Charité*, p. 93; Fischer, *Lexikon*, 1:211, 2:1036.

20. See *Journal of the American Medical Association* 100 (1933): 1783; Hoffmann, *Ringen*, p. 19; Julius Bauer's attack in "Gefährliche Schlagworte" and the Nazis' furious reaction in *Ziel und Weg* 5 (1935): 379, 453. Also see ibid. 3 (1933): 351–52.

21. As an example, Dr. Julius Citron, associate professor of internal medicine at Berlin University, went into private practice in Tel Aviv in 1934. See Fischer, *Lexikon*, 1:250–51; *List*, p. 67; *250 Jahre Charité*, p. 90.

22. Engelmann, *Deutschland*, p. 76; Krebs, "Wie ich," pp. 376–77; *List*, p. 61.

23. Drüll, *Gelehrtenlexikon*, pp. 174–75; Bürger-Prinz, *Psychiater*, p. 68; *List*, p. 74.

24. Krebs, "Wie ich," p. 376; Nissen, *Blätter*, p. 303.

25. See below in Chapter 6.

26. Nissen, *Blätter*, pp. 249, 254–55; Schönberg, "Geschichte," p. 75; Fischer, *Lexikon*, 2:1559; Drüll, *Gelehrtenlexikon*, p. 267; *List*, p. 71.

27. Fischer, *Lexikon*, 1:641; *Wer ist's?* p. 691; Hartshorne, *German Universities*, pp. 55–56; *List*, p. 81.

28. Fischer, *Lexikon*, 2:1038; Drüll, *Gelehrtenlexikon*, p. 180; Engelmann, *Deutschland*, p. 78; Krebs, "Wie ich," pp. 358–59.

29. Stoeckel, *Erinnerungen*, p. 225. Deservedly or not, Stoeckel takes credit for facilitating Meyer's transfer to America. See vita Meyer in Fischer, *Lexikon*, 2:1036.

30. Nissen, *Blätter*, pp. 256–309; Neumark, *Zuflucht am Bosporus*, esp. pp. 101, 105; *Wer ist's?* p. 737; *List*, pp. 65, 75, 84; Fischer, *Lexikon*, 1:222.

31. Examples are Alfred Storch (Giessen-Switzerland): Jakobi et al., *Aeskulap*, pp. 51–52; *List*, p. 74; Ferdinand Blumenthal (Berlin-Yugoslavia): *List*, p. 66; *250 Jahre Charité*, p. 90; Brugsch, *Arzt*, p. 122—Brugsch wrongly writes "Bulgaria."

32. BDC, RÄK Löning. See Fischer, *Lexikon*, 2:932.

33. Der Reichskommissar für die Wiedervereinigung Österreichs mit dem Deutschen Reich to Reichsminister des Innern, Vienna, January 24, 1940, DAÖW, 4101.

34. *250 Jahre Charité*, pp. 90, 95; Rosenstein, *Narben*, p. 206; Büchner, *Pläne*, p. 62. See Fischer, *Lexikon*, 1:205–6; 2:1214, 1527–28.

35. Hoffmann, *Ringen*, pp. 57, 178; Jakobi et al., *Aeskulap*, p. 49.

36. This figure is confirmed for 1938, in percent of faculty in 1931. See Ferber,

Entwicklung, p. 145. Also see Kümmel, "Ausschaltung," p. 77; Kater, "Medizinische Fakultäten," p. 83.

37. Schneider, "Widerstand," pp. 243–44. See Fischer, *Lexikon*, 1:445–46.

38. "Stellungnahme der Medizinischen Fakultät der Universität Heidelberg vom 5. April 1933," doc. 97 in Sauer, *Dokumente*, 1:118. See also Fischer, *Lexikon*, 2:1452; Vezina, *Heidelberg*, pp. 28–29, 78.

39. Schadewaldt, *Universität Düsseldorf*, p. 68.

40. Weitbrecht, *Psychiatrie*, pp. 21–23; Fischer, *Lexikon*, 1:545; Drüll, *Gelehrtenlexikon*, pp. 93–94. On Pohlisch, also see *Wer ist's?* pp. 1226–27. He was tried after the war but acquitted (Mitscherlich and Mielke, *Medizin ohne Menschlichkeit*, p. 289).

41. Bumke, *Erinnerungen*, p. 149.

42. Ibid.

43. Catel, *Leben*, pp. 63–65. Catel's account is questionable because till the end, he enjoyed an excellent relationship with de Crinis and his ministry. See BDC, Research Catel; also Kater, "Burden," pp. 45–46.

44. Kretschmer, *Gestalten*, pp. 150–59; idem, "Konstitutionslehre und Rassenhygiene," pp. 184, 185 (quotation); Fischer, *Lexikon*, 2:820; *Wer ist's?* p. 887; Cocks, *Psychotherapy*, esp. pp. 105, 108–9.

45. Schultz, *Lebensbilderbuch*, pp. 138–39; Cocks, *Psychotherapy*, pp. 115–16, 164–65 (Cocks alleges that Schultz may have wanted to join the party formations because his first wife had been Jewish); Fischer, *Lexikon*, 2:1418; *Wer ist's?* p. 1455.

46. Facsimile of Krause's suicide note dated Münster, May 7, 1934, published in Luther, "Durchsetzung," p. 114. Also see ibid., p. 113; Fischer, *Lexikon*, 2:817.

47. Luther, "Durchsetzung," pp. 113–31, quotation on p. 115. See the one-sided characterization in Hoffmann, *Ringen*, p. 31.

48. N. 20, above; quotation from Bauer, *Irrwege*, p. 46. See Fischer, *Lexikon*, 1:80.

49. See the telling examples in Weizsäcker, *Arzt*, p. 209; Gruber, *Einführung*, pp. 201–2; Krehl, *Arzt*, p. 44; Hoff, *Erlebnis*, pp. 317–18.

50. Schumann and Werner, *Menschenrecht*, pp. 193–94; Werle, "Formen," pp. 31–35; Kühn, "Mediziner," pp. 218–24. It is typical of the bigotry of East German historians like Kühn that they have elected to delete the name of Dr. Robert Havemann from the story of Groscurth because he ended up as a persecuted dissident in the DDR. By contrast, see Pross in Pross and Winau, *nicht misshandeln*, pp. 227–41.

51. Schumann and Werner, *Menschenrecht*, pp. 428–30; Biernat and Kraushaar, *Schulze-Boysen/Harnack-Organisation*, pp. 132–34; Werle, "Formen," pp. 39–41; Cocks, *Psychotherapy*, pp. 65–68, 165–68. See Rittmeister's article, "Augenblickliche Stand."

52. Nissen, *Blätter*, p. 68.

53. According to West German medical historians Johanna Bleker et al. in *Die Zeit*, November 6, 1987, p. 47.

54. See Büchner, *Pläne*, pp. 80–82, also pp. 55, 70–73; Platen-Hallermund, *Tötung*, p. 126; Pueschel, *Seenotverbände*, pp. 106–8. Rascher's remarks are not

contained in the published minutes of that meeting (for internal use only), but Büchner explains that they were not, formally, a part of the proceedings—for obvious reasons. See *Bericht über eine wissenschaftliche Besprechung*. Mitscherlich's and Mielke's initial charge that Büchner never put in a protest (*Diktat*, p. 42) was legally untenable and had to be changed to infer that no protest resulted at the actual convention (see their *Wissenschaft*, pp. 49–52, 280, 282–83, 285, 287–89, 291, 294; Büchner, *Grösse*, pp. 150–52). Hence Shirer was on shaky ground in claiming, as he did in the 1960s with regard to this convention, that "there were no questions put as to this and no protests therefore made" (*Rise and Fall*, p. 987, also see p. 979). In my own book, "*Ahnenerbe*," I adopted Shirer's unqualified verdict without scrutiny (p. 262).

55. Heubner to geschäftsführender Sekretär, Berlin, December 12, 1938, AAWG, Pers. 65/49. I owe my knowledge of this document to Professor H.-G. Herrlitz, Göttingen. Also see Fischer, *Lexikon*, 1:625; *Wer ist's?* p. 668–69, and, on Willstätter, born in 1872, p. 1735; Fischer, *Lexikon*, 2:1689. Willstätter's further fate under Nazism is not known.

56. Kühn, "Mediziner," p. 218.

57. Klinger, *Wege*, p. 36; Fischer, *Lexikon*, 2:1415.

58. Fischer, *Lexikon*, 2:828; *Wer ist's?* p. 896; Forssmann, *Selbstversuch*, p. 133; Ostrowski, "Schicksal," p. 337.

59. BDC, PK Degkwitz (1943); Oberreichsanwalt, "Anklageschrift," Berlin, [September 1943], BDC, Research Degkwitz; Hochmuth and Meyer, *Menschenrecht*, pp. 294–301; Giles, "University Government," p. 215; Werle, "Formen," pp. 42–52. Also see Kater, "Hitler's Early Doctors," p. 25; Fischer, *Lexikon*, 1:299.

60. Platen-Hallermund, *Tötung*, p. 126; Blasius, *Umgang mit Unheilbarem*, p. 112.

61. *Der Erbarzt*, no. 3 (1935): 41; Blasius, *Umgang mit Unheilbarem*, pp. 111–12; Bock, *Zwangssterilisation*, pp. 56, 192–93, 292; Bonhoeffer, "Rückblick." Cf. Lifton, *Nazi Doctors*, pp. 26, 81–82, 121. See Fischer, *Lexikon*, 1:145.

62. Fischer, *Lexikon*, 1:772; *Wer ist's?* p. 825; Platen-Hallermund, *Tötung*, p. 42; Klee, "*Euthanasie*," p. 47; Cocks, *Psychotherapy*, pp. 105–6; Lifton, *Nazi Doctors*, p. 39.

63. Büchner, *Grösse*, pp. 148–49; *Wer ist's?* p. 104.

64. Lifton, *Nazi Doctors*, p. 82; Fischer, *Lexikon*, 1:275.

65. Ewald was born in 1888 in Leipzig, studied in Erlangen and Heidelberg, and was *Assistenzarzt* at various universities. His *Habilitation* occurred in Erlangen in 1920. In 1923 he became an associate professor in Greifswald. After 1934 he was full professor in Göttingen. Fischer, *Lexikon*, 1:381; *Wer ist's?* p. 379. Also see Mitscherlich and Mielke, *Medizin ohne Menschlichkeit*, pp. 204, 287; Weitbrecht, *Psychiatrie*, p. 37; Dörner, "Nationalsozialismus," p. 143.

66. *Wer ist's?* p. 379; Lifton, *Nazi Doctors*, pp. 82–87, quotation on p. 85. Lifton's interpretation is supported by personnel files in BDC, PK Ewald. Also the sober evaluation by Klee, "*Euthanasie*," pp. 91, 223–26. On Strassburg, see de Crinis to Ewald, Berlin, November 10, 1944, BDC, Research Ewald.

67. See Stoeckel, *Erinnerungen*, p. 247; *Wer ist's?* p. 1448. Also see Groh to

Reich interior minister, Berlin, June 9, 1938, BA, R 21/485; Diepgen to Reich education minister, Berlin, June 30, 1938, BDC, Research Heischkel; entry for October in *Deutschland-Berichte* (1936), 3:1342; "Jahreslagebericht 1938" in *Meldungen aus dem Reich*, 2:110; Bumke, *Erinnerungen*, pp. 151–52.

68. See text in this chapter, section 1, at n. 31; memorandum Groh, Berlin, January 27, 1939, BA, R 21/485.

69. Thomas to Reich education minister, as well as appendix signed by Kleinschmidt, Leipzig, September 9, 1939; Chudoba to Bach, Bonn, November 21, 1939; Seifert to Bach, Würzburg, November 24, 1939, BA, R 21/484.

70. Seifert to Bach, Würzburg, November 24, 1939, BA, R 21/484; Schönberg, "Geschichte," pp. 87, 107; Büchner, *Pläne*, p. 79. As much as was possible, formerly dismissed non-Jewish instructors, as under the law of April 7, 1933, were reinstated. See the example of Otto Buchinger (*Deutsche Kolonialschule Witzenhausen*): Buchinger, *Marinearzt*, p. 147.

71. See Kater, "*Ahnenerbe*," pp. 285–86; entry for November 24, 1939, in *Meldungen aus dem Reich*, 3:493.

72. Memorandum Klingelhöfer for Scheer and de Crinis, Berlin, February 6, 1941, including appendix; memorandum for Schaller, Berlin, February 18, 1941, including appendix; appendix to letter Scheer to Streit, [Berlin], March 12, 1941, BA, R 21/476. Also see Aly, "Posener Tagebuch."

73. Memorandum for Schaller, Berlin, February 18, 1941, BA, R 21/476. Further correspondence regarding Strassburg (1940–41), ibid.

74. [Rostock] to Mentzel, Berlin, June 12, 1944, BDC, Research Rostock.

75. Memorandum, Berlin, September 10, 1940; memorandum for Breuer, Berlin, January 20, 1942; memorandum for Breuer, Berlin, July 7, 1942; memorandum Rostock for Breuer, Berlin, July 30, 1942; Klingelhöfer to Breuer, Berlin, June 30, 1942; memorandum, Berlin, June 23, 1944; memorandum Kuhnert, Berlin, July 12, 1944, BA, R 21/476. Regarding difficulties with the medical faculty of Prague, see [dean of Prague medical faculty] to Buntru, Prague, April 7, 1942, memorandum [de Crinis] for Kuhnert, Berlin, February 7, 1944, BA, R 21/476.

76. Memorandum Rostock for Breuer, Berlin, July 30, 1942, BA, R 21/476.

77. [Guertler], "Schweigen hiesse Verrat," Berlin, November 1939; memorandum Niedermayer, n.p., April 20, 1940, BA, R 43II/940b. Also see Seier, "Niveaukritik"; Kater, "Professoren und Studenten," p. 474; Popitz to Lammers et al., Berlin, June 1, 1940, BA, R 21/484.

78. See Schönberg, "Geschichte," p. 112; Hoff, *Erlebnis*, p. 355; example of casualty Professor Heinrich Lottig in *Deutsches Ärzteblatt* 71 (1941): 245; case of Dr. Paul Eduard Kyrle, Vienna (February 1941), DAÖW, 4100; case of Dr. Karl von Chiari, Vienna (March 1941), DAÖW, 4099; Stoeckel, *Erinnerungen*, pp. 247–49; Klee, "*Euthanasie*," p. 397 (regarding psychiatry).

79. Rostock to de Crinis, Berlin, July 9, 1942, BDC, Research Rostock; memorandum [de Crinis], [Berlin], n.d. [after 1939], BA, R 21/485; entry for August 27, 1942, in *Meldungen aus dem Reich*, 11:4141–42.

80. "Schnellbrief" Südhof, Berlin, September 18, 1942; Reich education minister to rectors et al., Berlin, December 14, 1942, BA, R 21/484.

81. Rostock to de Crinis, [Berlin], November 10, 1942, BDC, Research Rostock.

82. Entry for January 14, 1943, in *Meldungen aus dem Reich*, 12:4674; example of Schöne in Hoff, *Erlebnis*, p. 379; Stoeckel, *Erinnerungen*, pp. 253–54; example of Heilmeyer in Schönberg, "Geschichte," p. 24; example of consulting specialists in Seidler, *Prostitution*, pp. 50–51.

83. Those consequences are vividly described in Stoeckel, *Erinnerungen*, pp. 249–50. See memorandum for Berger, Berlin, November 5, 1943, BA, R 21/476; Rostock to Münster rector, Berlin, December 28, 1943; memorandum de Crinis for Kuhnert, Berlin, February 22, 1944, BDC, Research Rostock.

84. De Crinis to Kuhnert, Berlin, February 15, 1944, BA, R 21/477; Rostock to Berlin rector, February 19, 1944, BDC, Research Rostock. Vita Trendelenburg in Fischer, *Lexikon*, 2:1581.

85. Report [de Crinis], Berlin, April 11, 1944, BDC, Research Rostock. Vitae are in Fischer, *Lexikon*, 1:697, 2:1019.

86. Memorandum [de Crinis] for Frey, Berlin, June 12, 1944, BDC, Research Rostock. See Fischer, *Lexikon*, 1:369.

87. Rostock's observation according to "Dienstbesprechung der Dekane der Medizinischen Fakultäten in Halle am 28. Juli 1944," BA, R 21/476.

88. Memorandum [de Crinis], Berlin, February 5, 1943, BDC, Research Bach; de Crinis to Spectabilität, [Berlin], February 28, 1944, BA, R 21/477; Bergmann, *Rückschau*, p. 282; Schönberg, "Geschichte," pp. 23, 79.

89. Rostock to de Crinis, Berlin, September 13, 1944, BDC, Research Rostock.

90. See Hastings, *Overlord*, pp. 418–19; Abraham et al., "Historical Introduction," pp. 636–37, 657–61; Fleming, "Preface," in Fleming, *Penicillin*, pp. iv–v; Fleming, "History and Development," pp. 14–15; Chain, "Development," pp. 220–26; Macfarlane, *Howard Florey*, pp. 280–82, 284–85, 294–95, 304–6, 308–9, 327, 336, 358–59.

91. Research on penicillin had begun at Hoechst in 1942; by 1943 Hoechst was producing small quantities. By 1944, penicillin was available for "a limited number of patients." In March 1945 U.S. troops occupied the plant. Hobby, *Penicillin*, p. 208; and Bickel, *Rise up to Life*, pp. 295–98. Also *List*, p. 61; Engelmann, *Deutschland*, p. 75.

Chapter 5

1. The Development of the Medical Discipline in Peace and in War

1. Detailed background is in Kater, "Krisis des Frauenstudiums," Table 3, p. 214; idem, *Studentenschaft*, pp. 70–71, Table 4, p. 210–11; idem, "Physicians in Crisis." Also see Hadrich, "Voraussichtliche Angebot," p. 568.

2. Table 4 in Kater, *Studentenschaft*, pp. 210–22; Table 5.1 in this book.

3. The decline from summer semester 1934 to summer semester 1935 was from 23,028 to 19,974, according to Lorenz, *Zehnjahres-Statistik*, 1:152–53. For the other figures, see Tornau, "Medizinstudium und Berufsüberfüllung," *Deutsches Ärzteblatt* 64 (1934): 1201; *Ziel und Weg* 6 (1936): 649.

4. Dekanat medical faculty Marburg to Bach, Marburg, October 16, 1939, BA, R 21/484; Greifswald rector to Rust, February 2, 1940, BA, R 21/439.

5. [De Crinis] to Huber, Berlin, November 15, 1939, BA, R 21/484. The SD calculated 35 percent more medical students of all semesters for nine medical schools, from an enrollment at thirty universities open earlier (entry for November 8, 1939, in *Meldungen aus dem Reich*, 2:431). On the temporary closings, see de Crinis to Amtschef W, Berlin, September 15, 1939, BA, R 21/484.

6. Entry for February 2, 1940, in *Meldungen aus dem Reich*, 3:716–17. Also see entry for February 5, 1940, ibid., 726–27; entry for November 14, 1940, ibid., 5:1765; Erlangen rector to Bavarian ministry of education, Erlangen, January 16, 1940; Jena rector to Rust, Jena, February 8, 1940; Marburg rector to Rust, Marburg, February 12, 1940; Kiel rector to Rust, Kiel, February 14, 1940; memorandum Huber, Berlin, April 2, 1940, BA, R 21/439.

7. These results according to report of anon. SS-Sturmbannführer, n.p., January 10, 1944, BA, Schumacher/270, III. Also see entry for April 1, 1940, in *Meldungen aus dem Reich*, 4:942; and for March 25, 1941, in ibid., 6:2140; "Denkschrift an RFSS. Erziehernachwuchs 1942. Abgeschlossen 15.3.42," BA, NS 19 Neu/1531; Giles, *Students*, p. 283; Jakobi et al., *Aeskulap*, p. 68.

8. As in n. 7, but not Giles, and Jakobi et al.; but see text below at n. 21.

9. The latter connection becomes manifest after reading the memoirs of Güstrow, *Tödlicher Alltag*.

10. An updated version of "Reichsarbeitsdienstgesetz" of June 26, 1935, is in Schönfelder, *Deutsche Reichsgesetze*, section 18, pp. 1–4a. For the "Wehrgesetz" of May 21, 1935, see ibid., section 17a, pp. 1–8.

11. Winkler, "Frage," p. 278; Kreuser, "Erneuerung," p. 377; [Reich interior minister] to Rust, Berlin, January 29, 1936, BA, R 21/485; *Reichsstudentenwerk: Kurzberichte, 1938*, p. 16.

12. Tornau, "Schulzeitverkürzung"; *Ziel und Weg* 7 (1937): 125; Lottmann, "Ausbildungsdauer," p. 420; *Reichsstudentenwerk: Kurzberichte, 1938*, p. 16; Zschintzsch to Herren Vorsteher, Berlin, February 21, 1939, BA, R 21/485.

13. Bach to Schultze, [Berlin], November 15, 1939; Zschintzsch to Herren Rektoren, Berlin, October 25, 1940, BA, R 21/484; entries for November 22 and 29, 1939, in *Meldungen aus dem Reich*, 3:483, 507; Kater, "Medizinische Fakultäten," p. 99.

14. See the examples mentioned in Klee, *Was sie taten*, p. 114; Lifton, *Nazi Doctors*, pp. 103, 108. Regarding *Notapprobation* also see [Cropp?] to Bach, Berlin, November 2, 1939, BA, R 21/484.

15. Entry for October 25, 1939, in *Meldungen aus dem Reich*, 2:391; Rudolphi to Reichsfachgruppe Volksgesundheit, Berlin, October 23, 1939; dean of medical faculty Marburg to Bach, Marburg, October 16, 1939; [Cropp?] to Bach, Berlin, November 2, 1939, memorandum Herrmann for Huber, Berlin, November 22, 1939, BA, R 21/484; Leipzig rector to Rust, Leipzig, February 16, 1940, BA, R 21/439.

16. Case of Heinz Bello in Leber, *Gewissen*, pp. 25–26; Franze, *Studentenschaft*, p. 370; entry for June 4, 1942, in *Meldungen aus dem Reich*, 10:3794.

17. According to the reliable letter of anon. Wehrmacht *Stabsarzt*, appended to letter Meins to de Crinis, Berlin, May 13, 1942, BA, R 21/484.

18. Memorandum [de Crinis], Berlin, [after 1939], BA, R 21/485. Cf. the opinion of Prof. Wachholder (Rostock) expressed in "Tagung der Dekane der Medizinischen Fakultäten im Reichserziehungsministerium am 6. Mai," BDC, Research Rudolf Mentzel. The transfer tactic is also mentioned in entry of November 11, 1939, in *Meldungen aus dem Reich*, 2:431–32; and, especially in regard to law students, in the anonymous letter mentioned in n. 17.

19. Marburg dean of medicine to Bach, Marburg, October 16, 1939, BA, R 21/484.

20. [Cropp?] to Bach, Berlin, November 2, 1939; memorandum for Huber, Berlin, November 15, 1939, BA, R 21/484; Leipzig rector to Rust, Leipzig, February 16, 1940, BA, R 21/439.

21. Entry for December 12, 1939, in Boelcke, *Kriegspropaganda*, p. 241.

22. Entry for February 5, 1940, in *Meldungen aus dem Reich*, 3:726; Himmler to Heydrich, Berlin, December 9, 1939, doc. 55 in Heiber, *Reichsführer*, p. 69.

23. See Melior to Regierungen der Hochschulländer et al., Berlin, September 27, 1940, BA, R 18/3764; entry for June 4, 1942, in *Meldungen aus dem Reich*, 10:3794; Kurt Steude's testimony in Albrecht and Hartwig, *Ärzte*, p. 439.

24. Cropp to Vorsitzenden der Ausschüsse für die ärztliche Prüfung, Berlin, February 11, 1942, BA, R 18/3764.

25. Cropp to Herren Vorsitzenden der Ausschüsse, Berlin, July 2, 1943, BA, R 18/3764. Also see "Merkblatt" Diepgen, Berlin, July 9, 1943, BA, R 21/484.

26. [De Crinis], "Bericht über die Beratung zwecks Unterbringung der Charité und der Universitätskliniken," Berlin, August 27, 1943, BA, R 21/476.

27. Schultze's remarks, "Dienstbesprechung der Dekane der Medizinischen Fakultäten in Halle am 28. Juli 1944," BA, R 21/476.

28. Ebner, "Bestallungsordnung," p. 502; Diepgen, *Heilkunde*, p. 269; Mersmann, "Ausbildung," pp. 86, 98, 118–19. The complex evolution of *medizinische Studienordnung* is described in Opitz, *Bestallungsordnung*, pp. 1–7. For a more thorough, critical treatment from a modern perspective see Claudia Huerkamp's enlightening volume, *Aufstieg der Ärzte*.

29. Ebner, "Bestallungsordnung"; Kreuser, "Erneuerung"; Lottmann, "Ausbildungsdauer," pp. 418, 420; text in Chapter 1, 2, near n. 22, section 4, near n. 1. The *Bestallungsordnung* is printed in Opitz, *Bestallungsordnung*, pp. 7–40. According to this ordinance, some of the Latin-based terminology was changed to make it sound more German. The traditional *Physikum* was altered to *ärztliche Vorprüfung*, and *Approbation* (licensure) was changed to *Bestallung*.

30. "Studien- und Bestallungsordnung für Ärzte," effective April 1, 1939, BA, R 18/3764. See *Deutsches Ärzteblatt* 69 (1939): 78–79; "Fünfte Verordnung zur Durchführung und Ergänzung der Reichsärzteordnung," July 17, 1939, *Reichsgesetzblatt* (1939), I, 1273–89; Bestvater, "Gedanken und Anregungen."

31. "Erläuterungen zur Bestallungsordnung für Ärzte," [summer 1939], BA, R 18/3764; Ramm, *Standeskunde*, p. 37; Klein, *Amtsarzt*, 9:16.

32. Ramm, *Standeskunde*, p. 35; text above at n. 23.

33. Cropp to Regierungen der Hochschulländer et al., Berlin, November 7, 1940, BA, R 18/3764; Klingelhöfer to Unterrichtsverwaltungen der Länder et al., Berlin, May 10, 1941, BA, R 21/484. See Mersmann, "Ausbildung," p. 120, who points out

that the 1940 summer trimester was to serve merely practical training purposes to offset this effect.

34. "Ärztliche Vorprüfung," May 24, 1943, BA, R 18/3764.

35. "Bestallungsordnung," Berlin, January 26, 1944, BA, R 18/3764.

36. Conti to Reichsstatthalter der Reichsgaue et al., Berlin, November 22, 1944, BA, 18/3764.

37. See Gruber, *Einführung*, pp. 125–26; Wagner's remarks at Weimar on May 24, 1934, in *Deutsches Ärzteblatt* 64 (1934): 587; Vahlen to Universitätskurator et al., Berlin, December 1934, BA, R 21/485; Winkler, "Frage"; Ebner, "Bestallungsordnung," p. 502; Haag, "Krankenträgerausbildung," p. 416; Zschintzsch to Herren Vorsteher et al., Berlin, February 21, 1939, BA, R 21/485; "Erläuterungen zur Bestallungsordnung für Ärzte," [summer 1939], BA, R 18/3764.

38. Ebner, "Bestallungsordnung," p. 502; *Deutsches Ärzteblatt* 69 (1939): 79; "Erläuterungen zur Bestallungsordnung für Ärzte," [summer 1939], BA, R 18/3764; Ramm, *Standeskunde*, pp. 34–35; "Studien- und Bestallungsordnung für Ärzte," effective April 1, 1939, BA, R 18/3764; "Medizinische Studienordnung," effective October 1, 1944, BA, R 21/484. Also see text in section 3 after n. 39.

39. Zschintzsch to Herren Vorsteher et al., Berlin, February 21, 1939, BA, R 21/485; "Studien- und Bestallungsordnung für Ärzte," effective April 1, 1939, BA, R 21/3764; Ramm, *Standeskunde*, p. 35; "Medizinische Studienordnung," effective October 1, 1944, BA, R 21/484.

40. Mersmann, "Ausbildung," p. 84.

41. Wagner, "Volksgesundheit," p. 138; "Studien- und Bestallungsordnung für Ärzte," effective April 1, 1939, BA, R 18/3764; *Ärzteblatt für Norddeutschland* 2 (1939): 463–64; *Deutsches Ärzteblatt* 70 (1940): 43; "Praktische Ausbildung der Studierenden der Medizin im Krankenpflegedienst, Land- und Fabrikdienst und als Famulus," January 11, 1940, BA, R 18/3764; Ramm, *Standeskunde*, p. 34; "Medizinische Studienordnung," effective October 1, 1944, BA, R 21/484.

42. "Erläuterungen zur Bestallungsordnung für Ärzte," [summer 1939], BA, R 18/3764.

2. Implications of Politics and Social Class

1. Giles, *Students*; Kater, "Professoren und Studenten."

2. Scheel, "Rede des Reichsstudentenführers," esp. pp. 14, 16.

3. The pre-1933 origins of departmental *Fachschaften* and their organizational status in the Third Reich are touched upon in Giles, *Students*, pp. 75, 189–90.

4. Diepgen, *Heilkunde*, p. 29. On political reliability as an official desiderate see Kreuser, "Erneuerung," p. 375; par. 16 (2), 2 in "Fünfte Verordnung zur Durchführung und Ergänzung der Reichsärzteordnung (Bestallungsordnung für Ärzte)," July 17, 1939, *Reichsgesetzblatt* (1939), I, 1276; Klein, *Amtsarzt*, 3:3.

5. "Allgemeiner Bericht," n.p., [1933–34], ARW, I, 03 p 356; report Lindgens, Fachschaft Medizin Würzburg, summer semester 1934; Schenk, "Anordnung der Studentenschaft," Würzburg, June 25, 1934; "Fachschaftsbericht für die Vorklinikerschaft im W.S. 1936/37," Würzburg, December 16, 1936, ARW, IV, 1-31/10.

6. Report Keller, Würzburg, January 22, 1934; Keller, "Zusammenfassender Be-

richt über das W.-S. 1933/34," Würzburg, February 26, 1934, ARW, IV, 1-31/10.

7. Zink, activities report for Fachschaft Kliniker for summer semester 1937, Würzburg, June 17, 1937, ARW, IV, 1-31/10; report of medical Fachschaft Heidelberg, winter semester 1935–36, ARW, I, 80 g 581/2. On Hirt see Kater, "*Ahnenerbe*," pp. 245–55.

8. See "Fachschaftsmitteilungen der Klinikerschaft für das Sommer-Semester 1936 [Würzburg]"; Zink, activities report for Fachschaft Kliniker for summer semester 1937, Würzburg, June 17, 1937, ARW, IV, 1-31/10.

9. Hauptamtsleiter to Lindgens, [Würzburg], November 23, 1933, ARW, IV, 1-31/10; Wolff, "Bericht über das III. Reichslager," p. 164.

10. *Ziel und Weg* 5 (1935): 276–77; Prägert, "Krankenpflegerausbildung"; Lemberger, "Unsere praktischen Erfahrungen."

11. Report of medical Fachschaft Heidelberg, winter semester 1935–36, ARW, I, 80 g 581/2; Medizinerschaft Würzburg to Schriftleitung, Würzburg, February 4, 1937, ARW, IV, 1-31/10.

12. "Berichte der einzelnen Fachschaftsleiter über die bisher geleistete Arbeit," n.p., [March 1936], ARW, I, 80 g 581/1; Peterson to university senate, [Würzburg], October 10, 1933; Medizinische Fachschaft Würzburg to Studentenschaft Freiburg, April 4, 1936; "Fachschaftsmitteilungen der Klinikerschaft [Würzburg] für das Sommer-Semester 1936," ARW, IV, 1-31/10; Vowinkel to Liess, Krefeld, October 23, 1935; report of medical Fachschaft Heidelberg, winter semester 1935–36; report of medical Fachschaft Hamburg, Berlin, April 17, 1936, ARW, I, 80 g 581/2.

13. Zink, activities report for Fachschaft Kliniker for summer semester 1937, Würzburg, June 17, 1937, ARW, IV, 1-31/10.

14. See Gauwerky, "Tätigkeitsbericht," p. 1079; report Seifert, Berlin, April 17, 1934, ARW, I, 80 g 581/2.

15. Medizinische Fachschaft Munich to Medizinische Fachschaft Würzburg, Munich, November 15, 1935; Klinikerschaft Würzburg to Rieth, Würzburg, June 24, 1936; "Bestätigung," [Würzburg], November 4, 1936, and February 17, 1937; Fachschaftsleiter to Stahl, Würzburg, February 1, 1937; "Dienstleistungszeugnis," Würzburg, February 17, 1937; Zink, activities report for Fachschaft Kliniker for summer semester 1937, Würzburg, June 17, 1937, ARW, IV, 1-31/10.

16. Agreement Wagner and Stäbel, Munich, January 26, 1934, ARW, I, 11 p 71; text in Chapter 4, 2, before n. 2.

17. *Ziel und Weg* 6 (1936): 160.

18. Hoos to Reichsstudentenführung and to Führerschule Alt-Rehse, Würzburg, January 30 and February 20, 1937, ARW, IV, 1-31/10; Gauwerky, "Reichsfachgruppe Medizin"; Wolff, "Bericht über das III. Reichslager," p. 164.

19. Gauwerky, "Tätigkeitsbericht," p. 1079.

20. Ibid., pp. 1078–79.

21. For a listing of about two dozen of the medical topics for this competition, see ARW, III. Also see Gauwerky, "Reichsfachgruppe Medizin," p. 376.

22. *Ziel und Weg* 8 (1938): 231 (quotations); ibid., p. 413; Gauwerky, "Tätigkeitsbericht"; Kater, " 'Gesundheitsführung.' "

23. See *Ziel und Weg* 7 (1937): 508; Röder, "Lehrgang," p. 518.

24. Röder, "Lehrgang," p. 522; Kittel, "Einsatz von Medizinstudenten im Rassenpolitischen Amt der NSDAP," November 27, 1937, ARW, I, 20 g 670.

25. See the insidious role of *Fachschaft* in the intrigues against Professor Krause at Münster, as outlined in Luther, "Durchsetzung" (also see text in Chapter 4, 3, at n. 47).

26. Correspondence of Vollmann-Simon-Klein (spring–summer 1934), ARW, I, 33 g 178/4. Quotations Klein to Simon, [Berlin], June 28, 1934.

27. *Kameradschaften* were organized within the Nazi student administration similar to the *Fachschaften*, but they appear to have been much further removed from the influence of the Reich physician (health) leadership. At Heidelberg, the prototype of a medical *Kameradschaft* had existed since November 1934, under the aegis of Gustav Adolf Scheel, who was then the local student leader. See *Deutsches Ärzteblatt* 66 (1936): 1259; *Münchener Medizinische Wochenschrift* 83 (1936): 1950.

28. "Entwurf zu einem Artikel über 'Das Studium der Medizin während des Krieges,'" [November 1939], BA, R 21/484; entry for February 5, 1940, in *Meldungen aus dem Reich*, 3:727; *Reichsstudentenwerk: Bericht, 1941*, pp. 90–93; Ramm, *Standeskunde*, p. 80; "Verfügungsdurchschrift," Leitender Oberstaatsanwalt beim Landgericht Hamburg to Arbeitsgemeinschaft Neuengamme, Hamburg, August 24, 1967, DAÖW, 4748; Klee, "*Euthanasie*," p. 254; Lifton, *Nazi Doctors*, p. 67.

29. Kater, *Studentenschaft*, pp. 56–73; idem, "Professionalization," pp. 679–80; Huerkamp, *Aufstieg der Ärzte*, pp. 61–78.

30. Kater, *Studentenschaft*, pp. 56–73; *Deutsches Ärzteblatt* 65 (1935): 1212. Cf. Jarausch, *Studenten*, pp. 129–40.

31. The data in Lorenz, *Zehnjahres-Statistik*, 1:356–71, for winter trimester 1941 suggest this development but are incomplete and therefore not foolproof. See, however, Jarausch, *Studenten*, pp. 182–83, who makes this argument convincingly. An increase in the upper-middle-class portion, especially in medicine, would be likely in view of the inflated number of female students, who tended to hail from the upper classes more than men (and increasingly entered medicine).

32. This projection is based on the deliberations expressed in n. 31.

33. The Reichsstudentenwerk (RSW) collection, a voluminous file with two sets of data cards, each in alphabetical order, is accessible in BA, but not as part of the regular student material rubricized under R 149. See Granier et al., *Bundesarchiv und seine Bestände*, p. 458. It is to the credit of Konrad H. Jarausch that he saved this file from being shredded. For a preliminary analysis of the file, see Arminger's useful pilot study, "Involvement."

34. Cf. *Reichsstudentenwerk: Kurzberichte, 1935*, p. [16]; ibid., *1936*, p. [27].

35. The percentage figures for female medical students are as follows:

	(A) WS 34–35	(B) SS 1938	(C) W Trim. 41	(D) WS 43–44
1. Percentage of female medical students (census)	19.1	16.6	26.5	35.2
2. Percentage of female medical students (Kater sample)	12.9	9.6	17.0	37.3

These figures are taken from Kater loan-student sample for row 2 and calculated on the basis of figures in Lorenz, *Zehnjahres-Statistik*, 1:364; *Statistisches Handbuch*, p. 623, for row 1. The percentage of women students in Arminger's pilot sample (1933–45) is only 8.1 (Table 7, Arminger, "Involvement," p. 20).

36. See *Frankfurter Zeitung*, January 1, 1937; *Reichsstudentenwerk: Bericht, 1941*, pp. 47–48.

37. See *Reichsstudentenwerk: Bericht, 1941*, pp. 40, 48–49.

38. According to the complete loan-student data of 3,693 *N*, in the three disciplines of medicine, dentistry, and law a combined average of 424 students were supported annually from 1933 to 1940, inclusive. This annual average dropped to 76 *N* for the four-year period from 1941 to 1944. Unfortunately, Arminger, in "Involvement," neglected to demonstrate such a decline since he was using his sample based on the total of academic disciplines.

39. This translated into over 900 marks per semester for medical students. Mine is an approximate judgment based on figures in *Deutsches Ärzteblatt* 69 (1939): 186–87; and *Reichsstudentenwerk: Bericht, 1941*, p. 42. Also see "Richtlinien für das Verfahren bei den ärztlichen Vorprüfungen und Prüfungen sowie bei der Behandlung als Arzt," [1942], BA, R 18/3764.

40. See Kater, "Quantifizierung," pp. 479–80.

41. Figure 1, Kater, *Nazi Party*, p. 263.

42. *Reichsstudentenführung: Kurzberichte, 1936*, pp. [37]–[38]. According to my statistical analysis of 2,019 medical students, 1,210 law students, and 464 dental students, contained in the loan-student sample for 1933–45, the average amount allotted to the medical students was 729.61 marks, while to the law students it was 626.09 marks and to the dental students 590.47 marks. The average single grant made till 1937, and probably thereafter, was about 545 marks (*Reichsstudentenwerk: Kurzberichte, 1937*, p. 68). Hardly anyone ever received more than altogether 1,200 marks. See *Reichsstudentenwerk: Kurzberichte, 1937*, pp. 7, 68; *Reichsstudentenwerk: Bericht, 1941*, p. 47.

43. Report Lindgens, Fachschaft Medizin Würzburg, summer semester 1934, ARW, IV, 1-31/10; Bulitta to Führer der Studentenschaft Würzburg, December 2, 1933, and January 12, 1934; memorandum Remer, [Würzburg], December 5, 1933, ARW, IV, 1-31/9.

44. In 1933 it was stated that 28 percent of all students at universities and THs were in medicine, but only 21 percent of all the loan students were there. The figures for law were 21 and 20 percent respectively ("Umschau in der Arbeit der studentischen Selbsthilfe," Dresden, October 9, 1933, ARW, I, 6 p 359). For summer 1935 these statistics were 34 and 31 percent (medicine), 18 and 17 percent (law) (*Reichsstudentenwerk: Kurzberichte, 1936*, p. [37]. Also see p. [38]).

45. Table 5.4: cols. A and E vs. G: 40.3 percent and 39.5 percent vs. 32.5 percent; 3.5 percent and 4.4 percent vs. 6.2 percent; cols. B and F vs. H: 18.5 percent and 16.1 percent vs. 27.3 percent; 10.3 percent and 11.5 percent vs. 8.8 percent.

46. Table 5.4 (cols. C and D. vs. G and H respectively): 23.3 percent < 32.5 percent; 10.9 percent < 27.3 percent; 73.2 percent > 61.2 percent; 78.9 percent > 63.9 percent; 4.5 percent < 6.2 percent; 10.2 percent > 8.8 percent.

47. The correlation coefficient (Pearson's R) for the percentage columns A and C

in Table 5.5 is 0.99, for columns A and B it is only 0.82, and for columns B and C only 0.86. But since we are not dealing with interval data, this test has only an illustrative value.

48. Giles, *Students*, pp. 139–42; Franze, *Studentenschaft*, p. 219; Faust, *Studentenbund*, 2:128. On the unpopularity of the SA-Hochschulamt see "Allgemeiner Bericht," n.p., [1933–34]; report Göller, Munich, July 3, 1934, ARW, I, 03 p 356.

49. Text in Chapter 3, 3, after n. 27; Table 3.7.

50. Personal files in SA Fleischmann, BDC; Reiche, "SA Terror in Nuremberg," pp. 257–58 (quotation); Reiche, *Development*, p. 184.

51. Kater, "Professoren und Studenten," pp. 477–86; idem, *Nazi Party*, pp. 97–100, 127–28 (the figure of 40 percent student NSDAP members in 1944–45 mentioned on p. 128 now has to be revised downward). See Jarausch, *Studenten*, pp. 165–211. More recently Giles has shown that Hamburg students continued to favor the NSDAP until 1942, at which time new membership suddenly fell off. Unfortunately, his figures, limited to Hamburg, are not suitable for mapping out a trend for the entire Reich (*Students*, pp. 246–47).

52. Report of medical Fachschaft Rostock for winter semester 1935–36, ARW, I, 80 g 581/2; Kuntzmüller, activities report of preclinicians' Fachschaft, [Würzburg], winter semester 1936–37; Zink, activities report for Fachschaft Kliniker for summer semester 1937, Würzburg, June 17, 1937, ARW, IV, 1-31/10; "Jahreslagebericht 1938," in *Meldungen aus dem Reich*, 2:110.

53. "Berichte der einzelnen Fachschaftsleiter über die bisher geleistete Arbeit," n.p., [March 1936], ARW, I, 80 g 581/1.

54. Activities report of preclinicians [Würzburg] for winter semester 1936–37; Zink, activities report for Fachschaft Kliniker for summer semester 1937, Würzburg, June 17, 1937; summer semester 1937, report of preclinicians' Fachschaft [Würzburg]; Bartels, semester report of Fachgruppe Medizin, Würzburg, June 29, 1937, ARW, IV, 1-31/10.

55. Simon to Klein, Freiburg, June 18, 1934, ARW, I, 33 g 178/4.

56. Report about the work of medical Fachschaft Rostock for winter semester 1935–36, ARW, I, 80 g 581/2.

57. Spender, *European Witness*, pp. 20–21.

58. Entry for October 9, 1939, in *Meldungen aus dem Reich*, 2:332–33; entry for November 24, 1939, ibid., 3:494; entry for December 12, 1939, in Boelcke, *Kriegspropaganda*, p. 241.

59. Mutschmann to Rust, Dresden, December 18, 1943, appended to letter Kock to Groh et al., Berlin, January 1, 1944, BA, R 21/476. Also see entry for June 4, 1942, in *Meldungen aus dem Reich*, 10:3794 (cf. entry for December 20, 1943, ibid., 15:6176).

60. Hämel to Rust, Jena, July 15, 1943; Staatsrat to Rust, Jena, August 12, 1943, BA, R 21/439.

61. Güstrow, *Tödlicher Alltag*, pp. 187–203.

62. Hoffmann, *Ringen*, p. 14.

63. Schneider, "Widerstand," pp. 230–32.

64. Kurt Steude's testimony in Albrecht and Hartwig, *Ärzte*, pp. 434–38.

65. Mitscherlich, *Leben*, pp. 96, 98–101, 104, 115, 117.

66. Weisenborn, *Aufstand*, p. 94; Petry, *Studenten*; Hans Scholl's letters, April 1939–February 1943, esp. that to Rose Nägele, January 5, 1943 (pp. 113–14), in Scholl and Scholl, *Briefe*, pp. 23–116; Giles, *Students*, pp. 299–305; Hochmuth and Meyer, *Streiflichter*, pp. 387–421; Bittner, "Widerstand," pp. 1533–34.

67. Büchner, *Pläne*, pp. 72–76.

68. File Karl Groeger, DAÖW, 540.

69. Leber, *Gewissen*, pp. 25–26.

3. The So-called Jewish Question and the Quality of Medical Instruction

1. Düning, *SA-Student*; Feickert, *Studenten*; Faust, *Studentenbund*, 1:89–92.

2. Kümmel, "Ausschaltung," p. 72; Götz von Olenhusen, "'Nichtarischen' Studenten," pp. 176–82; Bracher et al., *Machtergreifung*, p. 318; Ellersdorfer, "Auswirkungen," pp. 25–26; Richarz, *Leben*, p. 14; Adam, *Judenpolitik*, pp. 69–70. See Schulz, "Entwicklung," p. 484, for the percentage decline. The Nazis claimed that in summer 1934, the percentage of Jewish students was 1.44, including baptized and partial Jews (*Ziel und Weg* 5 [1935]: 467).

3. Greis, "Tätigkeitsbericht der Zahnärztlichen Fachschaft," [Würzburg, winter semester 1933–34], ARW, IV, 1-31/2.

4. Table 11 in Kater, *Studentenschaft*, p. 218.

5. See Richarz, *Leben*, pp. 93–94; Faust, *Studentenbund*, 1:93; Grill, *Nazi Party in Baden*, pp. 30–31; Leonardo Conti, "Verraten und verkauft? Streiflichter aus dem Berliner Standesleben," in *Mitteilungsblatt der Arbeitsgemeinschaft Gross-Berlin des Nationalsozialistischen Deutschen Ärztebundes* 1 (September 1931), BA, NSD 53/2.

6. Schulze to DSt.-Vorstand, Hamburg, March 31, 1933, ARW, II, 288.

7. Examples for Düsseldorf (May 1933) and Würzburg (November 1933) in Schadewaldt, *Universität Düsseldorf*, p. 68; Starrek, "Bericht der Würzburger Vorklinikerschaft über die bisherige Tätigkeit," [Würzburg, November 1933], ARW, IV, 1-31/10.

8. *Das Schwarzbuch*, pp. 254–55.

9. Doc. 348 of February 2, 1934, in Walk, *Sonderrecht*, p. 72; Götz von Olenhusen, "'Nichtarischen' Studenten," p. 191.

10. Doc. 477 of November 13, 1934, in Walk, *Sonderrecht*, p. 97; doc. 193 of November 13, 1934, in Sauer, *Dokumente*, 1:238–40.

11. Götz von Olenhusen, "'Nichtarischen' Studenten," p. 192.

12. *Ziel und Weg* 5 (1935): 282; Götz von Olenhusen, "'Nichtarischen' Studenten," p. 190; Adam, *Judenpolitik*, p. 115. This stipulation was anchored in the Reich Physicians' Ordinance of December 13, 1935: par. 3 (5), BA, R 18/5574.

13. *Reichsstudentenwerk: Kurzberichte, 1937*, p. 23.

14. Ibid.

15. Götz von Olenhusen, "'Nichtarischen' Studenten," p. 184. See, as well, Zschintzsch to nachgeordnete Dienststelle der preussischen Hochschulverwaltung et al., Berlin, June 18, 1936, BA, R 21/485.

16. Winheim to [Studentenschaft Universität Würzburg], Würzburg, August 20, 1935, ARW, IV, 1-31/10.

17. Report on the Reichslager of Jena Fachschaft from June 23 to 25, 1935, ARW, II, 531.

18. "Berichte der einzelnen Fachschaftsleiter über die bisher geleistete Arbeit," n.p., [March 1936], ARW, I, 80 g 581/1; report of medical Fachschaft Hamburg, Berlin, April 17, 1936; report of medical Fachschaft Jena, Jena, April 17, 1936; report of medical Fachschaft Heidelberg, winter semester 1935–36, ARW, I, 80 g 581/2.

19. Report of medical Fachschaft Rostock for winter semester 1935–36, ARW, I, 80 g 581/2.

20. Winheim to Bavarian ministry of education, Würzburg, October 1, 1935, ARW, IV, 1-31/10. Also see Zink, activities report for Fachschaft Kliniker for summer semester 1937, Würzburg, June 17, 1937, ARW, IV, 1-31/10.

21. Zschintzsch to Frick, Berlin, February 18, 1938, BA, R 21/485. The decline in the number of Jewish medical students is difficult to measure because only figures for Mosaic (not for baptized or partial) Jews are available. Judging by those, there were 1,893 Jewish medical students in summer 1932, 916 in summer 1933, and 366 in winter 1933–34 (Reich citizens only). Expressed in percent of the total of Reich citizen medical students, the values were as follows: 7.6 percent Jews in 1932, 3.8 percent Jews in 1933, and 1.6 percent Jews in 1933–34, according to figures in Tornau, "Medizinstudium und Berufsüberfüllung," *Deutsches Ärzteblatt* 64 (1934): 1096.

22. Wagner, *Judengesetze*; *Deutsches Ärzteblatt* 65 (1935): 896–99; Schleunes, *Twisted Road*, pp. 119–20, 123–24, 127; Adam, *Judenpolitik*, pp. 126, 129–30, 135–42. See Chapter 6.

23. Stab, Stellvertreter des Führers, to Rust, Munich, August 4, 1937, included in letter Zschintzsch to Frick, Berlin, February 18, 1938, BA, R 21/485.

24. Zschintzsch to Frick, Berlin, February 28, 1938, R 21/485. Regarding *Mischlinge*, see doc. 362 of October 20, 1937, in Walk, *Sonderrecht*, pp. 202–3.

25. Wagner to Reich interior ministry, BA, R 21/485.

26. Ordinance of April 4, 1939, BA, R 21/485; "Fünfte Verordnung zur Durchführung und Ergänzung der Reichsärzteordnung," July 17, 1939, par. 15 (3), *Reichsgesetzblatt* (1939), I, 1275; "Bestallungsordnung für Ärzte, Runderlass," August 17, 1939, BA, R 18/3764; Klein, *Amtsarzt*, 3:2.

27. Götz von Olenhusen, " 'Nichtarischen' Studenten," pp. 199–201; Zschintzsch to Unterrichtsverwaltungen et al., Berlin, June 22, 1942, BA, R 22/1183. Conti was an old friend of Bormann, and loyal to the end. See Kater, "Doctor Leonardo Conti," pp. 311–13, 318–20; Conti to Rust, Berlin, February 23, 1944, BA, R 21/484.

28. Medical students' complicity in the persecution of medical teachers is reported for Würzburg, Düsseldorf, and Giessen, as described in "Berichte der einzelnen Fachschaftsleiter über die bisher geleistete Arbeit," n.p., [March 1936], ARW, I, 80 g 581/1; Schadewaldt, *Universität Düsseldorf*, p. 68; Jakobi et al., *Aeskulap*, p. 51.

29. As expressed by medical student Vollmann, [report Freiburg, spring 1934], ARW, I, 33 g 178/4.

30. An example of several such documents in the file: Königsberg dean of medicine, dispensation for Hans Porrmann, Königsberg, July 17, 1933, ARW, I, 05 g 353/2. Also see the petition by medical student Erhard Rathke, to Reichsamt Ostland für

Arbeitsdienst der Deutschen Studentenschaft, Danzig-Langfuhr, August 3, 1933, ibid.

31. "Allgemeiner Bericht," n.p., [1933–34], ARW, I, 03 p 356; Bumke, *Erinnerungen*, p. 152.

32. Keller, "Zusammenfassender Bericht über das W.-S. 1933/34," Würzburg, February 26, 1934, ARW, IV, 31/10.

33. Lindgens to Schenk [in Würzburg], [hospital at] Mülheim-Ruhr, August 26, 1934, ARW, IV, 31/10.

34. As overheard and recorded by Bella Fromm. See entry for February 10, 1935, in her *Blood and Banquets*, pp. 187–88.

35. Wagner, "Volksgesundheit," p. 138; *Deutsches Ärzteblatt* 69 (1939): 78; "Erläuterungen zur Bestallungsordnung für Ärzte," [summer 1939], BA, R 18/3764.

36. Zschintzsch to Herren Rektoren et al., Berlin, November 23, 1939; Bach to Otto, [Berlin], December 4, 1939; Mentzel to deans of medical faculties, Berlin, December 5, 1939; de Crinis to Ehlich, Berlin, May 15, 1942; "Auszug aus dem Protokoll über die Dekanbesprechung am 13. und 14.4.1943"; de Crinis to Kock, Berlin, July 13, 1943, BA, R 21/484; entry for December 4, 1939, in *Meldungen aus dem Reich*, 3:525.

37. Memorandum [de Crinis], Berlin, [after 1939], BA, R 21/485; memoranda de Crinis, Berlin, December 10 and 22, 1942, BA, R 21/484; "Dienstbesprechung der Dekane der Medizinischen Fakultäten in Halle am 28. Juli 1944," BA, R 21/476.

38. See the characteristic report of an anonymous *Stabsarzt*, appended to letter Meins to de Crinis, Berlin, May 13, 1942, BA, R 21/484.

39. Stark to Stadler, Weiden, May 17, 1941, BA, R 18/3781; Vienna dean of medicine to ministry of education, Vienna, June 26, 1942, BA, R 21/476; memorandum [de Crinis], [Berlin], February 24, 1941; Guleke to de Crinis, Jena, December 29, 1942; Guleke to Rostock, Jena, December 30, 1942, BA, R 21/484; "Tagung der Dekane der Medizinischen Fakultäten im Reichserziehungsministerium am 6. Mai 1941," BDC, Research Rudolf Mentzel; Fischer, *Erfahrungsberichten*, p. 6.

40. See *Reichsstudentenwerk: Kurzberichte, 1938*, p. 40; Burgschweiger, "Humangenetische und anthropologische Arbeiten." Also Chapter 4, 1, at n. 28. Further see case of Dr. med., Dr. med. dent. Richard Schöndorf, BDC, PÄ Schöndorf.

41. Blome, "Freiheit," p. 248; Kater, "Reich Vocational Contest," pp. 256–57.

42. Par. 68 (2) in "Fünfte Verordnung zur Durchführung und Ergänzung der Reichsärzteordnung (Bestallungsordnung für Ärzte)," July 22, 1939, *Reichsgesetzblatt* (1939), I, 1285; "Erläuterungen zur Bestallungsordnung für Ärzte," [summer 1939], BA, R 18/3764.

43. Conti to Rust, Berlin, February 23, 1944; and attached to this letter, memorandum de Crinis, Berlin, March 6, 1944; "Medizinische Studienordnung," effective October 1, 1944, BA, R 21/484.

44. Adam, *Hochschule*, p. 158. These figures will have to be modified somewhat because Adam included dental students in his count.

45. Munich dean of medicine to rector, Munich, October 6, 1939; "Auszug aus Bericht des Kurators der Universität Berlin vom 18.11.1940," BA, R 21/484; entry for February 16, 1942, in *Meldungen aus dem Reich*, 9:3321.

46. Entry for January 11, 1943, in *Meldungen aus dem Reich*, 12:4659; de Crinis to

Amtschef W and Klingelhöfer, Berlin, June 16, 1943, BA, R 21/484; "Forschung, Lehre und zivile Krankenversorgung im 4. Kriegsjahr," [Munich, 1943], BA, R 21/476.

47. Diepgen to Herren Mitglieder des Ausschusses, Berlin, February 5, 1945, BA, R 21/484.

48. In 1932–33, the percentage of medical students disrupting their course of studies (meaning about to fail) in Prussia was 16.8, in 1935–36 it was 13.8, and in 1938–39 it was 13.5. The corresponding percentages for examination finalists with the mark of "very good" were 7.7, 13.0, and 12.2. A Pearson's R coefficient of -.975 indicates an almost perfect negative correlation. My computations are on the basis of figures in lists for premedical and medical examinations in Prussia, 1932–39, BA, R 18/3764. On the Reich as a whole, see Lorenz, *Zehnjahres-Statistik*, 2:18. On the faculty judgments, see "1. Vierteljahreslagebericht 1939," in *Meldungen aus dem Reich*, 2:271.

49. Conti to Regierungen der Hochschulländer et al., Berlin, November 29, 1940, BA, R 18/3764.

50. Entry for July 16, 1942, in *Meldungen aus dem Reich*, 10:3959.

51. Entry for October 5, 1942, ibid., 11:4283.

52. Guleke to de Crinis, Jena, December 29, 1942; Guleke to Rostock, Jena, December 30, 1942, BA, R 21/484. On Guleke see Fischer, *Lexikon*, 1:552.

53. Remarks of anonymous *Stabsarzt*, appended to letter Meins to de Crinis, Berlin, May 13, 1942, BA, R 21/484.

54. Memorandum de Crinis, Berlin, December 22, 1942, BA, R 21/484.

55. De Crinis to Ehlich, Berlin, May 15, 1942; memorandum de Crinis for Klingelhöfer, December 10, 1942; de Crinis to Amtschef W and Klingelhöfer, Berlin, June 16, 1943, BA, R 21/484.

56. Himmler to Brandt, Feld-Kommandostelle, July 13, 1944, BA, R 18/3810.

Chapter 6

1. The Medicalization of the "Jewish Question"

1. *Nazi Doctors*, p. 17.

2. Daim, *Mann*; Mosse, *Toward the Final Solution*, p. 99.

3. Kater, "Hitler's Early Doctors," pp. 42–43.

4. See Hitler, *Mein Kampf*, pp. 53–54, 224, 277, 286, 512. Robert Lifton, to whom, next to George Mosse, I owe the inspiration for this approach, mentions the same or similar examples, culled from a different edition of *Mein Kampf*, on p. 16 of *Nazi Doctors*. For 1941, see *Nach Hitler*, p. 199, n. 20.

5. Kater, "Hitler's Early Doctors," p. 41.

6. Letter to *Chefarzt* Dr. B., Scheidegg, March 31, 1933, in Klare, *Briefe*, p. 73.

7. *Deutsches Ärzteblatt* 65 (1935): 896.

8. Amende, "Arzt," p. 60. On Amende's early Nazi career see Kudlien, "Ärzte als Anhänger," p. 25.

9. Wagner, "Ziele," p. 488; idem, "Rasse und Volksgesundheit," pp. 515–16.

10. Meier, "Ende des jüdischen Arzttums," p. 112.

11. Hiemer, *Pudelmopsdackelpinscher*, pp. 89–90. See Showalter, *Little Man, What Now?*.

12. See Hobohm, "Nationalsozialismus," p. 43.

13. Reichert, "Juden und jüdische Mischlinge," p. 322; Ruppert, "Seucheninsel," p. 28.

14. Ramm, *Standeskunde*, p. 46.

15. Conti, "Leistung," p. 18; Klein as quoted in Lifton, *Nazi Doctors*, pp. 15–16.

16. Hitler, *Mein Kampf*, pp. 295, 512.

17. See Mosse, *Toward the Final Solution*, pp. 101, 111.

18. Dinter, *Sünde wider das Blut*, pp. 265–67, 400. Also see Mosse, *Toward the Final Solution*, pp. 176–77; and, on Dinter's early Nazi career, Tyrell, *Führer*. Hitler did not consider the copulation between Jewish men and "Aryan" women as the typical method of race defilement. According to him, it was more common for Jewish women to marry "Aryan" (often aristocratic) men (*Mein Kampf*, p. 286).

19. Fischer, *Begriff*, p. 14.

20. Gross, "Arzt und Judenfrage," p. 188.

21. Viehweg, "Grundgesetze," p. 1117; Wagner, "Unser Reichsärzteführer spricht," p. 434.

22. Dr. Nitzsche in *Münchener Medizinische Wochenschrift* 85 (1938): 1943. Opportunistically, Nitzsche was referring here to the Sudetenland, which was in the process of being annexed.

23. Meier, "Ende des jüdischen Arzttums," p. 112.

24. Ramm, *Standeskunde*, p. 131.

25. Lifton, *Nazi Doctors*, pp. 123–24, 271–77, 280–83; testimony of witness Joseph Czarny at trial of John Demjanjuk, Jerusalem, Israel, as reported in *Globe and Mail* (Toronto), March 4, 1987.

26. See, for instance, *Mein Kampf*, pp. 55, 224–25.

27. Wagner, "Unser Reichsärzteführer spricht," pp. 433–34; idem, "Rasse und Volksgesundheit," p. 515. On the reputed criminality of Jews, see also Mosse, *Toward the Final Solution*, pp. 219–20.

28. *Mein Kampf*, pp. 53–54, 274 (quotation). Also see Chapter 4, 1, at n. 23.

29. Wagner, "Unser Reichsärzteführer spricht," pp. 432–33; Schulz, "Judentum und Degeneration."

30. Conti, "Stand der Volksgesundheit im 5. Kriegsjahr" [address of January 1944], BA, R 18/3805 (p. 4); quotations from Ruppert, "Seucheninsel," pp. 24, 28. Also see Browning, "Genocide and Public Health."

31. Entries for May 19 and June 8, 1942, in Voss's diary, partially reproduced in Aly, "Posener Tagebuch," p. 55.

32. Lifton, *Nazi Doctors*, p. 14.

33. Gross as cited in "Aufgaben der Ärztin," [Rittmarshausen, 1936], ARW, I, 80 g 581/1.

34. Amende, "Arzt," p. 56.

35. Wagner as reported in *Ärzteblatt für Berlin und Kurmark* 43 (1938): 521, facsimile in Goldschmidt, *Meine Arbeit*, p. 68.

36. Meier, "Ende des jüdischen Arzttums," p. 112; Conti's remarks at meeting of NSÄB in Berlin on April 24, 1942, in *Deutsches Ärzteblatt* 72 (1942): 200; Ramm, *Standeskunde*, pp. 130–32.

37. *Ziel und Weg* 3 (1933): 78. See Chapter 1, 2, at n. 9.

38. Lösener, "Rassereferent," pp. 280, 284, 296; Adam, *Judenpolitik*, pp. 31–36, 99–100, 105–6, 126, 129–30, 135–42, 224; Schleunes, *Twisted Road*, pp. 119–20, 123–24, 127.

39. Wagner, *Judengesetze*; Gütt et al., *Gesetz*. In addition, Wagner, "Unser Reichsärzteführer spricht," pp. 434–35; Viehweg, "Grundgesetze," pp. 1118–19; Helmreich, "Rassen- und Erbhygiene"; Ramm, *Standeskunde*, pp. 130–32. Also see Rühle, *Dritte Reich, 1935*, pp. 277–92.

40. Kluge and Krüger, *Verfassung*, pp. 135, 240–43; Ramm, *Standeskunde*, pp. 76–77.

41. *Ziel und Weg* 7 (1937): 611; ibid. 9 (1939): 209.

42. Schmidt, *Selektion*, pp. 42–43; Schmuhl, *Rassenhygiene*, pp. 197, 199, 215–16. Also see Adler, *Mensch*, pp. 235–37, 240–48; Klee, "*Euthanasie*," pp. 258–63; Friedlander, "Jüdische Anstaltspatienten."

43. Lifton, in *Nazi Doctors*, has driven this point home forcefully and eloquently.

44. Ramm, *Standeskunde*, p. 132.

45. Dr. C/Ka.[Kauffmann], unsigned memorandum [in Conti's office], Berlin, August 18, 1944, BA, R 18/3806.

2. Precarious Legality: Till September 1935

1. See Kater, "Everyday Anti-Semitism." The latest pronouncement on this problem so far is Kershaw, "German Popular Opinion."

2. Letter to Dr. D., Scheidegg, February 8, 1933, in Klare, *Briefe*, p. 46.

3. *Völkischer Beobachter*, February 28, 1933. Also see Adam, *Judenpolitik*, p. 49.

4. The article is significantly entitled "To German physicians. . . . Sweep away those who refuse to recognize the signs of our times!"

5. "Fort mit den jüdischen Vertrauensärzten!," *Völkischer Beobachter*, April 4, 1933.

6. Gütt, "Arzt," p. 81; Reiter, "Revolution," pp. 424–25. Moreover, see Kötschau, *Umbruch*, pp. 27–28. Quotation from Gross, "Arzt und Judenfrage," p. 188.

7. Blum and Teutsch to Oberlandesgericht Nürnberg, Nuremberg, December 7, 1937, UK, 130/123.02.

8. Müller, *Geschichte*, p. 212. See Reiche, *Development*, p. 53. Stöcker was born in 1882, joined the NSDAP in 1930, and by 1936 was said to be in the SA and NSÄB (BDC, "Fragebogen," Nuremberg, September 23, 1936, PK Stöcker; BDC, RÄK Stöcker).

9. File of Dr. Eduard Oppenheimer (Mannheim, 1933–35), UK, 217.

10. *Schwarzbuch*, p. 206.

11. *Deutsches Ärzteblatt* 62 (1933): 141–42. Also see *Schwarzbuch*, pp. 201–3; Michaelis et al., *Kultur*, pp. 260–61; Zapp, "Untersuchungen," pp. 89–90, 94.

12. Streicher acknowledged his authorship in a public speech on May 25, 1935, "The Physician and the People," reprinted as doc. 82 in Wuttke-Groneberg, *Medizin*, p. 151.

13. "Deutsche, kauft nicht beim Juden! Deutsche, lehnt es ab, Euer Geld zu jüdischen Rechtsanwälten und Ärzten zu tragen!," n.d., doc. 197 ibid., p. 343. Cf. Kater, "Everyday Anti-Semitism," pp. 139–41.

14. "Informationsbericht der NSF (Deutscher Frauenorden)," no. 11, Munich, April 8, 1933, HIS, 13/254.

15. Doc. of April 3, 1933, in Broszat et al., *Bayern*, p. 434. For a similar practice in Berlin, see entry for April 1, 1933, in *Tagebuch Nathorff*, p. 38.

16. Müller, *Geschichte*, p. 213; Gumpert, *Hölle*, p. 241.

17. Roth, " 'Auslese,' " p. 155. Also see entry for April 14, 1933, in *Tagebuch Nathorff*, p. 39.

18. Gordon, *Hitler*, p. 168; Hanke, *Geschichte*, p. 84.

19. *Ziel und Weg* 3 (1933): 132.

20. Gumpert, *Hölle*, p. 251.

21. Aretin, *Krone*, pp. 206–7.

22. Winter, *Benjamin*, pp. 22–23; Müller, *Geschichte*, p. 218; Ophir and Wiesemann, *Gemeinden*, pp. 208–9; Gilbert, *Holocaust*, pp. 40–41. Aretin's claim, *Krone*, p. 309, that Katz was killed while still in prison is probably spurious.

23. *Schwarzbuch*, pp. 197–98, 209; Adam, *Judenpolitik*, p. 49.

24. Müller, *Geschichte*, p. 214.

25. Doc. 24 of March 31, 1933; doc. 39 of April 4, 1933; doc. 53 of April 11, 1933, in Walk, *Sonderrecht*, pp. 8, 10, 13; Kümmel, "Ausschaltung," pp. 64–66.

26. See docs. 112 and 113 of March 30 and April 7, 1933, in Sauer, *Dokumente*, 1:131–32; Fliedner, *Judenverfolgung*, p. 173; *Schwarzbuch*, pp. 213–14.

27. *Schwarzbuch*, pp. 210–12.

28. Haedenkamp, "Gesamtvorstände," p. 310.

29. As an example of many see file of Professor Erich Seligmann (1880–1954), LBINY, Erich Seligmann Collection, AR-C.1640, Box 1, Folder 3. I owe my knowledge of this file to Howard Margolian, Toronto.

30. Seldte, "Verordnung über die Zulassung von Ärzten zur Tätigkeit bei den Krankenkassen," April 22, 1933, *Ziel und Weg* 3 (1933): 79–80. Also see Kümmel, "Ausschaltung," pp. 67–69.

31. Facsimile reproduction of April 1933 form letter in *Schwarzbuch*, p. 205; also see Michaelis et al., *Kultur*, pp. 261–62. Facsimile of cancellation notice dated June 12, 1933, is in Franke, *Geschichte*, p. 115. Further see *Tagebuch Nathorff*, passim.

32. See docs. 126, 152, 157, 162, 203, 207, 213, 278, all of 1933, in Walk, *Sonderrecht*, pp. 27, 32–34, 43–45, 58.

33. *Schwarzbuch*, p. 235.

34. Correspondence of Markus-Reich labor ministry-KVD Waldenburg (1933–35), UK, 235. Quotation is from Stellvertretender Amtsleiter, KVD Waldenburg, to KVD Provinzstelle Niederschlesien, Waldenburg, September 5, 1935.

35. This fear by the KVD is expressed in the letter cited in n. 34, above.

36. See the illuminating articles in Rebentisch and Teppe, *Verwaltung contra Menschenführung*.

37. Karstedt, "Durchführung," Also see Tennstedt and Leibfried, "Sozialpolitik," pp. 217–23; Jaffé to Korach, Amsterdam, January 21, 1939, partially printed in Leibfried, "Stationen der Abwehr," p. 5.

38. The calculations of the most recent scholar in this area seem to me the most reliable. See Kümmel, "Ausschaltung," pp. 69–71. Tennstedt and Leibfried write 2,800 ("Sozialpolitik," p. 217. Cf. Leibfried, "Stationen der Abwehr," p. 12). Schleunes's figure of about 1,150 (*Twisted Road*, p. 109) appears too low, and Richarz's of 3,000 (*Leben*, p. 42) too high.

39. Wagner to Engel, Munich, July 27, 1933, as quoted in Tennstedt and Leibfried, "Sozialpolitik," p. 219. On Grote's role see *Deutsches Ärzteblatt* 68 (1938): 144.

40. According to testimony of Dr. Fritz Goldschmidt, in Goldschmidt, *Meine Arbeit*, p. 45.

41. Testimonies of Dr. Ruth Aron, Dr. Jean Birnbaum, and Dr. Fritz Goldschmidt, in ibid., pp. 22–34, 38–43. See *Schwarzbuch*, pp. 225–26. Diels's self-perception is in his *Lucifer ante Portas*. See the realistic description of his "sinister quality" in Dodd, *Through Embassy Eyes*, pp. 52–56, 134–37.

42. *Schwarzbuch*, pp. 197, 222; *Deutsche Führerlexikon*, pp. 235–36; Pross in Pross and Winau, *nicht misshandeln*, pp. 183–90; Ostrowski, "Schicksal," p. 321 (Ostrowski's claim that Klein had one Jewish grandparent is almost certainly spurious).

43. Ostrowski, "Schicksal," pp. 323–24.

44. Ruppin to Wagner, Neubabelsberg, November 17, 1934; Wagner to Kube, Munich, December 3, 1934, BDC, OPG Ruppin; "Lebenslauf" Ruppin, Neubabelsberg, January 14, 1937, BDC, SS Ruppin; Ostrowski, "Schicksal," p. 325; Michaelis et al., *Kultur*, p. 266; *Wer ist's?* p. 1343.

45. Birnbaum, *Staat*, p. 225, n. 2; testimony of Max Reiner in Richarz, *Leben*, p. 116; Gumpert, *Hölle*, p. 251. It is important to point out that suicides of physicians appear to have started forming a pattern under the boycott of spring 1933. See entry for May 15, 1933, in *Tagebuch Nathorff*, p. 43.

46. Aretin, *Krone*, pp. 213–14.

47. Swoboda to Bapopo, Munich, October 13, 1933, SAM/LRA 30656.

48. See the advertisements referring to Jewish doctors "about to be taken down" in *Ziel und Weg* 3 (1933): 101, 205; and the Austrian letter to the editor openly accusing Nazi physicians of this (ibid., p. 304).

49. Stähle, *Geschichte*, p. 15.

50. Doc. 294 of November 20, 1933, in Walk, *Sonderrecht*, p. 61.

51. Zelzer, *Weg*, p. 167; Ellersdorfer, "Auswirkungen," pp. 96–97; Ostrowski, "Schicksal," p. 320; Huss to Arbeitsgericht Berlin, Berlin, March 19, 1935, UK, 207. Cf. Leibfried, "Stationen der Abwehr," p. 12.

52. Martha Krause's letter to the editor, *Ziel und Weg* 3 (1933): 472; Krüger, *Haus*, p. 18; testimony of Carl Schwabe in Richarz, *Leben*, p. 162.

53. Richarz, *Leben*, p. 43; testimony of Alexander Szanto, ibid., p. 223; testimony of Ernst Loewenberg, ibid., p. 247; Ostrowski, "Schicksal," p. 336.

54. Doc. 391 dated May 17, 1934, in Walk, *Sonderrecht*, pp. 80–81. Kümmel, "Ausschaltung," p. 73, heavily overinterprets this law when he writes that all the "Hindenburg exemptions" of 1933 were deleted, thereby implying the instant creation

of a mass of Jewish physicians bereft of panel practice privileges. This was not so. The May 17 decree merely repeated the contents of article 1 (1) and article 5 (2) stipulating that Jewish physicians with front-fighter status applying for panel practice would no longer be admitted. See Seldte, "Verordnung über die Zulassung von Ärzten zur Tätigkeit bei den Krankenkassen," April 22, 1933, *Ziel und Weg* 3 (1933): 79–80. An ordinance of November 20, 1933, excluded "Aryan" physicians with Jewish spouses from panel practice in cities with more than one hundred thousand inhabitants. See Jentzsch to Kulemann, Berlin, January 20, 1934, UK, 199; and case of Dr. Wilhelm Brandt, ibid.

55. Adam, *Judenpolitik*, p. 116, n. 14.

56. Klinger, *Wege*, p. 99; Witter, "Es hat doch auch."

57. An example of the latter is in doc. 9, dated March 5, 1934, in Sauer, *Dokumente*, 1:20–21.

58. Hoffmann, *Ringen*, p. 55.

59. Benn to Oelze, [Berlin], July 24, 1934, in Benn, *Briefe*, p. 36. See entry for July 12, 1933, in *Tagebuch Nathorff*, p. 47.

60. Entry for May 1935 in *Deutschland-Berichte* (1935), 2:534.

61. See doc. 114 of August 13, 1935, in Sauer, *Dokumente*, 1:132–33; entry for August in *Deutschland-Berichte* (1935), 2:924; Kulka, "Nürnberger Rassengesetze," pp. 594–95.

62. Entry for August in *Deutschland-Berichte* (1935), 2:928. See Ostrowski, "Schicksal," pp. 320–21.

63. Anonymous memorandum, [NSÄB office], Wiesbaden, September 20, 1934, HHSAW, 483/3159.

64. Adam, *Judenpolitik*, p. 120.

65. Doc. 587 of June 20, 1935, in Walk, *Sonderrecht*, p. 118; doc. 117 of September 14, 1935, in Sauer, *Dokumente*, 1:135–36.

66. Gumpert, *Hölle*, pp. 251–52. The account in Rosenstein, *Narben*, pp. 274–76, is somewhat different, and the timing seems wrong. For Cologne doctor Bruno Kisch's experience, see his *Wanderungen*, pp. 269–70.

67. Gumpert, *Hölle*, 241–42. Also entry for January in *Deutschland-Berichte* (1936), 3:32; Rosenstein, *Narben*, p. 275.

68. Toland, *Hitler*, pp. 517–18.

69. Althen to members of NSÄB Wiesbaden, Wiesbaden, August 30, 1934, HHSAW, 483/3159. My calculations are based on "Auszug aus der Arzt-Liste des neuen Kurvereins, Wiesbaden," appended to circular D 33/34, Wiesbaden, September 18, 1934, ibid.; and *Adressbuch der Stadt Wiesbaden*, pp. 15–17.

70. [Circular] Staeckert, Erfurt, October 20, 1934, UK, 215.

71. For example, decorated World War I veteran Dr. X in Spandau was expelled from the fund system despite his preferred status and never spoken to again by his "Aryan" colleagues (Stresau, *Jahr*, pp. 95–96). But a counterexample is in *Deutschland-Berichte* (1934), 1:115.

72. See Kater, "Everyday Anti-Semitism," pp. 147–55; Paucker, *Juden*.

73. Niedermeyer, *Wahn*, p. 285. On Hirsch, see Fischer, *Lexikon*, 1:633. Similar case recorded in entry for May 19, 1934, in *Tagebuch Nathorff*, p. 57.

74. Hanke, *Geschichte*, p. 115; Bessel, *Violence*, p. 136.

75. Ortsgruppenleiter to Bezirkswohlfahrtsamt, Berlin, November 14, 1934; Komm. Bezirksstadtrat to NSDAP-Gaugeschäftsstelle, Berlin-Lichtenberg, November 23, 1934, BA R 56I/100. Lazarus, born in 1873 in Czernowitz and by religion a Catholic, had been a professor since 1907 (Fischer, *Lexikon*, 2:875; *Wer ist's?* p. 940).

76. See entry for October 11, 1934, in *Tagebuch Nathorff*, p. 62; entries for July and August in *Deutschland-Berichte* (1935), 2:801, 931.

77. See the revealing letter by KVD central's lawyer Clemens Bewer to Dr. Brandes of KVD Vogtland, Berlin, January 5, 1935, UK, 200.

78. Adam, *Judenpolitik*, p. 117, n. 20.

79. Klipp to Gestapo Erfurt, Weimar, November 10, 1934; [unsent letter] Bewer to Klipp, Berlin, May 31, 1935, UK, 215. Also see Goldschmidt, *Meine Arbeit*, pp. 70–73.

80. *Deutsches Ärzteblatt* 65 (1935): 681.

81. For the image of Jewish doctors as calculating sexual race defilers see Kümmel, "Ausschaltung," p. 60; Lifton, *Nazi Doctors*, p. 41. For the mutual interaction of sexual and racial charges against Jewish doctors in 1933 see *Schwarzbuch*, pp. 196, 207–8; Reiter, "Revolution," pp. 424–25; Stähle, *Geschichte*, p. 7; Ackermann, "Nachwuchs," p. 125; Ostrowski, "Schicksal," p. 322; Kümmel, "Ausschaltung," p. 66.

82. Kater, "Everyday Anti-Semitism," pp. 148–50, 157–58.

83. *Ziel und Weg* 5 (1935): 314; entries for March, July, August in *Deutschland-Berichte* (1935), 2:358, 808–10, 923; entry for January in ibid. (1936), 3:32–33.

84. "Das Raubtier," *Der Stürmer* (1935), reprinted as doc. 210-11 in Wuttke-Groneberg, *Medizin*, pp. 353–54.

3. Progressive Disfranchisement: From the 1935 Nuremberg Race Laws to Delicensure in September 1938

1. Rühle, *Dritte Reich, 1935*, pp. 253–58. Quotation on p. 253.

2. Hitler and Frick, "Reichsbürgergesetz vom 15. September 1935," in Wagner, *Judengesetze*, p. 20; "Erste Verordnung zum Reichsbürgergesetz," Berlin, November 14, 1935, ibid., pp. 21–22; Hitler, Frick, Gürtner, Hess, "Gesetz zum Schutze des deutschen Blutes und der deutschen Ehre vom 15. September 1935," ibid., pp. 23–24; "Erste Verordnung zur Ausführung des Gesetzes zum Schutze des deutschen Blutes und der deutschen Ehre," n.d., ibid., pp. 24–31.

3. What these laws meant for the everyday life of the Jews may be gleaned from the general commentary in Rühle, *Dritte Reich, 1935*, pp. 277–92. In a book flawed by many mistakes of research and speciously argued (that anti-Semitism under Hitler was much less popular with the German people than has previously been believed; Gerhart Hauptmann was a Jew; Goebbels was not really anti-Semitic—see the justly critical review by Jill Stephenson in *History* 71 [1986]: 338–39; and George Steiner's indictment in *Times Literary Supplement*, July 13, 1984, questioning if the author, with all her errors, actually knows German), Sarah Gordon wrongly maintains that the Ger-

man Jews welcomed the Nuremberg Laws because they conveyed a sense of order (*Hitler*, p. 122). This opinion is based on a complete misreading of information in Meier, *Kirche und Judentum*, pp. 12–13.

4. Doc. 87 of December 21, 1935, in Walk, *Sonderrecht*, p. 148; Blau, *Ausnahmerecht*, p. 34; Adam, *Judenpolitik*, p. 149.

5. Ordinance Wagner, Berlin, February 13, 1936, *Deutsches Ärzteblatt* 66 (1936): 207–8.

6. Ibid.; par. 3 (5), "Reichsärzteordnung," December 13, 1935, BA, R 18/5574; Stuckart to minister [Frick], Berlin, December 3, 1935, BA, R 18/5574; Adam, *Judenpolitik*, p. 149.

7. Par. III and IV of ordinance Wagner, Berlin, February 13, 1936, *Deutsches Ärzteblatt* 66 (1936): 208.

8. See letter Jaffé to Korach, Amsterdam, January 21, 1939, partially printed in Leibfried, "Stationen der Abwehr," p. 6; entry for February in *Deutschland-Berichte* (1938), 5:194.

9. See letter Jaffé (as in n. 8, above); entry for August in *Deutschland-Berichte* (1936), 3:977; doc. 27 of May 5, 1937, in Sauer, *Dokumente*, 1:40; Ostrowski, "Schicksal," p. 326; Bielenberg, *Past*, p. 31.

10. File of Dr. Kurt Thomas (Berlin-Dahlem, 1936–38), UK, 243.

11. Entry for August in *Deutschland-Berichte* (1936), 3:982.

12. Entry for December, ibid., p. 1659.

13. Broszat et al., *Bayern*, p. 454, n. 18.

14. Doc. 301 of May 8, 1937, in Walk, *Sonderrecht*, p. 190.

15. Doc. 396 of January 1, 1938, ibid., pp. 209–10; *Ziel und Weg* 8 (1938): 50, 98; file of Dr. Georg Bernhardt, esp. Groote to Landgericht Berlin, Berlin, June 28, 1938; and [Bewer] to Kulemann, Berlin, August 20, 1938, UK, 130/131.02; file of Dr. Levisohn (Gelsenkirchen-Dortmund, June–July 1938), UK, 130/131.02. Also see entry for February in *Deutschland-Berichte* (1938), 5:190–91.

16. The following sources document the continued popularity of Jewish physicians and the resultant envy of their "Aryan" colleagues: doc. dated October 1, 1935, in Broszat et al., *Bayern*, p. 454; entry for January in *Deutschland-Berichte* (1936), 3:27; entries for July 25 and August 1, 1937, in Stresau, *Jahr*, pp. 140–41; Reichspropagandaministerium, Landesstelle Kurmark, to Spende "Künstlerdank," Berlin, October 5, 1937, BDC, RMK Fritz Goger-Sachs; Jaffé to Korach, Amsterdam, January 21, 1939, partially printed in Leibfried, "Stationen der Abwehr," p. 5; Hadda, "Als Arzt," p. 219; Rebentisch, "Beurteilung," p. 123.

17. Hanke, *Geschichte*, p. 146; entry for November in *Deutschland-Berichte* (1937), 4:1566.

18. Entry for January in *Deutschland-Berichte* (1936), 3:35.

19. Adam, *Judenpolitik*, p. 152, n. 44; Schütze, "Beamtenpolitik im Dritten Reich," p. 60; Kümmel, "Ausschaltung," p. 75; entry for December in *Deutschland-Berichte* (1936), 3:1655.

20. Entry for July in *Deutschland-Berichte* (1936), 3:870.

21. Entry for August in ibid., p. 984; on the legality see *Ziel und Weg* 7 (1937): 304. Also see entry for July in *Deutschland-Berichte* (1937), 4:933.

22. Entry for November in *Deutschland-Berichte* (1937), 4:1572.

23. See P. E. Rings, "Du—und Dein Arzt" (1937), printed as doc. 204-5 in Wuttke-Groneberg, *Medizin*, p. 349.

24. Excerpts from *Der Stürmer*, "Sie gehen zu Judenärzten" and "Brief aus Köln" (1938), as doc. 198, 1-2 reprinted ibid., p. 344.

25. See the examples in Stern, *Warum*, p. 206; Bielenberg, *Past*, p. 31. How things worked in practice is depicted in entries for March 1 and August 14, 1935; also June 28, 1938, in *Tagebuch Nathorff*, pp. 69, 72, 108–9. But also see the optimistic entry for October 10, 1936, p. 88. Further see example of Dr. Hanns Schwarz. His testimony is in Albrecht and Hartwig, *Ärzte*, p. 70.

26. Dr. Löllke and Dr. Sonnenberg, "In der Streitsache des praktischen Arztes Dr. med. Walter Schubert," [Berlin, June 6, 1939], UK, 130/118.02/4. The figure of 13,643 marks is mentioned for 1937 in text of Chapter 1, 3, at n. 45.

27. See entry for November in *Deutschland-Berichte* (1937), 4:1569; also Henry, *Victims and Neighbors*, p. 2.

28. See entries for September, *Deutschland-Berichte* (1935), 2:1037; August (1936), 3:987; February (1938), 5:185–86. See entry for New Year's Eve 1935, in *Tagebuch Nathorff*, pp. 77–78.

29. Testimony of Carl Schwabe in Richarz, *Leben*, pp. 164–65. Also see entry for January 4, 1937, in *Tagebuch Nathorff*, p. 93.

30. Entry for February in *Deutschland-Berichte* (1938), 5:186.

31. *Ziel und Weg* 5 (1935): 519. Cf. entries for June 5 and September 6, 1937, in *Tagebuch Nathorff*, pp. 95, 97.

32. *Ziel und Weg* 8 (1938): 574.

33. See the entries for August in *Deutschland-Berichte* (1936), 3:987, 989; February (1938), 5:185.

34. See the examples of Dr. Boas and Dr. Fels, entries for August, ibid. (1936), 3:1022; May (1937), 4:698, 706.

35. See entry for November, ibid. (1937), 4:1569.

36. Fliedner, *Judenverfolgung*, p. 63; doc. 491 of June 22, 1938, in Walk, *Sonderrecht*, p. 230. No Jews were admitted to Hamburg hospitals after January 1936 or to Düsseldorf hospitals after June 1936, only as outpatients (Lindemann, *140 Jahre*, p. 64; doc. 178 of June 29, 1936, in Walk, p. 166).

37. Docs. 116 and 117 of December 6, 1935, and March 6, 1936, in Sauer, *Dokumente* 1:133–35; Fliedner, *Judenverfolgung*, p. 186.

38. See entry for November in *Deutschland-Berichte* (1937), 4:1571–72; Müller-Hill, *Tödliche Wissenschaft*, pp. 39–40; Weingart, "Eugenik," p. 334.

39. Example of Dr. Crull in *Ziel und Weg* 7 (1937): 333.

40. Wagner as quoted in *Deutsches Ärzteblatt* 67 (1937): 906.

41. Doc. 349 of September 8, 1937, in Walk, *Sonderrecht*, p. 200; Haedenkamp, "Änderungen," p. 410; "Zum Recht der jüdischen Mischlinge nach dem Stande vom Mai 1938," June 10, 1938, BA, R 56I/114.

42. For example, see BDC, RÄK Hans Oppenheimer (Berlin), Berthold Krevet (Stolpen), Otto Sonnenfeld (Magdeburg), Konrad Grein (Halle).

43. As in n. 41.

44. Entry for July in *Deutschland-Berichte* (1937), 4:947.

45. Example of Dr. Hanns Schwarz (Berlin), married to a Jewish woman, was first

believed to be an "Aryan" by birth, then a half Jew, and finally reinstated as an "Aryan." See his testimony on this point in Albrecht and Hartwig, *Ärzte*, pp. 70–71.

46. Example: BDC, RÄK Georg Bolte.

47. Example of physician from Ketsch in entry for January in *Deutschland-Berichte* (1936), 3:31–33.

48. *Ziel und Weg* 7 (1937): 537; Hanns Schwarz's testimony in Albrecht and Hartwig, *Ärzte*, p. 68.

49. *Central-Verein-Zeitung* of October 21, 1937, as quoted in *Ziel und Weg* 7 (1937): 558; Ostrowski, "Schicksal," p. 332; Rosenstein, *Narben*, p. 267. On Seligmann, see n. 29 of section 2; Fischer, *Lexikon*, 2:1438.

50. Testimony of Alexander Szanto in Richarz, *Leben*, p. 223.

51. Taute et al., *Entwicklung*, p. 32.

52. Lindemann, *140 Jahre*, pp. 61–62.

53. Lindemann mentions the Jewish hospitals of Berlin, Breslau, Frankfurt, Hanover, Leipzig, Hamburg, and Cologne (ibid., pp. 61–66), but there were still others, such as the ones in Würzburg and Munich. See the memoirs of Ostrowski, "Schicksal"; Hadda, "Als Arzt"; Rosenstein, *Narben*.

54. Ophir and Wiesemann, *Gemeinden*, p. 264.

55. Entry for July in *Deutschland-Berichte* (1937), 4:942.

56. Such examples are recorded for December, ibid. (1936), 3:1658–59; July and November (1937), 4:944, 1573; and in Brugsch, *Arzt*, pp. 294–95; Ostrowski, "Schicksal," p. 333. Also see text in Chapter 2, 3, at n. 39.

57. Entries for July and November in *Deutschland-Berichte* (1937), 4:932–33, 1564.

58. One such case was that of the Nuremberg physicians' association functionary Dr. Ludwig Steinheimer (see text in section 2 at n. 7), who in January 1938 won a court case for a pension owed to him by the KVD since his wrongful dismissal (1933) by the Hartmannbund (Dr. Klipp, KVD Landesstelle Bayern, to KVD chapter Nuremberg, Munich, June 3, 1938; "Fragebogen wegen der laufenden Pensionen," Nuremberg, October 28, 1938, UK, 130/123.02).

59. Behrendt (KVD) to Schulz, Berlin, February 10, 1938, countersigned by KVD's lawyer Clemens Bewer February 11, 1938, UK, 243.

60. Dr. Pychlau, KVD Landesstelle Baden, to Hauptamt für Volksgesundheit, Mannheim, December 29, 1937, UK, 234.

61. Deuel, *Compassion*, pp. 212–13; Gilbert, *Holocaust*, p. 50.

62. Entry for January in *Deutschland-Berichte* (1936), 3:29; testimony of Hanns Schwarz in Albrecht and Hartwig, *Ärzte*, p. 70.

63. Entry for January in *Deutschland-Berichte* (1936), 3:35; doc. of February 8, 1936, in Broszat et al., *Bayern*, p. 459; Frei, *Provinzpresse*, p. 217.

64. Ophir and Wiesemann, *Gemeinden*, p. 254; Winter, *Benjamin*, p. 23.

65. Botz, *Wien*, pp. 93–105, 243–59; idem, *Wohnungspolitik*; Moser, *Judenverfolgung*, pp. 5–8; Gilbert, *Holocaust*, pp. 58–62; entry for July in *Deutschland-Berichte* (1938), 5:732–39.

66. See Carsten, *Rise of Fascism*, pp. 32–41; idem, *Fascist Movements*, pp. 9–39; Pulzer, *Rise of Political Anti-Semitism*, pp. 128–270; Johnston, *Austrian Mind*, pp.

27–29, 65–66. For pre-1914 Hungary see Deak's brilliant articles, "Could the Hungarian Jews," p. 24; and "Convert," p. 41.

67. Hitler, *Mein Kampf*, pp. 47–115.

68. Entry for July in *Deutschland-Berichte* (1938), 5:736; Gilbert, *Holocaust*, p. 59; Botz, *Wien*, p. 103.

69. *Ziel und Weg* 7 (1937): 391; 8 (1938): 631. Percentage calculations according to figures ibid. 9 (1939): 21. This is corroborated in Kann, "Zahl, 1942," p. 300. See also Ternon and Helman, *Les médecins allemands*, p. 92. Ramm's figure of 67 percent for Vienna is exaggerated (*Standeskunde*, p. 46), and Tennstedt's of 80 percent is even more so (*Selbstverwaltung*, p. 213).

70. See Table 3 in Botz, *Wien*, p. 102, and p. 103.

71. Gilbert, *Holocaust*, p. 59.

72. Ibid.; Botz, *Wien*, p. 105.

73. Botz, *Wien*, p. 243.

74. *Journal of the American Medical Association* 112 (1939): 2546.

4. The End of the Jewish Doctors

1. Adam, *Judenpolitik*, p. 157, n. 72. The regional SD order for Württemberg-Hohenzollern is printed in Sauer, *Dokumente*, 1:137.

2. Adam, *Judenpolitik*, p. 168.

3. "Vierte Verordnung zum Reichsbürgergesetz," July 25, 1938, signed Hitler, Frick, Hess, Gürtner, *Reichsgesetzblatt* (1938), I, 969–70.

4. "Die Bestallungen jüdischer Ärzte erlöschen mit dem 30. September," *Frankfurter Zeitung*, August 4, 1938, reprinted in Goldschmidt, *Meine Arbeit*, p. 62; *Journal of the American Medical Association* 111 (1938): 1674–75; and esp. the (left-wing underground oppositional) criticism in *Deutschland-Berichte* (1938), 5:742–43.

5. *Ziel und Weg* 8 (1938): 572.

6. Doc. 120 of October 11, 1938, in Sauer, *Dokumente*, 1:138–39; doc. of October 11, 1938, in Franke, *Geschichte*, p. 280; Zelzer, *Weg*, pp. 189–90; Ophir and Wiesemann, *Gemeinden*, p. 58; Tennstedt and Leibfried, "Sozialpolitik," p. 225. Also the critical commentary, entry for November in *Deutschland-Berichte* (1938), 5:1283–84. For Cologne (approximately six physicians for thirty thousand Jews), see Kisch, *Wanderungen*, p. 277.

7. Wagner, "Sicherung," p. 23; idem, "Gesundes Leben," p. 554; *Völkischer Beobachter*, October 16, 1938; "Das Ende der jüdischen Aerzte," in *Der Heilpraktiker* (1938), reprinted as doc. 200 in Wuttke-Groneberg, *Medizin*, p. 346.

8. See the example for the Prussian province of Pomerania in Zacke, "Bericht über die Prüfung bei der RÄK, Ärztekammer Pommern in Stettin," Berlin, August 24, 1939, UK, 156/RÄK, Revisionsamt.

9. Doc. 560 of October 6, 1938, in Walk, *Sonderrecht*, p. 245.

10. Hadda, "Als Arzt," p. 220.

11. Entry for December in *Deutschland-Berichte* (1938), 5:1330.

12. Ibid., p. 1344; *Deutsches Ärzteblatt* 69 (1939): 401. For the Sudetenland see *Ziel und Weg* 9 (1939): 392.

13. Doc. 241 of June 16, 1939, in Blau, *Ausnahmerecht*, p. 75; Adam, *Judenpolitik*, p. 221, n. 102.

14. For details other than those affecting Jewish physicians, see Rühle, *Dritte Reich, 1938*, pp. 394–404 (from the official Nazi vantage point); Bracher, *German Dictatorship*, pp. 366–68; Graml, *9. November 1938*; Genschel, *Verdrängung der Juden*, pp. 177–217; Schleunes, *Twisted Road*, pp. 214–54; Adam, *Judenpolitik*, pp. 204–16.

15. "Schicksal," p. 340. See also entries between November 10 and December 16, 1938, in *Tagebuch Nathorff*, pp. 121–40.

16. That doctor was Werner Forssmann. See his memoirs, *Selbstversuch*, pp. 211–12.

17. Ostrowski, "Schicksal," pp. 340–42. Also see the example for Breslau in Hadda, "Als Arzt," p. 220.

18. Testimony of Hans Berger in Richarz, *Leben*, pp. 332–33; Hadda, "Als Arzt," p. 221; entries for November and December in *Deutschland-Berichte* (1938), 5:1198, 1348; entry for July in ibid. (1939), 6:921; Henry, *Victims and Neighbors*, p. 74; Boveri, *Verzweigungen*, p. 338.

19. Suicide case of Frankfurt physician Dr. Bernard Rosenthal according to testimony of Hans Berger in Richarz, *Leben*, p. 324. Case of Goldberg in Bruss, *Bremer Juden*, pp. 186–87, 288; Stokes, *Kleinstadt*, p. 970, n. 4. Goldberg's name also appears in Gestapo list "of all Jews living in Bremen as of May 1, 1936," appended to letter Gestapa Bremen to Bremen NSDAP Kreispersonalamt, Bremen, June 3, 1936, BA, Schumacher/241.

20. Ophir and Wiesemann, *Gemeinden*, p. 212; entry for July in *Deutschland-Berichte* (1939), 6:920; Hadda, "Als Arzt," p. 221; Deich, "Jüdische Mediziner," p. 82; Ostrowski, "Schicksal," p. 342.

21. Ostrowski, "Schicksal," pp. 342–43.

22. Verschuer as quoted in Müller-Hill, *Tödliche Wissenschaft*, p. 40.

23. Richarz, *Leben*, p. 66; testimony of Bruno Blau, ibid., pp. 459–73; Ostrowski, "Schicksal," pp. 343–51; Lindemann, *140 Jahre*, pp. 67–70; Hadda, "Als Arzt," pp. 222–33; Fliedner, *Judenverfolgung*, p. 64; entry for April in *Deutschland-Berichte* (1940), 7:260.

24. Testimony of Camilla Neumann in Richarz, *Leben*, p. 418; testimony of Hermann Pineas, ibid., pp. 432–33; testimony of Bruno Blau, ibid., pp. 459–73; Hadda, "Als Arzt," pp. 226–30; entry for July in *Deutschland-Berichte* (1939), 6:923; Kwiet and Eschwege, *Selbstbehauptung*, pp. 206–7; Ostrowski, "Schicksal," pp. 344–51; Ophir and Wiesemann, *Gemeinden*, p. 298.

25. Robinsohn, *Justiz*, p. 66. Also see Adam, *Hochschule*, p. 187, n. 215; entry for July in *Deutschland-Berichte* (1939), 6:905.

26. See entries for July in *Deutschland-Berichte* (1939), 6:932, 936.

27. Winter, *Benjamin*, p. 23. Benjamin's case is, however, paralleled by that of his SPD colleague Julius Moses, who also perished in a concentration camp in 1942 (Tennstedt, "Sozialgeschichte," p. 407).

28. Ostrowski, "Schicksal," p. 348; *Deutsches Ärzteblatt* 70 (1940): 513 (quotation); speech by Conti at convention of Hauptamt für Volksgesundheit in Munich, March 28, 1942, "Gesundheitsführung—Volksschicksal," BDC, OPG Emil Ketterer

(p. 13). One must remember that Conti's mother, Nanna, was in charge of German midwives.

29. Conti's remarks at meeting of NSÄB in Berlin on April 24, 1942, in *Deutsches Ärzteblatt* 72 (1942): 201.

30. See doc. 143 of 1943 in Wuttke-Groneberg, *Medizin*, p. 250. Also Streicher's vituperative remarks (1939), in doc. 91, ibid., p. 169.

31. Adam, *Judenpolitik*, p. 210; text in section 3 near n. 36.

32. Docs. 337 and 338 of December 19 and 20, 1938, in Sauer, *Dokumente*, 2:79–81; Bruss, *Bremer Juden*, p. 134. Also see Knipping, *Geschichte*, pp. 66–67; docs. 14 and 15 of January 17 and 23 and March 18, 1939, in ibid., pp. 175–77.

33. Gestapo Dortmund to Herren Landräte et al., Dortmund, April 19, 1939, doc. 16 in Knipping, *Geschichte*, p. 178; Dr. Lochmann's announcement in *Ärzteblatt für Norddeutschland* 3 (1940): 51–52.

34. File of Dr. Karl Ritter von Steyskal (September–November 1941), DAÖW, 4491.

35. Partei-Kanzlei to Reich interior minister, Munich, July 6, 1942, BA, R 18/3764.

36. Doc. 393 of July 14, 1942, in Walk, *Sonderrecht*, p. 381.

37. Lösener, "Rassereferent," p. 286; Hilberg, *Destruction*, pp. 268–74; Adam, *Judenpolitik*, pp. 224–25; Müller-Hill, *Tödliche Wissenschaft*, p. 22. See Goebbels's confusion expressed in entry for March 7, 1942, in *Goebbels Diaries*, p. 140; "Vermerk: Behandlung jüdischer Mischlinge," October 30, 1944, BA, R 22/1183.

38. See BDC, RÄK Hans-Florian Hahn, Adolf Hahn, Johann Schöfer, Elisabeth Mietke, Martina Drucker, Johannes Malejka.

39. Chapter 1, 1, text at n. 49.

40. Reichsgesundheitsführer, information 2/43, Berlin, December 20, 1943, BA, R 18/3766a.

41. Klinger, *Wege*, p. 99; Witter, "Es hat doch auch." On the problem of mixed marriages after 1938 from the Nazi perspective see Hilberg, *Destruction*, pp. 274–77.

42. Testimony of Hermann Pineas in Richarz, *Leben*, pp. 433, 441–42, n. 13.

43. Gilbert, *Holocaust*, p. 213. Also see Krausnick, "Judenverfolgung," pp. 381–91; Hilberg, *Destruction*, pp. 298–99.

44. Cf. Lösener, "Rassereferent," p. 294.

45. Example of Dr. Erwin Korte, in entries for July 7 and September 29, 1941, in Hohenstein, *Wartheländisches Tagebuch*, pp. 145–46, 179–80; Hagen, *Auftrag*, pp. 221–22.

46. See Deich, "Mediziner," pp. 82–83; Ostrowski, "Schicksal," p. 345; Hadda, "Als Arzt," pp. 233–37; testimony Oskar Moos in Franke, *Geschichte*, pp. 238–39; and the cases from Stuttgart mentioned in Zelzer, *Weg*, pp. 460–62.

47. Kümmel, "Ausschaltung," p. 76. Also see Adler, *Theresienstadt*, p. 191.

48. See Gross, *Versteckt*, p. 254; Bruss, *Bremer Juden*, p. 231; testimony of Herta Pineas in Richarz, *Leben*, p. 430; Fliedner, *Judenverfolgung*, p. 186–87; Ophir and Wiesemann, *Gemeinden*, p. 186; Behrend-Rosenfeld, *Allein*, p. 90.

49. Lifton, *Nazi Doctors*, pp. 250–53.

5. A Chronicle of Exile and a Demographic Reckoning

1. Entry for August 12, 1936, in *Tagebuch Nathorff*, p. 87 (quotation), and passim. This was a general phenomenon, not just valid in the specialized case of the physicians. See Dawidowicz, *War*, p. 256.

2. Gumpert, *Hölle*, pp. 266–67. Also see Richarz, *Leben*, p. 51; entry for March 12, 1939, in *Tagebuch Nathorff*, p. 151.

3. Dawidowicz, *War*, p. 254; Richarz, *Leben*, p. 53. For very informative details within a broader context relating to Jewish emigration, and taking account of all potential host countries, the reader is referred to the excellent studies by Strauss, "Jewish Emigration from Germany," (I) and (II).

4. See the following: Hans Dornedden in *Deutsches Ärzteblatt* 65 (1935): 515; *Journal of the American Medical Association* 102 (1934): 1241–42; Leibfried, "Stationen der Abwehr," pp. 17, 20; Gumpert, *Hölle*, pp. 263–68; Bielenberg, *Past*, pp. 31–32; entry for September 5, 1937, in Stresau, *Jahr*, p. 150; testimony of Hanns Schwarz in Albrecht and Hartwig, *Ärzte*, p. 76; Sauer, *Schicksale*, p. 118; Zelzer, *Weg*, pp. 158, 460; Richarz, *Leben*, p. 52; entry for January 4, 1938, in *Tagebuch Nathorff*, p. 102; Niederland, "Deutsche Ärzte-Emigration," p. 157; and the second table in Davie, *Refugees*, p. 260.

5. *Ziel und Weg* 5 (1935): 229, 383, 498; Schulz, "Entwicklung," p. 484; Wagner, "Unser Reichsärzteführer spricht," p. 435; Aron, "Nichtarischen Ärzte"; entry for July in *Deutschland-Berichte* (1938), 5:749; Jaffé to Korach, Amsterdam, January 21, 1939, partially printed in Leibfried, "Stationen der Abwehr," p. 5; Fliedner, *Judenverfolgung*, pp. 50–51; Ostrowski, "Schicksal," p. 323; Leibfried, "Stationen der Abwehr," p. 14; Richarz, *Leben*, p. 82; Dawidowicz, *War*, pp. 254–55; Gilbert, *Holocaust*, pp. 44–45.

6. Richarz, *Leben*, p. 53.

7. Leibfried, "Stationen der Abwehr," p. 20.

8. Friedman, *No Haven*, pp. 56–65; Gilbert, *Holocaust*, p. 64; Strauss, "Jewish Emigration from Germany (II)," p. 362.

9. Entries for February, July, November, December in *Deutschland-Berichte* (1938), 5:182, 749, 1195, 1332; Sauer, *Schicksale*, p. 126; Richarz, *Leben*, p. 55; Frankenthal, *Dreifache Fluch*, pp. 197, 200; Strauss, "Jewish Emigration from Germany (I)," pp. 343–44; Wolfgang Benz in *Tagebuch Nathorff*, p. 13.

10. Before 1938, Rosenstein was also "blackmailed" for currency transfer infractions he had never committed (*Narben*, pp. 269–71, 281–82). His vita is in Fischer, *Lexikon*, 2:1325.

11. Entries for December in *Deutschland-Berichte* (1936), 3:1653; and for February, ibid. (1938), 5:182–83; Bruss, *Bremer Juden*, pp. 118–19.

12. The case of KVD versus Dr. Weill (Leipzig-Haifa) was won by the KVD only at a higher appellate court (January–April 1937) (UK, 248).

13. Entry for August 20, 1934, in *Tagebuch Nathorff*, p. 60; Gumpert, *Hölle*, p. 263.

14. Entry for November in *Deutschland-Berichte* (1937), 4:1566–67; entries for February and July 1938, ibid. (1938), 5:183, 749; Jaffé to Korach, Amsterdam, January 21, 1939, partially printed in Leibfried, "Stationen der Abwehr," p. 6;

Rosenstein, *Narben*, pp. 273–74. Also see text in section 3 at n. 8.

15. Henry, *Victims and Neighbors*, pp. 74–75.

16. Gumpert, *Hölle*, p. 258; Rosenstein, *Narben*, p. 110; entry for November 15, 1938, in Stresau, *Jahr*, p. 172.

17. Jaffé to Korach, Amsterdam, January 21, 1939, partially printed in Leibfried, "Stationen der Abwehr," p. 5; Boveri, *Verzweigungen*, p. 338.

18. Frankenthal, *Dreifache Fluch*, pp. 198–99.

19. Plesch, *János*, p. 291; Fischer, *Lexikon*, 2:1226; *List*, p. 70; testimony of Elisabeta Bihalji, Belgrade, March 11, 1962, DAÖW, 2962.

20. Davie, *Refugees*, p. xix.

21. Calculations on the basis of the list in Zelzer, *Weg*, pp. 460–62.

22. See Richarz, *Leben*, pp. 53–54; Boveri, *Verzweigungen*, p. 331; Strauss, "Jewish Emigration from Germany (II)," p. 345; entry for Easter 1934 in *Tagebuch Nathorff*, p. 56.

23. Friedman, *No Haven*, pp. 20–21 (Tincher as cited on p. 21); Strauss, "Jewish Emigration from Germany (II)," p. 358; Hempel, "*Wenn ich schon ein Fremder*," pp. 20–21.

24. Strauss, "Jewish Emigration from Germany (II)," pp. 359–61; Friedman, *No Haven*, pp. 21–27. Also see Edsall, "Emigré Physician," p. 1069; Kisch, *Wanderungen*, pp. 279–81.

25. Strauss, "Jewish Emigraton from Germany (II)," Table 4 on p. 359, and p. 361. With specific reference to physicians, see Edsall, "Program," p. 1986.

26. Strauss, "Jewish Emigration from Germany (II)," pp. 361–62; Friedman, *No Haven*, pp. 65–66.

27. Strauss, "Jewish Emigration from Germany (II)," Table 4 on p. 359, and p. 362.

28. Ibid.; Wyman, *Abandonment*, passim.

29. My calculation is based on figures for the total of Jews as indicated in Strauss, "Jewish Emigration from Germany (II)," p. 362, and the figure of just over three thousand Jewish-German, German-Sudeten, and Austrian émigré physicians as mentioned by Professor Eric D. Kohler, University of Wyoming, currently the leading expert on the subject of German-Jewish physicians in the United States, in his letter to me, Laramie, January 3, 1988. In a dated treatment of the problem, Sauer, *Schicksale*, p. 218, mentions twenty-five hundred German-Jewish refugee physicians in the United States (this would have lowered the percentage to 1.9).

30. Edsall, "Program," p. 1986; idem, "Emigré Physician," p. 1069.

31. Above all, see Table 2 of Edsall, "Emigré Physician," p. 1071, also pp. 1069–70, 1072. Also Edsall and Putnam, "Emigré Physician," p. 1885. For New York, Pearle, "Ärzteemigration nach 1933," pp. 115–16; Aron, "Wie geht es."

32. *Journal of the American Medical Association* 112 (1939): 735; *Medical Economics* 16, no. 5 (February 1939): 28; Edsall and Putnam, "Emigré Physician," pp. 1885–86; Pearle, "Ärzteemigration nach 1933," pp. 115–21, 126–28; Davie, *Refugees*, pp. 267–69. But see the favorable interpretation in Nissen, *Blätter*, pp. 251–52.

33. *Journal of the American Medical Association* 112 (1939): 735; Edsall, "Program," p. 1986; Edsall and Putnam, "Emigré Physician," pp. 1882, 1884–85, 1888; Pearle, "Ärzteemigration nach 1933," p. 113.

34. Compare the values for those states in Table 6 of Edsall and Putnam, "Emigré Physician," p. 1884, with the corresponding ones in Table 2 of Edsall, "Emigré Physician," p. 1071.

35. Edsall, "Program," p. 1987; Edsall and Putnam, "Emigré Physician," p. 1882; *Medical Economics* 16, no. 5 (February 1939): 96, 98, 100, 102.

36. *Medical Economics* 16, no. 5 (February 1939): 25. Also see McIntyre, "Citizenship and Medical Licensure."

37. Davie, *Refugees*, p. 167.

38. See Pearle, "Ärzteemigration nach 1933," pp. 128–30; see the example of Dr. Paul Rosenstein, below.

39. Eric D. Kohler, "Between Dr. Pinkham's Dilemma and Dr. Mumey's Jerusalem: German Jewish Physicians in California and Colorado," paper delivered at the annual meeting of the German Studies Association, Albuquerque, N.M., September 1986.

40. Pearle, "Ärzteemigration nach 1933," p. 115; Milch, "Expatriated Elite," p. 15.

41. Sauer, *Schicksale*, p. 218; Edsall, "Emigré Physician," p. 1069. See, however, the more realistic assessment by Edsall and Putnam, in "Emigré Physician," pp. 1883–84 and n. 278.

42. Müller, *Geschichte*, p. 214; Bruss, *Bremer Juden*, p. 40; Zelzer, *Wege*, p. 460.

43. File card of Ahronheim, RSW collection, BA (see n. 33 of Chapter 5, 2).

44. Obituary for Dr. Frederick Simōn Aron of 1962 reprinted in Goldschmidt, *Meine Arbeit*, p. 37.

45. Zelzer, *Wege*, p. 460. Also see entry for May 3, 1940, in *Tagebuch Nathorff*, p. 197.

46. Henry, *Victims and Neighbors*, p. 2. Dr. Hertha Nathorff was called "lousy Nazispy" (entry for March 7, 1940, in *Tagebuch Nathorff*, p. 171). Other testimonies of this nature are in Albrecht and Hartwig, *Ärzte*, pp. 72–76 (Hanns Schwarz); Gumpert, *Hölle*, p. 267.

47. Schwarz in Albrecht and Hartwig, *Ärzte*, p. 76.

48. Hagen, *Auftrag*, pp. 151, 247. See Fischer, *Lexikon*, 2:1554; *Wer ist's?* p. 1593.

49. Rosenstein, *Narben*, pp. 285–91.

50. Frankenthal, *Dreifache Fluch*, pp. 238–45. Also see Pearle's and Leibfried's postscript, ibid., pp. 249–58; and the parallels in *Tagebuch Nathorff*, pp. 166–212.

51. Pearle and Leibfried in Frankenthal, *Dreifache Fluch*, p. 258. For the comparable case of Dr. Hertha Nathorff, see Wolfgang Benz in *Tagebuch Nathorff*, p. 15. For all German Jews, see Strauss, "Immigration."

52. Official wording as quoted in Strauss, "Jewish Emigration from Germany (II)," p. 344.

53. Ibid., pp. 344–45. Wasserstein qualifies this by pointing out that approximately fifty-three thousand German and Austrian Jews went to Palestine until 1939 (*Britain*, p. 7).

54. Strauss, "Jewish Emigration from Germany (II)," pp. 345–55; Richarz, *Leben*, pp. 44–45, 51, 53. On youth, also see Angress, *Generation*.

55. Wasserstein, *Britain*, pp. 12–16; Strauss, "Jewish Emigration from Germany (II)," pp. 355–56.

56. Quotation from Wasserstein, *Britain*, p. 18.

57. Ibid., pp. 17–20.

58. Ibid., p. 26.

59. Richarz, *Leben*, p. 54; Strauss, "Jewish Emigration from Germany (II)," pp. 345, 349.

60. To practice medicine in Palestine in a dependent or self-employed capacity, a candidate had to satisfy academic and personal prerequisites. The academic requirement included the bestowing of a license by the Palestinian public health authorities upon proof of at least five years of regular studies at a recognized foreign medical school and possession of a medical diploma or doctorate. The personal requirement entailed proof of good character and residency papers for Palestine (Kalisch, "Regelung"; Dr. Siegfried Kanowitz [Tel Aviv] as paraphrased in *Ziel und Weg* 5 [1935]: 228).

61. *Deutsches Ärzteblatt* 64 (1934): 180–81; Dr. Hans Dornedden, ibid. 5 (1935): 515; Dr. Siegfried Kanowitz (Tel Aviv) as paraphrased in *Ziel und Weg* 5 (1935): 228; Aron, "Wie geht es."

62. Niederland, "Deutsche Ärzte-Emigration," p. 155. Dr. Siegfried Kanowitz (Tel Aviv) as paraphrased in *Ziel und Weg* 5 (1935): 228, mentions a ratio of 1:250 for 1935.

63. Dr. Siegfried Kanowitz as paraphrased in *Ziel und Weg* 5 (1935): 228; ibid., p. 58.

64. Trusted, "Draft: An Ordinance to Amend the Medical Practitioners Ordinance, 1928," [Jerusalem], July 18, 1935, *Palestine Gazette*, July 25, 1935, pp. 637–40, ISA, Record Group M/74/35. Also see *Palestine Post*, July 25, 1935. I owe my knowledge of this document and the other ones from Palestine (below) to Professor William E. Seidelman, McMaster University, whose help is greatly appreciated.

65. Shertok to chief secretary, Government Offices Jerusalem, Jerusalem, August 15, 1935, ISA, Record Group M/74/35.

66. J. Hathorn Hall, "Medical Practitioners (Amendment) Ordinance, No. 44 of 1935," [Jerusalem], October 30, 1935, ISA, Record Group 2, M/74/35; Kalisch, "Die Regelung"; *Ziel und Weg* 6 (1936): 110.

67. See Table 1 in Niederland, "Deutsche Ärzte-Emigration," on p. 156, and p. 157.

68. For the principle of this, see ibid., p. 162.

69. Franke, *Geschichte*, pp. 82–83; Zelzer, *Weg*, pp. 158–59, 460. Also see Sauer, *Schicksale*, pp. 228–29.

70. Zelzer, *Weg*, p. 460.

71. Birnbaum, *Staat*, p. 38 (n. 92), pp. 189–90 (n. 163). The work of German-Jewish physicians in Palestine as a group has been detailed by Niederland, "Deutsche Ärzte-Emigration," pp. 157–84.

72. Rosenstein, *Narben*, p. 251.

73. File cards of Georg Peysack and Max Sadger, RSW collection, BA (see n. 33 of Chapter 5, 2).

74. Ostrowski, "Schicksal," p. 351. See his medical paper, "Progressive Infectious Skin-Necrosis." The fate of other Jewish Berlin doctors in Palestine is depicted by Pross in Pross and Winau, *nicht misshandeln*, pp. 171–72, 174–76.

75. On this tragic and ever-recurring phenomenon, see, among others, Wyman, *Abandonment*, for example, p. 158.

76. Sauer, *Schicksale*, p. 369.

77. Director of medical services, Department of Health, to chief secretary, Government Offices, Jerusalem, October 29, 1940; Commissioner for migration and statistics, acting director, Department of Immigration, to chief secretary, Jerusalem, December 20, 1940, ISA, Record Group 2, M/7/40.

78. *Deutsches Ärzteblatt* 64 (1934): 180; Wasserstein, *Britain*, p. 7.

79. See Friedman, *No Haven*, p. 71.

80. Wasserstein, *Britain*, pp. 9–10, 82, 93. Also see Cole, *Lord Haw-Haw*, p. 180; Strauss, "Jewish Emigration from Germany (II)," p. 357; Richarz, *Leben*, p. 54. The argument regarding unemployment and economics was presented internationally in 1934 and by Britain's representative at the Evian conference in 1938. See *Journal of the American Medical Association* 102 (1934): 1861; Friedman, *No Haven*, p. 60.

81. *Journal of the American Medical Association* 100 (1933): 1784; ibid. 102 (1934): 1861; ibid. 107 (1936): 49; ibid. 111 (1938): 636–37; Aron, "Wie geht es"; *Medical Economics* 16, no. 5 (February 1939): 27. Also see Berghahn, *Refugees*, pp. 83–85; and the testimony of Hadda, "Als Arzt," pp. 219–20.

82. Plesch, *János*, pp. 292–96. Also see *Journal of the American Medical Association* 100 (1933): 2029–30; ibid. 107 (1936): 49.

83. Documentation in the order of listing: Zelzer, *Weg*, p. 462; Angress, *Generation*, p. 81; Bruss, *Bremer Juden*, p. 40, n. 88; Klinger, *Wege*, p. 82; file card of Rudolf Friedländer, RSW collection, BA (see n. 33 of Chapter 5, 2).

84. Edsall and Putnam, "Emigré Physician," p. 1884.

85. Strauss, "Jewish Emigration from Germany (I)," pp. 354–55; Dornedden in *Deutsches Ärzteblatt* 64 (1934): 180.

86. File cards of Werner Sandelowski and Dorothea Futter, RSW collection, BA (see n. 33 of Chapter 5, 2).

87. Aron, "Wie geht es"; Voigt, "Refuge," p. 14.

88. File card of Dorothea Futter, RSW collection, BA (see n. 33 of Chapter 5, 2).

89. Voigt, "Refuge," pp. 14–15.

90. Quotation according to *Medical Economics* 16, no. 5 (February 1939): 27. Also see Strauss, "Jewish Emigration from Germany (I)," p. 354. For anti-Semitism in Italy generally, see Cassels, *Fascism*, pp. 165–66.

91. As in n. 88 and Strauss, "Jewish Emigration from Germany (I)," p. 355; Sauer, *Schicksale*, p. 369.

92. See Aron, "Wie geht es."

93. See Leibfried, "Stationen der Abwehr," pp. 18, 20; *Medical Economics* 16, no. 5 (February 1939): 27; Plesch, *János*, p. 251; file card of Alfred Stern, RSW collection, BA (see n. 33 of Chapter 5, 2).

94. Strauss, "Jewish Emigration from Germany (I)," p. 354; Dornedden in *Deutsches Ärzteblatt* 64 (1934): 180.

95. Strauss, "Jewish Emigration from Germany (I)," p. 354. Wasserstein's figure

of altogether forty thousand European Jewish refugees in France before hostilities commenced in 1939 appears somewhat high (*Britain*, p. 7).

96. Strauss, "Jewish Emigration from Germany (I)," p. 353; *Ziel und Weg* 5 (1935): 79–81, 174; Aron, "Wie geht es"; Dornedden in *Deutsches Ärzteblatt* 64 (1934): 180; Plesch, *János*, p. 291; *Medical Economics* 16, no. 5 (February 1939): 26; Zelzer, *Weg*, p. 462; Frankenthal, *Dreifache Fluch*, pp. 209–17. Wolf is mentioned in Fischer, *Lexikon*, 2:1702.

97. Marrus and Paxton, *Vichy France*, pp. 4, 48–51, 98–99, 124–25; Liebling, *Republic of Silence*, p. 218; file cards of Kurt Schachtel and Bruno Meyerowitz, RSW collection, BA (see n. 33 of Chapter 5, 2).

98. Frankenthal, *Dreifache Fluch*, pp. 217–26. See also Strauss, "Jewish Emigration from Germany (I)," p. 355; Dornedden in *Deutsches Ärzteblatt* 64 (1934): 180; Wasserstein, *Britain*, p. 7; Richarz, *Leben*, p. 54; Franke, *Geschichte*, p. 207. For general background, see Pfanner, "Role."

99. See Wasserstein, *Britain*, p. 7; Friedman, *No Haven*, p. 68; Strauss, "Jewish Emigration from Germany (I)," p. 354; Rosenstein, *Narben*, pp. 283–84; Jaffé's testimonies in Leibfried, "Stationen der Abwehr," pp. 6–9 and 38, n. 60; also n. 60 on p. 38 in Leibfried; Franke, *Geschichte*, pp. 238–39; Gebhard, *Strom*, pp. 46–47; Haas, *Doctor*, pp. 9–10.

100. Strauss, "Jewish Emigration from Germany (I)," pp. 352, 354; Frankenthal, *Dreifache Fluch*, pp. 226–38; file card of Heinrich Löwenfeld, RSW collection, BA (see n. 33 of Chapter 5, 2).

101. Strauss, "Jewish Emigration from Germany (II)," pp. 384–89; Abella and Troper, *None Is Too Many*, esp. pp. x–xi, 54; Friedman, *No Haven*, pp. 59–60; Gilbert, *Holocaust*, p. 64; Blakeney, *Australia*, pp. 188–92.

102. Strauss, "Jewish Emigration from Germany (II)," pp. 363–82; Gilbert, *Holocaust*, p. 64; Friedman, *No Haven*, pp. 61–63, 68; Richard Roeder's testimony in Leibfried, "Stationen der Abwehr," p. 7; Leibfried, ibid., p. 20; Sauer, *Schicksale*, p. 238; file card of Hildegard Friedländer, RSW collection, BA (see n. 33 of Chapter 5, 2).

103. See Boveri, *Verzweigungen*, p. 331; Strauss, "Jewish Emigration from Germany (II)," pp. 383–84; *Ziel und Weg* 5 (1935): 283, 496; Sauer, *Schicksale*, pp. 244–47; Zelzer, *Weg*, p. 460; Berg-Pan, "Shanghai Chronicle."

104. Doc. 8 of February 16, 1934, in Sauer, *Dokumente*, 1:19. Also note the mindless repetition in Mass, *Jahr*, p. 24.

105. Hadrich, "Nichtarischen Ärzte," p. 1243; *Ziel und Weg* 8 (1938): 438; Grote as quoted in *Journal of the American Medical Association* 111 (1938): 1118; Ramm, *Standeskunde*, p. 46; Ellersdorfer, "Auswirkungen," p. 100. Cf. Strauss, "Jewish Emigration from Germany (I)," p. 340. The qualified figures are in Tennstedt and Leibfried, "Sozialpolitik," p. 224; Sauer, *Schicksale*, p. 81; and Kümmel, "Ausschaltung," p. 76.

106. *Ziel und Weg*, 5 (1935): 172; Hadrich, "Nichtarischen Ärzte," p. 1243; Kümmel, "Ausschaltung," p. 76; Aron, "Nichtarischen Ärzte." The figure of two to three thousand for Jewish émigré physicians by the end of 1934 quoted by Tennstedt and Leibfried, "Sozialpolitik," pp. 223–24, seems too high.

107. Gilbert, *Holocaust*, p. 44.

108. *Ziel und Weg* 7 (1937): 225; ibid. 8 (1938): 438; Strauss, "Jewish Emigration from Germany (I)," p. 340; Tennstedt and Leibfried, "Sozialpolitik," p. 224.

109. Strauss, "Jewish Emigration from Germany (I)," p. 340; Leibfried, "Stationen der Abwehr," Table 1 on p. 11; Tennstedt and Leibfried, "Sozialpolitik," p. 225; Sauer, *Schicksale*, p. 81; Kümmel, "Ausschaltung," p. 76.

110. These estimates are according to Kümmel, "Ausschaltung," pp. 78–79; Leibfried, "Stationen der Abwehr," p. 14.

111. Kümmel, "Ausschaltung," p. 78.

Conclusion

1. Fischer-Homberger, *Geschichte*, p. 119. For a more universal explication of those "norms," see Konner, *Becoming a Doctor*, pp. 365–66.

2. Ivy, "Nazi War Crimes," p. 268; Mitscherlich and Mielke, *Medizin ohne Menschlichkeit*, p. 13; Gunter Mann, "Medizin im Dritten Reich," paper presented to the Frankfurt Rotary Club on August 24, 1987.

3. *Wer ist Wer?* (1986), p. 1371; quotations from Vilmar in a contrived interview conducted by a journalist employed by the Vilmar-controlled *Deutsches Ärzteblatt* 84 B (1987): 849.

4. *Wer ist Wer?* (1986), pp. 1126–27; *Deutsches Ärzteblatt* 83 B (1986): 1187; Schadewaldt, *Hartmannbund*, p. 143. Also see the apologetic Bittner as early as 1961, "Widerstand," p. 1532; and *Deutsches Ärzteblatt* 82 B (1985): 1381.

5. Kater, *Politiker*, p. 164; BDC, MF, and Research Huwer; Huwer's letter to the editor in *Deutsches Ärzteblatt* 84 B (1987): 1453–54 (quotations).

6. Sons, " 'Wurzeln' "; example of Dr. Wagenfeld in Schönberg, "Geschichte," p. 103; Kater, "Burden," p. 41. See Stobrawa, *Ärztlichen Organisationen*, pp. 32–36.

7. Kater, "Burden," pp. 41–52. For background, idem, "Problems of Political Reeducation." Also Rohland, "Zur Rolle"; Berger, "Sozialversicherungsreform," p. 83; and the admission of West German physicians' functionary and former SS man Ernst Fromm, in "Berufsvertretung," p. 268.

8. Kiesselbach (born in 1907), a professor of anatomy since 1955 and rector of the University of Düsseldorf in 1963–64, at that very time was questioned by police for murder. In the end, the authorities decided not to proceed against him. Full documentation on all three persons named is in Kater, "*Ahnenerbe*," pp. 248, 255, 426, 428; idem, "Burden," pp. 43–44, 51–52; *Wer ist Wer?* (1970), p. 621. See text below at n. 115.

9. As has been so aptly expressed by Johanna Bleker et al., "Sich der Wahrheit stellen: Medizinhistoriker kritisieren Vilmar," *Die Zeit*, November 6, 1987, p. 47.

10. Henderson, *Rise*, pp. 173–242; Stürmer, *Reich*, pp. 89–91, 129–33; Jarausch, *Students*, pp. 24, 76, 180–81; Schieder, "Kultur," esp. p. 27, 30–31; Beyerchen, *Scientists under Hitler*, p. 3. Critical regarding Germany's rise to a highly capitalistic industrial nation is Wehler, *Kaiserreich*, pp. 41–59.

11. Huerkamp, *Aufstieg der Ärzte*; Jarausch, *Students*, pp. 144–46; Burchardt, "Wissenschaftsförderung"; Fischer, *Lexikon*, 1:352–54, 637, 784–86; Guthrie, *History*, pp. 286–87, 365, 384.

12. Schreiber, *Wissenschaftspolitik.*

13. Kocka, *Klassengesellschaft*, pp. 21–33; Rürup, *Wissenschaft*; Fischer, *Lexikon*, 2:1365; Sauerbruch, *Leben*, pp. 159–85.

14. Taute et al., *Entwicklung*, pp. 126–28; Roth, "Schöner neuer Mensch," passim. Also see Nachtsheim, "Warum Eugenik," p. 712; Klee, "*Euthanasie*," pp. 29–33.

15. Kisskalt, *Theorie*, pp. 124–41; Just, "Agnes Bluhm," pp. 519–20, 523–24. See Jonas, "Philosophical Reflections."

16. Professor Hans Nachtsheim's remarks printed in *Die Ärztin* 19 (1943): 215; Gruber, *Einführung*, pp. 61–63; Bergmann, *Rückschau*, p. 53; Kisskalt, *Theorie*, p. 135; Karlson quoting Domagk in "Versammlungen," p. 63; Aschoff, "93. Naturforscher-Versammlung," p. 1373. See Oehme, "Medizinische Experiment," pp. 489–90; Läuppi, "Experimente am Menschen."

17. Moll, *Ärztliche Ethik*, pp. 553–79; Fischer, *Lexikon*, 2:1059.

18. Baader, "Menschenexperimente," p. 186.

19. Kisskalt, *Theorie*, pp. 134–35; Fischer, *Lexikon*, 1:116; Oehme, "Medizinische Experiment," p. 490; Vogeler, *Bier*, pp. 31–32; Fischer-Homberger, *Geschichte*, p. 117.

20. Sauerbruch's address at the ninety-fourth meeting of Gesellschaft Deutscher Naturwissenschaftler und Ärzte, in *Mitteilungen der Gesellschaft Deutscher Naturforscher und Ärzte* 94 (1937): VII. See also Baader, "Menschenexperimente," p. 196.

21. On this general principle, see Weingart, "Eugenik," p. 315. More specifically Baader, "Menschenexperimente," p. 189 (case of Rose).

22. See Gruber, *Einführung*, p. 63.

23. Kürten, "Tagung," p. 409.

24. Mitscherlich and Mielke, *Medizin ohne Menschlichkeit*, pp. 39–41; Kater, "*Ahnenerbe*," pp. 231–33; Kreienberg and Winter, "Höhenfestigkeit"; Kreienberg and Schenkel, "Über die beschleunigte Blutgerinnung." Also see *Deutsches Ärzteblatt* 72 (1942): 158.

25. Grawitz to Himmler, Berlin, September 30, 1943, BDC, Research HO 2097; Mitscherlich and Mielke, *Medizin ohne Menschlichkeit*, pp. 93–95; Baader, "Menschenexperimente," p. 187; Clauberg to Himmler, Königshütte, May 30, 1942, BDC, Research HO 52/53.

26. Professors Sauerbruch, Wolfgang Heubner, and Friedrich Hermann Rein knew about concentration camp experiments to make seawater potable; surgeon Erwin Gohrbandt knew and approved of Rascher's freezing experiments; pathologist Julius Hallervorden obtained and used for research hundreds of human brains from "euthanasia" killing centers. See Mitscherlich and Mielke, *Wissenschaft*, pp. 279–97; Alexander, "Science," p. 40; Nowak, "*Euthanasie*," p. 86; Gohrbandt, "Auskühlung"; Mann, "Medizin im Dritten Reich" (as in n. 2); and list of no less than ninety-five highly specialized participants in a closed convention dealing with, among others, results of freezing experiments (Rascher) in October 1943 (*Bericht über eine wissenschaftliche Besprechung*, pp. 3–4). Also see Freund, "Ethical Problems," p. 692.

27. For contemporary examples, see Blome, *Arzt*, p. 87; Kühle, "Lehrgang," p. 525. Critical is Schmuhl, *Rassenhygiene*, pp. 83–84.

28. Stumpfl, "Untersuchungen"; idem, *Ursprünge*, esp. pp. 9–23, 170–76; Müller, *Lehrbuch*, pp. 278–79.

29. On the former, see Mueller, "Gegenwärtige Lage," p. 20; Pfreimbter, "Knabenmordprozess"; *Münchener Medizinische Wochenschrift* 84 (1937): 919; Plant, *Pink Triangle*, pp. 106–49. (For intellectual depth, see Mosse, *Nationalism and Sexuality*, pp. 133–80.) On the latter, see n. 85 of Chapter 4, 2.

30. See the shaky argument throughout in Stumpfl, "Untersuchungen"; Jakobi et al., *Aeskulap*, pp. 32–39, and esp. 153. In general, see Schmuhl, *Rassenhygiene*, p. 86; Kater, "Medizin und Mediziner," pp. 348–49.

31. See Mosse, *Crisis of German Ideology*; idem, *Toward the Final Solution*; Stern, *Politics of Cultural Despair*.

32. Liek died in February 1935. See Liek, *Gedanken eines Arztes*, p. 121; Werner Zabel's eulogy, ibid., p. 254; Liek, *Krebsverbreitung*, pp. 219–20; and the racist items in Liek's bibliography for *Arzt*, p. 171.

33. See Chapter 1, 3, at n. 2; Chapter 4, 1, at n. 53; Much, *Homöopathie*; Guthrie, *History*, pp. 50, 61, 76, 110, 114, 169, 176, 219–20, 283; Ackerknecht, *Short History*, pp. 61–62, 143; Fischer-Homberger, *Geschichte*, pp. 27, 78.

34. See Guthrie, *History*, p. 335; Sigerist, *Man and Medicine*, pp. 93–94.

35. Jünger, "Über den Schmerz." Also see Dahrendorf, *Gesellschaft*, p. 387. Dahrendorf aptly describes the specifically German attitude to pain but as a modern phenomenon cannot trace it to Liek's naturalist school.

36. Kötschau, "Zur nationalsozialistischen Revolution" (quotation p. 14); idem, *Umbruch*, pp. 26, 40–44, 48, 57; Hobohm, "Nationalsozialismus," p. 42. On Jews specifically, see Härtel, "Rasse und Chirurgie," pp. 248, 250; and the physician Fritz Lenz in Baur et al., *Menschliche Erblichkeitslehre*, p. 561.

37. Liek, *Welt*, pp. 101–11; idem, *Gedanken eines Arztes*, p. 132; Kötschau, *Umbruch*, pp. 36, 40–41, 47, 57, 66, 86; Knoll, "Arzt," p. 438; Schenck, "Wie sollen wir," p. 1093.

38. See Kötschau, "Zur nationalsozialistischen Revolution," p. 12; Kater, " 'Gesundheitsführung,' " p. 351.

39. Bumke, *Erinnerungen*, p. 145.

40. Wagner as quoted in *Deutsches Ärzteblatt* 64 (1934): 587; Grote, "KVD," p. 12; Mrugowsky, *Ethos*, p. 14. Also see Klare to Dr. K., Scheidegg, April 22, 1933, in Klare, *Briefe*, p. 119; *Deutsches Ärzteblatt* 64 (1934): 965; Wagner's eulogy for Liek as quoted by Anna Liek in Liek, *Bannkreis*, p. 10; Schenck, "Das Gesundheitshaus der Deutschen Ärzteschaft in Kempfenhausen," Munich, May 21, 1939, BA, R 18/3786; Schenck, "Wie sollen wir"; Wuttke-Groneberg, "Leistung," pp. 38, 52; and Chapter 4, 1, nn. 55–60.

41. Wirz, "Hochschule und Fortbildung," p. 48.

42. On the last phenomenon see Kater, "*Ahnenerbe*," passim.

43. See text of Conti's speech of April 24, 1942, in *Deutsches Ärzteblatt* 72 (1942): 201. When in 1941 two obstetricians published articles in favor of deleting pain during childbirth, Conti protested vehemently to leading university gynecologists. Details in Franken, "Schmerzbekämpfung"; Fuchs, "Erfahrungen"; Conti to Schröder, Berlin, May 2, 1941, BA, R 18/3781. Also see Conti to Siebke, Berlin, May 5, 1941; and to Blome et al., Berlin, July 25, 1941, ibid.; *Ziel und Weg* 9 (1939): 336;

Schenck, "Wie sollen wir," p. 1093. Conti had some pre-1933 training as a pediatrician.

44. Schenck, "Die Mitwirkung des 'Reichsgesundheitsführers' bei der Verwirklichung des 'Deutschen Gesundheitswerkes,'" enclosed with Schenck to Conti, January 9, 1941, BA, R 18/3786; "Betrifft: Hauptamtliche Ärzte für die NSDAP," enclosed with Röhrs to Schrepfer, Munich, November 25, 1943, BA, R 18/3810; Dietrich, "Entwicklung"; Kisskalt, *Theorie*, p. 237; Kötschau, "Sinnforschung."

45. Bluhm, *Aufgaben*, pp. 25–26; Achelis, "Physiologie der Schmerzen." On Achelis, see *Wer ist's?* p. 4.

46. Stoeckel to Conti, Berlin, March 6, 1941, BA, R 18/3781. Similar letters to Conti from Runge (Heidelberg, February 21, 1941), Mikulicz-Radecki (Königsberg, February 22, 1941), Schröder (Leipzig, May 7, 1941), Siebke (Bonn, May 15, 1941), ibid. A complete list of fourteen supportive gynecologists is in Stadler to Conti, Munich, July 25, 1941, BA, R 18/3806. In his memoirs, Stoeckel stresses his various differences with Conti. But in the matter of Liek's philosophy, the two men were of one mind. See Stoeckel, *Erinnerungen*, pp. 242–43, 257–58. Stoeckel's ultraconservative view regarding right to life is depicted on pp. 285–92. Liek's admiration for Stoeckel is expressed in *Gedanken eines Arztes*, p. 131.

47. Sauerbruch, *Leben*, p. 369.

48. See text in Chapter 4, 2, at n. 97.

49. Pfannenstiel, "Gedanken" (quotations on p. 124).

50. This quotation from 1944 reissued in Weizsäcker, *Natur*, p. 202. Also, with regard to Liek, see idem, "'Euthanasie,'" p. 88. Vita Weizsäcker is in Fischer, *Lexikon*, 2:1663.

51. Wuttke-Groneberg, "Von Heidelberg," p. 122.

52. Gay, *Freud*, p. 92. See obituary in *Deutsche medizinische Wochenschrift*, June 7, 1957, p. 926.

53. Tabulated vita Mollison, BDC, Research Mollison; Drüll, *Gelehrtenlexikon*, p. 183. For Bluhm in Zurich see Chapter 3, 1, at n. 22; for Rüdin see Fischer, *Lexikon*, 2:1340. On the significance of the "Zurich Circle" in the development of German *Rassenkunde* see Schmuhl, *Rassenhygiene*, p. 90.

54. On the latter, see Parlow, "Über einige kolonialistische."

55. Chapter 4, 1, at n. 11.

56. Quotation from Mollison, "Körperproportionen," p. 250. Also see idem, "Beitrag"; idem, "Maori."

57. Fischer and Mollison in Fischer et al., *Anthropologie*, p. 88.

58. *Wer ist's?* p. 408; Fischer, *Lexikon*, 1:410. For 1908 the personal friendship between Fischer and Mollison is documented in Mollison, "Beitrag," p. 529.

59. Fischer, *Rehobother Bastards*, quotation on p. 304.

60. Idem in Fischer et al., *Anthropologie*, pp. 189–90.

61. As in n. 58.

62. Tabulated vita Mollison; Mollison to Munich dean, January 16, 1942; research log Mollison, BDC, Research Mollison.

63. See Mosse, *Toward the Final Solution*, p. 76; Müller-Hill, *Tödliche Wissenschaft*, p. 124.

64. Fischer as quoted in Koester, "Grundlagen," p. 504.

65. Fischer, *Begriff*, p. 7; idem, "Fortschritte," p. 1071.
66. Fischer as quoted in Ericksen, *Theologians*, p. 65.
67. See Fischer, *Begriff*, p. 11; Lemser, "Untersuchungsergebnisse."
68. Müller-Hill, *Tödliche Wissenschaft*, pp. 34–35, 48; Pommerin, *Sterilisierung*, pp. 78–79.
69. To document that strong connection, see Verschuer, "Aufgaben und Ziele," p. 1000; idem, "Ehemalige Kaiser-Wilhelm-Institut." Also see Scholz, "Otmar Frhr. von Verschuer." Fischer himself frequently acknowledged Verschuer, as in "Fortschritte," p. 1069.
70. *Deutsche Führerlexikon*, p. 505; "Personalblatt" Verschuer, Berlin-Dahlem, November 4, 1942, BDC, PK Verschuer; Selchow, *Hundert Tage*, p. 326; Mosse, *Crisis of German Ideology*, pp. 194, 198; Zmarzlik, "Sozialdarwinismus," p. 265; Kater, *Studentenschaft*, pp. 27, 146.
71. *Deutsche Führerlexikon*, pp. 454, 505; Selchow, *Hundert Tage*, pp. 309–56. On Prussian Bogislav Freiherr von Selchow, born in 1877, see *Wer ist's?* p. 1488. His pre-1933 Nazism is documented in *Mitteilungen des Kampfbundes für deutsche Kultur* 1 (1929): 137, 143–44, 166. After 1933, Selchow joined the Nazi Academy for German Law but never was a formal party member ("Fragebogen," Berlin, April 16, 1937, BDC, RSK Selchow).
72. BDC, RÄK Verschuer; *Deutsche Führerlexikon*, p. 505; Verschuer, "Aufgaben und Ziele."
73. E.g. Verschuer, "Soziale Umwelt und Vererbung"; idem, "Qualitätsproblem."
74. Verschuer, *Erbpathologie*; Loeffler, "Auslesegedanke," p. 674; Liebenam, "Zwillingsforschung"; *Die Ärztin* 17 (1941): 320.
75. *Journal of the American Medical Association* 106 (1936): 308–9; ibid. 110 (1938): 59–60; Roth, "Schöner neuer Mensch," pp. 12–13; Seidelman, "Mengele Medicus," pp. 224–25.
76. *Wer ist's?* p. 1643.
77. BDC, MF Verschuer. Paul Weindling's observation in his otherwise perceptive piece "Race, Blood and Politics," p. 13, that Verschuer "joined the Nazi Party only in September 1941, when the 'final solution' was to provide new opportunities for research," is factually incorrect and, in its projection of Verschuer into Holocaust activities, undocumented.
78. Thomann, "Rassenhygiene"; Müller-Hill, *Tödliche Wissenschaft*, pp. 39–40.
79. Verschuer's lecture "Die körperlichen Rassenmerkmale des Judentums," as paraphrased in *Frankfurter Zeitung*, January 17, 1939.
80. Verschuer, "Vier Jahre," p. 63.
81. See Lechler, "Erkennung," p. 297; Kaupen-Haas, "Bevölkerungsplaner," p. 116; Roth, "Schöner neuer Mensch," p. 41; Seidelman, "Mengele Medicus," p. 225.
82. Verschuer, "Bevölkerungs- und Rassenfragen," p. 11. In the same article, there are deprecating references to Gypsies and "French colonials" (Negroes).
83. See Chapter 4, 1, at n. 38.
84. *Wer ist's?* p. 877.
85. Chapter 4.
86. See Kranz and Koller, "*Gemeinschaftsunfähigen*," pp. 40, 46; Verschuer,

"Ehemalige Kaiser-Wilhelm-Institut," pp. 134, 141, 150–51, 168.

87. Kranz, " 'Einkehr' und 'Umkehr.' "

88. Idem, "Entwicklung," p. 289. On Fischer see Verschuer in "Ehemalige Kaiser-Wilhelm-Institut," pp. 129–30.

89. Verschuer, "Ehemalige Kaiser-Wilhelm-Institut," p. 133.

90. As told by former Verschuer assistant Hans Grebe to Müller-Hill: *Tödliche Wissenschaft*, p. 158. Also see Verschuer, "Vier Jahre."

91. "Stammkarte" Mengele; "Lebenslauf" Mengele, January 1, 1939, BDC, SS Mengele; Mollison, "Rassenkunde und Rassenhygiene," p. 47 (quotation).

92. Mengele, "Rassenmorphologische Untersuchungen," esp. p. 111.

93. Teixeira, "Mengele Report"; "Ärztlicher Untersuchungsbogen" Mengele, sign. Dr. med. Schwarzweller, Frankfurt-Niederrad, February 26, 1938, BDC, SS Mengele. Also see Roth, "Schöner neuer Mensch," pp. 40, 62, n. 92. According to periodontist Dr. Mark Richardson, Oakville, Canada, it is most likely that Mengele was born without the bicuspids and that as a result a diastema between the upper central incisors widened as he grew up (personal communication, December 8, 1987).

94. Mengele, "Sippenuntersuchungen"; "Lebenslauf" Mengele, January 1, 1939, BDC, SS Mengele. Also see Verschuer's positive reaction to Mengele's M.D. research in "Vier Jahre," pp. 59–60. Schmieden, born in 1874, had been in Frankfurt since 1919 (Fischer, *Lexikon*, 2:1398–99).

95. See Chapter 2, 2, at n. 78; Chapter 4, 1, at n. 101.

96. Müller-Hill, *Tödliche Wissenschaft*, p. 72; idem, "Genetics after Auschwitz," pp. 5–6.

97. Nyiszli, *Auschwitz*, e.g., pp. 101–3; Lifton, *Nazi Doctors*, pp. 347–69.

98. See *Globe and Mail* (Toronto), February 7, 1985; Müller-Hill, *Tödliche Wissenschaft*, pp. 72–75; Lifton, *Nazi Doctors*, pp. 357–58, 362, 369; Kater, "Burden," pp. 48–49.

99. Verschuer, "Aufgaben und Ziele," p. 999; idem, "Vier Jahre," pp. 58–59. See *Klinische Wochenschrift* 5 (1926): 2237.

100. Lifton, *Nazi Doctors*, pp. 347–56; Nomberg-Przytyk, *Auschwitz*, pp. 89–93; *Globe and Mail* (Toronto), February 6, 1985.

101. See the case of Gypsy twins sewn together back to back, in *Globe and Mail* (Toronto), June 12, 1985.

102. Mengele's former secretary Ernst Cohn as quoted in ibid., January 29, 1985.

103. See ibid., February 7, 1985.

104. Lifton, "Medicalized Killing in Auschwitz," p. 289. In the same vein see the sobering article by Canadian geneticist David Suzuki in *Toronto Star*, November 16, 1985.

105. Jürgens, "Ohrmerkmale," p. 253, cites Mengele, "Zur Vererbung." See Seidelman, "Mengele Medicus," pp. 228–29. On Verschuer, see Verschuer, "Ehemalige Kaiser-Wilhelm-Institut"; Scholz, "Otmar Frhr. von Verschuer"; Thomann, "Rassenhygiene"; Thomann, "Otmar Freiherr von Verschuer," pp. 63–65. The baron was one of the honored guests at the Second International Conference of Human Genetics in Rome, September 6–12, 1961. See his photograph in *Acta Geneticae Medicae et Gemellologiae* 10 (1961): picture no. 19.

106. See text in Chapter 5, 3, at n. 40.

107. Entry for January 15, 1942, in *Meldungen aus dem Reich*, 9:3176. See Schmuhl, *Rassenhygiene*, p. 192.

108. Verschuer, "Vier Jahre," p. 62.

109. See the revealing letter, Simon to Klein, Freiburg, July 2, 1934, ARW, I, 33 g 178/4. For Schneider's own subsequent killer role see Klee, "*Euthanasie*," passim; Schmuhl, *Rassenhygiene*, passim after p. 146.

110. "Aufgaben der Ärztin," Rittmarshausen, 1936, ARW, I, 80 g 581/1.

111. See Herrmann, "Ist das Gesetz"; Engel, "Ärztliche Forderungen"; Müller-Meernach, "Fall"; and text in Chapter 5, 3, at nn. 40–43.

112. Müller, *Lehrbuch*; Gruber, *Einführung*.

113. See Kater, "Professionalization," pp. 684–88.

114. On Clauberg, see Zörner et al., *Ravensbrück*, pp. 132–35; Schübelin, "Expansionspolitik"; Klee, *Was sie taten*, pp. 280, 300–301. On Hirt, see Roth to REM, Berlin, January 6, 1945 (with enclosed), BA, R 21/366; Kater, "*Ahnenerbe*," pp. 245–55.

115. See n. 8 of this chapter and Chapter 5, 2, at n. 7.

116. Delmer, *Black Boomerang*, pp. 257–58.

117. Ebermayer, *Deutschland*, pp. 108–10; *Deutschland-Berichte* (1935), 2:162; ibid. (1936), 3:1300.

118. Paradigmatic for such excesses is the example of patient Katharina Beer, at the hands of Reit-im-Winkl Dr. Adolf Heiler, in Friedrich Beer to Reichsärztekammer, Munich, August 27, 1943, BDC, PÄ Heiler.

119. Bamm, *Flagge*, p. 114; Forssmann, *Selbstversuch*, p. 168. For the brutalizing effect of the war on all German soldiers see the powerful testimonies in *True to Type*, pp. 5–78. On the numbing of medics see p. 42.

120. Valentin, *Krankenbataillone*; Baader, "Militarisierung," p. 92.

121. For examples see *Deutschland-Berichte* (1937), 4:692; Siegert, "Flossenbürg," pp. 472–73; Lifton, *Nazi Doctors*, pp. 210, 265.

122. Bock, *Zwangssterilisation*, pp. 232–33, 241–42, and Schmuhl, *Rassenhygiene*, pp. 129–30, supersede Weitbrecht, *Psychiatrie*, p. 12; Nowak, "Euthanasie," p. 65.

123. See Ternon and Helman, *Les médecins allemands*, pp. 155–80; Bock, *Zwangssterilisation*, pp. 178–298; Kollath, *Grundlagen*, p. 387; Mayer, "Arzttum," p. 786; Lifton, *Nazi Doctors*, p. 29; Schwarz, *Gutachten*; Schmuhl, *Rassenhygiene*, pp. 157–58.

124. See Schiersmann, "Beitrag"; Gruber, *Einführung*, p. 203; Loehr, *Über die Stellung*, p. 33; *Ziel und Weg* 6 (1936): 134; Leibbrand, "Eugenik und Sterilisation"; Gütt, "Einführung," p. 128; Weitbrecht, *Psychiatrie*, pp. 12–14. Cases of sterilization with complications or death are recorded in *Deutschland-Berichte* (1936), 3:1042–43.

125. Unschuld, "Professionalisierung," pp. 265–72.

126. Fromm, "Berufsvertretung," p. 268; Bussche and Krähe, "Prognose," p. 365; Deneke, *Freien Berufe*, p. 202; Mausbach, "Vorstellungen," p. 154.

127. See photographs of physicians in sundry party uniforms in professional journals like *Deutsches Ärzteblatt* 65 (1935): 569; 71 (1941): 245.

128. See Kater, "Hitler's Early Doctors," pp. 47–49; Cocks, *Psychotherapy*, pp. 44–45; Wilhelm Josenhans in *Ziel und Weg* 3 (1933): 156; Ramm, *Standeskunde*, p. 116.

129. See Kater, " 'Gesundheitsführung' "; Schmiedebach, "Arzt."

130. See *Ziel und Weg* 5 (1935): 100, 312; Ramm, *Standeskunde*, pp. 101–2.

131. This complex issue is viewed much too simplistically by Geuter, *Professionalisierung*, pp. 325, 383, who, on the whole, decides on professional progress for the doctors. On a similar note but much less exhaustive see Prinz, *Vom neuen Mittelstand*, p. 324. On the pre-1933 anticipation of *Reichsärzteordnung*, see Stobrawa, *Ärztlichen Organisationen*, p. 29.

132. Unschuld, "Professionalisierung," p. 270.

133. "Auszug aus dem Protokoll über die Dekanbesprechung am 13. und 14.4. 1943," BA, R 21/484.

134. The Hippocratic Oath has been reprinted in Guthrie, *History*, p. 54.

135. Ibid.

Sources

Archival Documents

Archiv der Akademie der Wissenschaften Göttingen (AAWG):
Pers. 65/49.
Archiv der Reichsstudentenführung und des Nationalsozialistischen Deutschen Studentenbundes, Universität Würzburg (ARW):
I
03 p 356; 05 g 353/2; 6 p 154; 6 p 359; 11 g 218/1; 11 g 218/2; 11 g 218/3; 11 p 71; 20 g 670; 33 g 178/4; 80 g 581/1; 80 g 581/2.
II
280; 288; 531.
III.
IV
1-31/2; 1-31/9; 1-31/10.
Berlin Document Center (BDC):
MF; NSF; OPG; PÄ; PK; RÄK; Research; RMK; RSK; SA; SS; TF.
Bundesarchiv Koblenz (BA):
NS 19 Neu/1531.
NS 22/860; 1177; 1183; 1193; 4203.
NSD, 53/2.
R 18/1309; 1504; 2956; 2958; 3122; 3638; 3686; 3715; 3764; 3766; 3766a; 3781; 3783; 3785; 3786; 3789; 3791; 3792; 3797; 3805; 3806; 3809; 3810; 3813; 3814; 5574; 5575; 5576; 5582; 5583.
R 21/366; 439; 475; 476; 477; 484; 485.
R 43II/940b.
R 56I/83; 89; 100.
R 58/145; 146; 193.
RSW.
Schumacher/213; 241; 270, III.
Dokumentationsarchiv des Österreichischen Widerstandes Wien (DAÖW):
540; 957; 2962, 3136; 3996; 4100; 4101; 4491; 4748; 4799.
Generallandesarchiv Karlsruhe (GLAK):
465d/1419.
Hessisches Hauptstaatsarchiv Wiesbaden (HHSAW):
483/3159; 191.
Hoover Institution on War, Revolution, and Peace, Stanford (HIS):
13/254; 258.

Institut für Zeitgeschichte München (IfZ):
- Dc. 01.06.
- NO-864.

Israel State Archives, Jerusalem (ISA):
- Record Group M/74/35.
- Record Group 2/M/7/40.

Leo Baeck Institute, New York (LBINY):
- AR-C. 1640. Box 1, Folder 3.

National Archives, Washingon, D.C. (NA):
- T-253/23.
- T-580/154/248.

Niedersächsisches Hauptstaatsarchiv Hannover (NHSA):
- Hann. 122a, XII, 32 m.
- Hann. 122a, XII, 126.

Staatsarchiv München (SAM):
- LRA/30656.
- NSDAP/27 (SA); 28 (SA); 31; 122; 371.

Staatsarchiv Münster (SAMs):
- Gauleitung Westfalen-Nord, Gauamt für Volkswohlfahrt, 7.
- Polit. Polizei, 3. Reich, 109.

United Nations Archives, New York (UNANY):
- CROWCASS Central Registry File.

Unterlagen der Kassenärztlichen Vereinigung Deutschlands (KVD) und der Reichsärztekammer (RÄK), Berlin (photocopies in York University Archives) (UK):
- 100; 106; 112; 130/118.02; 130/118.02/3; 130/118.02/4; 130/123.02; 130/131.02; 156/RÄK Revisionsamt; 190; 196/1; 199; 200; 207; 213; 215; 217; 234; 235; 243; 248.

Newspapers, Journals, and Serials

Acta Geneticae Medicae et Gemellologiae, 1961.
Ärzteblatt für Norddeutschland, 1939, 1940.
Ärztliche Mitteilungen, 1933, 1961.
Ärztliches Vereinsblatt, 1929.
Archiv für Sozialgeschichte, 1982, 1983, 1987.
B.Z., Hamburg, 1955.
Bremer Nachrichten, 1936.
Bulletin of the History of Medicine, 1987.
Der Chirurg, 1943.
Der Erbarzt, 1935.
Der Freiwillige, 1967.
Der Führer, 1932.
Der Öffentliche Gesundheitsdienst, 1937.
Der SA-Mann (Munich), 1932.

Der Spiegel, 1976–79, 1984, 1986, 1988.
Der Tagesspiegel (Berlin), 1986.
Deutsche medizinische Wochenschrift, 1957.
Deutsche Zeitschrift für Nervenheilkunde, 1935.
Deutsches Ärzteblatt, 1933–37, 1939–43, 1985–87.
Die Ärztin, 1936–37, 1939, 1941, 1943–44.
Die medizinische Welt, 1933.
Die Wandlung, 1947.
Die Zeit (Hamburg), 1987.
Frankfurter Allgemeine Zeitung (Frankfurt am Main), 1985, 1988.
Frankfurter Zeitung (Frankfurt am Main), 1937, 1939.
Globe and Mail (Toronto), 1985–88.
Hastings Center Report, 1976.
History, 1986.
Journal of the American Medical Association, 1933–34, 1936, 1938–39.
Journal of the History of Medicine, 1986.
Klinische Wochenschrift, 1926.
Medical Economics, 1939.
Mitteilungen der Gesellschaft Deutscher Naturforscher und Ärzte, 1937.
Mitteilungen des Kampfbundes für deutsche Kultur, 1929.
Münchener Medizinische Wochenschrift, 1930, 1936, 1938.
Nationalsozialistisches Jahrbuch, 1943, 1944.
New York Review of Books, 1987.
Palestine Post (Jerusalem), 1935.
Reichsgesetzblatt, 1937–39, 1942.
Rundbrief: Ärzte warnen vor dem Atomkrieg, 1987.
Soziale Medizin: Zentralblatt für Reichsversicherung und Reichsversorgung, 1933.
Süddeutsche Zeitung (Munich), 1986–87.
taz (Berlin), 1985.
Times Literary Supplement (London), 1984.
Toronto Star, 1985.
Völkischer Beobachter, 1933, 1938–40.
Ziel und Weg, 1932–39.

Books (up to and including 1987), Articles, and Dissertations

Abella, Irving, and Harold M. Troper. *None Is Too Many: Canada and the Jews of Europe, 1933–1948*. Toronto, 1982.

Abraham, E. P., et al. "Historical Introduction." In Howard W. Florey et al., eds. *Antibiotics: A Survey of Penicillin, Streptomycin, and Other Antimicrobial Substances from Fungi, Actinomycetes, Bacteria, and Plants*. Vol. 2. London, 1949, pp. 631–71.

Achelis, Johann D. "Die Physiologie der Schmerzen," *Der Nervenarzt* 9 (1936): 559–68.

Ackerknecht, Erwin H. *A Short History of Medicine*. Baltimore, 1982.

Ackermann, Wilhelm. "Der ärztliche Nachwuchs zwischen Weltkrieg und nationalsozialistischer Erhebung." M.D. dissertation, Cologne, 1940.

Adam, Uwe Dietrich. *Hochschule und Nationalsozialismus: Die Universität Tübingen im Dritten Reich*. Tübingen, 1977.

———. *Judenpolitik im Dritten Reich*. Düsseldorf, 1979.

Adler, H. G. *Theresienstadt 1941–1945: Das Antlitz einer Zwangsgemeinschaft: Geschichte, Soziologie, Psychologie*. Tübingen, 1955.

———. *Der verwaltete Mensch: Studien zur Deportation der Juden aus Deutschland*. Tübingen, 1974.

Adolf Hitler: Monologe im Führerhauptquartier 1941–1944: Die Aufzeichnungen Heinrich Heims. Edited by Werner Jochmann. Hamburg, 1980.

Adressbuch der Stadt Wiesbaden und Umgebung 1934/35. Vol. 43. N.d., IV.

Albisetti, James C. "The Fight for Female Physicians in Imperial Germany." *Central European History* 15 (1982): 99–123.

———. "Women Students in the Third Reich." *Review of Education* 11 (1985): 33–36.

Albrecht, Günter, and Wolfgang Hartwig, eds. *Ärzte: Erinnerungen, Erlebnisse, Bekenntnisse*. 3d ed. Berlin (DDR), 1973.

Alexander, Leo. "Medical Science under Dictatorship." *New England Journal of Medicine* 241, no. 2 (1949): 39–47.

Der alltägliche Faschismus: Frauen im Dritten Reich. Berlin, 1981.

Althaus, Hermann. "Nationalsozialistische Volkswohlfahrt." In Paul Meier-Benneckenstein, ed., *Das Dritte Reich im Aufbau: Übersichten und Leistungsberichte*. Vol. 2. Berlin, 1939, pp. 9–59.

Altstädter, Wilfried. "Sippe und berufliche Herkunft der Studierenden an der Universität München im Winterhalbjahr 1935/36." *Bavaria: Statistisches Landesamt: Zeitschrift des Bayerischen Statistischen Landesamtes* 69 (1937): 237–62.

Aly, Götz, ed. "Das Posener Tagebuch des Anatomen Hermann Voss." In Götz Aly et al., *Biedermann und Schreibtischtäter: Materialien zur deutschen Täter-Biographie*. Berlin, 1987, pp. 15–66.

Aly, Götz, and Karl Heinz Roth. *Die restlose Erfassung: Volkszählen, Identifizieren, Aussondern im Nationalsozialismus*. Berlin, 1984.

Amann, Ursula. "Der antifaschistische Kampf deutscher Ärzte und Angehöriger des Sanitätsdienstes im national-revolutionären Krieg in Spanien 1936–1939." In Achim Thom and Horst Spaar, eds., *Medizin im Faschismus: Symposium über das Schicksal der Medizin in der Zeit des Faschismus in Deutschland 1933–1945*. Berlin (DDR), 1985, pp. 209–13.

Amende, Dietrich. "Arzt und Nationalsozialismus, Idealismus und Glaube." *Ziel und Weg* 7 (1937): 56–61.

Angress, Werner T. *Generation zwischen Furcht und Hoffnung: Jüdische Jugend im Dritten Reich*. Hamburg, 1985.

Arendt, Hannah. *Eichmann in Jerusalem: A Report on the Banality of Evil*. New York, 1963.

Aretin, Erwein von. *Krone und Ketten: Erinnerungen eines bayerischen Edelmannes*. Edited by Karl Buchheim and Karl Otmar von Aretin. Munich, 1955.

Arminger, Gerhard. "Involvement of German Students in NS Organisations Based on the Archive of the Reichsstudentenwerk." *Historical Social Research—Historische Sozialforschung*, no. 30 (April 1984): 3–34.

Aron, Fritz. "Wie geht es den ausgewanderten jüdischen Ärzten?" *C.V.-Zeitung*, June 6, 1935 [nonpaginated].

———. "Die nichtarischen Ärzte in Deutschland." *C.V.-Zeitung*, January 4, 1935 [nonpaginated].

Aschoff, Ludwig. "93. Naturforscher-Versammlung: Verbundenheit der Medizin mit der nationalen und übernationalen naturwissenschaftlichen Forschung." *Deutsche medizinische Wochenschrift* 60 (1934): 1371–73.

Atzbach, Ernst. "Grundfragen der ärztlichen Kammergesetzgebung und Berufsgerichtsbarkeit und ihr Verhältnis zum Grundgesetz unter besonderer Berücksichtigung der historischen Entwicklung des ärztlichen Berufsrechts." LL.D. dissertation, Marburg, 1960.

Auerbach, Hellmuth. "Volksmeinung und veröffentlichte Meinung in Deutschland zwischen März und November 1938." In Franz Knipping and Klaus-Jürgen Müller, eds., *Machtbewusstsein in Deutschland am Vorabend des II. Weltkrieges*. Paderborn, 1984, pp. 273–93.

Baader, Gerhard. "Menschenexperimente." In Fridolf Kudlien, ed., *Ärzte im Nationalsocialismus*. Cologne, 1985, pp. 175–97.

———. "Militarisierung des Gesundheitswesens im Nationalsozialismus und heute." *Jahrbuch für kritische Medizin* 9 (1983): 85–94.

Baecker-Vowinkel, Elisabeth. "8. Schulungslehrgang für Ärztinnen in Alt-Rehse vom 5.-15. Juli 1939." *Die Ärztin* 15 (1939): 260–62.

Bähr, Walter, and Hans W. Bähr, eds. *Kriegsbriefe gefallener Studenten 1939–1945*. Tübingen, 1952.

Bambach, Gertrud. "Wie wir Alt-Rehse erlebten: Eine Erinnerung an den 2. Ärztinnenlehrgang, 23. bis 30. September 1937." *Die Ärztin* 13 (1937): 334–37.

Bamm, Peter [Dr. Curt Emmrich]. *Eines Menschen Zeit: Memoiren eines Überheblichen*. Munich, 1980.

———. *Die unsichtbare Flagge: Ein Bericht*. 8th ed. Munich, 1957.

Bardua, Heinz. *Stuttgart im Luftkrieg 1939–1945: Mit Dokumentenanhang und 67 Abbildungen*. Stuttgart, n.d.

Bartel, Walter. "Zur Entlarvung von Theorie und Praxis der faschistischen Verbrechen: Der Kampf der Antifaschisten im Bereich der Medizin." In Achim Thom and Horst Spaar, eds., *Medizin im Faschismus: Symposium über das Schicksal der Medizin in der Zeit des Faschismus in Deutschland 1933–1945*. Berlin (DDR), 1985, pp. 204–8.

Bartels, Friedrich. "Die berufstätige Frau." *Ziel und Weg* 3 (1933): 13–17.

———. "Gesundheit und Wirtschaft." *Ziel und Weg* 8 (1938): 528–32.

Bastian, Till. *Von der Eugenik zur Euthanasie: Ein verdrängtes Kapitel aus der Geschichte der Deutschen Psychiatrie*. Bad Wörishofen, 1981.

Bauer, Curt. "Dem Arbeiter Ehestandsdarlehen—dem angestellten Arzt—das Coelibat?" *Ziel und Weg* 3 (1933): 542–45.

Bauer, Julius. "Gefährliche Schlagworte aus dem Gebiete der Erbbiologie."

Schweizerische Medizinische Wochenschrift 65 (1935): 633–35.
———. *Irrwege der menschlichen Gesellschaft: Medizin-psychologische Kritik sozialer Unzulänglichkeiten*. Liestal, 1959.
Baur, Erwin, et al. *Menschliche Erblichkeitslehre*. 3d ed. Munich, 1927.
Beckenbauer, Alfons. "Eine Landshuter Jugendfreundschaft und ihre Verwicklung in die NS-Politik: Der Arzt Dr. Karl Gebhardt und der Reichsführer-SS Heinrich Himmler." *Verhandlungen des Historischen Vereins für Niederbayern* 100 (1974): 5–22.
Becker, Sophinette, et al. "Einblicke in die Medizin während des Nationalsozialismus—Beispiele aus der Heidelberger Universität." In Karin Buselmeier et al., eds., *Auch eine Geschichte der Universität Heidelberg*. Mannheim, 1985, pp. 315–35.
Behrend-Rosenfeld, Else R. *Ich stand nicht allein: Erlebnisse einer Jüdin in Deutschland 1933–1944*. 2d ed. Frankfurt am Main, 1963.
Bekenntnisse der Professoren an den deutschen Universitäten und Hochschulen zu Adolf Hitler und dem nationalsozialistischen Staat. Dresden, [1934].
Below, Nicolaus von. *Als Hitlers Adjutant 1937–45*. Mainz, 1980.
Benn, Gottfried. *Briefe an F.W. Oelze 1932–1945*. Edited by Harald Steinhagen and Jürgen Schröder. 2d ed. Wiesbaden, 1977.
Berg-Pan, Renata. "Shanghai Chronicle: Nazi Refugees in China." In Jarrell C. Jackman and Carla M. Borden, eds., *The Muses Flee Hitler: Cultural Transfer and Adaptation, 1930–1945*. Washington, D.C., 1983, pp. 283–89.
Berger, Franz. "Einzelheiten zur Berufsgerichtsbarkeit." *Deutsches Ärzteblatt* 69 (1939): 81–84.
Berger, Hermann. *Kleiner Kulturspiegel des heutigen Arzttums nach Zeitschriftenstimmen des letzten Jahrzehnts*. Jena, 1940.
Berger, Michael. "Sozialversicherungsreform und Kassenarztrecht: Zur Verhinderung der Reform des Kassenarztrechtes in den Westzonen nach 1945." In *Entwicklung und Struktur des Gesundheitswesens: Argumente für eine soziale Medizin*. Berlin, 1974, pp. 73–93.
Berghahn, Marion. *German-Jewish Refugees in England: The Ambiguities of Assimilation*. London, 1984.
Berghahn, Volker R. "Meinungsforschung im 'Dritten Reich': Die Mundpropaganda-Aktion im letzten Kriegshalbjahr." *Militärgeschichtliche Mitteilungen* 1 (1967): 83–119.
Bergmann, Gustav von. *Rückschau: Geschehen und Erleben auf meiner Lebensbühne*. Munich, 1953.
Bericht über das Bayerische Gesundheitswesen für das Jahr 1939. Edited by Staatsministerium des Innern. Vol. 58. Munich, 1941.
Bericht über eine wissenschaftliche Besprechung am 26. und 27. Oktober 1942 in Nürnberg über Ärztliche Fragen bei Seenot und Winternot. (*Mitteilungen aus dem Gebiet der Luftfahrtmedizin*, *Tagungsbericht* 7/43). Edited by A. J. Anthony. N.p., n.d.
Berufszählung: Die berufliche und soziale Gliederung des Deutschen Volkes: Textliche Darstellungen und Ergebnisse. (*Statistik des Deutschen Reichs: Volks-, Berufs- und Betriebszählung vom 16. Juni 1933*, vol. 458). Berlin, 1937.

Bessel, Richard. *Political Violence and the Rise of Nazism: The Storm Troopers in Eastern Germany, 1925–1934*. New Haven, 1984.

Bestvater, Horst. "Gedanken und Anregungen zur Neuordnung des Medizinstudiums." *Deutsches Ärzteblatt* 69 (1939): 408–9.

Bethge, Eberhard. *Dietrich Bonhoeffer: Man of Vision, Man of Courage*. New York, 1970.

Bewer, Clemens. "Obrigkeitliche Befugnisse der Reichsärztekammer: Eine grundsätzliche Entscheidung des Reichsgerichts zu dem Fragenkomplex: Ärztekammer—Arzt—Ärztliche Verrechnungsstelle—Private Krankenversicherung." *Deutsches Ärzteblatt* 72 (1942): 221–27.

———. "Die Pflicht zur Hilfeleistung bei Unglücksfällen: Der neue Paragraph 330c StrGB in der Rechtsprechung des Reichsgerichts." *Deutsches Ärzteblatt* 71 (1941): 169–71.

Beyerchen, Alan D. *Scientists under Hitler: Politics and the Physics Community in the Third Reich*. New Haven, 1977.

Bickel, Lennard. *Rise up to Life: A Biography of Howard Walter Florey Who Gave Penicillin to the World*. New York, 1972.

Bielenberg, Christabel. *The Past Is Myself*. London, 1968.

Biernat, Karl Heinz, and Luise Kraushaar. *Die Schulze-Boysen/Harnack-Organisation im antifaschistischen Kampf*. Berlin (DDR), 1970.

Bilz, Josephine. "BDM.-Ärztin und BDM.-Führerin." *Die Ärztin* 17 (1941): 212–14.

Birnbaum, Max P. *Staat und Synagoge 1918–1938: Eine Geschichte des Preussischen Landesverbandes jüdischer Gemeinden (1918–1938)*. Tübingen, 1981.

Birnbaum, Walter. *Zeuge meiner Zeit: Aussagen zu 1912 bis 1972*. Göttingen, 1973.

Bittner, Georg. "Der deutsche Widerstand gegen Hitler: Ärzte in Opposition—Die sozial- und gesundheitspolitischen Vorstellungen des deutschen Widerstandes." *Ärztliche Mitteilungen* 46 (1961): 1529–35.

Blakeney, Michael. *Australia and the Jewish Refugees, 1933–1948*. Sydney, 1985.

Blank, Heinz, ed. *Augenzeugenberichte vom Kriegsende 1945 im Markt Gangkofen: Eine Dokumentation: Ein Beitrag zur Zeitgeschichte des Marktes Gangkofen*. Gangkofen, 1975.

Blasius, Dirk. *Umgang mit Unheilbarem: Studien zur Sozialgeschichte der Psychiatrie*. Bonn, 1986.

Blau, Bruno. *Das Ausnahmerecht für die Juden in Deutschland 1933–1945*. 3d ed. Düsseldorf, 1965.

Bleuel, Hans Peter, and Ernst Klinnert. *Deutsche Studenten auf dem Weg ins Dritte Reich: Ideologien—Programme—Aktionen 1918–1935*. Gütersloh, 1967.

Blome, Kurt. "Das ärztliche Fortbildungswesen in Deutschland: 3. Internationaler Kongress für ärztliche Fortbildung." *Ziel und Weg* 7 (1937): 437–39.

———. *Arzt im Kampf. Erlebnisse und Gedanken*. Leipzig, 1942.

———. "Freiheit der Forschung und Wissenschaft: Grundsätzliches zur Frage des ärztlichen und wissenschaftlichen Nachwuchses." *Deutsches Ärzteblatt* 68 (1938): 242–48.

———. "Neue Deutsche Heilkunde, Arzt und Fortbildung." *Ziel und Weg* 6 (1936): 246–51.

———. "Die Neuordnung der ärztlichen Fortbildung." *Deutsches Ärzteblatt* 66 (1936): 2–11.

———. "Rückblick und Ausblick unserer ärztlichen Fortbildung und Schulung." *Deutsches Ärzteblatt* 67 (1937): 2–12.

Bluhm, Agnes. *Die rassenhygienischen Aufgaben des weiblichen Arztes*. Berlin, 1936.

———. "Zur Frage nach der generativen Tüchtigkeit der deutschen Frauen und der rassenhygienischen Bedeutung der ärztlichen Geburtshilfe." *Archiv für Rassen- und Gesellschaftsbiologie* 9 (1912): 330–46.

Boberach, Heinz, ed. *Meldungen aus dem Reich: Auswahl aus den geheimen Lageberichten des Sicherheitsdienstes der SS 1939–1944*. Neuwied, 1965.

Bock, Gisela. *Zwangssterilisation im Nationalsozialismus: Studien zur Rassenpolitik und Frauenpolitik*. Opladen, 1986.

Boehnert, Gunnar C. "The Jurists in the SS-Führerkorps, 1925–1939." In Gerhard Hirschfeld and Lothar Kettenacker, eds., *Der "Führerstaat": Mythos und Realität: Studien zur Struktur und Politik des Dritten Reiches*. Stuttgart, 1981, pp. 361–73.

———. "A Sociography of the SS Officer Corps, 1925–1939." Ph.D. dissertation, London, 1977.

Boelcke, Willi A., ed. *Kriegspropaganda 1939–1941: Geheime Ministerkonferenzen im Reichspropagandaministerium*. Stuttgart, 1966.

Bölling, Rainer. *Volksschullehrer und Politik: Der Deutsche Lehrerverein 1918–1933*. Göttingen, 1978.

Böttcher, Alfred. "Wer ist Jude?" *Ziel und Weg* 5 (1935): 96–98.

Bonhoeffer, Karl. "Ein Rückblick auf die Auswirkung und die Handhabung des nationalsozialistischen Sterilisationsgesetzes." *Der Nervenarzt* 20 (1949): 1–5.

Borst, Max. "Forschung und Fortbildung." *Ziel und Weg* 7 (1937): 440–45.

Boschan, Siegfried. *Nationalsozialistische Rassen- und Familiengesetzgebung: Praktische Rechtsanwendung und Auswirkungen auf Rechtspflege, Verwaltung und Wirtschaft*. Berlin, 1937.

Botz, Gerhard. *Wien vom "Anschluss" zum Krieg: Nationalsozialistische Machtübernahme und politisch-soziale Umgestaltung am Beispiel der Stadt Wien 1938/39*. Vienna, 1978.

———. *Wohnungspolitik und Judendeportation in Wien 1938 bis 1945: Zur Funktion des Antisemitismus als Ersatz nationalsozialistischer Sozialpolitik*. Vienna, 1975.

Boveri, Margret. *Verzweigungen: Eine Autobiographie*. Edited by Uwe Johnson. Munich, 1982.

Bracher, Karl Dietrich. *The German Dictatorship: The Origins, Structure, and Effects of National Socialism*. New York, 1972.

———, et al. *Die nationalsozialistische Machtergreifung: Studien zur Errichtung des totalitären Herrschaftssystems in Deutschland 1933/34*. 2d ed. Cologne, 1962.

Brandenburg, Hans-Christian. *Die Geschichte der HJ: Wege und Irrwege einer Generation*. Cologne, 1968.

Bridenthal, Renate, and Claudia Koonz. "Beyond *Kinder, Küche, Kirche*: Weimar Women in Politics and Work." In Renate Bridenthal and Claudia Koonz, eds., *When Biology Became Destiny: Women in Weimar and Nazi Germany*. New York, 1984, pp. 33–65.

Bromberg, Norbert, and Verna Volz Small. *Hitler's Psychopathology*. New York, 1983.

Broszat, Martin. "Resistenz und Widerstand: Eine Zwischenbilanz des Forschungsprojekts." In Martin Broszat et al., *Bayern in der NS-Zeit IV: Herrschaft und Gesellschaft im Konflikt Teil C*. Munich, 1981, pp. 691–709.

———, et al., eds. *Bayern in der NS-Zeit: Soziale Lage und politisches Verhalten der Bevölkerung im Spiegel vertraulicher Berichte*. Munich, 1977.

Browning, Christopher R. "Genocide and Public Health: German Doctors and Polish Jews, 1939–41." *Holocaust and Genocide Studies* 3 (1988): 21–36.

Brugsch, Theodor. *Arzt seit fünf Jahrzehnten*. 2d ed. Berlin (DDR), 1958.

———. *Ganzheitsproblematik in der Medizin: Zugleich eine Einführung in die medizinische Erkenntnislehre*. Berlin, 1936.

Bruss, Regina. *Die Bremer Juden unter dem Nationalsozialismus*. Bremen, 1983.

Buchbender, Ortwin, and Reinhold Sterz, eds. *Das andere Gesicht des Krieges: Deutsche Feldpostbriefe 1939–1945*. Munich, 1982.

Buchinger, Otto. *Vom Marinearzt zum Fastenarzt: Metamorphosen eines Wandernden*. Freiburg i.Br., 1955.

Buchmann, Erika. *Frauen im Konzentrationslager*. Stuttgart, 1946.

———, ed. *Die Frauen von Ravensbrück*. Berlin (DDR), 1959.

Büchner, Franz. *Pläne und Fügungen: Lebenserinnerungen eines deutschen Hochschullehrers*. Munich, 1965.

———. *Von der Grösse und Gefährdung der modernen Medizin*. Freiburg i.Br., 1961.

Bürger-Prinz, Hans. *Ein Psychiater berichtet*. Munich, 1973.

Bumke, Oswald. *Erinnerungen und Betrachtungen: Der Weg eines deutschen Psychiaters*. Munich, 1952.

———. "Das Nichtordinarienproblem in den medizinischen Fakultäten." *Mitteilungen des Verbandes der deutschen Hochschulen* 12 (1932): 254–59.

———. "Der Staat und die Geisteskranken." In *Handbuch der Geisteskrankheiten: Ergänzungsband*. Edited by Oswald Bumke. Berlin, 1939, pp. 280–305.

Bunz, Fritz. *Was muss der praktische Arzt vom staatlichen Gesundheitswesen wissen*? Berlin, 1938.

Burchardt, Lothar. "Halbstaatliche Wissenschaftsförderung im Kaiserreich und in der frühen Weimarer Republik." In Gunter Mann and Rolf Winau, eds., *Medizin, Naturwissenschaft, Technik und das Zweite Kaiserreich: Vorträge eines Kongresses vom 6. bis 11. September 1973 in Bad Nauheim*. Göttingen, 1977, pp. 35–51.

Burgschweiger, Brigitte. "Humangenetische und anthropologische Arbeiten (Dissertationen) in der Medizinischen Fakultät der Universität Erlangen in den Jahren 1933–1945." M.D. dissertation, Erlangen-Nuremberg, 1970.

Bussche, Rik van den, and Horst Krähe. "Zur Prognose des Ärztebedarfs in der

BRD seit 1960: Eine Kritik ihrer Ansätze und die Analyse ihrer Folgen." In Volker Volkholz et al., *Analyse des Gesundheitssystems: Krankheitsstrukturen, ärztlicher Arbeitsprozess, Sozialstaat: Reader zur Medizinsoziologie*. Frankfurt am Main, 1974, pp. 341–67.

Carmon, Arye. "The Impact of the Nazi Radical Decrees on the University of Heidelberg: A Case Study." *Yad Vashem Studies* 11 (1976): 131–63.

Carsten, Francis L. *Fascist Movements in Austria: From Schönerer to Hitler*. London, 1977.

———. *The Rise of Fascism*. London, 1970.

Cassels, Alan. *Fascism*. New York, 1975.

Catel, Werner. *Leben im Widerstreit: Bekenntnisse eines Arztes*. Nuremberg, 1974.

Chain, Ernst Boris. "The Development of Bacterial Chemotherapy." *Antibiotics and Chemotherapy* 4 (1954): 215–41.

Childers, Thomas. *The Nazi Voter: The Social Foundations of Fascism in Germany, 1919–1933*. Chapel Hill, 1983.

Christian, Shirley. "In South America, Malpractice Has a Moral Dimension." *New York Times*, May 11, 1986, sec. 4, p. 22.

Chroust, Peter. "Friedrich Mennecke: Innenansichten eines medizinischen Täters im Nationalsozialismus: Eine Briefauswahl." In Götz Aly et al., *Biedermann und Schreibtischtäter: Materialien zur deutschen Täter-Biographie*. Berlin, 1987, pp. 67–122.

———. "Social Situation and Political Orientation—Students and Professors at Giessen University, 1918–1945, II." *Historical Social Research—Historische Sozialforschung*, no. 39 (July 1986): 36–85.

Cocks, Geoffrey. *Psychotherapy in the Third Reich: The Göring Institute*. New York, 1985.

Coermann, Wilhelm, and Fritz Wagner, eds. *Deutsches Ärzterecht: Ein Wegweiser für Ärzte, Zahnärzte und Krankenanstalten*. Stuttgart, 1938.

Cole, John Alfred. *Lord Haw-Haw—and William Joyce*. London, 1964.

Coleman, William. "The Physician in Nazi Germany: An Essay Review." *Bulletin of the History of Medicine* 60 (1980): 234–40.

Conrad-Martius, Hedwig. *Utopien der Menschenzüchtung: Der Sozialdarwinismus und seine Folgen*. Munich, 1955.

Conti, Leonardo. "Leistung und Aufgabe des deutschen Arztes im Kriege." In *Aus Deutscher Medizin: Ausländisch-Deutsches Medizinertreffen Innsbruck 1942*. Berlin, 1944, pp. 15–26.

———. "Rückschau und Ausblick." *Deutsches Ärzteblatt* 71 (1941): 1–3.

———. "Zum neuen Jahre." *Deutsches Ärzteblatt* 70 (1940): 1–3.

Conti, Nanna. "Des Hebammenwesen in Deutschland." *Die Ärztin* 13 (1937): 294–302.

———. "Die Mitarbeit der Hebammen in der Säuglingsfürsorge." *Die Ärztin* 17 (1941): 394–99.

Crome, Grete. "Der Gesundheitsdienst im Reichsarbeitsdienst: Arbeitsdienst für die weibliche Jugend." *Die Ärztin* 13 (1937): 140–42.

Cron, Helmut. "Die Studentin: Soziales Herkommen und Berufswahl." *Die Frau* 45 (1937–38): 249–52.

Dahrendorf, Ralf. *Gesellschaft und Demokratie in Deutschland*. Munich, 1968.
Daim, Wilfried. *Der Mann, der Hitler die Ideen gab: Von den religiösen Verirrungen eines Sektierers zum Rassenwahn des Diktators*. Munich, 1958.
Dammer, Anna. "Frauenstudium und Ausleseprinzip im Kriege." *Die Ärztin* 20 (1944): 81–83.
Davidson, Henry A. "Professional Secrecy." In E. Fuller Torrey, ed., *Ethical Issues in Medicine: The Role of the Physician in Today's Society*. Boston, 1968, pp. 181–94.
Davie, Maurice R. *Refugees in America: Report of the Committee for the Study of Recent Immigration from Europe*. New York, 1947.
Dawidowicz, Lucy S. *The War against the Jews, 1933–1945*. New York, 1976.
Deak, Istvan. "The Convert." *New York Review of Books*, March 12, 1987, pp. 39–44.
______. "Could the Hungarian Jews Have Survived?" *New York Review of Books*, February 4, 1982, pp. 24–27.
Decker, Hannah S. *Freud in Germany: Revolution and Reaction in Science, 1893–1907*. New York, 1977.
De Crinis, Max. *Gerichtliche Psychiatrie*. 2d and 3d eds. Berlin, 1943.
Deich, Friedrich. "Jüdische Mediziner in München." In Hans Lamm, ed., *Von Juden in München: Ein Gedenkbuch*. 2d ed. Munich, 1959, pp. 244–51.
Deicke-Busch, Grete. "BDM.-Ärztin und Elternhaus." *Die Ärztin* 17 (1941): 214–18.
______. "Soforteinsatz von Feldscheren und GD-Mädeln der Hitler-Jugend nach Terrorangriffen." *Die Ärztin* 20 (1944): 11–13.
Delmer, Sefton. *Black Boomerang: An Autobiography*. London, 1962.
Deneke, J. F. Volrad. "Deutsche Wissenschaftler vor dem Militärgericht in Lyon." *Ärztliche Mitteilungen* 39 (1954): 362–64.
______. *Die freien Berufe*. Stuttgart, 1956.
Deneke, J. F. Volrad, and Richard E. Sperber. *Einhundert Jahre Deutsches Ärzteblatt-Ärztliche Mitteilungen*. Lövenich, 1973.
Das Deutsche Führerlexikon 1934/35. Berlin, n.d.
Deutsche Hochschulstatistik: Sommerhalbjahr 1928. Edited by Hochschulverwaltungen. [Berlin, 1928].
Deutschland-Berichte der Sopade. 7 vols. (1934–40). 5th ed. Frankfurt am Main, 1980.
Dicks, Henry V. *Licensed Mass Murder: A Socio-Psychological Study of Some SS Killers*. Sussex, 1972.
Diels, Rudolf. *Lucifer ante Portas: Zwischen Severing und Heydrich*. Zurich, n.d.
Diepgen, Paul. *Die Heilkunde und der ärztliche Beruf: Eine Einführung*. Munich, 1938.
Dietrich, A. "Die Entwicklung des Krankheitsbegriffes." *Hippokrates* 12 (1941): 1222–26.
Dinter, Artur. *Die Sünde wider das Blut: Ein Zeitroman*. 3d ed. Leipzig, 1919.
Dodd, Martha. *Through Embassy Eyes*. New York, 1940.
Döring, Hans-Joachim. *Die Zigeuner im nationalsozialistischen Staat*. Hamburg, 1964.

Dörner, Klaus. "Nationalsozialismus und Lebensvernichtung." *Vierteljahrshefte für Zeitgeschichte* 15 (1967): 121–52.

Dohrmann, Fredegunde. "Aus dem Arbeitsgebiet des Betriebsarztes." *Die Ärztin* 20 (1944): 39–41.

"Ein Dokument der Schande: Das Tagebuch des SS-Arztes Johann Paul Kremer." *Der Widerstandskämpfer* 22 (1974): 71–74.

Domeinski, Heinz. "Zur Entnazifizierung der Ärzteschaft im Lande Thüringen." In Achim Thom and Horst Spaar, eds., *Medizin im Faschismus: Symposium über das Schicksal der Medizin in der Zeit des Faschismus in Deutschland 1933–1945*. Berlin (DDR), 1985, pp. 250–54.

Drexel, Emmi. "Über schulärztliche Arbeit." *Die Ärztin* 13 (1937): 206–11.

Drüll, Dagmar. *Heidelberger Gelehrtenlexikon 1803–1932*. Berlin, 1986.

Düning, Hans-Joachim. *Der SA-Student im Kampf um die Hochschule (1925–1935): Ein Beitrag zur Geschichte der deutschen Universität im 20. Jahrhundert*. Weimar, 1936.

Ebermayer, Erich. *Denn heute gehört uns Deutschland . . . : Persönliches und politisches Tagebuch: Von der Machtergreifung bis zum 31. Dezember 1935*. Hamburg, 1959.

Ebner, Franz. "Die Bestallungsordnung für Ärzte." *Deutsches Ärzteblatt* 66 (1936): 502–3.

Eckelmann, Christine, and Kristin Hoesch. "Ärztinnen—Emanzipation durch den Krieg?" In Johanna Bleker and Heinz-Peter Schmiedebach, eds., *Medizin und Krieg: Vom Dilemma der Heilberufe 1865 bis 1985*. Frankfurt am Main, 1987, pp. 153–70.

Edsall, David L. "The Emigré Physician in American Medicine." *Journal of the American Medical Association* 114 (1940): 1068–73.

———. "A Program for the Refugee Physician." *Journal of the American Medical Association* 112 (1939): 1986–87.

Edsall, David L., and Tracy J. Putnam. "The Emigré Physician in America, 1941: A Report of the National Committee for Resettlement of Foreign Physicians." *Journal of the American Medical Association* 117 (1941): 1881–88.

Eiber, Ludwig. "Frauen in der Kriegsindustrie: Arbeitsbedingungen, Lebensumstände und Protestverhalten." In Martin Broszat et al., eds., *Bayern in der NS-Zeit III: Herrschaft und Gesellschaft im Konflikt Teil B*. Munich, 1981, pp. 569–644.

Eichhoff, Theodore. "Nationalsozialistische Stimmen zur Frauenfrage." *Soziale Praxis* 43 (1934): 1244–48.

Ellersdorfer, Richard. "Auswirkungen der Machtergreifung des Nationalsozialismus auf das Gesundheitswesen in Deutschland im Spiegel der 'Münchner Neuesten Nachrichten' von 1933 bis 1938." M.D. dissertation, Munich, 1977.

Engel, Richard. "Ärztliche Forderungen zum Sterilisationsgesetz." M.D. dissertation, Erlangen, 1935.

Engelhardt, Dietrich von, and Heinrich Schipperges. *Die inneren Verbindungen zwischen Philosophie und Medizin im 20. Jahrhundert*. Darmstadt, 1980.

Engelmann, Bernt. *Deutschland ohne Juden: Eine Bilanz*. Munich, 1974.

Ericksen, Robert P. *Theologians under Hitler: Gerhard Kittel, Paul Althaus and Emanuel Hirsch*. New Haven, 1985.
Etziony, M. B. *The Physician's Creed: An Anthology of Medical Prayers, Oaths and Codes of Ethics Written and Recited by Medical Practitioners through the Ages*. Springfield, Ill., 1973.
Falkenberg, Friedrich. "Misstände im Gesundheitswesen." *Deutsches Ärzteblatt* 72 (1942): 38–41.
Falstein, Louis, ed. *The Martyrdom of Jewish Physicians in Poland*. New York, 1963.
Falter, Jürgen W. "Die Wähler der NSDAP 1928–1933: Sozialstruktur und parteipolitische Herkunft." In Wolfgang Michalka, ed., *Die nationalsozialistische Machtergreifung*. Paderborn, 1984, pp. 47–59.
______, et al. *Wahlen und Abstimmungen in der Weimarer Republik: Materialien zum Wahlverhalten 1919–1933*. Munich, 1986.
Faust, Anselm. *Der Nationalsozialistische Deutsche Studentenbund: Studenten und Nationalsozialismus in der Weimarer Republik*. 2 vols. Düsseldorf, 1973.
______. "Professoren für die NSDAP: Zum politischen Verhalten der Hochschullehrer 1932/33." In Manfred Heinemann, ed., *Erziehung und Schulung im Dritten Reich*. Vol. 2. Stuttgart, 1980, pp. 31–49.
Feickert, Andreas. *Studenten greifen an: Nationalsozialistische Hochschulrevolution*. Hamburg, 1934.
Feiten, Willi. *Der Nationalsozialistische Lehrerbund: Entwicklung und Organisation: Ein Beitrag zum Aufbau und zur Organisationsstruktur des nationalsozialistischen Herrschaftssystems*. Weinheim, 1981.
Ferber, Christian von. *Die Entwicklung des Lehrkörpers der deutschen Universitäten und Hochschulen 1864–1954*. Göttingen, 1956.
Feuchter, Georg W. *Der Luftkrieg*. 3d ed. Frankfurt am Main, 1964.
Finkenrath, Kurt. *Die Organisation der deutschen Ärzteschaft: Eine Einführung in die Geschichte und den gegenwärtigen Aufbau des wissenschaftlichen, standes- und wirtschaftspolitischen ärztlichen Vereinslebens*. Berlin, 1928.
Fischer, Conan. *Stormtroopers: A Social, Economic and Ideological Analysis, 1929–35*. London, 1983.
Fischer, Eugen. *Der Begriff des völkischen Staates, biologisch betrachtet: Rede bei der Feier zur Erinnerung an den Stifter der Berliner Universität, König Friedrich Wilhelm III. in der Alten Aula am 29. Juli 1933*. Berlin, 1933.
______. "Die Fortschritte der menschlichen Erblehre als Grundlage eugenischer Bevölkerungspolitik." *Deutsche medizinische Wochenschrift* 59 (1933): 1069–73.
______. *Die Rehobother Bastards und das Bastardierungsproblem beim Menschen: Anthropologische und ethnographische Studien am Rehobother Bastardvolk in Deutsch-Südwest-Afrika, ausgeführt mit Unterstützung der Kgl. preuss. Akademie der Wissenschaften*. Jena, 1913.
______, et al. *Anthropologie*. Leipzig, 1923.
Fischer, Hubert. *Aus den Erfahrungsberichten der Beratenden Chirurgen im Krieg 1939–1945*. Darmstadt, 1963.
Fischer, Isidor, ed. *Biographisches Lexikon der hervorragenden Ärzte der letzten*

fünfzig Jahre. Vol. 1: Berlin, 1932. Vol. 2: Berlin, 1933.
Fischer, Thora F. "Der nationalsozialistische Arzt." M.D. dissertation, Kiel, 1971.
Fischer-Homberger, Esther. *Geschichte der Medizin*. Berlin, 1975.
Fleming, Alexander. "History and Development of Penicillin." In Alexander Fleming, ed., *Penicillin: Its Practical Application*. London, 1946, pp. 1–23.
Fliedner, Hans-Joachim. *Die Judenverfolgung in Mannheim 1933–1945*. Vol. 1. Stuttgart, 1971.
Floud, Roderick. *An Introduction to Quantitative Methods for Historians*. London, 1974.
Forssmann, Werner. *Experiments on Myself*. New York, 1972.
———. *Selbstversuch: Erinnerungen eines Chirurgen*. Düsseldorf, 1972.
Franke, Hans. *Geschichte und Schicksal der Juden in Heilbronn: Vom Mittelalter bis zur Zeit der nationalsozialistischen Verfolgungen (1050–1945)*. Heilbronn, 1963.
Franken, Hermann. "Die Schmerzbekämpfung in der Geburtshilfe." *Geburtshilfe und Frauenheilkunde* 3 (1941): 153–65.
Frankenthal, Käte. *Der dreifache Fluch: Jüdin, Intellektuelle, Sozialistin: Lebenserinnerungen einer Ärztin in Deutschland und im Exil*. Edited by Kathleen M. Pearle and Stephan Leibfried. Frankfurt am Main, 1981.
Franze, Manfred. *Die Erlanger Studentenschaft 1918–1945*. Würzburg, 1972.
Frei, Norbert. *Nationalsozialistische Eroberung der Provinzpresse: Gleichschaltung, Selbstanpassung und Resistenz in Bayern*. Stuttgart, 1980.
Freund, Paul A. "Ethical Problems in Human Experimentation." *New England Journal of Medicine* 273 (1965): 687–92.
Friedländer, Saul. *Kurt Gerstein oder die Zwiespältigkeit des Guten*. Gütersloh, 1968.
Friedlander, Henry. "Jüdische Anstaltspatienten im NS-Deutschland." In Götz Aly, ed., *Aktion T4 1939–1945: Die "Euthanasie"-Zentrale in der Tiergartenstrasse 4*. Berlin, 1987, pp. 34–44.
Friedman, Saul S. *No Haven for the Oppressed: United States Policy toward Jewish Refugees, 1938–1945*. Detroit, 1973.
Fröhlich, Elke. *Bayern in der NS-Zeit IV: Die Herausforderung des Einzelnen: Geschichten über Widerstand und Verfolgung*. Munich, 1983.
Fromm, Bella. *Blood and Banquets: A Berlin Social Diary*. 2d ed. New York, 1942.
Fromm, Ernst. "Die Ärztliche Berufsvertretung im Wandel der Zeit." *Bayerisches Ärzteblatt* no. 8 (1960): 264–69.
Fuchs, H. "Erfahrungen mit dem geburtshilflichen Dämmerschlaf." *Die medizinische Welt*, no. 15 (1941): 371–73.
25 [Fünfundzwanzig] Jahre Medizinische Fakultät der Universität Münster. Münster, 1951.
Gasman, Daniel. *The Scientific Origins of National Socialism: Social Darwinism in Ernst Haeckel and the German Monist League*. London, 1971.
Gatz, Erwin. *Hospitäler und Krankenhäuser im Kreise Kempen-Krefeld*. Kempen, 1970.
Gauwerky, F. "Die Reichsfachgruppe Medizin in der Führerschule Alt-Rehse vom 10. bis 14. März 1937." *Deutsches Ärzteblatt* 67 (1937): 375–76.

———. "Tätigkeitsbericht der Reichsfachgruppe Medizin im Sommersemester 1937." *Deutsches Ärzteblatt* 67 (1937): 1078–79.

Gay, Peter. *Freud, Jews and Other Germans: Masters and Victims in Modernist Culture*. Oxford, 1979.

Gebhard, Bruno. *Im Strom und Gegenstrom 1919–1937*. Wiesbaden, 1976.

Geilen, Elisabeth. "Der erste Ärztinnen-Fortbildungslehrgang im Rudolf Hess-Krankenhaus." *Deutsches Ärzteblatt* 67 (1937): 46–47.

Geisler, Erika. "Ziel und Wege in der Gesundheitserziehung des Mädels." *Die Ärztin* 17 (1941): 200–206.

Gelwick, Robert Arthur. "Personnel Policies and Procedures of the Waffen-SS." Ph.D. dissertation, University of Nebraska, 1971.

Genschel, Helmut. *Die Verdrängung der Juden aus der Wirtschaft im Dritten Reich*. Göttingen, 1966.

Gersbach, Alfons, ed. *Der Bürgermeister und der öffentliche Gesundheitsdienst: Ein Leitfaden für die unteren Verwaltungsbehörden, Bürgermeister, Ortspolizeibehörden und Gesundheitsämter*. Berlin, 1939.

Gersdorff, Ursula von, ed. *Frauen im Kriegsdienst 1914–1945*. Stuttgart, 1969.

Geuter, Ulfried. *Die Professionalisierung der deutschen Psychologie im Nationalsozialismus*. Frankfurt am Main, 1984.

———. "Psychiatrisch-psychologische Folter in Chile und die psychosoziale Betreuung lateinamerikanischer Flüchtlinge: Ein Interview mit dem chilenischen Arzt Jorge Borudy." *Psychologie und Gesellschaftskritik*, no. 2 (1978): 89–107.

Geyer-Kordesch, Johanna. "Die Diskriminierung von Frauen in der Medizin." In Anne Schlüter and Annette Kuhn, eds., *Lila Schwarzbuch: Zur Diskriminierung von Frauen in der Wissenschaft*. Düsseldorf, 1986, pp. 225–33.

Gilbert, Martin. *The Holocaust: A History of the Jews of Europe during the Second World War*. New York, 1985.

Giles, Geoffrey J. *Students and National Socialism in Germany*. Princeton, 1985.

———. "University Government in Nazi Germany: Hamburg." *Minerva* 16 (1978): 196–221.

Gillmor, Don. *I Swear by Apollo: Dr. Ewen Cameron, the CIA, and the Canadian Mind-Control Experiments*. Montreal, 1987.

Glöcker, Heino. "Bestand und Entwicklung des berufsmässig tätigen deutschen Heil- und Pflegepersonals bis Anfang 1938." *Ärzteblatt für Norddeutschland* 3 (1940): 45.

Goebbels, Joseph. *Tagebücher 1945: Die letzten Aufzeichnungen*. Hamburg, 1977.

The Goebbels Diaries. Edited by Louis P. Lochner. New York, 1948.

Götz von Olenhusen, Albrecht von. "Die 'nichtarischen' Studenten an den deutschen Hochschulen: Zur nationalsozialistischen Rassenpolitik 1933–1945." *Vierteljahrshefte für Zeitgeschichte* 14 (1966): 175–206.

Goetze, Fritz, and Hellmut Meeske, eds. *Reichsgesundheitswesen: Eine Sammlung der wichtigeren Gesetze, Verordnungen und Verwaltungsvorschriften des Reichsrechts über das Gesundheitswesen*. Munich, 1937.

Gohrbandt, Erwin. "Auskühlung." *Zentralblatt für Chirurgie* 70 (1943): 1553–57.

Goldschmidt, Fritz. *Meine Arbeit bei der Vertretung der Interessen der jüdischen*

Ärzte in Deutschland seit dem Juli 1933. (*Arbeitsbericht zu verschütteten Alternativen in der Gesundheitspolitik*, no. 2.) Edited by Stephan Leibfried and Florian Tennstedt. Bremen, 1979.

Goldstein, Richard H., and Patrick Breslin. "Technicians of Torture: How Physicians Become Agents of State Terror." *Sciences* 26, no. 2 (March–April 1985): 14–19.

Golücke, Friedhelm. *Schweinfurt und der strategische Luftkrieg 1943: Der Angriff der US Air Force vom 14. Oktober 1943 gegen die Schweinfurter Kugellagerindustrie*. Paderborn, 1980.

Gordon, Sarah. *Hitler, Germans and the "Jewish Question."* Princeton, 1984.

Graetz-Menzel, Charlotte. "Über die rassenbiologische Wirkung der akademischen Frauenberufe mit besonderer Berücksichtigung der Ärztinnen und Zahnärztinnen." *Archiv für Rassen- und Gesellschaftsbiologie* 27 (1933): 129–50.

Graml, Hermann. *Der 9. November 1938: "Reichskristallnacht."* 6th ed. Bonn, 1958.

Granier, Gerhard, et al., eds. *Das Bundesarchiv und seine Bestände*. 3d ed. Boppard, 1977.

Grill, Johnpeter Horst. *The Nazi Party in Baden, 1920–1945*. Chapel Hill, 1983.

Grober, Julius. "Lehrstühle für Rassenhygiene." *Deutsches Ärzteblatt* 64 (1934): 337–38.

Gross, Leonard. *Versteckt: Wie Juden in Berlin die Nazi-Zeit überlebten*. Reinbek, 1983.

Gross, Walter. "Arzt und Judenfrage." *Ziel und Weg* 3 (1933): 186–89.

———. "Die Dresdener Versammlung der Deutschen Naturforscher und Ärzte: Rückblick und Kritik." *Ziel und Weg* 6 (1936): 538–42.

———. "Hütet die Flamme!" *Ziel und Weg* 3 (1933): 114–15.

———. "Von der politischen zur geistigen Revolution." *Deutsches Ärzteblatt* 64 (1934): 818–23.

Grossmann, Anton. "Milieubedingungen von Verfolgung und Widerstand: Am Beispiel ausgewählter Ortsvereine der SPD." In Martin Broszat and Hartmut Mehringer, eds., *Bayern in der NS-Zeit V: Die Parteien KPD, SPD, BVP in Verfolgung und Widerstand*. Munich, 1983, pp. 433–540.

Grossmann, Atina. "Abortion and Economic Crisis: The 1931 Campaign against Paragraph 218." In Renate Bridenthal et al., eds., *When Biology Became Destiny: Women in Weimar and Nazi Germany*. New York, 1984, pp. 66–86.

———. "Berliner Ärztinnen und Volksgesundheit in der Weimarer Republik: Zwischen Sexualreform und Eugenik." In Christiane Eifert and Susanne Rouette, eds., *Unter allen Umständen: Frauengeschichte(n) in Berlin*. Berlin, 1986, pp. 183–217.

Grote, Heinrich. "Die Entwicklung des Berufs- und Standeslebens der deutschen Ärzteschaft durch den Nationalsozialismus." *Deutsches Ärzteblatt* 66 (1936): 337–41.

———. "Kriegsbesoldung, Familienunterhalt und Zahlungen der KVD an einberufene Kassenärzte." *Deutsches Ärzteblatt* 70 (1940): 158–61.

———. "KVD und ärztliche Fortbildung." *Deutsches Ärzteblatt* 66 (1936): 11–13.

———. "Die Tätigkeit der KVD im Kriege." *Deutsches Ärzteblatt* 72 (1942): 56–60.

Gruber, Georg B. *Einführung in Geist und Studium der Medizin: Zwölf Vorlesungen*. Leipzig, 1934.

Gruchmann, Lothar. *Justiz im Dritten Reich 1933–1940: Verwaltung, Anpassung und Ausschaltung in der Ära Gürtner*. Munich, 1987.

Grunberger, Richard. *The 12-Year Reich: A Social History of Nazi Germany, 1933–1945*. New York, 1972.

Günther, Hans F. K. *Das Bauerntum als Lebens- und Gemeinschaftsform*. 2d ed. Leipzig, 1941.

Güse, Hans-Georg, and Norbert Schmacke. *Psychiatrie zwischen bürgerlicher Revolution und Faschismus*. Vol. 2. Kronberg, 1976.

Güstrow, Dietrich. *Tödlicher Alltag: Strafverteidiger im Dritten Reich*. Berlin, 1981.

Gütt, Arthur. "Der Aufbau des Gesundheitswesens im Dritten Reich." In Paul Meier-Benneckenstein, ed., *Das Dritte Reich im Aufbau: Übersichten und Leistungsberichte*. Vol. 2. Berlin, 1939, pp. 60–117.

———. "Der Deutsche Arzt im Dritten Reich." *Ziel und Weg* 3 (1933): 80–82.

———. "Einführung zum Blutschutz- und Ehegesundheitsgesetz." *Der Öffentliche Gesundheitsdienst* 2 A (1936): 121–31.

———, ed. *Der öffentliche Gesundheitsdienst: Erläuterungen zum Gesetz über die Vereinheitlichung des Gesundheitswesens vom 3. Juli 1934 nebst Durchführungsverordnungen, Gebührenordnung und Anhang mit Erlassen*. 2d ed. Berlin, 1939.

———, et al. *Gesetz zur Verhütung erbkranken Nachwuchses vom 14. Juli 1933 mit Auszug aus dem Gesetz gegen gefährliche Gewohnheitsverbrecher und über Massregeln der Sicherung und Besserung vom 24. Nov. 1933*. Munich, 1934.

Gumpert, Martin. *Heil Hunger! Health under Hitler*. New York, 1940.

———. *Hölle im Paradies: Selbstdarstellung eines Arztes*. Stockholm, 1939.

Guthrie, Douglas. *A History of Medicine*. London, 1960.

Haag, F. E. "Die Krankenträgerausbildung im ärztlichen Studium." *Ziel und Weg* 6 (1936): 414–17.

Haas, Albert. *The Doctor and the Damned*. New York, 1984.

Hadda, Siegmund. "Als Arzt am Jüdischen Krankenhaus zu Breslau 1906–1943." *Jahrbuch der Schlesischen Friedrich-Wilhelms-Universität zu Breslau* 17 (1972): 198–238.

Hadrich, Julius. "Das voraussichtliche Angebot von Ärzten in den kommenden Jahren." *Deutsches Ärzteblatt* 64 (1934): 568–69.

———. "Die Fachärzte für Orthopädie." *Deutsches Ärzteblatt* 64 (1934): 801–3.

———. "Die nichtarischen Ärzte in Deutschland." *Deutsches Ärzteblatt* 64 (1934): 1243–45.

———. "Die Zahl der Ärzte Deutschlands und ihre Gliederung im Jahre 1935." *Deutsches Ärzteblatt* 65 (1935): 696–700.

———. "Die Zahl der Allgemeinpraktiker und Fachärzte in den deutschen Gross- und Mittelstädten im Jahre 1929." *Ärztliche Mitteilungen* 30 (1929): 542–44.

———. "Die Zahl der Allgemeinpraktiker und Fachärzte in den deutschen Gross- und Mittelstädten im Jahre 1930." *Ärztliche Mitteilungen* 32 (1931): 386–88.
———. "Zahl und Verteilung der Kassenärzte im Jahre 1936." *Deutsches Ärzteblatt* 66 (1936): 1058–60.
———. "Zur sozialen und wirtschaftlichen Lage der angestellten Ärzte." *Deutsches Ärzteblatt* 65 (1935): 159–61.
Haedenkamp, Carl. "Änderungen der Zulassungsordnung für Ärzte." *Münchener Medizinische Wochenschrift* 85 (1938): 409–13.
———. "Die Gesamtvorstände zur Lage." *Ärztliche Mitteilungen* 34 (1933): 209–12.
———. "Grundlagen und Bedeutung des neuen Zulassungsrechtes." *Deutsches Ärzteblatt* 64 (1934): 558–62.
———. *Die Neuordnung der deutschen Sozialversicherung*. Munich, 1937.
Härtel, Fritz. "Rasse und Chirurgie." In Johannes Schottky, ed., *Rasse und Krankheit*. Munich, 1937, pp. 248–73.
Hagen, Louis. *Follow My Leader*. London, 1951.
Hagen, Wilhelm. *Auftrag und Wirklichkeit: Sozialarzt im 20. Jahrhundert*. Munich-Gräfelfing, 1978.
Hahn, Susanne. "Positionen der kommunistischen Partei Deutschlands zur lebensbewahrenden Aufgabe der Medizin in der Zeit der Weimarer Republik." *Zeitschrift für die gesamte Hygiene und ihre Grenzgebiete* 28 (1982): 468–71.
Hanauske-Abel, Hartmut M. "From Nazi Holocaust to Nuclear Holocaust: A Lesson to Learn?" *Lancet*, August 2, 1986, pp. 271–73.
———. "Die Unfähigkeit zu trauern: Erziehungsziel für junge deutsche Ärzte?" *Rundbrief: Ärzte warnen vor dem Atomkrieg*, special issue, November 1987, pp. 25–44.
Hanke, Peter. *Zur Geschichte der Juden in München zwischen 1933 und 1945*. Munich, 1967.
Hansen, Eckhard, et al. *Seit über einem Jahrhundert . . . : Verschüttete Alternativen in der Sozialpolitik: Sozialer Fortschritt, organisierte Dienstleistermacht und nationalsozialistische Machtergreifung: Der Fall der Ambulatorien in den Unterweserstädten und Berlin*. Cologne, 1981.
Harrison's Principles of Internal Medicine. Edited by Robert G. Petersdorf et al. 10th ed. New York, 1983.
Hartmann, Hans. "Der Mut zur Verantwortung: Eine Betrachtung zum Chirurgenkongress 1940." *Deutsches Ärzteblatt* 70 (1940): 169–72.
Hartshorne, Edward Yarnell, Jr. *The German Universities and National Socialism*. Cambridge, Mass., 1941.
Hassell, Ulrich von. *Vom Andern Deutschland: Aus den nachgelassenen Tagebüchern 1938–1944*. Frankfurt am Main, 1964.
Hastings, Max. *Overlord: D-Day and the Battle for Normandy*. London, 1985.
Hauer, Jakob Wilhelm, ed. *Paragraph 218: Eine sachliche Aussprache*. Leipzig, [1931].
Haug, Alfred. "Der Lehrstuhl für Biologische Medizin in Jena." In Fridolf Kudlien, ed., *Ärzte im Nationalsozialismus*. Cologne, 1985, pp. 130–38.
———. "Das Rudolf-Hess-Krankenhaus in Dresden." In Fridolf Kudlien, ed., *Ärzte*

im Nationalsozialismus. Cologne, 1985, pp. 138–45.
Hausen, Karin. "Unemployment Also Hits Women: The New and the Old Woman on the Dark Side of the Golden Twenties in Germany." In Peter D. Stachura, ed., *Unemployment and the Great Depression in Weimar Germany*. Basingstoke, 1986, pp. 78–120.
Heiber, Helmut. *Walter Frank und sein Reichsinstitut für Geschichte des neuen Deutschlands*. Stuttgart, 1966.
______, ed. *Reichsführer! . . . : Briefe an und von Himmler*. Stuttgart, 1968.
Heidepriem, Lore. "Der erste Ärztinnenlehrgang in Alt-Rehse." *Deutsches Ärzteblatt* 66 (1936): 1056–57.
Hellmann, Dr. med. "Besonderheiten der ärztlichen Landpraxis." *Ziel und Weg* 7 (1937): 368–74, 416–20.
Hellpap, Cläre. "Erholungspflege nach einfachen klimatischen Regeln: Aus der Müttererholungspflege der NSV." *Die Ärztin* 13 (1937): 143–47.
______. "Die NSV. verschickt die stillende Mutter." *Die Ärztin* 12 (1937): 33–35.
Helmreich, W. "Rassen- und Erbhygiene im neuen Eherecht." *Münchener Medizinische Wochenschrift* 83 (1936): 480–85.
Hempel, Henri Jacob, ed. *"Wenn ich schon ein Fremder sein muss . . ." : Deutsch-jüdische Emigranten in New York*. Frankfurt am Main, 1983.
Henderson, W. O. *The Rise of German Industrial Power, 1834–1914*. Berkeley and Los Angeles, 1975.
Henry, Frances. *Victims and Neighbors: A Small Town in Nazi Germany Remembered*. South Hadley, Mass., 1984.
Herf, Jeffrey. *Reactionary Modernism: Technology, Culture, and Politics in Weimar and the Third Reich*. Cambridge, Eng., 1984.
Herrmann, Gertraud, and Erwin Hermann. "Nationalsozialistische Agitation und Herrschaftspraxis in der Provinz: Das Beispiel Bayreuth." *Zeitschrift für Bayerische Landesgeschichte* 59 (1976): 201–50.
Herrmann, Martin. "Ist das Gesetz zur Verhütung erbkranken Nachwuchses imstande, die Huntington-Chorea-Familien zum Aussterben zu bringen?" M.D. dissertation, Erlangen, 1935.
Heston, Leonard L., and Renate Heston. *The Medical Casebook of Adolf Hitler*. London, 1979.
Hetzer, Gerhard. "Die Industriestadt Augsburg: Eine Sozialgeschichte der Arbeiteropposition." In Martin Broszat et al., eds., *Bayern in der NS-Zeit III: Herrschaft und Gesellschaft im Konflikt Teil B*. Munich, 1981, pp. 1–233.
Hiemer, Ernst. *Der Pudelmopsdackelpinscher und andere besinnliche Erzählungen*. Nuremberg, 1940.
Hilberg, Raul. *The Destruction of the European Jews*. Chicago, 1967.
His, Wilhelm. *Die Front der Ärzte*. Bielefeld, 1931.
Hitler, Adolf. *Mein Kampf*. Translated by Ralph Manheim. London, 1974.
Hobby, Gladys L. *Penicillin: Meeting the Challenge*. New Haven, 1985.
Hobohm, Johannes. "Der Nationalsozialismus als Überwinder des Zeitalters der Neurose." *Ziel und Weg* 4 (1934): 41–44.
Hochmuth, Ursel, and Gertrud Meyer. *Streiflichter aus dem Hamburger Widerstand 1933–1945: Berichte und Dokumente*. Frankfurt am Main, 1969.

Hoemberg, Elisabeth. *Thy People, My People*. London, 1950.
Höhne, Heinz. *Der Orden unter dem Totenkopf: Die Geschichte der SS*. Gütersloh, 1967.
Höss, Rudolf. *Kommandant in Auschwitz: Autobiographische Aufzeichnungen*. Edited by Martin Broszat. Munich, 1963.
Hoff, Ferdinand. *Erlebnis und Besinnung: Erinnerungen eines Arztes*. 4th ed. Frankfurt am Main, 1972.
Hoffa, Lizzie. "Das Frauenstudium." *Ärztliche Mitteilungen* 34 (1933): 203–5.
Hoffmann, Auguste. "Das sportärztliche Arbeitsgebiet." *Die Ärztin* 13 (1937): 211–15.
Hoffmann, Erich. *Ringen um Vollendung: Lebenserinnerungen aus einer Wendezeit der Heilkunde 1933–1946*. Hanover, 1949.
Hoffmann, Peter. *Widerstand, Staatsstreich, Attentat: Der Kampf der Opposition gegen Hitler*. 2d ed. Frankfurt am Main, 1974.
Hohenstein, Alexander. *Wartheländisches Tagebuch aus den Jahren 1941/42*. Munich, 1963.
Hohmann, Joachim S. *Zigeuner und Zigeunerwissenschaft: Ein Beitrag zur Grundlagenforschung und Dokumentation des Völkermordes im "Dritten Reich."* Marburg, 1980.
Huber, Ernst Rudolf. "Die Rechtsgestalt der NSDAP." *Deutsche Rechtswissenschaft* 4 (1939): 314–51.
Huerkamp, Claudia. *Der Aufstieg der Ärzte im 19. Jahrhundert: Vom gelehrten Stand zum professionellen Experten: Das Beispiel Preussens*. Göttingen, 1985.
Huerkamp, Claudia, and Reinhard Spree. "Arbeitsmarktstrategien der deutschen Ärzteschaft im späten 19. und frühen 20. Jahrhundert: Zur Entwicklung des Marktes für professionelle ärztliche Dienstleistungen." In Toni Pierenkemper and Richard Tilly, eds., *Historische Arbeitsmarktforschung: Entstehung, Entwicklung und Probleme der Vermarktung von Arbeitskraft*. Göttingen, 1982, pp. 77–116.
Ich studiere: Ein Überblick über die Arbeit des deutschen Studententums. N.p., 1940.
Ivy, Andrew C. "Nazi War Crimes of a Medical Nature." In Stanley Joel Reiser et al., eds., *Ethics in Medicine: Historical Perspectives and Contemporary Concerns*. Cambridge, Mass., 1977, pp. 267–72.
Jaeckel, Gerhard. *Die Charité: Die Geschichte des berühmtesten deutschen Krankenhauses*. Bayreuth, 1963.
Jakobi, Helga, et al. *Aeskulap und Hakenkreuz: Zur Geschichte der Medizinischen Fakultät in Giessen zwischen 1933 und 1945*. Giessen, 1982.
Jamin, Mathilde. *Zwischen den Klassen: Zur Sozialstruktur der SA-Führerschaft*. Wuppertal, 1984.
Jarausch, Konrad H. "The Crisis of German Professions, 1918–33." *Journal of Contemporary History* 20 (1985): 379–98.
———. *Deutsche Studenten 1800–1970*. Frankfurt am Main, 1984.
———. "The Perils of Professionalism: Lawyers, Teachers, and Engineers in Nazi Germany." *German Studies Review* 9 (1986): 107–37.
———. *Students, Society, and Politics in Imperial Germany: The Rise of Academic Illiberalism*. Princeton, 1982.

Jaspers, Karl. "Heidelberger Erinnerungen." *Heidelberger Jahrbücher* 5 (1961): 1–10.

Jess, F. "Wie lange noch 'Chirurgogynäkologen'?" *Ziel und Weg* 5 (1935): 167–69.

Johanny, Carl, and Oskar Redelberger. *Volk, Partei, Reich*, 2d ed. Berlin, 1943.

Johe, Werner. *Die gleichgeschaltete Justiz: Organisation des Rechtswesens und Politisierung der Rechtsprechung 1933–1945 dargestellt am Beispiel des Oberlandesgerichtsbezirks Hamburg*. Frankfurt am Main, 1967.

Johnston, William M. *The Austrian Mind: An Intellectual and Social History, 1848–1938*. Berkeley, 1983.

Jonas, Hans. "Philosophical Reflections on Experimenting with Human Subjects." *Daedalus* 98 (1969): 219–47.

Jonas, Wolfgang. *Das Leben der Mansfeld-Arbeiter 1924 bis 1945*. Berlin (DDR), 1957.

Jünger, Ernst. "Über den Schmerz." In Ernst Jünger, *Werke*. Vol. 5. Stuttgart, n.d. (first published 1934), pp. 151–98.

Jürgens, Hans W. "Ohrmerkmale." In Luigi Gedda, ed., *De Genetica Medica*. Vol. 2. Rome, 1961, pp. 243–54.

Jungmann, Gerhard. "Von der Fürsorge zur Vorsorge." *Deutsches Ärzteblatt* 69 (1972): 831–35.

Just, Günther. "Agnes Bluhm und ihr Lebenswerk." *Die Ärztin* 17 (1941): 516–26.

Kalb, Renate. "Facheinsatz Ost 1940 der deutschen Studentinnen." *Die Ärztin* 17 (1941): 19–23.

Kalisch, Hans. "Die Regelung des Ärztewesens in Palästina." *Central-Verein-Zeitung*, November 22, 1935, nonpaginated.

Kann, Edmund van. "Der Altersaufbau der deutschen Ärzteschaft im Jahre 1937." *Deutsches Ärzteblatt* 68 (1938): 208–11.

______. "Die Zahl der Ärzte 1942 und ein Rückblick bis 1937." *Deutsches Ärzteblatt* 72 (1942): 300–303.

______. "Zahl und Gliederung der Fachärzte Deutschlands im Jahre 1940." *Deutsches Ärzteblatt* 70 (1940): 283–86.

Kardorff, Ursula von. *Berliner Aufzeichnungen: Aus den Jahren 1942 bis 1945*. 3d ed. Munich, 1962.

Karlson, Peter. "Die Versammlungen der Gesellschaft Deutscher Naturforscher und Ärzte 1920–1960." In Hans Querner and Heinrich Schipperges, eds., *Wege der Naturforschung 1922–1972 im Spiegel der Versammlungen Deutscher Naturforscher und Ärzte*. Berlin, 1972, pp. 39–67.

Karstedt, Oskar. "Die Durchführung der Arier- und Kommunistengesetzgebung bei den Kassen-Ärzten, -Zahnärzten usw." *Reichsarbeitsblatt* 2 (Nichtamtlicher Teil, 1934): 179–83.

Kater, Hermann, ed. *Politiker und Ärzte: 600 Kurzbiographien und Portraits*. 3d ed. Hameln, 1968.

Kater, Michael H. "Ärzte und Politik in Deutschland, 1848–1945." *Jahrbuch des Instituts für Geschichte der Medizin der Robert Bosch Stiftung* 5 (1987): 34–48.

______. *Das "Ahnenerbe" der SS 1935–1945: Ein Beitrag zur Kulturpolitik des Dritten Reiches*. Stuttgart, 1974.

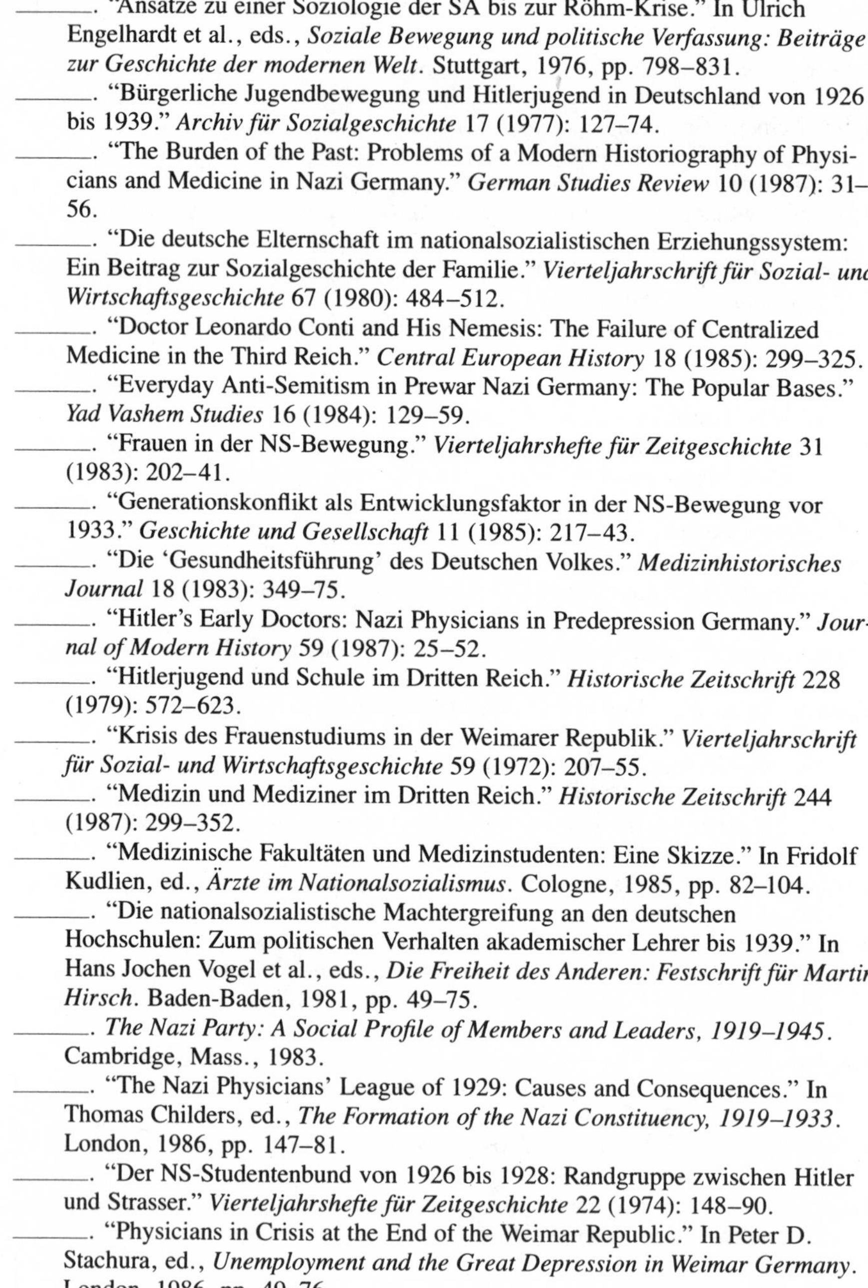

———. "Ansätze zu einer Soziologie der SA bis zur Röhm-Krise." In Ulrich Engelhardt et al., eds., *Soziale Bewegung und politische Verfassung: Beiträge zur Geschichte der modernen Welt*. Stuttgart, 1976, pp. 798–831.

———. "Bürgerliche Jugendbewegung und Hitlerjugend in Deutschland von 1926 bis 1939." *Archiv für Sozialgeschichte* 17 (1977): 127–74.

———. "The Burden of the Past: Problems of a Modern Historiography of Physicians and Medicine in Nazi Germany." *German Studies Review* 10 (1987): 31–56.

———. "Die deutsche Elternschaft im nationalsozialistischen Erziehungssystem: Ein Beitrag zur Sozialgeschichte der Familie." *Vierteljahrschrift für Sozial- und Wirtschaftsgeschichte* 67 (1980): 484–512.

———. "Doctor Leonardo Conti and His Nemesis: The Failure of Centralized Medicine in the Third Reich." *Central European History* 18 (1985): 299–325.

———. "Everyday Anti-Semitism in Prewar Nazi Germany: The Popular Bases." *Yad Vashem Studies* 16 (1984): 129–59.

———. "Frauen in der NS-Bewegung." *Vierteljahrshefte für Zeitgeschichte* 31 (1983): 202–41.

———. "Generationskonflikt als Entwicklungsfaktor in der NS-Bewegung vor 1933." *Geschichte und Gesellschaft* 11 (1985): 217–43.

———. "Die 'Gesundheitsführung' des Deutschen Volkes." *Medizinhistorisches Journal* 18 (1983): 349–75.

———. "Hitler's Early Doctors: Nazi Physicians in Predepression Germany." *Journal of Modern History* 59 (1987): 25–52.

———. "Hitlerjugend und Schule im Dritten Reich." *Historische Zeitschrift* 228 (1979): 572–623.

———. "Krisis des Frauenstudiums in der Weimarer Republik." *Vierteljahrschrift für Sozial- und Wirtschaftsgeschichte* 59 (1972): 207–55.

———. "Medizin und Mediziner im Dritten Reich." *Historische Zeitschrift* 244 (1987): 299–352.

———. "Medizinische Fakultäten und Medizinstudenten: Eine Skizze." In Fridolf Kudlien, ed., *Ärzte im Nationalsozialismus*. Cologne, 1985, pp. 82–104.

———. "Die nationalsozialistische Machtergreifung an den deutschen Hochschulen: Zum politischen Verhalten akademischer Lehrer bis 1939." In Hans Jochen Vogel et al., eds., *Die Freiheit des Anderen: Festschrift für Martin Hirsch*. Baden-Baden, 1981, pp. 49–75.

———. *The Nazi Party: A Social Profile of Members and Leaders, 1919–1945*. Cambridge, Mass., 1983.

———. "The Nazi Physicians' League of 1929: Causes and Consequences." In Thomas Childers, ed., *The Formation of the Nazi Constituency, 1919–1933*. London, 1986, pp. 147–81.

———. "Der NS-Studentenbund von 1926 bis 1928: Randgruppe zwischen Hitler und Strasser." *Vierteljahrshefte für Zeitgeschichte* 22 (1974): 148–90.

———. "Physicians in Crisis at the End of the Weimar Republic." In Peter D. Stachura, ed., *Unemployment and the Great Depression in Weimar Germany*. London, 1986, pp. 49–76.

———. "Problems of Political Reeducation in West Germany, 1945–1960." *Simon Wiesenthal Center Annual* 4 (1987): 99–123.

———. "Professionalization and Socialization of Physicians in Wilhelmine and Weimar Germany." *Journal of Contemporary History* 20 (1985): 677–701.

———. "Professoren und Studenten im Dritten Reich." *Archiv für Kulturgeschichte* 67 (1985): 465–87.

———. "Quantifizierung und NS-Geschichte: Methodologische Überlegungen über Grenzen und Möglichkeiten einer EDV-Analyse der NSDAP-Sozialstruktur von 1925 bis 1945." *Geschichte und Gesellschaft* 3 (1977): 453–84.

———. "The Reich Vocational Contest and Students of Higher Learning in Nazi Germany." *Central European History* 7 (1974): 225–61.

———. "Sozialer Wandel in der NSDAP im Zuge der nationalsozialistischen Machtergreifung." In Wolfgang Schieder, ed., *Faschismus als soziale Bewegung: Deutschland und Italien im Vergleich*. 2d ed. Göttingen, 1983, pp. 25–67.

———. *Studentenschaft und Rechtsradikalismus in Deutschland 1918–1933: Eine sozialgeschichtliche Studie zur Bildungskrise in der Weimarer Republik*. Hamburg, 1975.

———. "Zum gegenseitigen Verhältnis von SA und SS in der Sozialgeschichte des Nationalsozialismus von 1925 bis 1939." *Vierteljahrschrift für Sozial- und Wirtschaftsgeschichte* 62 (1975): 339–79.

Kaul, Friedrich Karl. *Ärzte in Auschwitz*. Berlin (DDR), 1968.

Kaupen-Haas, Heidrun. "Die Bevölkerungsplaner im Sachverständigenbeirat für Bevölkerungs- und Rassenpolitik." In Heidrun Kaupen-Haas, ed., *Der Griff nach der Bevölkerung: Aktualität und Kontinuität nazistischer Bevölkerungspolitik*. Nördlingen, 1986, pp. 103–20.

Kelchner, Mathilde. "Ärztliche Berufstätigkeit der Frau und Muttertum." *Die Ärztin* 12 (1936): 115–25.

———. *Die Frau und der weibliche Arzt: Eine psychologische Untersuchung auf Grund einer Umfrage*. Leipzig, 1934.

Keller, Karl. "Dozenten der Medizin und Zahnheilkunde an den deutschen Hochschulen." *Deutsches Ärzteblatt* 65 (1935): 695–96.

Kelly, Reece Conn. "National Socialism and German University Teachers: The NSDAP's Efforts to Create a National Socialist Professoriate and Scholarship." Ph.D. dissertation, University of Washington, 1973.

Kelting, Kristin. "Das Tuberkuloseproblem im Nationalsozialismus." M.D. dissertation, Kiel, 1974.

Kershaw, Ian. "German Popular Opinion and the 'Jewish Question,' 1939–1943: Some Further Reflections." In Arnold Paucker, ed., *Die Juden im Nationalsozialistischen Deutschland: The Jews in Nazi Germany, 1933–1943*. Tübingen, 1986, pp. 365–85.

———. *The "Hitler Myth": Image and Reality in the Third Reich*. Oxford, 1987.

———. *Popular Opinion and Political Dissent in the Third Reich: Bavaria, 1933–1945*. Oxford, 1983.

Kirkpatrick, Clifford. *Nazi Germany: Its Women and Family Life*. Indianapolis, 1938.

Kisch, Bruno. *Wandlungen und Wanderungen: Die Geschichte eines Arztes im 20. Jahrhundert*. Cologne, 1966.

Kisskalt, Karl. *Theorie und Praxis in der Medizinischen Forschung*. Munich, 1942.

Klare, Kurt. *Briefe von Gestern für Morgen: Gedanken eines Arztes zur Zeitenwende*. Stuttgart, 1934.

———. *Soll ich Medizin studieren? Ein Brief*. Leipzig, 1941.

Klecker, Erika. "Frauenvorbildung und Frauenstudium an den deutschen Universitäten." *Die Ärztin* 17 (1941): 499–505.

Klee, Ernst. *"Euthanasie" im NS-Staat: Die "Vernichtung lebensunwerten Lebens."* 2d ed. Frankfurt am Main, 1983.

———. "Geldverschwendung an Schwachsinnige und Säufer." *Die Zeit*, April 25, 1986, pp. 41–42, 45.

———. *Was sie taten—Was sie wurden: Ärzte, Juristen und andere Beteiligte am Kranken- oder Judenmord*. Frankfurt am Main, 1986.

Klein, Ulrich. "SA-Terror und Bevölkerung in Wuppertal 1933/34." In Detlev Peukert and Jürgen Reulecke, eds., *Die Reihen fast geschlossen: Beiträge zur Geschichte des Alltags unterm Nationalsozialismus*. Wuppertal, 1981, pp. 45–61.

Klein, Wilhelm, ed. *Der Amtsarzt: Ein Nachschlagewerk für Medizinal- und Verwaltungsbeamte*. 2d ed. Jena, 1943.

Klinger, Heinz. *Wege und Nebenwege: Erinnerungen eines Hamburger Arztes*. Hamburg, 1976.

Klinksiek, Dorothee. *Die Frau im NS-Staat*. Stuttgart, 1982.

Kluge, Heinrich. "Die wirtschaftliche Lage der Ärzte im Deutschen Reich." *Deutsches Ärzteblatt* 66 (1936): 1206–9.

Kluge, Rudolf, and Heinrich Krüger, eds. *Verfassung und Verwaltung im Dritten Reich (Reichsbürgerkunde)*. Berlin, 1937.

Knipping, Ulrich. *Die Geschichte der Juden in Dortmund während der Zeit des Dritten Reiches*. Dortmund, 1977.

Knoll, Wilhelm. "Arzt und Hochschullehrer." *Ziel und Weg* 6 (1936): 436–39.

Knüpling, Harm. "Untersuchungen zur Vorgeschichte der Deutschen Ärzteordnung von 1935." M.D. dissertation, Berlin, 1965.

Kocka, Jürgen. *Klassengesellschaft im Krieg: Deutsche Sozialgeschichte 1914–1918*. Göttingen, 1973.

Koehl, Robert Lewis. *The Black Corps: The Structure and Power Struggles of the Nazi SS*. Madison, Wisc., 1983.

Koester, Fritz. "Grundlagen und Bedeutung des Gesetzes zur Verhütung erbkranken Nachwuchses vom 14. Juli 1933." *Deutsches Ärzteblatt* 64 (1934): 500–504.

Kötschau, Karl. "Die nationalsozialistische Revolution in der Medizin." *Ziel und Weg* 3 (1933): 292–96.

———. "Sinnforschung in ihrer wissenschaftlichen und praktischen Bedeutung für den Arzt." *Deutsches Ärzteblatt* 74 (1944): 72–76.

———. "Vorsorge und Fürsorge im Rahmen einer Neuen Deutschen Heilkunde." *Ziel und Weg* 6 (1936): 240–46.

———. *Zum nationalsozialistischen Umbruch in der Medizin*. Stuttgart, 1936.

———. "Zur nationalsozialistischen Revolution in der Medizin." *Ziel und Weg* 5 (1935): 11–14, 132–35.

Kohte, Gisela. "Als Obergauärztin im Wartheland." *Die Ärztin* 17 (1941): 207–11.

Kollath, Werner. *Grundlagen, Methoden und Ziele der Hygiene: Eine Einführung für Mediziner und Naturwissenschaftler, Volkswirtschaftler und Techniker*. Leipzig, 1937.

Konner, Melvin. *Becoming a Doctor: A Journey of Initiation in Medical School*. New York, 1987.

Koonz, Claudia. *Mothers in the Fatherland: Women, the Family, and Nazi Politics*. New York, 1987.

Kovács, Mária. "Luttes professionnelles et antisemitisme: Chronique de la montée du fascisme dans le corps médical hongrois, 1920–1944." *Actes de la Recherche en Sciences Sociales*, March 1985, pp. 31–44.

———. *The Politics of the Legal Profession in Interwar Hungary*. Published by the Institute on East Central Europe, Columbia University. [New York], 1987.

Kramarz, Joachim. *Claus Graf Stauffenberg: 15. November 1907–20. Juli 1944: Das Leben eines Offiziers*. Frankfurt am Main, 1965.

Krannhals, Paul. *Das organische Weltbild: Grundlagen einer neuentstehenden deutschen Kultur*. 2 vols. 2d ed. Munich, 1936 (first published 1928).

Kranz, Heinrich Wilhelm. *"Die Gemeinschaftsunfähigen": (Ein Beitrag zur wissenschaftlichen und praktischen Lösung des sog. "Asozialenproblems")*. Giessen, [1939].

———. " 'Einkehr' und 'Umkehr.' " *Ziel und Weg* 4 (1934): 38–40.

———. "Zur Entwicklung der Rassenhygienischen Institute an unseren Hochschulen." *Ziel und Weg* 9 (1939): 286–90.

Kranz, Heinrich Wilhelm, and Siegfried Koller. *"Die Gemeinschaftsunfähigen": (Ein Beitrag zur wissenschaftlichen und praktischen Lösung des sog. "Asozialenproblems")*. Giessen, 1941.

Krausnick, Helmut. "Judenverfolgung." In Hans Buchheim et al., *Anatomie des SS-Staates*. Vol. 2. Freiburg i.Br., 1965, pp. 283–448.

Krebs, Hans. "Wie ich aus Deutschland vertrieben wurde: Dokumente mit Kommentaren." *Medizinhistorisches Journal* 15 (1980): 357–77.

Krehl, Ludolf von. *Der Arzt*. 2d ed. Stuttgart, 1938.

Kreienberg, Walter. "Die Auswirkungen des Gesetzes zur Verhütung erbkranken Nachwuchses an dem Krankenbestand der Psychiatrischen und Nervenklinik Erlangen." M.D. dissertation, Erlangen, 1937.

Kreienberg, Walter, and J. Schenkel. "Über die beschleunigte Blutgerinnung beim Aufenthalt in grossen Höhen." *Luftfahrtmedizin* 8 (1943): 196–200.

Kreienberg, Walter, and A. Winter. "Die Höhenfestigkeit von Hyper- und Hypotonikern." *Luftfahrtmedizin* 5 (1941): 119–26.

Krenzlin, Hans-Helmuth. "Das NSKK: Wesen, Aufgaben und Aufbau des Nationalsozialistischen Kraftfahrkorps, dargestellt an einem Abriss seiner geschichtlichen Entwicklung." In Paul Meier-Benneckenstein, ed., *Das Dritte Reich im Aufbau: Übersichten und Leistungsberichte*. Vol. 3. Berlin, 1939, pp. 266–87.

Kretschmer, Ernst. *Gestalten und Gedanken: Erlebnisse*. 2d ed. Stuttgart, 1971.

———. "Konstitutionslehre und Rassenhygiene." In Ernst Rüdin, ed., *Erblehre und Rassenhygiene im völkischen Staat*. Munich, 1934, pp. 184–93.

Kreuser, F. "Erneuerung des Studiums der Heilkunde." *Ziel und Weg* 8 (1938): 373–79.

Die Kriminalität der Ärzteschaft: Eine Sammlung von Kriminalfällen der approbierten Ärzteschaft. Edited by Zentralverband der Volksgesundheit und Freiheit des Heilwesens Berlin. Essen, 1929.

Krüger, Horst. *Das zerbrochene Haus: Eine Jugend in Deutschland*. 2d ed. Munich, 1967.

Kubach, Fritz, ed. *Studenten bauen auf! Der 3. Reichsberufswettkampf der deutschen Studenten 1937/38: Ein Rechenschaftsbericht*. N.p., n.d.

Kudlien, Fridolf. "Ärzte als Anhänger der NS-'Bewegung.'" In Fridolf Kudlien, ed., *Ärzte im Nationalsozialismus*. Cologne, 1985, pp. 18–34.

———. "Ärzte als Helfer von Verfolgten: Kritiker von NS-Massnahmen, Gegner des Dritten Reiches." In Fridolf Kudlien, ed., *Ärzte im Nationalsozialismus*. Cologne, 1985, pp. 209–45.

———. "Widerstand deutscher Ärzte gegen das Dritte Reich." In Gerhard Baader and Ulrich Schultz, eds., *Medizin und Nationalsozialismus: Tabuisierte Vergangenheit—Ungebrochene Tradition?* Berlin, 1980, pp. 212–18.

———, ed. *Ärzte im Nationalsozialismus*. Cologne, 1985.

Kudlien, Fridolf, and Christian Andree. "Sauerbruch und der Nationalsozialismus." *Medizinhistorisches Journal* 15 (1980): 201–22.

Kühle, L. "Der erste Lehrgang des Hauptamtes für Volksgesundheit auf der Ordensburg Vogelsang vom 26. Sept. bis 4. Okt. 1937." *Ziel und Weg* 7 (1937): 524–31.

Kühn, Kurt. "Deutsche Mediziner im Kampf gegen den Faschismus—dargestellt an Lebensbildern antifaschistischer Ärzte." In Kurt Kühn, ed., *Ärzte an der Seite der Arbeiterklasse: Beiträge zur Geschichte des Bündnisses der deutschen Arbeiterklasse mit der medizinischen Intelligenz*. Berlin (DDR), 1973, pp. 212–48.

Kümmel, Werner F. "Die Ausschaltung rassisch und politisch missliebiger Ärzte." In Fridolf Kudlien, ed., *Ärzte im Nationalsozialismus*. Cologne, 1985, pp. 56–81.

Kürten, Heinz. "Die 47. Tagung der Deutschen Gesellschaft für Innere Medizin." *Deutsches Ärzteblatt* 65 (1935): 407–10.

Kuhlo, Ulla. "Gesundheitsdienst im Bund Deutscher Mädel." *Die Ärztin* 17 (1941): 193–200.

———. "Zum Jahre 1944." *Die Ärztin* 20 (1944): 1–2.

Kuhn, Helmut. "Die deutsche Universität am Vorabend der Machtergreifung." In Helmut Kuhn et al., *Die deutsche Universität im Dritten Reich: Acht Beiträge*. Munich, 1966, pp. 13–43.

Kulka, Otto Dov. "Die Nürnberger Rassengesetze und die deutsche Bevölkerung im Lichte geheimer NS-Lage- und Stimmungsberichte." *Vierteljahrshefte für Zeitgeschiche* 32 (1984): 582–624.

Kwiet, Konrad, and Helmut Eschwege. *Selbstbehauptung und Widerstand: Deutsche Juden im Kampf um Existenz und Menschenwürde 1933–1945*. Hamburg, 1984.

Labisch, Alfons, and Florian Tennstedt. *Der Weg zum "Gesetz über die Vereinheitlichung des Gesundheitswesens" vom 3. Juli 1934: Entwicklungslinien und -momente des staatlichen und kommunalen Gesundheitswesens in Deutschland.* 2 vols. Düsseldorf, 1985.

Läuppi, E. "Experimente am Menschen als medizinisch-rechtliches Grenzproblem." *Praxis* 60 (1961): 837–41.

Langbein, Friedrich. "Die Entstehung und Entwicklung der ärztlichen Organisationen in Deutschland seit Einführung der Sozialversicherung." *Südwestdeutsches Ärzteblatt* 4 (1949): 81–90.

Langbein, Hermann. . . . *wir haben es getan: Selbstportraits in Tagebüchern und Briefen 1939–1945.* Vienna, 1964.

Leber, Annedore, ed. *Das Gewissen steht auf: 64 Lebensbilder aus dem deutschen Widerstand 1933–1945.* 9th ed. Berlin, 1960.

Lechler, Karl Ludwig. "Erkennung und Ausmerze der Gemeinschaftsunfähigen." *Deutsches Ärzteblatt* 70 (1940): 293–97.

Leibbrand, W. "Eugenik und Sterilisation." *Fortschritte der Medizin* 81 (1963): 718.

Leibfried, Stephan. "Stationen der Abwehr: Berufsverbote für Ärzte im Deutschen Reich 1933–1938 und die Zerstörung des sozialen Asyls durch die organisierten Ärzteschaften des Auslands." *Leo Baeck Institute Bulletin* 62 (1982): 3–39.

Leiter, Anna. "Über bisherige Tätigkeit und Erfolg des Jugendpsychiaters im BDM." *Die Ärztin* 17 (1941): 218–23.

Lemberger, Fritz. "Unsere praktischen Erfahrungen in der Krankenpflegeausbildung der Vorkliniker in München." *Ziel und Weg* 7 (1937): 421–23.

Lemser, H. "Untersuchungsergebnisse an diabetischen Zwillingen." *Münchener Medizinische Wochenschrift* 85 (1938): 1811–15.

Leuner, H. D. *When Compassion Was a Crime: Germany's Silent Heroes, 1933–45.* London, 1966.

Liebenam, Leonore. "Zwillingsforschung." *Die Ärztin* 17 (1941): 100–106.

Liebling, A. J., ed. *The Republic of Silence.* New York, 1947.

Liek, Erwin. *Der Arzt und seine Sendung: Gedanken eines Ketzers.* 4th ed. Munich, 1927.

———. *Gedanken eines Arztes: Aus 30 Jahren Praxis.* 3d ed. Berlin, 1942.

———. *Im Bannkreis des Arztes: Aus dem Nachlass.* Dresden, 1935.

———. *Krebsverbreitung, Krebsbekämpfung, Krebsverhütung.* Munich, 1932.

———. *Die Welt des Arztes: Aus 30 Jahren Praxis.* Dresden, 1933.

Lifton, Robert Jay. "Medicalized Killing in Auschwitz." *Psychiatry* 45 (1982): 283–97.

———. *The Nazi Doctors: Medicalized Killing and the Psychology of Genocide.* New York, 1986.

Lilienthal, Georg. *Der "Lebensborn e.V.": Ein Instrument nationalsozialistischer Rassenpolitik.* Stuttgart, 1985.

———. "Rassenhygiene im Dritten Reich: Krise und Wende." *Medizinhistorisches Journal* 14 (1979): 114–34.

———. "Zum Anteil der Anthropologie an der NS-Rassenpolitik." *Medizinhistorisches Journal* 19 (1984): 148–60.

Lindemann, Mary. *140 Jahre Israelitisches Krankenhaus in Hamburg: Vorgeschichte und Entwicklung*. Hamburg, 1981.
List of Displaced German Scholars. 2d ed. Stockholm, 1975 (first published 1936).
Loeffler, Lothar. "Der Auslesegedanke als Forderung in der Medizin." *Münchener Medizinische Wochenschrift* 83 (1936): 673–76.
Loehr, Hanns. *Über die Stellung und Bedeutung der Heilkunde im nationalsozialistischen Staate*. Berlin, 1934.
Lölhöffel, Edith von. "Die Ärztin in der Front der Heimat." *Die Ärztin* 15 (1939): 267–68.
———. "Frauensport und Frauentum." *Die Ärztin* 12 (1936): 10–15.
Lösener, Bernhard. "Als Rassereferent im Reichsministerium des Innern." *Vierteljahrshefte für Zeitgeschichte* 9 (1961): 264–313.
Lorenz, Charlotte. *Zehnjahres-Statistik des Hochschulbesuchs und der Abschlussprüfungen*. 2 vols. Berlin, 1943.
Lottmann, Werner. "Die Ausbildungsdauer auf den Hochschulen: Ein Problem der Bevölkerungspolitik und Begabtenförderung." *Das Junge Deutschland*, 1938, pp. 413–26.
Lubarsch, Otto. *Ein bewegtes Gelehrtenleben: Erinnerungen und Erlebnisse: Kämpfe und Gedanken*. Berlin, 1931.
Ludwig, Karl-Heinz. *Technik und Ingenieure im Dritten Reich*. Düsseldorf, 1974.
———. "Der VDI als Gegenstand der Parteipolitik 1933 bis 1945." In Karl-Heinz Ludwig, ed., *Technik, Ingenieure und Gesellschaft: Geschichte des Vereins Deutscher Ingenieure 1856–1981*. Düsseldorf, 1981, pp. 407–27.
Lüth, Paul. "Die Subkultur der Ärzte: Am Beispiel ihrer Körperschaften und Verbände." In Volker Volkholz et al., eds., *Analyse des Gesundheitssystems: Krankheitsstruktur, ärztlicher Arbeitsprozess, Sozialstaat: Reader zur Medizinsoziologie*. Frankfurt am Main, 1974, pp. 368–96.
Luther, Ernst. "Die Durchsetzung des faschistischen Führerprinzips an der Medizinischen Fakultät Münster." *Wissenschaftliche Beiträge der Martin-Luther-Universität Halle-Wittenberg*, 1967, pp. 113–31.
Luther, Ernst, and Burchard Thaler, eds. *Das hippokratische Ethos: Untersuchungen zu Ethos und Praxis in der deutschen Ärzteschaft*. Halle, 1967.
Luther, Irmgart. "Landdienst—Gesundheitsdienst." *Die Ärztin* 15 (1939): 230–31.
Maassen, Willy. "Die Lebensverhältnisse der Jungärzte in Schleswig-Holstein." *Ziel und Weg* 9 (1939): 292–96.
Macfarlane, Gwyn. *Howard Florey: The Making of a Great Scientist*. Oxford, 1979.
Macrakis, Kristie. "Wissenschaftsförderung durch die Rockefeller-Stiftung im 'Dritten Reich': Die Entscheidung, das Kaiser-Wilhelm-Institut für Physik finanziell zu unterstützen." *Geschichte und Gesellschaft* 12 (1986): 348–79.
Mäding, Erhard. "Ergebnisse einer Erhebung über die Lebensverhältnisse der Jungakademiker in Sachsen." *Ziel und Weg* 7 (1937): 62–64.
———. "Nachwuchspflege: Bericht über erbbiologisch bestimmte Selbsthilfebestrebungen für Akademiker." *Ziel und Weg* 6 (1936): 444–47.
Maerz, Barbara. "Die 'Münchener Neuesten Nachrichten' als Quelle zur medizinischen Lokalgeschichte für die Zeit von 1933 bis 1938 unter bevorzugter Berücksichtigung der medizinischen Veranstaltungen und der Bericht-

erstattung über Personen und Institutionen des Gesundheitswesens." M.D. dissertation, Munich, 1977.

Mammach, Klaus. "Zum antifaschistischen Kampf der KPD." In Dietrich Eichholz and Karl Gossweiler, eds., *Faschismusforschung: Positionen, Probleme, Polemik*. Berlin (DDR), 1980, pp. 323–54.

Mann, Erika. *School for Barbarians*. New York, 1938.

Mann, Gunter. "Rassenhygiene—Sozialdarwinismus." In Gunter Mann, ed., *Biologismus im 19. Jahrhundert: Vorträge eines Symposiums vom 30. bis 31. Oktober 1970 in Frankfurt am Main*. Stuttgart, 1973, pp. 73–93.

———. "Sozialbiologie auf dem Wege zur unmenschlichen Medizin des Dritten Reiches." In Marina Elisabeth Pfeffer-Küppers, ed., *Unmenschliche Medizin: Geschichtliche Erfahrungen, Gegenwärtige Probleme und Ausblick auf die zukünftige Entwicklung: Seminar*. Mainz, 1983, pp. 22–43.

Manthey, Gerda. "Aus der medizinischen Fachgruppenarbeit der Universität Berlin." *Die Ärztin* 13 (1937): 51–55.

Marks, Sally. "Black Watch on the Rhine: A Study in Propaganda, Prejudice and Prurience." *European Studies Review* 13 (1983): 297–334.

Marrus, Michael R., and Robert O. Paxton. *Vichy France and the Jews*. New York, 1981.

Maršalek, Hans. "Eine teuflische 'Initiative': Die medizinischen Versuche im Konzentrationslager Mauthausen." *Der Widerstandskämpfer* 18, no. 11 (1970): 49–52.

Martin, Rolf Ludwig. "Rasse und Verbrechen." M.D. dissertation, Giessen, 1937.

Mason, Timothy W. *Arbeiterklasse und Volksgemeinschaft: Dokumente und Materialien zur deutschen Arbeiterpolitik 1936–1939*. Opladen, 1975.

———. "Arbeiteropposition im nationalsozialistischen Deutschland." In Detlev Peukert and Jürgen Reulecke, eds., *Die Reihen fast geschlossen: Beiträge zur Geschichte des Alltags unterm Nationalsozialismus*. Wuppertal, 1981, pp. 293–313.

Mass, Konrad. *Das erste Jahr der Regierung Hitler*. Munich, 1934.

Mausbach, Hans. "Gesundheits- und sozialpolitische Vorstellungen der deutschen Ärzteschaft." In *Entwicklung und Struktur des Gesundheitswesens: Argumente für eine soziale Medizin*. Vol. 5. Berlin, 1974, pp. 152–63.

Mausbach, Hans, and Barbara Mausbach-Bromberger. "Anmerkungen zu den Formen, dem Spektrum und dem Wesen des antifaschistischen Widerstandes unter den Ärzten." In *Volk und Gesundheit: Heilen und Vernichten im Nationalsozialismus*. Tübingen, 1982, pp. 222–29.

Mayer, August. "Arzttum im Dritten Reich: Ärztliches Berufsgeheimnis, Tötung von missgebildeten Neugeborenen, Euthanasie." *Deutsches Ärzteblatt* 63 (1966): 785–87.

———. *50 [Fünfzig] Jahre selbst erlebte Gynäkologie: Abschiedsvorlesung vom 25.7.1950*. Munich, 1961.

Mayr-Weber, Vilma. "Die Aufgabe der Reichsarbeitsdienstärztin an der Volksgesundheit." *Die Ärztin* 19 (1943): 174–76.

McClelland, Charles. *State, Society and University in Germany, 1700–1914*. Cambridge, Eng., 1980.

McIntyre, J. Earl. "Citizenship and Medical Licensure." *Journal of the American Medical Association* 112 (1939): 1075–77.
McIntyre [Stephenson], Jill. "Women and the Professions in Germany, 1930–1940." In Anthony Nicholls and Erich Matthias, eds., *German Democracy and the Triumph of Hitler: Essays in Recent German History*. London, 1971, pp. 175–213.
Mehringer, Hartmut. "Die KPD in Bayern 1919–1945." In Martin Broszat and Hartmut Mehringer, eds., *Bayern in der NS-Zeit V: Die Parteien KPD, SPD, BVP in Verfolgung und Widerstand*. Munich, 1983, pp. 1–286.
Meier, H. "Das Ende des jüdischen Arzttums." *Ziel und Weg* 9 (1939): 110–12.
Meier, Kurt. *Kirche und Judentum: Die Haltung der evangelischen Kirche zur Judenpolitik des Dritten Reiches*. Göttingen, 1968.
Meinberg, Wilhelm. "Gesundheitsbetreuung der Belegschaft der Reichswerke Hermann Göring." *Ziel und Weg* 8 (1938): 524–28.
Meldungen aus dem Reich: Die geheimen Lageberichte des Sicherheitsdienstes der SS 1938–1945. Edited by Heinz Boberach. 17 vols. Herrsching, 1984.
Mengele, Josef. "Rassenmorphologische Untersuchungen des vorderen Unterkieferabschnittes bei vier rassischen Gruppen." *Morphologisches Jahrbuch* 79 (1937): 60–117.
———. "Sippenuntersuchungen bei Lippen-Kiefer-Gaumenspalte." *Zeitschrift für menschliche Vererbungslehre- und Konstitutionslehre* 23 (1938): 17–42.
———. "Zur Vererbung der Ohrfisteln." *Der Erbarzt*, no. 8 (1940): 59–60.
Mersmann, Ingrid. "Medizinische Ausbildung im Dritten Reich." M.D. dissertation, Munich, 1978.
Meyer, Ernie. "Deathly Science." *Jerusalem Post Magazine*, January 23, 1987, pp. 6–9.
Meyerhoff, Hermann. *Herne 1933–1945: Die Zeit des Nationalsozialismus: Ein kommunalhistorischer Rückblick*. Herne, 1963.
Michaelis, Cassie, et al. *Die braune Kultur: Ein Dokumentenspiegel*. Zurich, 1934.
Middlebrook, Martin. *The Battle of Hamburg: Allied Bomber Forces against a German City in 1943*. London, 1980.
Miedzinski, Herta. "Kriegseinsatz der deutschen Studentinnen." *Die Ärztin* 17 (1941): 256–60.
Milch, Isabella. "The Expatriated Elite: The Emigration of Scholars during the Third Reich." *Kultur Chronik*, no. 2 (1985): 14–16.
Mitscherlich, Alexander. *Ein Leben für die Psychoanalyse: Anmerkungen zu meiner Zeit*. Frankfurt am Main, 1980.
Mitscherlich, Alexander, and Fred Mielke. *Das Diktat der Menschenverachtung: Eine Dokumentation*. Heidelberg, 1947.
———. *Medizin ohne Menschlichkeit: Dokumente des Nürnberger Ärzteprozesses*. Frankfurt am Main, 1962.
———. *Wissenschaft ohne Menschlichkeit: Medizinische und Eugenische Irrwege unter Diktatur, Bürokratie und Krieg*. Heidelberg, 1949.
Modersohn, Wolf J. "Das Führerprinzip in der Deutschen Medizin 1933–1945." M.D. dissertation, Kiel, 1982.

Moe, Kristine. "Should the Nazi Research Data Be Cited?" *Hastings Center Report*, December 1984, pp. 5–7.
Moll, Albert. *Ärztliche Ethik: Die Pflichten des Arztes in allen Beziehungen seiner Thätigkeit*. Stuttgart, 1902.
Mollison, Theodor. "Beitrag zur Kraniologie und Osteologie der Maori." *Zeitschrift für Morphologie und Anthropologie* 11 (1908): 529–95.
______. "Die Körperproportionen der Primaten." *Gegenbaurs Morphologisches Jahrbuch* 42 (1911): 79–302.
______. "Die Maori in ihren Beziehungen zu verschiedenen benachbarten Gruppen." *Korrespondenzblatt: Deutsche Gesellschaft für Anthropologie, Ethnologie und Urgeschichte* 38 (1907): 147–52.
______. "Rassenkunde und Rassenhygiene." In Ernst Rüdin, ed., *Erblehre und Rassenhygiene im völkischen Staat*. Munich, 1934, pp. 34–48.
Moser, Jonny. *Die Judenverfolgung in Österreich 1938–1945*. Vienna, 1966.
Mosse, George L. *The Crisis of German Ideology: Intellectual Origins of the Third Reich*. New York, 1964.
______. *Germans and Jews: The Right, the Left, and the Search for a "Third Force" in Pre-Nazi Germany*. New York, 1971.
______. *Nationalism and Sexuality: Respectability and Abnormal Sexuality in Europe*. New York, 1985.
______. *Toward the Final Solution: A History of European Racism*. New York, 1978.
Mrugowsky, Joachim, ed. *Das ärztliche Ethos: Christoph Wilhelm Hufelands Vermächtnis einer fünfzigjährigen Erfahrung*. Munich, 1939.
Much, Hans. *Homöopathie: Kritische Gänge hüben und drüben*. Leipzig, 1926.
Müller, Arnd. *Geschichte der Juden in Nürnberg 1146–1945*. Nuremberg, 1968.
Mueller, B. "Die gegenwärtige Lage der Strafrechtsreform, vom medizinischen Standpunkt aus gesehen." *Münchener Medizinische Wochenschrift* 83 (1936): 20–23.
Müller, Ingo. *Furchtbare Juristen: Die unbewältigte Vergangenheit unserer Justiz*. Munich, 1987.
Müller, Reiner. *Lehrbuch der Hygiene für Ärzte und Biologen*. Munich, 1935.
Müller-Hill, Benno. "Genetics after Auschwitz." *Holocaust and Genocide Studies* 2, no. 1 (1987): 3–20.
______. *Tödliche Wissenschaft: Die Aussonderung von Juden, Zigeunern und Geisteskranken 1933–1945*. Reinbek, 1984.
Müller-Meernach, Wolfgang. "Ein Fall von Missbildungen bei Zwillingen und seine erbgesundheitliche Bedeutung." M.D. dissertation, Erlangen, 1937.
Nabielek, Rainer. "Anmerkungen zu Paul Diepgens Selbsteinschätzung seiner Tätigkeit an der Berliner Universität während des NS-Regimes." *Zeitschrift für die gesamte Hygiene und ihre Grenzgebiete* 31 (1985): 309–14.
Nach Hitler: Der schwierige Umgang mit unserer Geschichte: Beiträge von Martin Broszat. Edited by Hermann Graml and Klaus-Dieter Henke. 2d ed. Munich, 1987.
Nachtsheim, Hans. "Warum Eugenik?" *Fortschritte der Medizin* 81 (1963): 711–13.

Naschold, Frieder. *Kassenärzte und Krankenversicherungsreform: Zu einer Theorie der Statuspolitik*. Freiburg i.Br., 1967.

Nau, Elisabeth. "Die jugendgerichtsärztliche Tätigkeit in ihren vorbeugenden und fürsorgerischen Auswirkungen." *Die Ärztin* 19 (1943): 138–46.

Nazi Medicine: Doctors, Victims and Medicine in Auschwitz. New York, 1986.

Neubert, Rudolf. *Mein Arztleben: Erinnerungen*. Rudolstadt, 1974.

Neumaier, Hugo. "Krisis der Medizin und Ausbildung des Ärztenachwuchses." *Ziel und Weg* 6 (1936): 16–18.

Neumann, Bernd. *Auschwitz: Bericht über die Strafsache gegen Mulka und andere vor dem Schwurgericht Frankfurt*. Frankfurt am Main, 1965.

Neumark, Fritz. *Zuflucht am Bosporus: Deutsche Gelehrte, Politiker und Künstler in der Emigration 1933–1953*. Frankfurt am Main, 1980.

Neumeister, H. "Die gegenwärtige Lage der akademischen Berufe." *Soziale Praxis* 45 (1936): 1263–70.

Niederland, Doron. "Deutsche Ärzte-Emigration und gesundheitspolitische Entwicklungen in 'Eretz Israel' (1933–1948)." *Medizinhistorisches Journal* 20 (1985): 149–84.

Niedermeyer, Albert. *Wahn, Wissenschaft und Wahrheit: Lebenserinnerungen eines Arztes*. Innsbruck, 1956.

Nissen, Rudolf. *Helle Blätter—dunkle Blätter: Erinnerungen eines Chirurgen*. Stuttgart, 1969.

Nomberg-Przytyk, Sara. *Auschwitz: True Tales from a Grotesque Land*. Edited by Eli Pfefferkorn and David H. Hirsch. Chapel Hill, 1985.

Novikov, Jouri. *Politische Psychiatrie in der UdSSR: Gastvortrag*. Berlin, 1981.

Nowak, Kurt. *"Euthanasie" und Sterilisierung im "Dritten Reich": Die Konfrontation der evangelischen und katholischen Kirche mit dem "Gesetz zur Verhütung erbkranken Nachwuchses" und der "Euthanasie"-Aktion*. 2d ed. Göttingen, 1980.

Nyiszli, Miklos. *Auschwitz: An Eyewitness Account of Mengele's Infamous Death Camp*. New York, 1986.

Oehme, Curt. "Das medizinische Experiment am Menschen." *Die Wandlung* 2 (1947): 484–91.

Oettingen, Eberhard Notger von. "Wir Assistenzärzte: Eine zeitgemässe Betrachtung." *Ziel und Weg* 7 (1937): 601–4.

Ophir, Baruch Zvi, and Falk Wiesemann, eds. *Die jüdischen Gemeinden in Bayern 1918–1945: Geschichte und Zerstörung*. Munich, 1979.

Opitz, Kurt, ed. *Bestallungsordnung für Ärzte und Prüfungsordnung für Zahnärzte*. 4th ed. Berlin, 1936.

Orlopp-Pleick, Erna. "Organisation der Bezirksgruppe Ostpreussen des Bundes Deutscher Ärztinnen." *Die Ärztin* 12 (1936): 30–34.

Orlow, Dietrich. *The History of the Nazi Party, 1933–1945*. Pittsburgh, 1973.

Ostler, Fritz. *Die deutschen Rechtsanwälte 1871–1971*. Essen, 1971.

Ostrowski, Siegfried. "Progressive Infectious Skin-Necrosis and Hospital-Gangrene (with a Report of an Epidemic of Hospital Gangrene)." *Acta Medica Orientalia* 9 (1950): 139–52.

———. "Vom Schicksal jüdischer Ärzte im Dritten Reich: Ein Augenzeugenbericht aus den Jahren 1933–1939." *Leo Baeck Institute Bulletin* 6 (1963): 313–51.

Padover, Saul K. *Experiment in Germany: The Story of an American Intelligence Officer*. New York, 1946.

Panhuizen, Anneliese. "Wie mache ich die Schularzttätigkeit fruchtbar für die ärztliche Tätigkeit im Bund Deutscher Mädel?" *Die Ärztin* 12 (1936): 7–10.

Parlow, Siegfried. "Über einige Aspekte der politisch-ideologischen Haltung deutscher Ärzte in der November-Revolution 1918 bis zum Eisenacher Ärztetag im September 1919 unter besonderer Berücksichtigung der medizinischen Fachpresse." *Wissenschaftliche Beiträge der Martin-Luther-Universität Halle-Wittenberg*, 1967, pp. 49–74.

———. "Über einige kolonialistische und annexationistische Aspekte bei deutschen Ärzten von 1884 bis zum Ende des 1. Weltkrieges." *Wissenschaftliche Zeitschrift der Universität Rostock: Mathematisch-Naturwissenschaftliche Reihe* 15 (1966): 537–49.

———. "Zum Faschisierungsprozess innerhalb der deutschen Ärzteschaft (1933–1945)." In Iris Ganzke et al., *Medizin, Menschenbild und sozial-biologisches Problem: Ein Beitrag zu den philosophischen Grundlagen der Medizin in der sozialistischen Gesellschaft*. Berlin (DDR), 1974, pp. 163–73.

———. "Zur Integration ärztlicher Standesorganisationen in das faschistische Machtgefüge." In Achim Thom and Horst Spaar, eds., *Medizin im Faschismus: Symposium über das Schicksal der Medizin in der Zeit des Faschismus in Deutschland 1933–1945*. Berlin (DDR), 1985, pp. 77–84.

Partei-Statistik. Edited by Reichsorganisationsleiter der NSDAP. Vol. 1. Munich, [1935].

Pascher, Joseph. "Das Dritte Reich, erlebt an drei deutschen Universitäten." In Helmut Kuhn et al., *Die deutsche Universität im Dritten Reich: Acht Beiträge*. Munich, 1966, pp. 47–69.

Paucker, Arnold, ed. *Die Juden im Nationalsozialistischen Deutschland/The Jews in Nazi Germany, 1933–1945*. Tübingen, 1986.

Paul, Helmut A., and Hans Stirn. "Die fachärztliche Versorgung." In Maria Blohmke et al., eds., *Handbuch der Sozialmedizin*. Vol. 3. Stuttgart, 1976, pp. 193–211.

Pauwels, Jacques R. *Women, Nazis, and Universities: Female University Students in the Third Reich, 1933–1945*. Westport, Conn., 1984.

Pearle, Kathleen M. "Ärzteemigration nach 1933 in die USA: Der Fall New York." *Medizinhistorisches Journal* 19 (1984): 112–37.

Pechel, Rudolf. *Deutscher Widerstand*. Erlenbach-Zurich, 1947.

Petersilie, Paul. "Die Honorarverteilung der KVD während des Krieges." *Deutsches Ärzteblatt* 70 (1940): 26–32.

Petry, Christian. *Studenten aufs Schafott: Die Weisse Rose und ihr Scheitern*. Munich, 1968.

Petzina, Dieter. *Autarkiepolitik im Dritten Reich: Der nationalsozialistische Vierjahresplan*. Stuttgart, 1968.

Peukert, Detlev. *Volksgenossen und Gemeinschaftsfremde: Anpassung, Ausmerze*

und Aufbegehren unter dem Nationalsozialismus. Cologne, 1982.
Pfannenstiel, Wilhelm. "Gedanken über das Wertproblem in der Medizin." *Ziel und Weg* 5 (1935): 122–28.
Pfanner, Helmut F. "The Role of Switzerland for the Refugees." In Jarrell C. Jackman and Carla M. Borden, eds., *The Muses Flee Hitler: Cultural Transfer and Adaptation, 1930–1945*. Washington, D.C., 1983, pp. 235–48.
Pfreimbter, Richard. "Der Schweriner Knabenmordprozess." *Münchener Medizinische Wochenschrift* 83 (1936): 448–50.
Piechocki, Werner, and Wolfram Kaiser. "Jüdische Gelehrtenschicksale 1933 bis 1945." *Wissenschaftliche Zeitschrift der Humboldt-Universität zu Berlin: Mathematisch-Naturwissenschaftliche Reihe* 19 (1970): 383–88.
Plant, Richard. *The Pink Triangle: The Nazi War against Homosexuals*. New York, 1986.
Platen-Hallermund, Alice. *Die Tötung Geisteskranker in Deutschland*. Frankfurt am Main, 1948.
Plesch, János. *János: Ein Arzt erzählt sein Leben*. Munich, 1949.
Ploetz, Alfred. *Die Tüchtigkeit unsrer Rasse und der Schutz der Schwachen*. Berlin, 1895.
Pommerin, Reiner. *"Sterilisierung der Rheinlandbastarde": Das Schicksal einer farbigen deutschen Minderheit 1918–1937*. Düsseldorf, 1979.
Ponsold, Albert. *Der Strom war die Newa: Aus dem Leben eines Gerichtsmediziners*. St. Michael, 1980.
Prägert, Hans. "Die Krankenpflegerausbildung für Vorkliniker in München." *Ziel und Weg* 6 (1936): 417–18.
Preuss, Ulrich K. "Die Perversion des Rechtsgedankens." In Jörg Tröger, ed., *Hochschule und Wissenschaft im Dritten Reich*. 2d ed. Frankfurt am Main, 1986, pp. 116–18.
Pridham, Geoffrey. *Hitler's Rise to Power: The Nazi Movement in Bavaria, 1923–1933*. London, 1973.
Prinz, Michael. *Vom neuen Mittelstand zum Volksgenossen: Die Entwicklung des sozialen Status der Angestellten von der Weimarer Republik bis zum Ende der NS-Zeit*. Munich, 1986.
Prokop, Otto, and Ehrenfried Stelzer. "Die Menschenexperimente des Dr. med. Heissmeyer (Medizinische und kriminalistische Erhebungen)." *Kriminalistik und forensische Wissenschaften* 3 (1970): 67–104.
Pross, Christian, and Rolf Winau, eds. *nicht misshandeln: Das Krankenhaus Moabit*. Berlin, 1984.
Pueschel, Erich. *Die Seenotverbände der deutschen Luftwaffe und ihr Sanitätsdienst 1939–1945*. Düsseldorf, 1978.
Pulzer, Peter. *The Rise of Political Anti-Semitism in Germany and Austria*. New York, 1964.
Quinn, Susan. *A Mind of Her Own: The Life of Karen Horney*. New York, 1987.
Ramm, Rudolf. *Ärztliche Rechts- und Standeskunde: Der Arzt als Gesundheitserzieher*. Berlin, 1942.
Rauschning, Hermann. *Men of Chaos*. 1942. Reprint. Freeport, N.Y., 1971.
Rebentisch, Dieter. "Die 'politische Beurteilung' als Herrschaftsinstrument der

NSDAP." In Detlev Peukert and Jürgen Reulecke, eds., *Die Reihen fast geschlossen: Beiträge zur Geschichte des Alltags unterm Nationalsozialismus*. Wuppertal, 1981, pp. 107–25.

Rebentisch, Dieter, and Karl Teppe, eds. *Verwaltung contra Menschenführung: Studien zum politisch-administrativen System*. Göttingen, 1986.

Reck-Malleczewen, Friedrich Percyval. *Diary of a Man in Despair*. London, 1970.

Reich-Ranicki, Marcel, ed. *Meine Schulzeit im Dritten Reich: Erinnerungen deutscher Schriftsteller*. Munich, 1984.

Reiche, Eric G. *The Development of the SA in Nürnberg, 1922–1934*. Cambridge, Eng., 1986.

______. "From 'Spontaneous' to Legal Terror: SA, Police, and the Judiciary in Nürnberg, 1933–34." *European Studies Review* 9 (1979): 237–64.

Reichert, F. "Juden und jüdische Mischlinge im Deutschen Reich: Umfang und zeitliche Entwicklung des jüdischen Einbruchs in die deutschen Reichsteile." *Deutsches Ärzteblatt* 70 (1940): 322–25.

Reichsstudentenwerk: Bericht über die Arbeit im Kriege. Edited by Otto Reise. Berlin, 1941.

Reichsstudentenwerk: Kurzberichte aus der Arbeit des Jahres 1935 [–1939]. [Berlin-Charlottenburg, 1935–39].

Reinmöller, Johannes. *Ins Dritte Reich: Antrittsrede des neuen Rektors Professor Dr. Johannes Reinmöller am 4. November 1933: Rede am Reichsgründungstage, am 18. Januar 1934*. Erlangen, 1934.

Reiter, Hans. "Ärzte—Forscher—Pfuscher: Vortrag, gehalten auf der Tagung des NS-Ärztebundes des Gaues Madgeburg in Schierke i.H., am 29. September 1933." *Deutsches Ärzteblatt* 65 (1935): 1014–18.

______. "Nationalsozialistische Revolution in Medizin und Gesundheitspolitik." *Ziel und Weg* 3 (1933): 422–27.

______. "Vorschläge zur Neugestaltung des Hygieneunterrichts und zur Sicherung des Nachwuchses auf dem Gebiet der Hygiene." *Münchener Medizinische Wochenschrift* 85 (1938): 16–19.

______, ed. *Ziele und Wege des Reichsgesundheitsamtes im Dritten Reich: Zum 60jährigen Bestehen des Reichsgesundheitsamtes*. Leipzig, 1936.

Repgen, Konrad. "Ein KPD-Verbot im Jahre 1933?" *Historische Zeitschrift* 240 (1985): 67–99.

Richarz, Monika, ed. *Jüdisches Leben in Deutschland: Selbstzeugnisse zur Sozialgeschichte 1918–1945*. Stuttgart, 1982.

Ring, Friedrich. *Zur Geschichte der Militärmedizin in Deutschland*. Berlin (DDR), 1962.

Ringer, Fritz K. *The Decline of the German Mandarins: The German Academic Community, 1890–1933*. Cambridge, Mass., 1969.

Rissom, Renate. *Fritz Lenz und die Rassenhygiene*. Husum, 1983.

Rittmeister, John. "Der augenblickliche Stand der Poliklinik und ihre künftigen Aufgaben." *Zentralblatt für Psychotherapie und ihre Grenzgebiete* 12 (1940): 88–96.

Robinsohn, Hans. *Justiz als politische Verfolgung: Die Rechtsprechung in "Rassenschandefällen" beim Landgericht Hamburg 1936–1943*. Stuttgart, 1977.

Rodenwaldt, Ernst. "Die Rückwirkung der Rassenmischung in den Kolonialländern auf Europa." *Archiv für Rassen- und Gesellschaftsbiologie* 32 (1938): 385–96.

———. *Ein Tropenarzt erzählt sein Leben*. Stuttgart, 1957.

Rodenwaldt, Ernst, and Heinz Zeiss. *Einführung in die Hygiene und Seuchenlehre*. 5th ed. Stuttgart, 1943.

Rodnick, David. *Postwar Germans: An Anthropologist's Account*. New Haven, 1948.

Röder, Hans. "Der erste Lehrgang der Reichsfachgruppe Medizin auf der Ordensburg Vogelsang." *Ziel und Weg* 7 (1937): 518–24.

Röhrs, Hans-Dietrich. *Hitlers Krankheit: Tatsachen und Legenden: Medizinische und psychische Grundlagen seines Zusammenbruchs*. Neckargemünd, 1966.

Röpke, Erna. "Die Ärztin im Reichsmütterdienst." *Die Ärztin* 12 (1936): 39–46.

Rohland, Brigitte. "Zur Rolle des Hartmannbundes in Vergangenheit und Gegenwart: Bemerkungen zu einem fragwürdigen Jubiläum." *Humanitas: Zeitung für Medizin und Gesellschaft* 26 (1980): 9.

Romann, Ursula. "Die Ärztin." *Frauenkultur*, no. 11 (November 1937): 8–9.

———. "Die Sondertagung der Studentinnen auf dem Lager der Reichsfachgruppe Medizin vom 16.–26. Sept. 1937 auf der Ordensburg Vogelsang." *Die Ärztin* 13 (1937): 306–11.

———. "Zweites Medizinerinnenlager in Kiel: Über die Betreuung des gesunden und kranken Kindes." *Die Ärztin* 13 (1937): 243–44.

Rosenstein, Paul. *Narben bleiben zurück: Die Lebenserinnerungen des grossen jüdischen Chirurgen*. Munich, 1954.

Roth, Karl Heinz. " 'Auslese' und 'Ausmerze': Familien- und Bevölkerungspolitik unter der Gewalt der nationalsozialistischen 'Gesundheitsfürsorge.' " In Gerhard Baader and Ulrich Schultz, eds., *Medizin und Nationalsozialismus: Tabuisierte Vergangenheit—Ungebrochene Tradition?* Berlin, 1980, pp. 152–64.

———. "Schöner neuer Mensch: Der Paradigmenwechsel der klassischen Genetik und seine Auswirkungen auf die Bevölkerungsbiologie des 'Dritten Reichs.' " In Heidrun Kaupen-Haas, ed., *Der Griff nach der Bevölkerung: Aktualität und Kontinuität nazistischer Bevölkerungspolitik*. Nördlingen, 1986, pp. 11–63.

Roth, Karl Heinz, and Götz Aly. "Die Diskussion über die Legalisierung der nationalsozialistischen Anstaltsmorde in den Jahren 1938–1941." *Recht und Psychiatrie* 1–2 (1983–84): 51–64 (1983), 36–47 (1984).

Rothfels, Hans. "Augenzeugenbericht zu den Massenvergasungen." *Vierteljahrshefte für Zeitgeschichte* 1 (1953): 177–94.

Rüdiger, Jutta, ed. *Die Hitler-Jugend und ihr Selbstverständnis im Spiegel ihrer Aufgabengebiete*. Lindhorst, 1983.

Rühle, Gerd. *Das Dritte Reich: Dokumentarische Darstellung des Aufbaues der Nation*. Vols. 1, 3, 6. Berlin, 1933, 1935, 1938.

Rürup, Reinhard. *Emanzipation und Antisemitismus: Studien zur "Judenfrage" der bürgerlichen Gesellschaft*. Göttingen, 1975.

———, ed. *Wissenschaft und Gesellschaft: Beiträge zur Geschichte der Technischen Universität Berlin 1879–1979*. 2 vols. Berlin, 1979.

Ruppert, Joseph. "Die Seucheninsel Polen: Allgemeine Gesundheitspflege unter deutscher Ärzteführung." In Jost Walbaum, ed., *Deutsche Ärzte—Einsatz im*

Osten: Die Aufbauarbeit im Gesundheitswesen des Generalgouvernements. Cracow, 1941, pp. 23–38.

Sadji, Amadou Booker. *Das Bild des Negro-Afrikaners in der Deutschen Kolonialliteratur (1884–1945): Ein Beitrag zur literarischen Imagologie Schwarzafrikas.* Berlin, 1985.

Saller, Karl. *Die Rassenlehre des Nationalsozialismus in Wissenschaft und Propaganda.* Darmstadt, 1961.

Sauer, Paul. *Die Schicksale der jüdischen Bürger Baden-Württembergs während der nationalsozialistischen Verfolgungszeit 1933–1945: Statistische Ergebnisse der Erhebungen der Dokumentationsstelle bei der Archivdirektion Stuttgart und zusammenfassende Darstellung.* Stuttgart, 1969.

______, ed. *Dokumente über die Verfolgung der jüdischen Bürger in Baden-Württemberg durch das nationalsozialistische Regime 1933–1945.* 2 vols. Stuttgart, 1966.

Sauerbruch, Ferdinand. *Das war mein Leben.* 2d ed. Munich, 1979.

Schadewaldt, Hans. *75 [Fünfundsiebzig] Jahre Hartmannbund: Ein Kapitel deutscher Sozialpolitik.* Bonn-Bad Godesberg, 1975.

______, ed. *Von der Medizinischen Akademie zur Universität Düsseldorf 1923–1973: Festschrift anlässlich des 50jährigen Jubiläums der Gründung der Medizinischen Akademie am 13. Mai 1923.* Berlin, 1973.

Schadt, Jörg, ed. *Verfolgung und Widerstand unter dem Nationalsozialismus in Baden: Die Lageberichte der Gestapo und des Generalstaatsanwalts Karlsruhe 1933–1940.* Stuttgart, 1976.

Schäfer, Hans Dieter. *Das gespaltene Bewusstsein: Über deutsche Kultur und Lebenswirklichkeit 1933–1945.* 2d ed. Munich, 1982.

Schallwig, Volker. "Paracelsus' Bedeutung in der Medizin des Nationalsozialismus." M.D. dissertation, Kiel, 1974.

Scheda, Karl, ed. *Deutsches Bauerntum: Sein Werden, Niedergang und Aufstieg.* Konstanz, [1935].

Scheel, Gustav-Adolf. "Rede des Reichsstudentenführers zum Abschluss des Deutschen Studententages 1938." In *Wille und Weg der nationalsozialistischen Studenten.* (*Die Studentische Kameradschaft*, special issue), 1939, pp. 13–19.

Schellenberg, Walter. *Aufzeichnungen: Die Memoiren des letzten Geheimdienstchefs unter Hitler.* Edited by Gita Petersen. Wiesbaden, 1979.

Schenck, Ernst Günther. *Grundlagen und Vorschriften für die Regelung der Krankenernährung im Kriege.* 4th ed. Berlin, 1942.

______. *Ich sah Berlin sterben: Als Arzt in der Reichskanzlei.* Herford, 1970.

______. *Das menschliche Elend im 20. Jahrhundert: Eine Pathologie der Kriegs-, Hunger- und politischen Katastrophen Europas.* Herford, 1965.

______. "Wie sollen wir uns zur Schulmedizin stellen?" *Hippokrates* 10 (1939): 1089–96.

Scherler, Johannes. *Querschnitt durch die deutsche Sozialversicherung: Zum praktischen Gebrauch des Arztes.* Berlin, 1937.

Schieder, Theodor. "Kultur, Wissenschaft und Wissenschaftspolitik im Deutschen Kaiserreich." In Gunter Mann and Rolf Winau, eds., *Medizin, Naturwissenschaft, Technik und das Zweite Kaiserreich: Vorträge eines Kongresses vom 6.*

bis 11. September 1973 in Bad Nauheim. Göttingen, 1977, pp. 9–34.

Schiersmann, Otto. "Ein Beitrag zur praktischen Auswirkung des Gesetzes zur Verhütung erbkranken Nachwuchses." *Deutsches Ärzteblatt* 64 (1934): 30–31.

Schleunes, Karl A. *The Twisted Road to Auschwitz: Nazi Policy toward German Jews, 1933–1939*. Urbana, Ill., 1970.

Schmidt, Gerhard. *Selektion in der Heilanstalt 1939–1945*. Stuttgart, 1965.

Schmidt, Dr. med. "Nochmals: Der ledige Assistenzarzt." *Ziel und Weg* 3 (1933): 575–77.

Schmiedebach, Heinz-Peter. "Der Arzt als Gesundheitsoffizier—die systematische Militarisierung der Medizin von 1933 bis zum Zweiten Weltkrieg." In Johanna Bleker and Heinz-Peter Schmiedebach, eds., *Medizin und Krieg: Vom Dilemma der Heilberufe 1865 bis 1985*. Frankfurt am Main, 1987, pp. 191–208.

Schmuhl, Hans-Walter. *Rassenhygiene, Nationalsozialismus, Euthanasie: Von der Verhütung zur Vernichtung "lebensunwerten Lebens," 1890–1945*. Göttingen, 1987.

Schneeberger, Guido, ed. *Nachlese zu Heidegger: Dokumente zu seinem Leben und Denken*. Berne, 1962.

Schneider, Ulrich. "Widerstand und Verfolgung an der Marburger Universität 1933–1945." In Dieter Kramer and Christina Vanja, eds., *Universität und demokratische Bewegung: Ein Lesebuch zur 450-Jahrfeier der Philipps-Universität Marburg*. Marburg, 1977, pp. 219–56.

Schönberg, Volker. "Die Geschichte der I. Medizinischen Klinik A und B an der Universität Düsseldorf von der Begründung im Jahre 1907 bis zum Jahre 1973." M.D. dissertation, Düsseldorf, 1973.

Schönfeld, Walther. "Die Einstellung der Heidelberger Medizinischen Fakultät in den achtziger Jahren zum Medizinstudium der Frauen." *Ruperto-Carola* 29 (1961): 198–205.

Schönfelder, Heinrich, ed. *Deutsche Reichsgesetze: Sammlung des Verfassungs-, Gemein-, Straf- und Verfahrensrechts für den täglichen Gebrauch*. 13th ed. Munich, 1943.

Scholl, Hans, and Sophie Scholl. *Briefe und Aufzeichnungen*. Edited by Inge Jens. Frankfurt am Main, 1984.

Scholz, Walter. "Otmar Frhr. von Verschuer zum 70. Geburtstag." *Münchener Medizinische Wochenschrift* 108 (1966): 1469–70.

Schreiber, Georg. *Deutsche Wissenschaftspolitik von Bismarck bis zum Atomwissenschaftler Otto Hahn*. Cologne, 1954.

Schröder, Gerald. "Die 'Wiedergeburt' der Pharmazie—1933 bis 1934." In Herbert Mehrtens and Steffen Richter, eds., *Naturwissenschaft, Technik und NS-Ideologie: Beiträge zur Wissenschaftsgeschichte des Dritten Reichs*. Frankfurt am Main, 1980, pp. 166–88.

Schübelin, Jürgen. "Expansionspolitik und Ärzteverbrechen: Das Beispiel Carl Clauberg." In *Volk und Gesundheit: Heilen und Vernichten im Nationalsozialismus*. Tübingen, 1982, pp. 187–204.

Schütze, Erwin. "Beamtenpolitik im Dritten Reich." In Hans Pfundtner, ed., *Dr. Wilhelm Frick und sein Ministerium: Aus Anlass des 60. Geburtstages des*

Reichs- und Preussischen Ministers des Innern Dr. Wilhelm Frick am 12. März 1937. Munich, 1937, pp. 47–65.

Schultz, Johannes Heinrich. *Lebensbilderbuch eines Nervenarztes: Jahrzehnte in Dankbarkeit*. Stuttgart, 1964.

Schultze, Walter. "Die Bedeutung der Rassenhygiene für Staat und Volk in Gegenwart und Zukunft." In Ernst Rüdin, ed., *Erblehre und Rassenhygiene im völkischen Staat*. Munich, 1934, pp. 1–21.

Schulz, Edgar. "Die Entwicklung der Berufsverhältnisse der Glaubensjuden in Preussen zwischen den Zählungen vom 16. Juni 1925 und 16. Juni 1933." *Ziel und Weg* 7 (1937): 460–73.

______. "Judentum und Degeneration." *Ziel und Weg* 5 (1935): 349–55.

Schumann, Heinz, and Gerda Werner, eds. *Erkämpft das Menschenrecht: Lebensberichte und letzte Briefe antifaschistischer Widerstandskämpfer*. Berlin (DDR), 1958.

Schwarberg, Günther. *Der SS-Arzt und die Kinder: Bericht über den Mord vom Bullenhuser Damm*. [Munich], n.d.

Schwarz, Hanns. *Ein Gutachten über die ärztliche Tätigkeit in sog. Erbgesundheitsverfahren*. Halle, 1950.

Das Schwarzbuch: Tatsachen und Dokumente: Die Lage der Juden in Deutschland 1933. Edited by Comité des Délégations Juives. Paris, 1934. 2d printing. Frankfurt am Main, 1983.

Seidelman, William E. "Mengele Medicus: Medicine's Nazi Heritage." *Milbank Quarterly* 66 (1988): 221–39.

Seidler, Franz W. "Das nationalsozialistische Kraftfahrkorps und die Organisation Todt im Zweiten Weltkrieg." *Vierteljahrshefte für Zeitgeschichte* 32 (1984): 625–36.

______. *Prostitution, Homosexualität, Selbstverstümmelung: Probleme der deutschen Sanitätsführung 1939–1945*. Neckargemünd, 1977.

Seier, Hellmut. "Niveaukritik und partielle Opposition: Zur Lage an den deutschen Hochschulen 1939/40." *Archiv für Kulturgeschichte* 58 (1976): 227–46.

______. "Der Rektor als Führer: Zur Hochschulpolitik des Reichserziehungsministeriums 1934–1945." *Vierteljahrshefte für Zeitgeschichte* 12 (1964): 105–46.

Seifert, Ernst. "Zur ärztlichen Ausbildung auf der Hochschule des Dritten Reiches." *Ziel und Weg* 8 (1938): 370–73.

Seifert, Johannes. "Die Krankenversicherung nach dem Stande von 1935 und 1936." *Deutsches Ärzteblatt* 68 (1938): 79–81.

Selchow, Bogislav von. *Hundert Tage aus meinem Leben*. Leipzig, 1936.

Senger, Valentin. *No. 12 Kaiserhofstrasse*. New York, 1980.

Shirer, William L. *The Rise and Fall of the Third Reich: A History of Nazi Germany*. New York, 1960.

Showalter, Dennis E. *Little Man, What Now?* Der Stürmer *in the Weimar Republic*. Hamden, 1982.

Siebert, Margret. "Studentinnen beim 'Medizinischen Facheinsatz Ost' vom Sommer 1940." *Die Ärztin* 17 (1941): 312–15.

Siegert, Toni. "Das Konzentrationslager Flossenbürg: Gegründet für sogenannte Asoziale und Kriminelle." In Martin Broszat and Elke Fröhlich, eds., *Bayern in der NS-Zeit II: Herrschaft und Gesellschaft im Konflikt Teil A*. Munich, 1979, pp. 429–91.

Sigerist, Henry E. *Man and Medicine: An Introduction to Medical Knowledge*. 1932. Reprint. College Park, Md., 1970.

Söken, Gertrud. "Rassenpolitische Erziehung in der Mütterschule." *Die Ärztin* 13 (1937): 94–96.

Sons, Hans-Ulrich. "'Bis in die psychologischen Wurzeln': Die Entnazifizierung der Ärzte in Nordrhein-Westfalen (britisches Besatzungsgebiet)." *Deutsches Ärzteblatt* C 79, no. 36 (1982): 60–62.

Speer, Albert. *Inside the Third Reich: Memoirs*. New York, 1970.

Spender, Stephen. *European Witness*. New York, 1946.

Stachura, Peter D. *Nazi Youth in the Weimar Republic*. Santa Barbara, 1975.

Stadler, Dr. med. "Unverheirateter Arzt gesucht!" *Ziel und Weg* 3 (1933): 339–41.

Stähle, Eugen. *Geschichte des Nationalsozialistischen Deutschen Ärztebundes e.V.: Gau Württemberg-Hohenzollern*. Stuttgart, 1940.

Staff, Ilse, ed. *Justiz im Dritten Reich: Eine Dokumentation*. Frankfurt am Main, 1964.

Stalherm, Dr. med. "Die Betriebsärztin." *Die Ärztin* 20 (1944): 37–39.

Statistisches Handbuch von Deutschland 1928–1944. Edited by Länderrat des Amerikanischen Besatzungsgebiets. Munich, 1949.

Statistisches Jahrbuch für das Deutsche Reich. Edited by Statistisches Reichsamt. Berlin, 1932, 1934, 1935, 1937.

Stein, George H. *The Waffen-SS: Hitler's Elite Guard at War, 1939–1945*. Ithaca, 1966.

Steinert, Marlis G. *Hitlers Krieg und die Deutschen: Stimmung und Haltung der deutschen Bevölkerung im Zweiten Weltkrieg*. Düsseldorf, 1970.

Stephenson, Jill. *The Nazi Organisation of Women*. London, 1981.

———. *Women in Nazi Society*. London, 1975.

Sterilization: Implications for Mentally Retarded and Mentally Ill Persons. Law Reform Commission of Canada, Working Paper 24. Ottawa, 1979.

Stern, Fritz. *The Politics of Cultural Despair: A Study in the Rise of the Germanic Ideology*. Garden City, N.Y., 1965.

Stern, Heinemann. *Warum hassen sie uns eigentlich? Jüdisches Leben zwischen den Kriegen: Erinnerungen*. Edited by Hans Ch. Meyer. Düsseldorf, 1970.

Stern, Karl. *The Pillar of Fire*. New York, 1951.

Steude, Kurt. "Prof. Dr. med. Karl Gelbke—ein Leben als Arzt und Kommunist." In Kurt Kühn, ed., *Ärzte an der Seite der Arbeiterklasse: Beiträge zur Geschichte des Bündnisses der deutschen Arbeiterklasse mit der medizinischen Intelligenz*. Berlin (DDR), 1973, pp. 192–201.

Stobrawa, Franz. *Die ärztlichen Organisationen in der Bundesrepublik Deutschland: Entstehung und Struktur*. Düsseldorf, 1979.

Stock, Ulrich. "Deutsche Ärzte und die Vergangenheit." *Die Zeit*, June 12, 1987, p. 56.

Stockhorst, Erich. *Fünftausend Köpfe: Wer war was im Dritten Reich.* Velbert, 1967.

Stoeckel, Walter. *Erinnerungen eines Frauenarztes.* Edited by Hans Borgelt. Munich, 1966.

Stokes, Lawrence D. "Das Eutiner Schutzhaftlager 1933/34: Zur Geschichte eines 'Wilden' Konzentrationslagers." *Vierteljahrshefte für Zeitgeschichte* 27 (1979): 570–625.

______. "Professionals and National Socialism: The Case Histories of a Small-Town Lawyer and Physician, 1918–1945." *German Studies Review* 8 (1985): 449–80.

———, ed. *Kleinstadt und Nationalsozialismus: Ausgewählte Dokumente zur Geschichte von Eutin 1918–1945.* Neumünster, 1984.

Strauss, Herbert A. "The Immigration and Acculturation of the German Jew in the United States of America." *Leo Baeck Institute Yearbook* 16 (1971): 63–94.

______. "Jewish Emigration from Germany: Nazi Policies and Jewish Responses (I)." *Leo Baeck Institute Yearbook* 25 (1980): 313–61.

______. "Jewish Emigration from Germany: Nazi Policies and Jewish Responses (II)." *Leo Baeck Institute Yearbook* 26 (1981): 343–409.

Stresau, Hermann. *Von Jahr zu Jahr.* Berlin, 1948.

Stürmer, Michael. *Das ruhelose Reich: Deutschland 1866–1918.* Berlin, 1983.

Stürzbecher, Manfred. "Die gesundheitspolitische Konzeption Arthur Gütts im Jahre 1924." *Berliner Ärzteblatt* 84 (1971): 1072–82.

Stumpfl, Friedrich. "Untersuchungen an kriminellen und psychopathischen Zwillingen." *Der Öffentliche Gesundheitsdienst* 2 B (1936): 409–13.

______. *Die Ursprünge des Verbrechens: Dargestellt am Lebenslauf von Zwillingen.* Leipzig, 1936.

Syroth, Max. "Das ärztliche Berufsgeheimnis." *Münchener Medizinische Wochenschrift* 83 (1936): 1469–73.

Szagunn, Ilse. "Dritte Wiener Medizinische Woche: Die Bekämpfung der Volkskrankheiten Krebs, Rheumatismus und Tuberkulose." *Deutsches Ärzteblatt* 71 (1941): 235–39.

______. "Edith von Lölhöffel zum Gedächtnis." *Die Ärztin* 17 (1941): 95–99.

______. "Sportärztliche Erfahrungen für den deutschen Frauensport: Ein ärztlicher Fortbildungskurs der Wiener Akademie für ärztliche Fortbildung über Sportschäden und Sportverletzungen." *Die Ärztin* 17 (1941): 50–54.

______. "Die Vierte Wiener Medizinische Woche." *Deutsches Ärzteblatt* 71 (1941): 402–4.

______. "Wandlungen im Krankheitsbegriff." *Deutsches Medizinisches Journal* 2 (1951): 328–32.

Das Tagebuch der Hertha Nathorff: Berlin-New York: Aufzeichnungen 1933 bis 1945. Edited by Wolfgang Benz. Munich, 1987.

Die Tagebücher von Joseph Goebbels: Sämtliche Fragmente. Vol. 4: *1.1.1940–8.7.1941.* Edited by Elke Fröhlich. Munich, 1987.

Taute, M., et al., eds. *Die Entwicklung des deutschen Gesundheitswesens: Kulturhistorische Schau über hundert Jahre.* Berlin, 1931.

Teixeira, Wilmes Roberto G. "The Mengele Report." *American Journal of Forensic Medicine and Pathology* 6 (1985): 279–83.

Tenfelde, Klaus. "Proletarische Provinz: Radikalisierung und Widerstand in Penzberg/Oberbayern 1900–1945." In Martin Broszat et al., eds., *Bayern in der NS-Zeit IV: Herrschaft und Gesellschaft im Konflikt Teil C*. Munich, 1981, pp. 1–382.

Tennstedt, Florian. *Geschichte der Selbstverwaltung in der Krankenversicherung von der Mitte des 19. Jahrhunderts bis zur Gründung der Bundesrepublik Deutschland*. Bonn, [1977].

———. "Sozialgeschichte der Sozialversicherung." In Maria Blohmke et al., eds., *Handbuch der Sozialmedizin*. Vol. 3. Stuttgart, 1976, pp. 385–492.

Tennstedt, Florian, and Stephan Leibfried. "Sozialpolitik und Berufsverbote im Jahre 1933: Die Auswirkungen der nationalsozialistischen Machtergreifung auf die Krankenkassenverwaltung und die Kassenärzte." *Zeitschrift für Sozialreform* 25 (1979): 129–53, 211–38.

Teppe, Karl. "Der Reichsverteidigungskommissar: Organisation und Praxis in Westfalen." In Dieter Rebentisch and Karl Teppe, eds., *Verwaltung contra Menschenführung im Staat Hitlers: Studien zum politisch-administrativen System*. Göttingen, 1986, pp. 278–301.

Ternon, Yves, and Socrate Helman. *Les médecins allemands et le national-socialisme: Les métamorphoses du darwinisme*. Tournai, 1973.

Thévoz, Robert, et al., eds. *Pommern 1934/35 im Spiegel von Gestapo-Lageberichten und Sachakten (Darstellung)*. Cologne, 1974.

Thimm, Lea. "Agnes Bluhm: Die rassenhygienischen Aufgaben des weiblichen Arztes." *Die Ärztin* 12 (1936): 135–39.

———. "Alt-Rehse." *Die Ärztin* 12 (1936): 187–88.

Thomann, Klaus-Dieter. "Otmar Freiherr von Verschuer—ein Hauptvertreter der faschistischen Rassenhygiene." In Achim Thom and Horst Spaar, eds., *Medizin im Faschismus: Symposium über das Schicksal der Medizin in der Zeit des Faschismus in Deutschland 1933–1945*. Berlin (DDR), 1985, pp. 57–67.

———. "Rassenhygiene und Anthropologie: Die zwei Karrieren des Prof. Verschuer." *Frankfurter Rundschau*, May 20, 1985, p. 20.

Toland, John. *Adolf Hitler*. New York, 1977.

The Torture Report. Published by the British Medical Association. London, 1986.

Trepper, Leopold. *Die Wahrheit: Autobiographie*. Munich, 1978.

True to Type: A Selection from Letters and Diaries of German Soldiers and Civilians Collected on the Soviet-German Front. London, n.d.

Tyrell, Albrecht, ed. *Führer befiehl . . . : Selbstzeugnisse aus der "Kampfzeit" der NSDAP: Dokumentation und Analyse*. Düsseldorf, 1969.

Über menschliches Mass: Opfer der Hölle Ravensbrück sprechen . . . Warsaw, 1970.

Ungern-Sternberg, Roderich von. "Wert und Bedeutung der weiblichen Berufstätigkeit." *Deutsches Ärzteblatt* 68 (1938): 44–46.

Unschuld, Paul Ulrich. "Professionalisierung im Bereich der Medizin: Entwurf zu einer historisch-anthropologischen Studie." *Saeculum* 25 (1974): 251–76.

Valentin, Rolf. *Die Krankenbataillone: Sonderformationen der deutschen Wehrmacht im Zweiten Weltkrieg*. Düsseldorf, 1981.

Verschuer, Otmar Freiherr von. "Aufgaben und Ziele der menschlichen

Erblichkeitslehre." *Münchener Medizinische Wochenschrift* 74 (1927): 999–1002.

______. "Bevölkerungs- und Rassenfragen in Europa." *Europäischer Wissenschafts-Dienst*, no. 1 (1944): 11–14.

______. "Das ehemalige Kaiser-Wilhelm-Institut für Anthropologie, menschliche Erblehre und Eugenik." *Zeitschrift für Morphologische Anthropologie* 55 (1964): 127–74.

______. *Erbpathologie: Ein Lehrbuch für Ärzte*. Dresden, 1934.

______. "Das Qualitätsproblem in der Bevölkerungspolitik." *Medizinische Welt*, no. 26 (1931): 934–35.

______. "Soziale Umwelt und Vererbung." In Alfred Grotjahn et al., eds., *Ergebnisse der Sozialen Hygiene und Gesundheitsfürsorge*. Vol. 2. Leipzig, 1930, pp. 1–33.

______. "Vier Jahre Frankfurter Universitäts-Institut für Erbbiologie und Rassenhygiene." *Der Erbarzt*, no. 5 (1939): 57–64.

Vescovi, Gerhard. "Die soziale Bedeutung und Funktion des ärztlichen Berufsrechts." In Maria Blohmke et al., eds., *Handbuch der Sozialmedizin*. Vol. 3. Stuttgart, 1976, pp. 211–44.

Vezina, Birgit. *Die "Gleichschaltung" der Universität Heidelberg im Zuge der nationalsozialistischen Machtergreifung*. Heidelberg, 1982.

Viehweg, Dr. med. "Die Nürnberger Grundgesetze." *Deutsches Ärzteblatt* 65 (1935): 1116–19.

Vogeler, Karl. *August Bier: Leben und Werk*. Munich, 1941.

Voigt, Klaus. "Refuge and Persecution in Italy, 1933–1945." *Simon Wiesenthal Center Annual* 4 (1987): 3–64.

Volz, Hans. *Daten der Geschichte der NSDAP*. 9th ed. Berlin, 1939.

Voswinckel, Peter. *50 Jahre Deutsche Gesellschaft für Hämatologie and Onkologie*. Würzburg, 1987.

Wagner, Gerhard. " 'Gesundes Leben—Frohes Schaffen': Rede zur Eröffnung der Ausstellung am 24. September 1938 in Berlin." *Ziel und Weg* 8 (1938): 549–55.

______. "Neue Deutsche Heilkunde." *Deutsches Ärzteblatt* 66 (1936): 419–21.

______. *Die Nürnberger Judengesetze: Nationalsozialistische Rassen- und Bevölkerungspolitik: Mit Erläuterungen zu den Nürnberger Rassegrundgesetzen*. 3d ed. Munich, 1939.

______. "Rasse und Volksgesundheit." *Ziel und Weg* 8 (1938): 515–21.

______. "Die Reichsärzteordnung, ein Instrument nationalsozialistischer Gesundheitspolitik." *Ziel und Weg* 6 (1936): 2–4.

______. "Sicherung der wirtschaftlichen Existenz des Kassenarztes." *Deutsches Ärzteblatt* 69 (1939): 23–24.

______. "Die Stellung des Arztes im neuen Deutschland." *Ziel und Weg* 7 (1937): 394–97.

______. "Stellung und Aufgaben des beamteten Arztes im neuen Reiche." *Deutsches Ärzteblatt* 64 (1934): 778–80.

______. "Unser Reichsärzteführer spricht: Rede, gehalten auf dem Reichsparteitag 1935." *Ziel und Weg* 5 (1935): 431–35.

———. "Volksgesundheit und Leistungsprinzip im nationalsozialistischen Staate: Die Aufhebung der Kurierfreiheit in Deutschland." *Ziel und Weg* 9 (1939): 137–40.

———. "Die Ziele der nationalsozialistischen Gesundheitspolitik." *Ziel und Weg* 7 (1937): 487–93.

Walk, Joseph, ed. *Das Sonderrecht für die Juden im NS-Staat: Eine Sammlung der gesetzlichen Massnahmen und Richtlinien—Inhalt und Bedeutung*. Heidelberg, 1981.

Wasserstein, Bernard. *Britain and the Jews of Europe, 1939–1945*. Oxford, 1979.

Wegner, Bernd. *Hitlers Politische Soldaten: Die Waffen-SS 1933–1945: Studien zu Leitbild, Struktur und Funktion einer nationalsozialistischen Elite*. Paderborn, 1982.

Wehler, Hans-Ulrich. *Das Deutsche Kaiserreich 1871–1918*. 4th ed. Göttingen, 1980.

Weindling, Paul. "Die preussische Medizinalverwaltung und die 'Rassenhygiene,' 1905–1933." In Achim Thom and Horst Spaar, eds., *Medizin im Faschismus: Symposium über das Schicksal der Medizin in der Zeit des Faschismus in Deutschland 1933–1945*. Berlin (DDR), 1985, pp. 48–56.

———. "Race, Blood and Politics." *Times Higher Education Supplement*, July 19, 1985, p. 13.

Weingart, Peter. "Eugenik—Eine angewandte Wissenschaft: Utopien der Menschenzüchtung zwischen Wissenschaftsentwicklung und Politik." In Peter Lundgreen, ed., *Wissenschaft im Dritten Reich*. Frankfurt am Main, 1985, pp. 314–49.

Weisenborn, Günther. *Der lautlose Aufstand: Bericht über die Widerstandsbewegung des deutschen Volkes 1933–1945*. Hamburg, 1953.

Weiss, Sheila Faith. *Race Hygiene and National Efficiency: The Eugenics of Wilhelm Schallmeyer*. Berkeley, 1987.

Weitbrecht, H. J. *Psychiatrie in der Zeit des Nationalsozialismus: Rede, gehalten am 10. Februar 1966 in der Rheinischen Friedrich-Wilhelms-Universität zu Bonn im Rahmen des Studium Universale*. Bonn, 1968.

Weizsäcker, Viktor von. *Arzt und Kranker*. Leipzig, 1941.

———. " 'Euthanasie' und Menschenversuche." *Psyche* 1 (1947–48): 68–102.

———. *Natur und Geist: Erinnerungen eines Arztes*. 2d ed. Göttingen, 1955.

Wer ist Wer? Das deutsche Who's Who. 16th ed. Edited by Walter Habel. Berlin, 1970.

Wer ist Wer? Das deutsche Who's Who. 25th ed. Lübeck, 1986.

Wer ist's? 10th ed. Edited by Herrmann A. L. Degener. Berlin, 1935.

Werle, Karl-Peter. "Formen des Widerstandes deutscher Ärzte 1933 bis 1945." M.D. dissertation, Kiel, 1974.

Werner, Andreas. "SA und NSDAP: SA: 'Wehrverband,' 'Parteitruppe' oder 'Revolutionsarmee'? Studien zur Geschichte der SA und der NSDAP 1920–1933." Ph.D. dissertation, Erlangen-Nuremberg, 1964.

Whalen, Robert Weldon. *Bitter Wounds: German Victims of the Great War, 1914–1939*. Ithaca, 1984.

Who's Who in Germany. 3d ed. Edited by Horst G. Kliemann and Stephen S. Taylor. Munich, 1964.

Winkler, Dörte. *Frauenarbeit im "Dritten Reich*." Hamburg, 1977.

Winkler, Ernst. "Zur Frage der Krankenausbildung der Medizinstudenten." *Ziel und Weg* 5 (1935): 277–78.

Winter, Irina, ed. *Georg Benjamin: Arzt und Kommunist*. Berlin (DDR), 1962.

Wirtschaftstaschenbuch für Ärzte. Edited by Julius Hadrich. Leipzig, 1926.

Wirz, Franz. "Hochschule und Fortbildung." *Deutsches Ärzteblatt* 67 (1937): 47–49.

Witter, Ben. "Es hat doch auch die anderen Deutschen gegeben." *Die Zeit*, July 19, 1981, p. 54.

Wolff, Inge. "Bericht über das III. Reichslager für medizinische Fachgruppenreferentinnen vom 31.3.–4.4.1937 auf der Reichsschule I der NS.-Frauenschaft in Coburg." *Die Ärztin* 13 (1937): 162–65.

______. "Die politische Erziehung der deutschen Studentin." In *Wille und Weg der nationalsozialistischen Studenten*. (*Die Studentische Kameradschaft*, special issue), 1939, pp. 66–69.

Wolff-Mönckeberg, Mathilde. *Briefe, die sie nicht erreichten: Briefe einer Mutter an ihre fernen Kinder in den Jahren 1940–1946*. Edited by Ruth Evans. Hamburg, 1980.

Wren, Christopher. "Salvaging Lives after Torture." *New York Times Magazine*, August 17, 1986, pp. 18–24.

Wuttke [-Groneberg], Walter. "Die Herrschaft von Künstlern: Zur ärztlichen Methodenlehre." In Martin Doehlemann, ed., *Wem gehört die Universität? Untersuchungen zum Zusammenhang von Wissenschaft und Herrschaft anlässlich des 50jährigen Bestehens der Universität Tübingen*. Lahn-Giessen, 1977, pp. 177–200.

______. "Leistung, Vernichtung, Verwertung: Überlegungen zur Struktur der Nationalsozialistischen Medizin." In *Volk und Gesundheit: Heilen und Vernichten im Nationalsozialismus*. Tübingen, 1982, pp. 6–59.

______. "Von Heidelberg nach Dachau." In Gerhard Baader and Ulrich Schultz, eds., *Medizin und Nationalsozialismus: Tabuisierte Vergangenheit—Ungebrochene Tradition?* Berlin, 1980, pp. 113–44.

______, ed. *Medizin im Nationalsozialismus: Ein Arbeitsbuch*. Tübingen, 1980.

Wyman, David S. *The Abandonment of the Jews: America and the Holocaust, 1941–1945*. New York, 1985.

Zapp, Albert. "Untersuchungen zum Nationalsozialistischen Deutschen Ärztebund (NSDÄB)." M.D. dissertation, Kiel, 1979.

Zelzer, Maria. *Weg und Schicksal der Stuttgarter Juden: Ein Gedenkbuch*. Stuttgart, n.d.

Der Zivile Luftschutz im Zweiten Weltkrieg: Dokumentation und Erfahrungsberichte über Aufbau und Einsatz. Edited by Erich Hampe. Frankfurt am Main, 1963.

Zmarzlik, Hans-Günter. "Der Sozialdarwinismus in Deutschland als geschichtliches Problem." *Vierteljahrshefte für Zeitgeschichte* 11 (1963): 246–73.

Zörner, G., et al. *Das Frauen-KZ Ravensbrück*. Berlin (DDR), 1971.

Zofka, Zdenek. "Der KZ-Arzt Josef Mengele: Zur Typologie eines NS-Ver-

brechers." *Vierteljahrshefte für Zeitgeschichte* 34 (1986): 245–67.
Zondek, Hermann. *Auf festem Fusse: Erinnerungen eines jüdischen Klinikers*. Stuttgart, 1973.
Zorn, Gerda. *Stadt im Widerstand*. Frankfurt am Main, [1965].
Zülch, Tilman, ed. *In Auschwitz vergast, bis heute verfolgt: Zur Situation der Roma (Zigeuner) in Deutschland und Europa*. Reinbek, 1979.
250 [Zweihundertfünfzig] Jahre Charité Berlin. Berlin (DDR), [1960].

Index